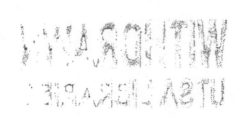

INFECTIOUS DISEASES OF THE CENTRAL NERVOUS SYSTEM

CONTEMPORARY NEUROLOGY SERIES AVAILABLE:

INFECTIOUS DISEASES OF THE CENTRAL NERVOUS SYSTEM

KENNETH L. TYLER, M.D.
Associate Professor
Departments of Neurology, Medicine,
and Microbiology-Immunology
University of Colorado Health Science
Center and Denver Veterans
Administration Medical Center
Denver, Colorado

JOSEPH B. MARTIN, M.D., Ph.D.
Professor of Neurology
Dean, School of Medicine
University of California, San Francisco
San Francisco, California

F. A. Davis Company
1915 Arch Street
Philadelphia, PA 19103

Copyright © 1993 by F. A. Davis Company

Printed in the United States of America

Last digit indicates print number: 10 9 8 7 6 5 4 3 2 1

Acquisitions Editor: Robert H. Craven
Developmental Editor: Bernice M. Wissler
Production Editors: Jody Gould and Arofan Gregory

As new scientific information becomes available through basic and clinical research, recommended treatments and drug therapies undergo changes. The author(s) and publisher have done everything possible to make this book accurate, up to date, and in accord with accepted standards at the time of publication. The authors, editors, and publisher are not responsible for errors or omissions or for consequences from application of the book, and make no warranty, expressed or implied, in regard to the contents of the book. Any practice described in this book should be applied by the reader in accordance with professional standards of care used in regard to the unique circumstances that may apply in each situation. The reader is advised always to check product information (package inserts) for changes and new information regarding dose and contraindications before administering any drug. Caution is especially urged when using new or infrequently ordered drugs.

Library of Congress Cataloging-in-Publication Data

Infectious diseases of the central nervous system / [edited by]
    Kenneth L. Tyler, Joseph B. Martin.
       p.   cm.—(Contemporary neurology series ; 41)
    Includes bibliographical references and index.
    ISBN 0-8036-8767-2 (alk. paper)
    1. Central nervous system—Infections. 2. Mycoses. 3. Parasitic
    Diseases. I. Tyler, Kenneth L., 1953– . II. Martin, Joseph B.,
    1938– . III. Series.
    [DNLM: 1. Central Nervous System Diseases. 2. Virus Diseases.
    3. Bacterial Infections. W1 C0769N v.41 1993 / WL 300 I434 1993]
    RC359.5.I55 1993
    616.8—dc20
    DNLM/DLC   93-4862
    for Library of Congress   CIP

We would like to dedicate this book to our wives and children: Lisa, Eric, and Max (KLT); and Rachel (JBM); for their continued support, good humor, and encouragement.

FOREWORD

Infectious diseases that localize in the CNS are among the most dramatic of all acute illnesses. In spite of a variety of antibiotic, antifungal, and antiviral drugs, prognosis is often poor. The spectrum of serious CNS infections has changed significantly in recent years, most dramatically with such newer diseases as HIV- and HTLV-1–related CNS syndromes. Treatments, especially antibiotics, have improved the outcome of some bacterial infections significantly.

Research on CNS infections has evolved over the years. The earliest phases of CNS research were clinical and involved classic descriptions of CNS infections. Subsequently, studies on pathogenesis provided critical insights into such features as tissue localization ("tropism"), pathways of spread (blood and neural), and the role of various immune components (including antibody, T cells, cytokines). Recent studies have attempted to understand CNS infections by using the recent burst of molecular biological and genetic studies to develop a profound understanding of the mechanisms of CNS infections in precise molecular terms. Insights on the molecular level should provide newer ways of interrupting the life cycles of microbes in the host and thus are likely to be of increasing importance in future therapeutic approaches.

The editors and authors of this book are all highly respected experts in the field. Several have been associated with Dr. Richard T. Johnson, who pioneered studies on viral pathogenesis using the fluorescent antibody technique and taught us much of what is known about many features of virus-CNS interactions.

The focus in this book on the diseases caused by infectious agents is especially important in the 1990s. As more and more researchers are trained in the disciplines of molecular biology, we tend to forget that modern science, especially molecular biology, is particularly meaningful when the power of modern technologies can be focused on solving disease problems. Since the study of CNS infections involves three levels of increasing complexity—the molecular, the cellular, and the host—it is critical to keep in perspective the idea that understanding disease ultimately requires a firm understanding of the cellular and host aspects of the process. As long as the diseases are clearly defined, we can anticipate that, with the use of newer technologies, our understanding of CNS infection will make major progress during the next several years. The scope of *Infectious Diseases of the Central Nervous System,* and the quality of the editors and the authors, will make this book a valuable source of information for years to come.

BERNARD N. FIELDS, M.D.
Harvard Medical School

PREFACE

Patients afflicted with central nervous system (CNS) infections often present a daunting array of diagnostic and therapeutic problems to the physicians who treat them. The list of potential pathogens is legion; the therapies are diverse and often effective only for particular agents. To the non-neurologist, the complexities of neurological diagnosis and neuroanatomy often seem Byzantine. Neurologists are often equally bewildered by the dazzling and ever-expanding array of new antimicrobial agents. These problems are made more intense by the fact that the overwhelming majority of CNS infections are in fact treatable or preventable diseases, and that their ultimate outcome may depend on the accuracy and speed with which diagnostic and therapeutic decisions are made.

Our book is directed primarily at the clinicians—neurological, medical, and pediatric—who initially come into contact with patients with CNS infections. We have tried to summarize in a concise and readable, rather than encyclopedic, format a number of selected, key topics related to CNS infections. The diagnosis and therapy of these infections has been dramatically altered by the widespread use and availability of new neuroimaging techniques, including computed tomography (CT) and magnetic resonance imaging (MRI). In addition, many molecular biological techniques, as exemplified by the polymerase chain reaction (PCR), have made their way from the benches of basic science laboratories to become standard tools in the diagnostic microbiology laboratories of hospitals and clinics. New antimicrobial therapies, exemplified by the antiviral agents utilized in the treatment of herpesviruses and the human immunodeficiency virus (HIV), are based on understanding at a cellular, molecular, and genetic level the pathogenesis and replication cycle of viruses. We have encouraged our authors to incorporate these various developments into the appropriate chapters of our book.

Our book begins with six chapters devoted to viral infections of the CNS. The first chapter provides an overview of the diagnosis and clinical management of acute viral encephalitis. For viral infections, the host's immune system can at times be a double-edged sword, in some cases contributing to recovery and in other cases mediating CNS injury as exemplified by syndromes of postinfectious immune-mediated encephalomyelitis. These issues are discussed in detail in Chapter 2. Chapters 3 to 5 deal individually with selected classes of viruses including HIV, herpesviruses, and enteroviruses. It was obviously impossible to include chapters dealing with every virus known to infect the CNS. We have selected these particular viruses because of the frequency with which they are encountered, their obvious epidemiological importance, and, in the case of HIV and herpesviruses, their responsiveness to specific antiviral therapy. This section of the book concludes with a review of chronic and slow infections of the CNS. These infections are among the most dramatic (and in some cases, exotic) neurological infections encountered by clinicians. Although the transmissible neurodegenerative diseases caused by prions are often reviewed as "slow virus" diseases, they are only briefly discussed in this chapter. Accumulating evidence indicates that prions are not conventional infectious agents, and that most human prion diseases are likely to be genetic rather than 'infectious' in a traditional sense.

The second section of the book (Chapters 7 to 13) deals with infections of the CNS caused by bacteria, fungi, and parasites. This section begins with chapters devoted to specific clinical types of CNS infection that clinicians commonly encounter, including focal suppurative infections (Chapter 7), bacterial meningitis (Chapter 8), and chronic meningitis (Chapter 9). The following three chapters deal with the syndromes produced by Lyme disease, neurosyphilis, and parasitic and rickettsial infections. The manifestations produced by these agents are protean, may involve virtually any region of the nervous system, and may pose significant diagnostic and therapeutic conundrums. We have selected these particular agents from among the many that can infect the nervous system because of the frequency and complexity of their diagnostic, clinical, and therapeutic problems. The final chapter of the book is a detailed review of antimicrobial drugs commonly used in the therapy of bacterial and fungal infections of the CNS. We felt that the increasing availability of large numbers of new antimicrobial and antifungal drugs made it important to synopsize in a single place an extensive body of information concerning their antimicrobial spectrum, pharmacological properties, dosing regimens, and complications. We intended this section in part to provide more detailed information on the antimicrobial agents discussed in the preceding chapters, but we did not try to impose uniformity of recommendations for drug use on our authors. Knowledge and experience concerning the use of newer antimicrobial agents in infections is increasing dramatically, yet in many cases therapeutic regimens are based on the personal experiences of the individual authors. We feel that this personal insight is important and valuable, even if not always identical between authors!

Writing this book has been both a gratifying and frustrating experience. We are gratified by the hard work that so many of our authors put into producing excellent chapters. We have been frustrated at times by the laggards, and by the fact that important contributions to knowledge of CNS infections appears on a daily basis and makes the current "state of the art" a constantly moving target that one tries to approach rather than achieve.

We hope that neurologists, internists, pediatricians, general practitioners, and indeed anyone with an interest in infections of the CNS will find this book valuable and interesting reading.

Kenneth L. Tyler, M.D.
Joseph B. Martin, M.D., Ph.D.

ACKNOWLEDGMENTS

We would be remiss if we did not acknowledge the mentors, friends, colleagues, and collaborators in neurology, virology, and infectious disease who provided support over the years and along the pathway leading up to the production of this book. Among those who served as teachers and mentors, Kenneth L. Tyler would like to thank his father, H. Richard Tyler, for initiating his interest in medicine and neurology, and Raymond D. Adams, E.P. Richardson, and C. Miller Fisher for continuing to challenge and nurture that interest at MGH. Our interest in neurovirology and infectious disease was fostered and encouraged by Louis Weinstein, Richard T. Johnson, and Bernard N. Fields.

The actual mechanics of putting together this book have been made immeasurably easier by the continued help and good will of many people at F. A. Davis. Our editor, Bernice M. Wissler, deserves special thanks for her help at every stage of book production. Secretarial and editorial support was provided by Karen Kaplan (KLT) and Leslie LaPiana (JBM). The editors could not have devoted the time required were it not for continued grant support over the years, for research and other activities, from the NINDS, NIAID, Alfred P. Sloan Foundation, and the Department of Veterans Affairs.

Finally, we would like to thank our wives and family members for unselfishly continuing to support us through all the many joys and frustrations of producing this book.

Kenneth L. Tyler, M.D.
Joseph B. Martin, M.D., Ph.D.

CONTRIBUTORS

James F. Bale, Jr., M.D.
Professor
Division of Pediatric Neurology
Departments of Pediatrics and
    Neurology
The University of Iowa College of
    Medicine
Iowa City, Iowa

Lydia Bayne, M.D.
Clinical Assistant Professor of
    Neurology
Department of Neurology
University of California, San Francisco
School of Medicine
San Francisco, California

William E. Bell, M.D.
Professor
Departments of Pediatrics and
    Neurology
Division of Child Neurology
The University of Iowa Hospitals and
    Clinics
Iowa City, Iowa

Joseph R. Berger, M.D.
Professor of Neurology and Internal
    Medicine
University of Miami School of Medicine
Miami, Florida

Jerrold J. Ellner, M.D.
Professor of Medicine and Pathology
Chief, Division of Infectious Diseases
Case Western Reserve University
University Hospitals of Cleveland
Cleveland, Ohio

Donald H. Gilden, M.D.
Professor and Chairman
Department of Neurology
Professor of Microbiology and
    Immunology
University of Colorado Health Sciences
    Center
Denver, Colorado

Diane Edmund Griffin, M.D., Ph.D.
Professor of Medicine and Neurology
Departments of Medicine and Neurology
The Johns Hopkins University School of
    Medicine
Baltimore, Maryland

John J. Halperin, M.D.
Chairman
Department of Neurology
North Shore University Hospital
Manhasset, New York
Associate Professor
Department of Neurology
Cornell University Medical College
New York, New York

Daniel F. Hanley, M.D.
Director
Neuroscience Critical Care Unit
Associate Professor
Departments of Neurology/
    Neurosurgery and Anesthesiology
Critical Care Medicine
The Johns Hopkins University
Baltimore, Maryland

David N. Irani, M.D.
Chief Resident
Department of Neurology
The Johns Hopkins Hospital
Baltimore, Maryland

Richard T. Johnson, M.D.
Professor and Director of Neurology
Professor of Microbiology and
    Neuroscience
Neurologist-in-Chief
Department of Neurology
The Johns Hopkins Hospital
Baltimore, Maryland

Burk Jubelt, M.D.
Professor and Chairman
Department of Neurology
Professor
Department of Microbiology and
    Immunology
State University of New York Health
    Science Center at Syracuse
Syracuse, New York

Robert M. Levy, M.D., Ph.D.
Associate Professor of Neurosurgery and
    Physiology
Northwestern University Medical
    School
Chicago, Illinois

Howard L. Lipton, M.D.
Professor of Neurology
University of Chicago School of
    Medicine
Chicago, Illinois
Evanston Hospital
Evanston, Illinois

Joseph B. Martin, M.D., Ph.D.
Professor of Neurology
Dean, School of Medicine
University of California, San Francisco
San Francisco, California

Gail A. McGuinness, M.D.
Professor
Department of Pediatrics
Division of Neonatology
University of Iowa Hospitals and Clinics
Iowa City, Iowa

W. Michael Scheld, M.D.
Professor of Internal Medicine and
    Neurosurgery
Departments of Medicine and
    Neurosurgery
Division of Infectious Diseases
University of Virginia Health Sciences
    Center
Charlottesville, Virginia

Roger Simon, M.D.
Professor and Vice Chair
Department of Neurology
University of California, San Francisco
Chief of Staff and Chief of Neurology
San Francisco General Hospital
San Francisco, California

Tarvez Tucker, M.D.
Associate Professor
Case Western Reserve University
School of Medicine
Department of Neurology
University Hospitals of Cleveland
Cleveland, Ohio

Kenneth L. Tyler, M.D.
Associate Professor
Departments of Neurology, Medicine,
    and Microbiology-Immunology
University of Colorado Health Science
    Center and Denver Veterans
    Administration Medical Center
Denver, Colorado

Leslie P. Weiner, M.D.
Richard Angus Grant, Sr. Chair in
    Neurology
Chairman, Department of Neurology
Professor of Neurology and Microbiology
University of Southern California
    School of Medicine
Los Angeles, California

CONTENTS

8. BACTERIAL MENINGITIS 176

*Joseph B. Martin, M.D., Ph.D., Kenneth L. Tyler, M.D.,
and W. Michael Scheld, M.D.*

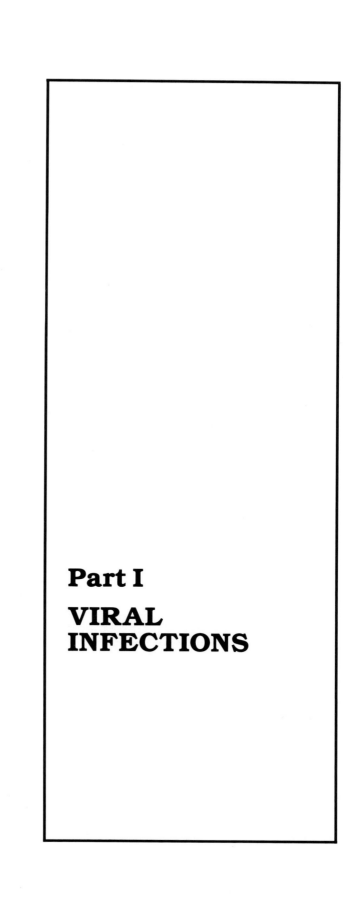

Part I

VIRAL INFECTIONS

Chapter 1

ACUTE VIRAL ENCEPHALITIS: DIAGNOSIS AND CLINICAL MANAGEMENT

David N. Irani, M.D.,
Daniel F. Hanley, M.D., and
Richard T. Johnson, M.D.

A broad range of viral pathogens can infect the human central nervous system (CNS), causing acute viral encephalitis.[36] The diagnosis and management of this condition present the clinician with an array of important decisions, many of which require urgent consideration. In the past, the specific cause of viral infection within the CNS for the most part has been difficult to identify rapidly, with the possible exception of herpes simplex encephalitis (HSE).[82,99] Only recently have more rapid diagnostic assays become available for a broader range of infectious agents. Additionally, nonviral conditions (either infectious or noninfectious) can present with similar clinical pictures and fur-

ther complicate the diagnostic dilemma of suspected viral encephalitis.[92] Epidemiologic data have demonstrated that HSE accounts for only 5% to 10% of the 20,000 annual reported cases of encephalitis in the United States,[8,13] and yet this particular condition has garnered increasing attention since recent advances in the antiviral therapy of herpesviruses have emphasized the need to secure a rapid and specific diagnosis of HSE. The overall untreated mortality rate of the disease exceeds 70%, whereas the institution of antiviral therapy before a complete loss of consciousness reduces this figure to 17%, and patients under 30 years of age have even better survival rates.[91] Conversely, delayed recognition and treatment of HSE is associated with a 35% mortality when symptoms have been present for longer than 4 days.[91] Other viral encephalitides vary widely in their mortality rates but to date have not been amenable to specific antiviral therapies. Furthermore, since many nonviral conditions that mimic viral encephalitis are also potentially treatable, rapid diagnostic efforts become even more important. With these data in mind, consideration of the pathogenesis, approach to diagnosis, and clinical management of suspected viral encephalitis will be discussed, with particular emphasis placed on HSE.

PATHOGENESIS

Most CNS viral infections represent uncommon sequelae of common systemic viral infections.[26,42] Typically either the meninges become involved, such as in aseptic meningitis, or brain parenchyma becomes involved to a mild degree, causing a benign meningoencephalitis. The degree of symptomatic involvement in encephalitis depends on the virus, the host, and the route and dose of viral inoculation. Viruses gain entry into the CNS by two primary routes: from the blood across the blood-brain barrier or within peripheral nerves by retrograde intraneuronal transport.[35–37,42,90] Hematogenous spread is the most common route, since transient or sustained viremias occur with a broad range of viral infections. Whether a CNS infection occurs depends on the capacity of the virus to avoid clearance from the blood by such immune mechanisms as antibodies or the complement system, as well as on its ability to circumvent the blood-brain barrier.[29,36] Viruses within the bloodstream can gain entry into the brain by directly infecting cerebral capillary endothelial cells,[20] by using established transendothelial transport mechanisms,[21] or by being sequestered within hematogenous cells that normally traffic across the blood-brain barrier.[23,45,97]

The alternative mechanism for entry into the CNS is retrograde axonal transport up neurons with centrally located cell bodies and axonal processes in the periphery. Viruses can use the bidirectional transport mechanisms that normally exist in neurons,[27] and this route is the primary mode of entry into the CNS for the rabies virus[61] and varicellazoster virus (VZV).[32] The cutaneous reactivation of VZV and herpes simplex virus (HSV) also uses this mechanism, and its importance for the entry of HSV into the CNS remains controversial but is strongly suspected.[5]

Once viruses gain entry into the CNS, the susceptibility of various cell types to infection determines both the clinical manifestations produced and the degree of intracranial spread.[36] Cortical neuron involvement may lead to seizures as well as to focal motor or sensory symptoms. Infection of oligodendroglia can produce demyelination. Ependymal cell infection may result in obstructive hydrocephalus caused by obliteration of cerebrospinal fluid (CSF) outflow from blockage of the aqueduct of Sylvius. Viruses with tropisms for ependymal cells as well as for the choroid plexus and meninges are likely to be shed into the CSF and potentially spread throughout the neuraxis. Those that are limited to replication in parenchymal cells probably spread on a cell-to-cell basis and are more likely to produce focal CNS disease.

CLINICAL PRESENTATION

The hallmarks of viral encephalitis include various manifestations of brain dysfunction accompanied by fever and evidence of CNS inflammation. Specific clinical signs and symptoms of acute viral infections within the CNS depend on which neural cells are infected, and as mentioned previously, individual cell populations of the nervous system have varying susceptibilities to different viruses. If infection is confined to the meninges covering the nervous system, clinical manifestations may be limited to headache, fever, nuchal rigidity, and a CSF pleocytosis. In addition to producing signs of meningeal irritation, infection that spreads to the parenchymal cells of the brain may produce a depressed level of consciousness, seizures, behavioral or speech disturbances, focal neurologic deficits, and evidence of increased intracranial pressure. The tropisms of viruses for different CNS cell types thus produce the spectrum of neurologic disease.[26,36,42] For example, polioviruses infect and destroy anterior horn cells, resulting in the characteristic clinical findings of acute meningitis with lower motor neuron paralysis. Rabies virus typically infects neurons of the brainstem and limbic system, producing behavioral changes, seizures, and disorientation, often accompanied by hydrophobia and aerophobia.[1] The predisposition of HSV to involve the temporal lobes can lead to bizarre behavior, aphasias, superior-quadrant visual field defects, hemiparesis with greater involvement of face and arm, and temporal lobe seizures.[24,96] However, despite these particular tendencies, the clinical presentations of various forms of encephalitis overlap

broadly, often precluding a specific diagnosis on clinical findings alone. In fact, the National Institute of Allergy and Infectious Diseases (NIAID) Collaborative Antiviral Study Group found no statistical differences in the presenting signs and symptoms of patients with biopsy-proven HSE that distinguished them from patients with suspected infection who did not have HSE (Table 1–1).[92,96]

Nevertheless, the presenting history in these patients can provide important epidemiologic trends that can facilitate a diagnosis. Information about potential exposures, the season during which disease occurs, geographic location, and the proximity to ongoing epidemic infections are all relevant. A history of an antecedent animal bite can suggest

Table 1–1 COMPARISON OF FINDINGS IN BIOPSY-POSITIVE AND BIOPSY-NEGATIVE PATIENTS WITH SUSPECTED HERPES SIMPLEX ENCEPHALITIS*

	No. (%) of Patients	
	Biopsy-Positive	*Biopsy-Negative*
HISTORICAL FINDINGS		
Alteration of consciousness	109/112 (97)	82/84 (98)
CSF pleocytosis	107/110 (97)	71/82 (87)
Fever	101/112 (90)	66/85 (78)
Headache	89/110 (81)	56/73 (77)
Personality change	62/87 (71)	44/65 (68)
Seizures	73/109 (67)	48/81 (59)
Vomiting	51/111 (46)	38/82 (46)
Hemiparesis	33/100 (33)	19/72 (26)
Memory loss	14/59 (24)	9/47 (19)
CLINICAL FINDINGS AT PRESENTATION		
Fever	101/110 (92)	64/79 (81)
Personality change	69/81 (85)	43/58 (74)
Dysphasia	58/76 (76)	36/54 (67)
Autonomic dysfunction	53/88 (60)	40/71 (56)
Ataxia	22/55 (40)	18/45 (40)
Hemiparesis	41/107 (38)	24/81 (30)
Seizures	43/112 (38)	40/85 (47)
Focal	28/112 (25)	13/85 (15)
Generalized	10/112 (9)	14/85 (17)
Both	5/112 (4)	13/85 (15)
Cranial neuropathy	34/105 (32)	27/81 (33)
Visual field loss	8/58 (14)	4/33 (12)
Papilledema	16/111 (14)	9/84 (11)

*None of the differences were significant at the $p < .05$ level by χ^2 tests.
Source: Adapted from Whitley RJ et al. JAMA 247:317–320, 1982, with permission. Copyright 1982, American Medical Association.

rabies; disease in a temperate climate during late summer or fall implicates enteroviral infection; and outbreaks in warm, damp regions with burgeoning mosquito populations increase the possibility of arthropod-borne viral infection. Centers for Disease Control (CDC) information regarding specific disease outbreaks can provide valuable diagnostic assistance throughout the differ-

ent geographic regions of the United States.

Likewise, although the physical examination of patients with suspected viral encephalitis is not diagnostic in the majority of cases, several factors remain relevant. Many viral infections are systemic illnesses with characteristic tropisms for nonneural tissue, and these can produce associated findings

Table 1–2 DISEASES THAT MIMIC HERPES SIMPLEX ENCEPHALITIS

Disease	No. of Patients (n = 432)	Percentage (%) of Patients
Herpes simplex encephalitis (biopsy-proven)	195	45
No diagnosis	142	33
Other diagnosis (see below)	95	22
TREATABLE CONDITIONS	38	9
Infection		
Abscess/subdural empyema		
Bacterial	5	
Listeria	1	
Fungal	2	
Mycoplasma	2	
Tuberculosis	6	
Cryptococcal	3	
Rickettsial	2	
Toxoplasmosis	1	
Mucormycosis	1	
Meningococcal meningitis	1	
Tumor	5	
Subdural hematoma	2	
Systemic lupus erythematosus	1	
Adrenal leukodystrophy	6	
NONTREATABLE CONDITIONS	57	13
Nonviral		
Vascular disease	11	
Toxic encephalopathy	5	
Reye's syndrome	1	
Viral		
Arbovirus infections		
St. Louis encephalitis	7	
Western equine encephalitis	3	
California encephalitis	4	
Eastern equine encephalitis	2	
Other herpesviruses		
Epstein-Barr virus	8	
Cytomegalovirus	1	
Others		
Echovirus	3	
Influenza A	4	
Mumps	3	
Adenovirus	1	
Progressive multifocal leukoencephalopathy	1	
Lymphocytic choriomeningitis	1	
Subacute sclerosing panencephalitis	2	

Source: Adapted from Whitley RJ et al,[92] pp 235–236.

that implicate particular causes. For example, parotitis and orchitis occur with mumps infection, and a mononucleosis syndrome is often produced by Epstein-Barr virus (EBV) and cytomegalovirus (CMV). Furthermore, focality in the neurologic examination is extremely important, because HSE is the most common cause of sporadic, focal encephalitis in the United States.[92,96] Despite this fact, however, more than half of the patients in the NIAID Collaborative Study who underwent brain biopsy for presumptive HSE turned out to have something other than the suspected diagnosis (Table 1–2).[92]

CSF FINDINGS

A complete evaluation of the CSF is critical in establishing the diagnosis of viral encephalitis. If focal neurologic signs or evidence of increased intracranial pressure is present on examination, a contrast-enhanced imaging study should precede the lumbar puncture to rule out a space-occupying lesion with a shift of midline structures. Typically, modest numbers of mononuclear cells are present in the CSF during encephalitis, although large numbers of polymorphonuclear cells can be seen on the first day or two of disease. Approximately 3% to 5% of patients with severe viral infections of the CNS, such as HSE, have no pleocytosis on the initial CSF examination,[96] and it should be noted that in animal models of arboviral encephalitis, the temporal profile of CSF inflammation does not necessarily reflect the degree of parenchymal involvement.[57] Red blood cells in the CSF are suggestive of HSE, but their presence does not clearly implicate herpetic encephalitis, nor does their absence exclude it (Table 1–3). The protein content is usually elevated, whereas the CSF glucose most commonly shows a normal ratio of 0.6 to 0.8 with the serum level. Mildly decreased CSF glucose can be seen with mumps or lymphocytic choriomeningitis (LCM) virus infections.[2,47,88] When there is an absence of cells or a preponderance of polymorphonuclear cells, another CSF examination in 12 to 24 hours usually shows a transition to more typical findings if the diagnosis of viral encephalitis is correct.

Culture of the CSF to isolate the offending agent is typically of minimal value in the acute management of viral encephalitis. Viral cultures of CSF for enteroviruses, mumps, and occasionally arboviruses may be positive, but herpes simplex virus type 1 (HSV-1) is seldom recovered from the CSF. A positive culture for one of the former agents, however, might allow the discontinuation of antiviral therapy for suspected HSE, as these viruses themselves are not currently amenable to specific antiviral therapy and management is therefore strictly supportive. Further laboratory confirmation of the specific cause of viral encephalitis is discussed later. Although it is not always helpful from a therapeutic standpoint, this information is generally of prognostic value.

NEURODIAGNOSTIC TECHNIQUES

A number of neurodiagnostic techniques can provide helpful information when evaluating a febrile patient who manifests evidence of brain dysfunction and in whom viral encephalitis is suspected. Computed tomography (CT) may demonstrate a contrast-enhanced lesion or mass effect, suggesting a tumor or an abscess, or may show a low-density abnormality in the inferior and mesial aspects of one or both temporal lobes, implicating HSE. The earliest CT findings during the course of HSE may frequently be normal or equivocal,[64] however, and it is important to determine rapidly with other techniques whether a localized abnormality exists when behavioral disturbances, seizures, or focal signs on examination suggest HSE. Electroencephalography (EEG) is a very sensitive test early in this disease. The EEG may

Table 1–3 INITIAL CSF FINDINGS WITHIN 3 DAYS OF BIOPSY FOR SUSPECTED HERPES SIMPLEX ENCEPHALITIS

	Biopsy-Positive Patients (n = 98)	Biopsy-Negative Patients (n = 75)	p Value*
PROTEIN			NS†
Median, mg/dL	80	53	
Range, mg/dL	7–755	12–492	
Quantity, no. of patients			
<40 mg/dL	18	25	
40–100 mg/dL	43	22	
>100 mg/dL	37	28	
WHITE BLOOD CELLS (WBC)			.0001
Median, WBC/mm^3	130	28	
Range, WBC/mm^3	0–1100	0–5500	
Quantity, no. of patients			
0–5/mm^3	4	17	
6–50/mm^3	18	28	
51–500/mm^3	68	24	
>500/mm^3	8	6	
RED BLOOD CELLS (RBC)			NS
Quantity, no. of patients			
0	16	9	
1–50/mm^3	37	26	
51–500/mm^3	23	23	
>500/mm^3	18	17	
GLUCOSE RATIO			NS
Quantity, no. of patients			
CSF:blood < 0.5	5	4	

*The median test and χ^2 test were used to test for differences between two medians and two frequency distributions, respectively.
†NS = not significant ($p > .05$).
Source: Adapted from Whitley RJ et al. JAMA 247:317–320, 1982, with permission. Copyright 1982, American Medical Association.

show only diffuse slowing, but often there are unilateral or bilateral periodic discharges in the temporal leads. In some patients, characteristic slow-wave complexes seen at regular intervals of 2 to 3 per second are highly suggestive of the diagnosis.[81] Radionuclide brain scans may show increased isotope uptake in one or both temporal lobes in HSE before an abnormality is seen on CT scans,[66] and this modality proved to be the most specific study in the NIAID antiviral trial (Table 1–4).[96] Angiographic findings are normal early in the disease and likely do not facilitate a diagnosis of encephalitis.[66] Angiography performed later in HSE can demonstrate evidence of temporal swelling, a prolongation of arterial filling, and hypervascularity in one or both tempo-ral areas.[66] The improved resolution as well as the greater sensitivity of magnetic resonance imaging (MRI) when compared with CT suggests a role for this modality as an early diagnostic tool in HSE. Several centers have in fact demonstrated this increased sensitivity in small groups of HSE patients.[64,77] Unfortunately, this test is not universally available, and it cannot always be performed on an urgent basis. Furthermore, agitated HSE patients do not do well in the claustrophobic MRI setting, and motion artifact often negates the promise of increased resolution. Nevertheless, improved imaging capacity should allow earlier detection of temporal lobe pathology in HSE than is seen with CT, and it should also facilitate the diagnosis of tumors or ab-

Table 1–4 DIFFERENCES IN NEURODIAGNOSTIC ASSESSMENTS BETWEEN BIOPSY-POSITIVE AND BIOPSY-NEGATIVE PATIENTS WITH SUSPECTED HERPES SIMPLEX ENCEPHALITIS

| Test Result | No. (%) of Patients | | p Value* |
	Biopsy-Positive	Biopsy-Negative	
Focal EEG abnormality	59/73 (81)	39/66 (59)	.005
Brain scan localization	37/74 (50)	6/44 (14)	.0001
CT scan localization	33/56 (59)	8/37 (22)	.0004
One or more localizations	83/101 (82)	47/75 (63)	.004
Two or more localizations	31/64 (48)	9/50 (18)	.001

*By χ^2 tests.
Source: Adapted from Whitley RJ et al. JAMA 247:317–320, 1982, with permission. Copyright 1982, American Medical Association.

scesses of the CNS that present as HSE. This imaging modality should be urgently obtained, if possible, in suspected viral encephalitis.

CONFIRMATION OF SPECIFIC CAUSES

The laboratory confirmation of the specific cause of viral encephalitis is of therapeutic value for only a few pathogens. Of primary concern should be the rapid distinction of HSE from other forms of viral encephalitis so that specific antiviral chemotherapy for this infection can be instituted and continued appropriately. In general, identification and quantification of antiviral antibodies both in the serum and in the CSF are not useful diagnostically unless the temporal profile of their titers is followed. Documentation of seroconversion or seroboosting with acute and convalescent serum does not affect the decision to institute therapy and is only helpful to confirm the cause of the infection retrospectively. Intrathecal synthesis of antibody is more specific for the demonstration of actual CNS infection, but again, the time course of this antiviral immune response is too slow to influence therapeutic decisions. One exception is the enzyme-linked immunosorbent assay (ELISA), which detects the specific antiviral immunoglobulin M (IgM) antibody response in the CSF of patients with Japanese encephalitis. This test is both sensitive and specific;

most patients demonstrate such antibodies at the time of hospitalization, and virtually all demonstrate them within 72 hours of illness.[11,12] Although not helpful to direct therapy, this test confirms the diagnosis and provides prognostic information. Similar antibody detection methods for other arboviral infections are becoming available and will certainly achieve greater use in the future.

Alternative strategies, particularly for HSV, have focused on methods for the rapid, noninvasive detection of viral enzymes, proteins, and even nucleic acids to confirm the diagnosis of encephalitis. One approach is to selectively image HSV-infected cell populations by administering the antiviral drug FMAU (2′-fluoro-5-methyl-1-β-D-arabinosyluracil) coupled to detectable gamma-emitting isotopes. This drug is specifically phosphorylated by the HSV thymidine kinase and thus should accumulate and be retained only in infected cells. To date, however, this method has been complicated by the detection of high concentrations of drug in both choroid plexus and in proliferating but uninfected cell populations, and it still requires that effective imaging and diagnostic sensitivity be demonstrated in humans.[74,86] Nevertheless, it would be a means to take advantage of the theoretical specificity of currently available antiviral drugs for the detection of HSV-infected cells.

A second technique is the rapid detection of a herpesvirus-specific glycoprotein in the CSF of patients with HSE. Preliminary data suggest that the method is 80% sensitive and 90% specific when performed within 72 hours after the onset of disease,[46] although it can still sometimes be negative in the earliest stages, when therapeutic decisions are being made. The latest efforts have centered on the detection of viral deoxyribonucleic acid (DNA) from samples using the polymerase chain reaction (PCR) amplification technique. Again, preliminary data have demonstrated the specific detection of HSV sequences in the CSF of patients with biopsy-proven HSE but not in specimens from other CNS infections or controls.[71] Despite some theoretical advantages over other rapid detection methods, the efficacy of this technique in the detection of the earliest cases of HSE remains to be evaluated in comparison to the standard of direct brain biopsy. Nevertheless, the pursuit of a rapid, noninvasive diagnostic method to obviate the need for brain biopsy in suspected HSE should be aggressively continued in clinical studies.

BRAIN BIOPSY

Brain biopsy is currently the most sensitive and specific means of establishing the diagnosis of HSE or of confirming one of the many conditions that can mimic it.[63,92,96] Most statistical models support this concept, because diagnostic certainty is unacceptably low when decision making in suspected HSE is based on non–biopsy-derived information.[7,63,83,96] A tissue sample should be obtained from the area of maximal involvement, because virus is found where the gross pathologic lesion is located. False-negative results of biopsy have been most frequently associated with an arbitrary surgical decision to limit the risk of postoperative deficit by selecting the frontal convexity or random sampling in the nondominant temporal lobe.[95] Biopsy should be done via open craniotomy, not by a needle aspiration (CT-guided or otherwise).[60,76]

Although needle biopsy through a burr hole seems a conservative approach, this procedure is probably more hazardous than open biopsy. In view of the increase in intracranial pressure often seen in acute encephalitis, craniotomy with decompression of the affected area may have a therapeutic effect, as well as allowing direct visualization of the brain for the selection of an optimal biopsy site. Furthermore, there is frequently a hemorrhagic component to HSE, and hemostasis can be achieved with greatest certainty under direct visualization. This is also of particular concern because prebiopsy angiography is not routinely performed, and a common postbiopsy diagnosis can be some form of vascular disease such as vasculitis or arteriovenous malformation. Both of these alternative diagnoses do not lend themselves well to the blind biopsy approach, because they tend to result in bleeding.

Tissue specimens obtained should be fixed for routine histology and electron microscopy, prepared for viral antibody staining, and inoculated into cell cultures for virus isolation. Frozen sections show inclusion bodies in only half of virus-positive tissue specimens, but they quickly confirm perivascular inflammation and effectively rule out many other diseases. Both electron microscopy and immunofluorescence can be rapid and useful in experienced hands but are limited by a high rate of false-negative results (45% and 37%, respectively) and a small number of false-positive results in HSE.[95] Virus isolation yields the most definitive results but may require up to 5 days to become positive.

Direct biopsy-related mortality has not been reported in the NIAID Collaborative Study Group experience, and the 1.4% morbidity incidence for the group's 432 biopsies since 1973 suggests that biopsy is a relatively safe procedure in practiced hands.[92] Specific complications of the procedure include worsening of local brain edema and hemorrhage at the biopsy site. Wound dehiscence occurred in one patient in this study. Nevertheless, with careful attention to achieving hemostasis and close postoperative monitoring, brain biopsy can be safely and rapidly performed to expedite a diagnosis of suspected HSE.

FEATURES OF SPECIFIC VIRAL ENCEPHALITIDES

Enteroviruses

The enterovirus group of the picornaviruses includes the polioviruses (3 types), coxsackieviruses (29 types), echoviruses (31 types), and several miscellaneous enteroviruses, including the hepatitis A virus. Almost all these agents are contracted by fecal-oral transmission and replicate initially in the gastrointestinal tract.[73] Spread to the CNS occurs primarily by hematogenous dissemination.[30,53] Infection is most common in the late summer and early fall but can occur sporadically throughout the year. Overall, the enteroviruses account for 70% to 80% of all cases of aseptic meningitis and 11% to 22% of viral encephalitis, but paralysis and cerebellar ataxia are also rarely associated with enteroviral infection.[30,59] Typical infection, however, is either asymptomatic or associated with mild constitutional symptoms; even when CNS spread occurs, meningitis is usually benign and symptoms typically resolve in several days. With poliovirus, frank paralysis occurs in approximately 1 in 1000 infections, although this disease has been essentially eradicated from the United States by the use of current vaccines. Coxsackievirus and echovirus infections result in sequelae when acquired in the perinatal period, producing up to 20% mortality with in utero infection.[44,56] These agents also cause a chronic meningoencephalitis in immunocompromised individuals, particularly children with defective antibody synthesis.[52]

Enteroviral CNS infection is often suspected based on epidemiologic data within a particular community. These infectious agents are readily recoverable, and isolation attempts should be made from the stool, urine, and throat, as well as from the CSF. There currently are two forms of vaccine for poliovirus: the oral, attenuated live-virus vaccine given routinely to infants; and the inactivated poliovirus vaccine given intramuscularly to unimmunized adults and immunocompromised individuals.[19] There is no currently available vaccine for the many serotypes of coxsackievirus and echovirus, but long-term sequelae from these infections are fortunately quite infrequent.

Arboviruses

The arthropod-borne viruses (arboviruses) are a common cause of both sporadic and epidemic encephalitis throughout the world. They include alphaviruses, flaviviruses, and bunyaviruses. These viruses replicate in both invertebrate and vertebrate hosts and are transmitted to humans by ticks and mosquitoes. Generally they are inoculated as infected saliva from the insect vector, replicate locally to produce a viremia, and spread to the CNS by hematogenous dissemination.[38] The incubation period for arboviral encephalitis is thought to be on the order of several days to several weeks, and clinical symptoms typically present as a prodrome of fever, headache, and malaise. This picture can progress to confusion, obtundation, and coma and is frequently complicated by seizures, especially in children. Although many arboviruses cause encephalitis, specific viruses are restricted geographically and seasonally by their particular vector, so that only a few exist in any one part of the world.

Important alphaviruses are those that cause eastern equine encephalitis (EEE), western equine encephalitis (WEE), and Venezuelan equine encephalitis (VEE). EEE is endemic along the eastern and Gulf coasts of the United States, in the Caribbean, and in South America. North American strains produce a fulminant disease with a case fatality rate of 50% to 75%, and survivors have a high incidence of neurologic sequelae.[25,72] WEE produces a similar clinical picture but is most common in the western and midwestern United States; its mortality rate is only 10%. VEE occurs in South and Central America as well as in the southwestern United States. Disease is typically mild, causing fever, headache, myalgias, and pharyngitis, with encephalitis occurring only rarely. Neurologic residua are rare, and mortality from the encephalitis is only about 1%.[72]

The flaviviruses are transmitted by both ticks and mosquitoes and can be found worldwide. In terms of overall morbidity and mortality, the most important flavivirus infection is Japanese B encephalitis, which causes disease throughout Asia from India to the Philippines.[58] In endemic areas, children are most commonly affected, although in epidemics that occur elsewhere throughout the year, individuals of all ages are equally susceptible. The infection may be asymptomatic or can present as fever, meningitis, or encephalitis. The typical onset of encephalitis is rapid and can be accompanied by abdominal pain, nausea, headache, and fever. Associated neurologic signs include a parkinsonian masklike facies, rigidity, and tremor, all suggesting basal ganglia involvement, along with altered consciousness, seizures in children, and a lower motor neuron polio-like clinical appearance.[39,69] St. Louis encephalitis is the most common disease caused by flavivirus in the United States and seems to occur widely throughout the country. Outbreaks occur usually in August through October, later in the year than is typical for most arboviruses.[84] Individual susceptibility increases with age, and encephalitis can frequently be accompanied by hyponatremia from inappropriate antidiuretic hormone secretion. The disease mortality rate is also age-related, ranging from 2% to 20%, and recovery is often protracted, with sequelae in 20% of survivors.[58,84]

Bunyaviruses constitute the largest group of the arboviruses, the most important of which are those in the California serogroup, including La Crosse, Jamestown Canyon, and California encephalitis viruses.[78] La Crosse virus is the most common cause of arboviral encephalitis in the United States, producing disease in which seizures and focal neurologic signs are often manifested, primarily in children. The mortality rate, however, is less than 1%, and sequelae are rare.[34]

Rabies

Rabies virus is an important pathogen primarily in developing countries where endemic canine infection still exists. It is also present in many wild animals in Europe and North America, however, where infection has been controlled in domestic animals by immunization requirements. In the United States, rabies is carried by skunks, foxes, raccoons, and bats, and infection is transmitted primarily by the bite of a rabid animal. Rare cases have developed from inhalation of virus shed by bats in caves, and at least one case has been described as resulting from a laboratory accident.[15,98] Virus is taken up by peripheral nerve endings and transported to the CNS, where it spreads transsynaptically.[61,62] The incubation period can be from days to years but typically lasts 20 to 60 days. Infection does not occur in every individual bitten by a rabid animal, but it is uniformly fatal when clinical disease develops.[9] Symptoms typically present as a prodrome of fever, headache, and malaise, which is then followed by neurologic disease. Seizures, behavioral abnormalities, hydrophobia, and aerophobia occur and commonly lead to coma and death in one to several weeks.[3,9] Specific diagnosis is usually retrospective at postmortem examination and requires immunofluorescent staining of infected tissue. Brain tissue is most definitive, although occasionally viral antigens can be detected during life in corneal smears, skin, or buccal mucosa.[3] Effective vaccines exist and are used as preexposure immunization for animal handlers at risk and as postexposure prophylaxis in individuals bitten by a potentially rabid animal. Postexposure treatment is ineffective, however, once symptoms develop.[4,14]

Retroviruses

Two human retroviruses, human immunodeficiency virus (HIV) and human T-cell lymphotropic virus type I (HTLV-I), are associated with neurologic disease. HTLV-I causes predominantly a spastic paraparesis.[89] HIV produces a broad spectrum of neurologic manifestations,[18,22,50] which can be the presenting signs and symptoms of HIV infection and include aseptic meningitis or meningoencephalitis. More chronic infection can cause a myelopathy and encephalopathy, among other neurologic syndromes. Infection results from intimate contact with infected individuals or exposure to contaminated blood products. The diagnosis and management of these conditions have been extensively reviewed elsewhere.[18,22,50]

Paramyxoviruses and Arenaviruses

Two paramyxoviruses, measles and mumps viruses, are commonly associated with neurologic disease. Several of the arenaviruses, LCM virus and Lassa fever virus in particular, can occasionally produce CNS infection. Both mumps and measles have been well controlled in the United States by means of vaccines but previously were major causes of viral meningoencephalitis.[55] When mumps meningoencephalitis occurs, it typically appears 3 to 10 days after the characteristic parotitis and generally resolves without sequelae, except when it occasionally results in hydrocephalus from ependymal cell involvement.[85] Measles infection in

its acute stages does not involve the CNS, but approximately 1 in 1000 cases can give rise to a postinfectious autoimmune encephalomyelitis. Direct CNS infection can rarely occur in immunodeficient patients who develop an inclusion-body encephalitis over weeks, and about one child per million normal children infected with measles goes on to manifest subacute sclerosing panencephalitis years after the original infection.[31,40,54]

Rodents are the natural reservoir for the arenaviruses, so LCM virus infection occurs most commonly in winter months, when mice are indoors and human contact with infected animals or their excreta is most likely to occur.[33] Typical disease is biphasic after a 5- to 10-day incubation period; an initial flu-like illness accompanied by leukopenia and thrombocytopenia is followed by an aseptic meningitis or meningoencephalitis. Recovery can be prolonged but is usually complete.[33,88] Lassa fever is a West African disease that begins as a nonspecific respiratory or gastrointestinal condition that can lead to a fulminant hemorrhagic shock.[33] Neurologic disease consists of acute mental status changes and the sequelae of unilateral or bilateral deafness in 5% of cases.[48] Diagnosis is made on the basis of geographic exposure and can be confirmed by immunocytochemical staining of conjunctival scrapings with anti-Lassa antiserums. Overall fatality during outbreaks can range from 8% to 52%, and it has recently been shown that the antiviral agent ribavirin can be effective in its treatment.[51]

Herpesviruses

Of the many species of herpesviruses, seven have been shown to infect humans, and six of these are currently recognized to be at least occasional causes of some form of CNS disease. Each of these agents can establish latency after the primary infection has occurred, and CNS involvement can develop with either a primary or a reactivated infection[43] (see Chap. 4). Most commonly HSV-1 is latent in sensory neurons within the trigeminal ganglia, HSV-2 is typically present in the sacral ganglia, VZV is probably present in the satellite cells of multiple sensory ganglia, and EBV is present in B lymphocytes.[43] The site of CMV and herpes B virus *(Herpesvirus simiae)* latency has not yet been clearly established.

HSE is the most common form of sporadic, acute, focal encephalitis in the United States, and more than 95% of adult cases are caused by infection with HSV-1.[5,63] As already mentioned, particular emphasis is placed on the specific diagnosis of HSE because it is the only CNS viral infection for which antiviral therapy has been proven beneficial in controlled studies.[91,95] Its consistency in temporal lobe localization suggests that the virus enters the CNS by specific neural routes, although virus isolated from a peripheral site may or may not be the same strain found in the brain of that individual.[94] Neonatal infection is distinct in that it may be caused by either HSV-1 or HSV-2. The latter is much more readily recoverable from the CSF of infected infants and is typically a disseminated CNS disease that does not demonstrate the specific temporal lobe involvement seen in adults.[93] Adult infection occurs with equal frequency throughout the year and predominantly affects patients younger than 20 years of age or older than 50 years of age.[24] Most cases occur in individuals without any antecedent illness, and the disease may have an insidious or fulminant onset. Many of the diagnostic features have been previously discussed, but ultimately, successful therapy depends on a high index of suspicion and the early institution of antiviral chemotherapy.

As mentioned, other herpesviruses can cause CNS infection that results in acute encephalitic syndromes. Acute EBV infection is associated with a 25% incidence of CSF abnormalities but produces a variety of neurologic manifestations as part of infectious mononucleosis in only about 1% of cases.[79] A diffuse meningitis or meningoencephalitis can occur, usually 1 to 3 weeks after the onset of mononucleosis. Occasionally, however, the disease is focal in nature and sometimes can be the only manifestation of EBV infection.[28,79] CMV is a rare cause of meningoencephalitis in normal individuals but is increasingly noted as the cause of a subacute encephalopathy in immunosuppressed patients.[17,49] VZV produces neurologic sequelae as a result of both primary and reactivated infection. Occasionally with varicella, a cerebellar ataxia and, rarely, a meningoencephalitis occur; both are thought to be mediated by the immune system, and the former is typically benign.[41] With zoster in older or immunocompromised patients, disseminated encephalitis, myelopathy, and granulomatous angiitis are the most common CNS manifestations seen among the many sequelae of this recurrent infection.[65,70]

MANAGEMENT

Current management of acute viral encephalitis has been facilitated by two recent advances: the improved monitoring and support provided by an intensive care unit (ICU) setting, and the development of effective antiviral chemotherapeutic agents. Therapeutic decisions in suspected viral encephalitis are often made in conjunction with diagnostic endeavors, and management of neurologic sequelae often require the most immediate attention. Presently, successful treatment of HSE appears to depend on the institution of antiviral chemotherapy in the shortest time from the onset of symptoms.[95] Thus consideration of the need for both of these interventions is an important factor when evaluating suspected encephalitis. Even though effective antiviral therapy is presently limited to treatment of the herpesviruses, rapid diagnostic efforts can lead to the confirmation of other potentially treatable conditions that mimic HSE.[92] Otherwise, management is strictly supportive and is directed toward prevention or rapid detection and treatment of both neurologic and systemic complications. Even without antiviral therapy, however, vigorous supportive care can dramatically improve outcome, because many of the complications that occur with encephalitis are what ultimately influence morbidity and mortality.[36]

When the history, physical and neurologic examinations, initial CSF analysis, and imaging studies suggest HSE, acyclovir therapy should be started and arrangements made for a brain biopsy. The NIAID Collaborative Antiviral Study Group has demonstrated the efficacy of acyclovir for documented HSE in a placebo-controlled trial.[91] The antiviral agent is given at a dose of 30 mg/kg per day, divided into three doses. Each dose is diluted in at least 100 mL of standard intravenous solution and administered over 1 hour. Diagnostic information can still routinely be obtained 24 to 48 hours after the institution of therapy, including viral isolation from biopsy material. In an open study of the previous antiviral agent, vidarabine, the critical determinants of outcome in HSE were patient age and level of consciousness at the onset of treatment.[95] Therefore, it seems advisable to start acyclovir even as the biopsy is being organized. If biopsy material is positive for HSV antigens by immunocytochemical methods, acyclovir therapy should continue for a full 10 days. If negative, viral cultures should be observed daily for cytopathic effect, and if at the end of 5 days the cultures are negative and other studies indicative of herpes infection are absent, acyclovir can be discontinued.

Failure to improve, or deterioration after stabilization or improvement, presents a difficult problem in management of patients with suspected HSE. If HSV has not been established as the etiologic agent in suspected encephalitis, an alternative diagnosis must be sought, because other causes are more likely under these circumstances. In biopsy-proven cases with late deterioration, repeated imaging studies can help confirm the presence of parenchymal hemorrhage, subdural hematoma, herniation, or other structural complications, which might mimic disease relapse. Rarely, patients treated with acyclovir have survived HSE but maintained high CSF titers of anti-HSV antibodies,[80] and others who have died after full courses of standard treatment have had virus isolated from brain tissue.[16,87] Both of these populations suggest that a small number of patients with HSE can relapse despite antiviral therapy. A relapse of the infection should be documented by a second biopsy, but it is suggested by a striking enhancement of the cortical ribbon with contrast CT studies or with MRI. Relapse may result either from failure to achieve adequate drug levels at the actual site of infection or from the selection of drug-resistant mutants. Because of its uncommon occurrence, controlled therapeutic trials for HSE relapse have not been performed. In vitro studies, however, suggest that a longer course of acyclovir is indicated with the addition of vidarabine, 15 mg/kg per day by continuous intravenous infusion.

Management of Precipitous Neurologic Deterioration

Patients with severe viral encephalitis often present with progressive symptoms that can rapidly be compounded by precipitous neurologic deterioration. Consequently, the most immediate decisions about patients who come to medical attention often involve management of the acute manifestations of encephalitis. Respiratory compromise, obtundation or coma, and seizures are the most severe of these acute complications. Organizing diagnostic procedures and defining the rate of progression of the encephalitis require frequent assessments of neurologic status, which are best conducted in a critical care environment. If airway reflexes and general level of consciousness mandate, intubation with subsequent tracheostomy is indicated.

Table 1–5 GLASGOW COMA SCALE

Eye opening	Spontaneous	4
	To verbal stimuli	3
	To pain	2
	None	1
Best verbal response	Oriented	5
	Confused and converses	4
	Inappropriate words	3
	Garbled sounds	2
	None	1
Best motor response	Obeys commands	6
	Localizes pain	5
	Withdrawal (flexion)	4
	Abnormal flexion	3
	Extension	2
	None	1

Source: Teasdale G and Jennett B: Assessment of coma and impaired consciousness. A practical scale. Lancet 2:81, 1974.

Agitated encephalitis patients also often require temporary sedation for neuroradiologic procedures or vascular cannulations. As this sedation can precipitate respiratory arrest, prophylactic airway protection is strongly suggested. The Glasgow Coma Scale (Table 1–5) and British Medical Research Council Strength Scale (Table 1–6) provide simple and reliable measures to assess disease progression that can be applied by all members of the critical care team. In a patient with a declining level of consciousness, the deterioration can result from ventilatory failure, seizures or postictal state, pharmacologic sedation, primary brainstem involvement, or brain edema with compartment shift. The last two most commonly result in prolonged obtundation and are

Table 1–6 BRITISH MEDICAL RESEARCH COUNCIL STRENGTH SCALE

Normal power	5
Active movement against gravity with resistance	4
Active movement against gravity	3
Active movement with gravity eliminated	2
Flicker or trace of contraction	1
No contraction	0

Source: Medical Research Council: Aids to the examination of the peripheral nervous system, Memorandum 45. Pendragon House, London, 1976.

best evaluated in a rapid manner with a careful cranial nerve examination and a CT scan. The primary temporal lobe involvement in HSE often causes a progressive encroachment on the perimesencephalic cistern, with a subsequent lateral shift of the midbrain and thalamus. Compartment shift is an ominous sign that is usually followed by uncal herniation and permanent impairment of consciousness or death.[67] Early fluid restriction to produce passive dehydration of the brain remains the most effective preventive measure in managing brain edema and is best instituted as quickly as possible. An overall restriction of fluid intake to 1000 to 1500 mL/day is tolerated well by most adults and produces a moderate hyperosmolarity (305 to 315 mOsm) depending on the degree of insensible fluid loss and renal concentrating abilities. Additional agents (steroids, osmotic agents, and barbiturates) useful in treating intracranial hypertension of other causes[10,68] are often used, but in our experience with HSE, they appear to have limited benefits. In a small study group of patients with encephalitis, increased intracranial pressure was associated with a poor outcome, perhaps indicative of a more fulminant infection.[6] Optimal results still seem to be associated with early diagnosis and institution of antiviral therapy in HSE; intracranial pressure monitoring in other encephalitides may be useful in facilitating the decision to use steroids or osmotic agents, can help in titrating these agents, and can provide prognostic information.[6]

Management of Seizures

Seizures probably increase the morbidity and mortality associated with HSE infection, and status epilepticus at presentation is a particularly poor prognostic factor for an undiagnosed encephalitis patient.[75] Intubation must be immediately followed by pharmacologic control of seizures, which often requires anesthetic levels of benzodiazepines and barbiturates. Fortunately, this is an exceedingly rare scenario that in our experience is encountered only in nonherpetic encephalitis (Johnson RT, personal communication, 1989). More commonly, the HSE patient will present with one or two seizures and a prolonged postictal state. This situation requires rapid, but not emergent, loading with an anticonvulsant such as phenytoin. Prophylactic anticonvulsants are not routinely given unless a biopsy has been performed, but if seizures occur before a diagnosis is made, an improvement of deficits or improved level of consciousness with anticonvulsants should not be confused with a remission of the encephalitis. Rather, the patient should be investigated by biopsy as quickly as possible when stable. Patients with biopsy-proven HSE should be treated with anticonvulsants for several months, but in other patients, medications can be discontinued once fever has abated. If seizures recur after the patient is afebrile, the patient can be treated with intravenous diazepam followed by phenobarbital or phenytoin.

General Support

General support is the most important part of the complete care of patients with encephalitis. Bed rest is indicated, but strict isolation procedures are not essential because most of the viruses that cause encephalitis are not readily spread from human to human. Enteric precautions should be instituted for suspected enteroviral infection, however, and if measles, chickenpox, rubella, or mumps virus infection is evident, the usual isolation of susceptible persons is recommended. Vigorous avoidance of hyperthermia may not be indicated, since most viruses are thermolabile and modest temperature elevations may serve as a natural defense mechanism. Headache can usually be managed by judicious doses of aspirin or acetaminophen.

More severe encephalitis often leads to coma, but because recovery is possible, aggressive support and avoidance of chronic complications are essential. Maintenance of adequate nutrition during this period often requires nasogastric tube feeding; hyperosmolar preparations are particularly useful, as they provide high caloric intake and facilitate dehydration of the patient. Extensive efforts should be made to maintain a positive nitrogen balance in febrile patients with high metabolic demands. Serum glucose and electrolytes should be checked frequently, because water, glucose, and salt regulation are not infrequently compromised during encephalitis. Paradoxical antidiuretic hormone secretion is particularly common in St. Louis encephalitis.[84] The respiratory tract, urinary tract, intravenous catheter sites, and skin all should be checked assiduously for evidence of secondary bacterial infection. These infections for the most part can be avoided by good pulmonary toilet, meticulous catheter care, and frequent turning of the patient. Prophylaxis for deep venous thrombosis and gastrointestinal ulceration is recommended, as these are other frequent complications seen in immobilized ICU patients. Recovery in HSE usually occurs over several weeks, with a substantial degree of somnolence, altered cognition, and focal deficits resolving only after a full course of antiviral therapy. CT scanning or MRI performed at this time can be useful in defining the presence of continued mass effect and brain edema and in determining the need for continued aggressive neurologic and systemic interventions.

SUMMARY

Although viral encephalitis remains an uncommon manifestation of systemic viral infection, its variability in clinical presentation and potential for fulminant neurologic deterioration provide the clinician with a broad range of both diagnostic and therapeutic considerations. To date, only the herpesviruses have proven amenable to specific antiviral therapy, and they account for only a small fraction of the total number of patients with encephalitis. Present noninvasive diagnostic techniques are imprecise, so that direct brain biopsy is necessary to secure the diagnosis of HSE. Nevertheless, rapid, noninvasive diagnostic techniques that will apply to a broader group of the viral encephalitides are being developed. It is also clear that vigorous supportive care and improved management of the specific neurologic complications are now improving the chances of survival and long-term outlook of today's encephalitis victims.

REFERENCES

1. Anderson LJ, Nicholson KG, Tauxe RV, and Winkler WG: Human rabies in the United States, 1960–1979: Epidemiology, diagnosis, and prevention. Ann Intern Med 100:728–735, 1984.
2. Azimi PH, Cramblett HG, and Haynes RE: Mumps meningoencephalitis in children. JAMA 207:509–512, 1969.
3. Baer GM, Bellini WJ, and Fishbein DB: Rhabdoviruses. In Fields BN and Knipe DM (eds): Virology, Ed 2, vol 1. Raven Press, New York, 1990, pp 883–930.
4. Baer GM and Fishbein DB: Rabies postexposure prophylaxis. N Engl J Med 316:1270–1272, 1987.
5. Baringer JR: Herpes simplex virus infection of nervous tissue in animals and man. Prog Med Virol 20:1–26, 1975.
6. Barnett GH, Ropper AH, and Romeo J: Intracranial pressure and outcome in adult encephalitis. J Neurosurg 68:585–588, 1988.
7. Barza M and Pauker SG: The decision to biopsy, treat, or wait in suspected herpes encephalitis. Ann Intern Med 92:641–649, 1980.
8. Beghi E, Nicolosi A, Kurland LT, Mulder DW, Hauser WA, and Shuster L: Encephalitis and aseptic meningitis, Olmsted County, Minnesota, 1950–1981: I. Epidemiology. Ann Neurol 16:283–294, 1984.
9. Bernard KW and Hattwick MAW: Rabies virus. In Mandell GL, Douglas RG Jr, and Bennett JE (eds): Principles and Practice of Infectious Diseases, Ed 2. John Wiley, New York, 1985, pp 897–909.
10. Borel C and Hanley DF: Neurologic intensive care unit monitoring. Crit Care Clin 1(2):223–239, 1985.
11. Burke DS, Lorsomrudee W, Leake CJ, et al: Fatal outcome in Japanese encephalitis. Am J Trop Med Hyg 34:1203–1210, 1985.
12. Burke DS, Nisalak A, Ussery MA, Laorakpongse T, and Chantavibul S: Kinetics of IgM and IgG responses to Japanese encephalitis virus in human serum and cerebrospinal fluid. J Infect Dis 151:1093–1099, 1985.
13. Centers for Disease Control: Summary of notifiable diseases, United States, 1987. MMWR 36:4–8, 1987.
14. Centers for Disease Control: Rabies vaccine, adsorbed: A new rabies vaccine for use in humans. MMWR 37:217–223, 1988.
15. Constantine DG: Rabies transmission by the non-bite route. Public Health Rep 77:287–292, 1962.
16. Davis LE and McLaren LC: Relapsing herpes simplex encephalitis following antiviral therapy. Ann Neurol 13:192–195, 1982.
17. Dorfman LJ: Cytomegalovirus encephalitis in adults. Neurology 23:136–144, 1973.
18. Elder GA and Sever JL: Neurologic disorders associated with AIDS retroviral infection. Rev Infect Dis 10:286–302, 1988.
19. Fox JP: Modes of action of poliovirus vaccines and relation to resulting immunity. Rev Infect Dis (Suppl) 6:S352–S355, 1984.
20. Friedman HM, Macarak EJ, MacGregor RR, Wolfe J, and Kefalides NA: Virus infection of endothelial cells. J Infect Dis 143:266–273, 1981.
21. Friedmann U: Permeability of the blood-brain barrier to neurotropic viruses. Arch Pathol 35:912–931, 1943.
22. Gabuzda DH and Hirsch MS: Neurologic manifestations of infection with human immunodeficiency virus. Ann Intern Med 107:383–391, 1987.

23. Gabuzda DH, Ho DD, de la Monte SM, Hirsch MS, Rota TR, and Sobel RA: Immunohistochemical identification of HTLV-III antigen in brains of patients with AIDS. Ann Neurol 20:289–296, 1986.

24. Goldsmith SM and Whitley RJ: Herpes simplex encephalitis. In Lambert HP (ed): Infections of the Central Nervous System. BC Decker, Philadelphia, 1991, pp 283–299.

25. Griffin DE: Alphavirus pathogenesis and immunity. In Schlesinger S and Schlesinger MJ (eds): The Togaviridae and Flaviviridae. Plenum, New York, 1986, pp 209–249.

26. Griffin DE: Viral infections of the central nervous system. In Galasso GJ, Whitley RJ, and Merrigan TC (eds): Antiviral Agents and Viral Diseases of Man, Ed 3. Raven Press, New York, 1990, pp 461–495.

27. Griffin JW and Watson DF: Axonal transport in neurologic disease. Ann Neurol 23:3–13, 1988.

28. Grose C, Henle W, Henle G, and Feorino PM: Primary Epstein-Barr virus infections in acute neurologic diseases. N Engl J Med 292:392–395, 1975.

29. Hirsch RL: The complement system: Its importance in the host response to viral infection. Microbiol Rev 46:71–85, 1982.

30. Horstmann DM and McCollum RW: Poliomyelitis virus in human blood during the "minor illness" and the asymptomatic infection. Proc Soc Exp Biol Med 82:434–437, 1953.

31. Horta-Barbosa L, Fucillo DA, and Sever JL: Subacute sclerosing panencephalitis: Isolation of measles virus from a brain biopsy. Nature 221:974, 1969.

32. Jemsek J, Greenberg SB, Taber L, Harvey D, Gershon A, and Couch RB: Herpes zoster–associated encephalitis: Clinicopathologic report of 12 cases and review of the literature. Medicine 62:81–87, 1983.

33. Johnson KM: Lymphocytic choriomeningitis virus, Lassa fever, tacaribe group of viruses and hemorrhagic fevers. In Mandell GL, Douglas RG Jr, and Bennett JE (eds): Principles and Practice of Infectious Diseases, Ed 2.

John Wiley, New York, 1985, pp 909–914.

34. Johnson KP, Lepow ML, and Johnson RT: California encephalitis. I. Clinical and epidemiological studies. Neurology 18:250–254, 1969.

35. Johnson RT: Virus invasion of the central nervous system: A study of Sindbis virus infection in the mouse using fluorescent antibody. Am J Pathol 46:929–943, 1965.

36. Johnson RT: Viral Infections of the Nervous System. Raven Press, New York, 1982.

37. Johnson RT: The pathogenesis of acute viral encephalitis and postinfectious encephalomyelitis. J Infect Dis 155:359–364, 1987.

38. Johnson RT: Arboviral encephalitis. In Warren KS and Mahmoud AAF (eds): Tropical and Geographical Medicine, ed 2. McGraw-Hill, New York, 1990, pp 691–700.

39. Johnson RT, Burke DS, Elwell M, et al: Japanese encephalitis: Immunocytochemical studies of viral antigen and inflammatory cells in fatal cases. Ann Neurol 18:567–573, 1985.

40. Johnson RT, Griffin DE, Hirsch RL, et al: Measles encephalomyelitis—clinical and immunologic studies. N Engl J Med 310:137–141, 1984.

41. Johnson RT and Milbourn PD: Central nervous system manifestations of chickenpox. Can Med Assoc J 102:831–834, 1970.

42. Johnson RT and Mims CA: Pathogenesis of viral infections of the nervous system. N Engl J Med 278:23–30, 84–92, 1968.

43. Jordan MC, Jordan GW, Stevens JG, and Miller G: Latent herpesviruses of humans. Ann Intern Med 100:866–880, 1984.

44. Kaplan MH, Klein SW, McPhee, J, and Harper RG: Group B coxsackie virus infections in infants younger than three months of age. Rev Infect Dis 5:1019–1032, 1983.

45. Keonig S, Gendelman HE, Orenstein JM, et al: Detection of AIDS virus in macrophages in brain tissue from AIDS patients with encephalopathy. Science 233:1089–1093, 1986.

46. Lakeman FD, Koga K, and Whitley RJ: Detection of antigen to herpes simplex virus in cerebrospinal fluid from patients with herpes simplex encephalitis. J Infect Dis 155:1172–1178, 1987.

47. Levitt LP, Rich TA, Kinde SW, et al: Central nervous system mumps: A review of 64 cases. Neurology (Minneapolis) 20:829–834, 1970.

48. Maiztegui JI, Fernandez NJ, and de Damilano AJ: Efficacy of immune plasma in treatment of Argentine hemorrhagic fever and association between treatment and a late neurological syndrome. Lancet 2:1216–1217, 1979.

49. Masdeu JC, Small CB, Weiss L, Elkin CM, Llena J, and Mesa-Tejada R: Multifocal cytomegalovirus encephalitis in AIDS. Ann Neurol 23:97–99, 1988.

50. McArthur JC: Neurologic manifestations of human immunodeficiency virus infection. Medicine 66:407–437, 1987.

51. McCormick JB, King IJ, Webb PA, et al: Lassa fever: Effective therapy with ribavirin. N Engl J Med 314:20–26, 1986.

52. McKinney RE, Katz SL, and Wilfert CM: Chronic enteroviral meningoencephalitis in agammaglobulinemic patients. Rev Infect Dis 9:334–356, 1987.

53. Melnick JL: Enteroviruses: Polioviruses, coxsackie viruses, echoviruses, and newer enteroviruses. In Fields BN and Knipe DM (eds): Virology, Ed 2, Vol 1. Raven Press, New York, 1990, pp 549–605.

54. Meulen V and Carter MJ: Measles virus persistency and disease. Prog Med Virol 30:44–61, 1984.

55. Meyer HM, Johnson RT, Crawford IP, et al: Central nervous syndromes of ''viral'' etiology: A study of 713 cases. Am J Med 29:334–347, 1960.

56. Modlin JF: Perinatal echovirus infection: Insights from a literature review of 61 cases of serious infection and 16 outbreaks in nurseries. Rev Infect Dis 8:918–926, 1986.

57. Moench TR and Griffin DE: Immunocytochemical identification and quantitation of the mononuclear cells in the cerebrospinal fluid, meninges, and brain during acute viral encephalitis. J Exp Med 159:77–88, 1984.

58. Monath TP: Flaviviruses. In Fields BN and Knipe DM (eds): Virology, Ed 2, Vol 1. Raven Press, New York, 1990, pp 763–814.

59. Moore M: Enteroviral disease in the United States, 1970–79. J Infect Dis 146:103–108, 1982.

60. Moweratz RB, Whitley RJ, and Murphy DM: Experience with brain biopsy for suspected herpes encephalitis: A review of forty consecutive cases. Neurosurgery 12:654–657, 1983.

61. Murphy FA: Rabies pathogenesis: A brief review. Arch Virol 54:279–297, 1975.

62. Murphy FA, Bauer SP, Harrison AK, et al: Comparative pathogenesis of rabies and rabies-like viruses: Viral infection and transit from inoculation site to the central nervous system. Lab Invest 28:361–376, 1973.

63. Nahimas AJ, Whitley RJ, Visintine AN, Takei Y, and Alford CA Jr: Herpes simplex virus encephalitis: Laboratory evaluations and their diagnostic significance. J Infect Dis 145:829–836, 1982.

64. Neils EW, Lukin R, Tomsick TA, and Tew JM: Magnetic resonance imaging and computerized tomography scanning of herpes simplex encephalitis: Report of two cases. J Neurosurg 67:592–594, 1987.

65. Peterson LR and Ferguson RM: Fatal central nervous system infection with varicella-zoster virus in renal transplant recipients. Transplantation 37:366–368, 1984.

66. Pexman JHW: Angiographic and brain scan features of acute herpes simplex encephalitis. Br J Radiol 47:179–184, 1974.

67. Ropper AH: Lateral displacement of the brain and level of consciousness in patients with acute hemispheral mass. N Engl J Med 314:953–958, 1986.

68. Ropper AH: Neurologic and Neurosurgical Critical Care. Aspen Press, New York, 1988.

69. Rosen L: The natural history of Japanese encephalitis virus. Annu Rev Microbiol 40:395–414, 1986.

70. Rosenblum WI and Hadfield MG: Granulomatous angiitis of the central nervous system in cases of herpes zos-

ter and lymphosarcoma. Neurology 22:348–354, 1972.

71. Rowley AH, Whitley RJ, Lakeman FD, and Wolinsky SM: Rapid detection of herpes simplex virus DNA in cerebrospinal fluid of patients with herpes simplex encephalitis. Lancet 335:440–441, 1990.

72. Russell PK: Alphavirus (Eastern, Western, and Venezuelan equine encephalitis). In Mandell GL, Douglas RG Jr, and Bennett JE (eds): Principles and Practice of Infectious Diseases, Ed 2. John Wiley, New York, 1985, pp 917–920.

73. Sabin AB and Ward R: The natural history of poliomyelitis: I. Distribution of virus in nervous and non-nervous tissues. J Exp Med 73:771–793, 1941.

74. Saito Y, Rubenstein R, Price RW, Fox JJ, and Watanabe KA: Diagnostic imaging of herpes simplex virus encephalitis using a radiolabeled antiviral drug: Autoradiographic assessment in an animal model. Ann Neurol 15:548–558, 1984.

75. Schlitt M, Bucker AP, Stroop WG, et al: Neurovirulence in an experimental focal herpes encephalitis: Relationship to observed seizures. Brain Res 440:293–298, 1988.

76. Schlitt MJ, Moweratz RB, Bonnin JM, Zieger HE, and Whitley RJ: Brain biopsy for encephalitis. Clin Neurosurg 33:591–602, 1986.

77. Schroth G, Kretzschmar K, Gawehn J, and Voigt K: Advantage of magnetic resonance imaging in the diagnosis of cerebral infections. Neuroradiology 29:120–126, 1987.

78. Shope RE: Bunyaviruses. In Fields BN and Knipe DM (eds): Virology, Ed 2, Vol 1. Raven Press, New York, 1990, pp 1195–1228.

79. Silverstein A, Steinberg G, and Nathanson M: Nervous system involvement in infectious mononucleosis: The heralding and/or major manifestation. Arch Neurol 26:353–358, 1972.

80. Skoldenberg B, Kalimo K, Carlstrom A, Forsgren M, and Halonen P: Herpes simplex encephalitis: A serological follow-up study. Acta Neurol Scand 63:273–285, 1981.

81. Smith JB, Westmoreland BF, Regan TJ, and Sandok BA: A distinctive clinical EEG profile in herpes simplex encephalitis. Mayo Clin Proc 50:469–474, 1975.

82. Smith MG, Lennette EH, and Reames HR: Isolation of the virus of herpes simplex and the demonstration of intranuclear inclusions in a case of acute encephalitis. Am J Pathol 17:55–68, 1941.

83. Soong SJ, Cuddell GR, Alford CA, Whitley RJ, and the NIAID Collaborative Study Group: Utilization of patients with herpes simplex encephalitis: A statistical model. 26th annual ICAAC meeting, 1986.

84. Southern PM, Smith JW, Luby JP, Barnett JA, and Sanford JP: Clinical and laboratory features of epidemic St. Louis encephalitis. Ann Intern Med 71:681–690, 1969.

85. Timmons GD and Johnson KP: Aqueductal stenosis and hydrocephalus after mumps encephalitis. N Engl J Med 283:1505–1507, 1970.

86. Tovell DR, Samuel J, Mercer JR, et al: The in vitro evaluation of nucleoside analogues as probes for use in the noninvasive diagnosis of herpes simplex encephalitis. Drug Des Deliv 3:213–221, 1988.

87. Van Landingham KE, Marsteller HM, Ross GW, and Hayden FG: Relapse of herpes simplex encephalitis after conventional acyclovir therapy. JAMA 259:2547, 1988.

88. Vanzee BE, Douglas RJ, Betts RF, et al: Lymphocytic choriomeningitis in university hospital personnel. Clinical features. Am J Med 58:803–809, 1975.

89. Vernant JC, Maurs L, Gessain A, et al: Endemic tropical spastic paraparesis associated with human T-lymphotropic virus type I: A clinical and seroepidemiological study of 25 cases. Ann Neurol 21:117–122, 1987.

90. Whitley RJ: Viral encephalitis. N Engl J Med 323:242–250, 1990.

91. Whitley RJ, Alford CA, Hirsch MJ, et al: Vidarabine versus acyclovir in herpes simplex encephalitis. N Engl J Med 314:144–149, 1986.

92. Whitley RJ, Cobbs CG, Alford CA Jr, et al: Diseases that mimic herpes simplex encephalitis: Diagnosis, presentation,

and outcome. JAMA 262:234–239, 1989.

93. Whitley RJ, Corey L, Arvin A, et al: Changing presentation of herpes simplex virus infection in neonates. J Infect Dis 158:109–116, 1988.

94. Whitley R, Lakeman AD, Nahmias A, and Roizman B: DNA restriction-enzyme analysis of herpes simplex virus isolates obtained from patients with encephalitis. N Engl J Med 307:1060–1062, 1982.

95. Whitley RJ, Soong SJ, Hirsch MS, et al: Herpes simplex encephalitis: Vidarabine therapy and diagnostic problems. N Engl J Med 304:313–318, 1981.

96. Whitley RJ, Soong SJ, Linneman C Jr, Liu C, Pazin G, and Alford CA: Herpes simplex encephalitis: Clinical assessment. JAMA 247:317–320, 1982.

97. Wiley CA, Schrier RD, Nelson JA, Lampert PW, and Oldstone MBA: Cellular localization of human immunodeficiency virus infection within brains of acquired immunodeficiency syndrome patients. Proc Natl Acad Sci USA 83:7089–7095, 1986.

98. Winkler WG, Fashinell TR, Leffingwell L, et al: Non–bite-transmitted rabies in a laboratory worker. JAMA 226:1219–1221, 1973.

99. Zarafonetis CJD, Smadel JE, Adams JW, and Haymaker W: Fatal herpes simplex encephalitis in man. Am J Pathol 20:429–445, 1944.

Chapter 2

THE IMMUNOLOGY OF CNS VIRAL INFECTIONS

Diane Edmund Griffin, M.D., Ph.D.

PATHOPHYSIOLOGIC MECHANISMS OF IMMUNE RESPONSES WITHIN THE CENTRAL NERVOUS SYSTEM
IMMUNE RESPONSES TO CNS VIRAL INFECTIONS
IMMUNOLOGICALLY MEDIATED ENCEPHALOMYELITIS

Virus infections may cause central nervous system (CNS) disease either by direct infection of CNS cells or by inciting an autoimmune response to CNS antigens. CNS disease caused by direct viral infection is usually due to virus-induced injury to neurons, glia, and ependymal or meningeal cells, but injury may also be mediated by the response of the immune system to the virus-infected cells. CNS disease caused by an immunologically mediated attack in the absence of virus-infected CNS cells is usually targeted toward myelin or myelin-forming cells and produces primarily monophasic demyelinating disease.

The basic components of any immune response are T lymphocytes, B lymphocytes, monocyte/macrophages, and the soluble products of these cells. T lymphocytes are subdivided into two basic groups based on function and surface markers. The helper/inducer or CD4-positive T cells are the primary producers of soluble products (cyto-

kines) important for cellular chemotaxis and for B- and T-cell expansion and differentiation and monocyte/macrophage activation. CD4 T cells recognize antigen only in association with major histocompatibility complex (MHC) class II antigens. Most cytokines act through their cellular receptors to transcriptionally activate sets of genes within the target cell. Cellular receptivity to such activation is dependent on regulated expression of the appropriate receptor resulting in a complex network of cellular interactions. The cytotoxic/suppressor or CD8-positive T cells appear to produce a more limited array of cytokines but have cytotoxic function. CD8 T cells recognize and lyse cells expressing antigen in association with MHC class I antigens. The primary product of B lymphocytes is antibody. Immunoglobulin M (IgM) is produced initially, followed by IgG and IgA as B cells mature, with the help of CD4 T cells, into plasma cells. Monocyte/macrophages are important phagocytic cells that do not have antigen-specificity but express MHC class II antigens and thus can present antigen to antigen-specific CD4 T cells. Macrophages also produce cytokines that contribute to T- and B-cell activation. Macrophages are the primary effector cells in immunologically mediated demyelination.

PATHOPHYSIOLOGIC MECHANISMS OF IMMUNE RESPONSES WITHIN THE CENTRAL NERVOUS SYSTEM

Immune responses occurring within the CNS may be initiated in lymphoid tissue outside the CNS or possibly within the CNS by infiltrating lymphoid cells. In either case, there are two areas of special consideration related to development of immune responses either to foreign or autologous antigens within the CNS: (1) the ability of cells and circulating soluble factors to cross the specialized capillaries of the blood-brain barrier, and (2) the existence of cells within the CNS capable of presenting antigen in an MHC-restricted fashion to lymphoid cells functioning as regulatory or effector cells of the immune response.

The basic components for development of immune reactions—T cells, B cells, and antigen-presenting cells (macrophages, dendritic cells, and so forth)—normally reside primarily in

peripheral lymphoid tissue. Classically, the CNS has not been thought to have a lymphatic circulation or to be subjected to routine immune surveillance. Current evidence suggests, however, that a normal pattern of fluid drainage exists from the interstitial fluid to cerebrospinal fluid (CSF) and into the deep cervical lymph nodes.[16] In fact, some studies have demonstrated that immunization by intracerebral inoculation of soluble antigen into CSF is more effective for eliciting a systemic antibody response than immunization by peripheral routes of inoculation.[63] If lymphocytes can routinely enter the CNS from the blood and follow a similar pathway back to lymphoid tissue,[110] then the essential elements exist for immune surveillance of the CNS by a recirculating population of cells.

Entry of Mononuclear Cells

T cells, B cells, and macrophages are represented in the blood by circulating subsets of cells that have the opportu-

Table 2–1 POTENTIAL RECEPTOR-LIGAND INTERACTIONS BETWEEN LEUKOCYTES, VASCULAR ENDOTHELIAL CELLS, AND EXTRACELLULAR MATRIX THAT MAY CONTRIBUTE TO THE DEVELOPMENT OF INFLAMMATION

Receptor Type	Receptor	Ligands	Ligand Type
Adhesive (β_2) integrins[12,127]	LFA-1[39a,127]	ICAM-1, ICAM-2[33,94,116]	Ig
	CR3[121]	iC3b, fibrinogen	Complement, ECM
	p150,95	?	?
Matrix (β_1) integrins[12,68,127]	VLA-1	Collagen, laminin	ECM
	VLA-2 (ECMR-II)	Collagen, laminin	ECM
	VLA-3 (ECMR-I)	Laminin, fibronectin, collagen	ECM
	VLA-4 (LPAM-1)[71a]	VCAM-1 (INCAM-110)[113b]	Ig
	VLA-5 (FNR, ECMR-VI)	Fibronectin	ECM
	VLA-6	Laminin	ECM
Selectins[113a]	mLHR (MEL-14)	Mannose-6-phosphate	Carbohydrate
	LAM-1 (Leu-8)[137a]	?	?
	ELAM-1[11,145a]	Sialyl-Le	Carbohydrate
	GMP140[82]		
Immunoglobulin (Ig) superfamily[127]	LFA-1 (CD2)[12]	LFA-3	Ig
Proteoglycan	Pgp-1 (CD44)[129a]	?	?
	ECMR-III	?	?

Key: ? = unknown. See Table 2–2 for definition of abbreviations.

nity to leave the circulation to participate in local immune responses. Tissue-based immune responses are probably initiated by a recirculating population of cells that enter organs and tissues across capillary endothelium and leave through efferent lymphatics.[50,126] Some of this lymphocyte recirculation is tissue-specific.[20,76] The initiating factors and mechanisms by which immunologically important cells cross the specialized endothelium of the blood-brain barrier either normally or during disease is not yet known but represents an active area of investigation (Table 2–1). Data suggest that activated, but not resting, T cells can cross cerebral capillaries into the CNS[107,147] and that antigen specificity is not important for initial entry but is important for retention of T cells in the tissue.[64,147]

To enter brain parenchyma and initiate the inflammatory response, T cells must cross the structural complex of endothelial cells connected by tight junctions, pericytes, basement membrane, and astrocytic foot processes. It is likely that changes in the surface characteristics of both the traversing cells and the traversed endothelium contribute to cell entry at various stages of the inflammatory response (Fig. 2–1).[127] Based on biochemical analysis and sequence information, receptor molecules belonging to five general molecular families—adhesive (β_2) integrins, matrix (β_1) integrins, selectins, immunoglobulins, and proteoglycans—have been identified (see Table 2–1). Combinations of receptors and ligands subserving the interactions of circulating leukocytes and vascular endothelial cells can be independently regulated. For instance, intercellular adhesion molecule 1 (ICAM-1) is constitutively expressed at low levels on endothelial cells and can be up-regulated by a variety of cytokines including interferon gamma (IFN-γ), interleukin 1 (IL-1), and tumor necrosis factor (TNF)[33,116] (Table 2–2). The high-avidity form of the receptor for this ligand, leukocyte function antigen 1 (LFA-1), is expressed, and can be up-regulated, on

many types of leukocytes including T and B lymphocytes and monocytes,[12,39a,94] increasing the likelihood that they will attach securely to and traverse the endothelium.[13] Other molecules such as endothelial-leukocyte adhesion molecule 1 (ELAM-1) and vascular cell adhesion molecule 1 (VCAM-1) are not normally expressed on endothelial cells but can be induced by soluble factors to greatly increase the binding and penetration of endothelial cells by leukocytes.[11,113a] There may be specialized homing receptor-addressin systems promoting specific entry into the CNS, as there are for other tissues.[20] The extent to which any of these systems are important for normal trafficking of lymphocytes and monocytes or for initiation and perpetuation of inflammatory reactions within the CNS is as yet unknown.

Once a cell has adhered to the vascular endothelium, the expression of receptors for relevant extracellular matrix proteins (laminin, fibronectin, and so forth), the very late antigens (VLAs) of lymphocytes (see Table 2–1), is important for entry of the adherent cell into tissue.[12,68,127] Binding to matrix proteins and production of matrix-degrading enzymes[107a,122] probably allow cells to enter and move into the brain parenchyma. In addition, macrophage expression of the complement receptor CR3 has been shown to be essential for

Table 2–2 GLOSSARY OF COMMON CYTOKINE AND ADHESION MOLECULE ABBREVIATIONS

CYTOKINES

IFN	Interferon
IL	Interleukin
TNF	Tumor necrosis factor

ADHESION MOLECULES

LFA	Leukocyte function–related antigen
ICAM	Intercellular adhesion molecule
ELAM	Endothelial-leukocyte adhesion molecule
VCAM	Vascular cell adhesion molecule
VLA	Very late antigen
CR	Complement receptor
ECMR	Extracellular matrix receptor
LHR	Lymphocyte homing receptor

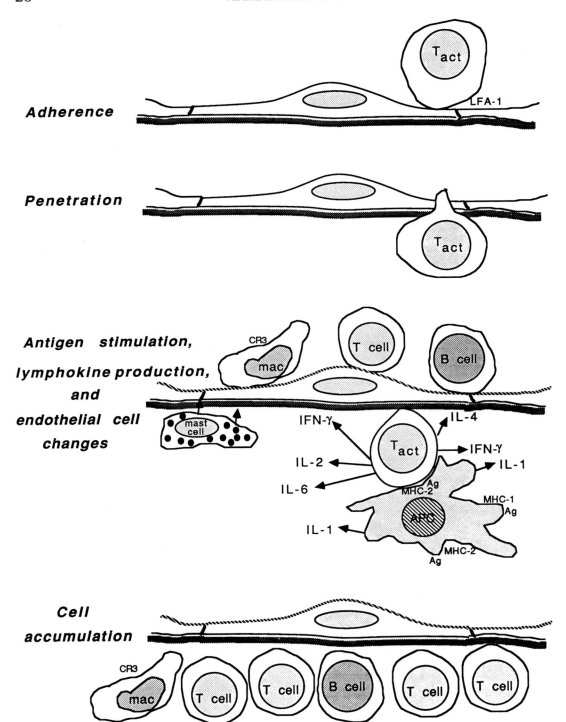

Figure 2–1. Postulated sequence of events involved in the initiation and amplification of immune response to CNS viral infections. T_{act} = activated T cell; APC = antigen presenting cell; Ag = viral antigen; CR3 = complement receptor, type 3.

entry of these cells into sites of inflammation (see Fig. 2–1).[121]

Expression of MHC Antigens

Expression of MHC antigens is required at two phases of the immune response: antigen presentation to lymphocytes, and lymphocyte recognition of antigen-bearing target cells.[123] Antigen presentation to lymphocytes for initiation of the immune response requires simultaneous expression of MHC class II (Ia) antigens and the foreign antigen by the antigen-presenting cell to provide a signal recognized by the helper/inducer CD4 T lymphocyte.[123] CD4 T cells provide helper function for B cells[60] and are the primary producers of a variety of lymphokines that activate and attract macrophages to an area of immune response.[104] CD8 T cells, which include cytotoxic T lymphocytes capable of eliminating virus-infected cells, recognize antigen (and therefore virus-infected cells) only in the context of MHC class I antigen.[27,123] Either endogenously synthesized antigen or antigen entering the cell by endocytosis can be degraded and presented with class II, whereas internal cellular synthesis of the protein (that is, virus replication) is required for class I presentation.

Neither MHC class I nor class II antigens are found in significant amounts in the normal CNS,[139,145,150] but both classes are often induced on microglia during immune responses within the CNS[98,132,139,144] and, in some instances, may also be induced on other glial, choroid plexus, and endothelial cells.[42,119,125,135,151] Neuronal expression of MHC antigens probably does not occur.[19a] Most potentially MHC-positive CNS cells are capable of presenting antigen to T cells in vitro,[39,69,97,151] and many can also be induced to secrete a variety of cytokines.[19,92] These cells alone may not be fully capable of activating T cells,[117a] however, and the relevance of in vitro observations to in vivo responses has yet to be demonstrated.[42]

Since class I and class II antigen expression by microglia is also induced after nonimmunologically mediated damage such as axotomy, this may be a generalized response of microglia to nervous system injury.[133]

IMMUNE RESPONSES TO CNS VIRAL INFECTIONS

Most viruses that infect the CNS replicate at some peripheral location (respiratory tract, subcutaneous tissue, gastrointestinal tract, and so forth) before entering the CNS. Even when infection is limited to the CNS, viral antigen may appear in cervical lymph nodes. It is, therefore, most likely that initial stimulation of the immune response occurs in the spleen and lymph nodes exposed to viral antigen by traditional routes; the earliest recognized immune events associated with *infection* in the CNS are initiated in the periphery, with subsequent entry of sensitized cells into the CNS. In this case, investigations seek to determine how inflammatory cells and antibodies enter into the area of CNS viral infection. For *autoimmune disease,* the earliest events in the induction of disease are less clear. The possibility that immune responses are initiated entirely within the CNS is an important area of study of the pathophysiology of these diseases.

Cell-Mediated Immunity

The inflammatory response to viral infection at any location is characteristically composed of mononuclear cells (lymphocytes, monocytes, and natural killer cells). Viral infections of the CNS induce inflammation in the meninges, the CSF, and the brain parenchyma. The infiltration of mononuclear cells into each of these locations is an immunologically specific event that is dependent on the presence of sensitized T cells[26,55] and on histocompatibility between T cells and brain cells.[28,31] The earliest event that initiates the mononuclear inflammatory process after infection is not clear. It is likely that changes in T cells in response to immune activation in the periphery and in endothelial cells in response to local tissue injury in the CNS will prove to be important in initiating the reaction. Pathologically, the earliest change seen in the brain parenchyma is the adherence of lymphocytes to vascular endothelial cells near the site of virus replication (see Fig. 2–1).[8] The cells that adhere to and cross the capillary endothelium first are probably those that have entered the circulation after having been activated by exposure to viral antigen in peripheral lymphoid tissue. These activated cells have increased numbers of surface receptors for endothelial cells and matrix proteins.

The secondary phase of the cell entry is partially dependent on the presence of local mast cells that facilitate the entry of cells by opening capillary endothelial tight junctions. Mast cells are probably stimulated to release vasoactive amines by lymphokines released locally by the initial virus-specific T cells (see Fig. 2–1).[6] Mice that are either pharmacologically depleted of vasoactive amines with reserpine or genetically deficient in mast cells have a reduced inflammatory response to viral infection of the CNS.[56,103]

Viruses may infect cells of the meninges or parenchyma of the brain or spinal cord. Within the parenchyma, certain regions of the CNS or particular cell types within the CNS may be more likely than others to be infected by a particular virus. Inflammation may also be focal or generalized, and the cells present in one CNS location may or may not be the same cells present in another location. Likewise, even though viral infections all induce a mononuclear inflammatory response, the types of cells responding to one type of virus may differ from those responding to another type of virus. The two primary locations for cell accumulation during viral infection are the CSF and the perivascular regions of the parenchyma of brain and spinal cord.

CEREBROSPINAL FLUID

Cells entering the CSF are primarily T cells and natural killer (NK) cells.* In experimental models of alphavirus meningoencephalitis, the numbers of cells in the CSF reach a peak before they do in the meninges or brain parenchyma.[101] NK cells are most abundant early.[54] The types of T cells that make up this CSF pleocytosis have been studied most thoroughly in humans and mice and vary with the virus (Table 2–3). During acute alphavirus- (e.g., Sindbis virus) and flavivirus- (e.g., Japanese encephalitis virus) induced meningo-

---

*References 3, 23, 25, 30, 32, 54, 74, 81, 96, 101, 106.

Table 2–3 IMMUNE CELLS IN CSF DURING CNS VIRAL INFECTION

| Virus Group | Virus | Percentage of Total Cells | | | |
| | | T Cells | | | |
		CD4	CD8	B Cells	Macrophage
Alphavirus[101]	Sindbis	45	23	1	1
Flavivirus[81]	Japanese encephalitis	48	15	8	9
Arenavirus[23,30]	Lymphocytic choriomeningitis	30	25	ND	45
Morbillivirus[25]	Measles (SSPE)	34	40	ND	ND
Poxvirus[32]	Vaccinia	58	55	1	12
Retrovirus[96]	Human immunodeficiency	20	35	9	6

Key: ND = not determined; SSPE = subacute sclerosing panencephalitis.

Table 2–4 SOLUBLE PRODUCTS OF LYMPHOCYTES AND MACROPHAGES FOUND IN CSF DURING ACUTE VIRAL MENINGITIS OR ENCEPHALITIS AND DURING POSTINFECTIOUS ENCEPHALOMYELITIS

Soluble Product	Viral Encephalitis	Postinfectious Encephalomyelitis
T CELLS		
Interferon-γ[57,84]	+ +	−
Soluble IL-2 receptor[15,58]	+ +	−
Soluble CD8[58]	+ + +	+ + +
Interleukin 6[44,71b]	+	−
β_2-microglobulin[17,58a]	+	+
B CELLS		
Antiviral antibody[81,142]	+ + +	−
MACROPHAGES		
Neopterin[40,57]	+ + +	+ +
Interleukin 1[44]	+	?

Key: + (+ +, + + +) = relative amounts of product; − = absent; ? = unknown.

encephalitis, the T cells are predominantly of the CD4 helper/inducer phenotype.[81,101] During acute arenavirus (e.g., lymphocytic choriomeningitis virus) infections and chronic infections caused by measles virus (i.e., subacute sclerosing panencephalitis) and retroviruses (e.g., human immunodeficiency virus), a larger proportion of the T cells are of the CD8 cytotoxic/suppressor phenotype.[23,25,30,96] These differences in cell type may relate to differences in the pathogenesis of CNS disease caused by these diverse agents, or to the types of cells preferentially stimulated in the periphery by infection with viruses with various primary sites of replication. T cells entering the CSF appear to be an activated population[64a,95a] with an increased proportion expressing MHC class II[41] and phagocyte glycoprotein 1 (Pgp-1)[93] antigens, compared with the cells in peripheral blood.

It is not clear why CD4 T cells in the CSF do not usually recruit monocytes and B cells into the CSF, but it is probably a manifestation of the MHC-restricted interaction of T lymphocytes with virus-infected cells.[28,29] Cell-associated viral antigen for T-cell recognition is found primarily in the brain parenchyma, while cell-free virus is most abundant in CSF. Monocytes and B cells may therefore be recruited into the

brain parenchyma by locally stimulated and locally produced lymphokines and then remain in situ.

There is often evidence in the CSF, however, of the secretory activity of T cells within the CNS (Table 2–4). T-cell products such as IFN-γ, IL-6, soluble IL-2 receptor, and soluble CD8 are increased in the CSF during acute and chronic viral infections of the CNS.[15,44,57,84] Macrophage products such as neopterin and IL-1 may also be increased in CSF during viral infection,[40,44] as is β_2-microglobulin, the α chain of the MHC class I molecule.[17]

BRAIN PARENCHYMA

Cells in the parenchymal perivascular cuffs are more varied and are composed of significant numbers of T cells, B cells, monocytes,[41,78,101] and probably NK cells.[54] Many of these inflammatory cells express MHC class II antigens.[139] In the earliest phase the primary cells present are T cells,[88,101] and MHC compatibility with CNS cells is necessary for initiation and development of the inflammatory response.[31] These observations suggest the importance of T-cell interaction with infected cells for initiation and amplification of cellular infiltration.[28,130] During many viral infections, CD4 T cells are the earliest cells to arrive at the site of virus replication and probably provide the immunologic specificity for the inflammatory response.[88,101,131] Upon antigenic stimulation in the local environment, CD4 T lymphocytes produce a variety of lymphokines, including chemotactic factors for monocytes and B cells, and factors promoting activation, proliferation, and differentiation of monocytes and lymphocytes (see Fig. 2–1).[46,87,101]

The delayed appearance of macrophages and B cells in the perivascular cuffs, and the fact that these cells do not appear in significant numbers in T-cell–deficient mice,[138] suggests that they are recruited to the area of virus replication secondarily by T cells stimulated by local viral antigen to produce relevant lymphokines. It is unclear which brain cell provides antigen presentation for this local lymphocyte stimulation, but there are several candidates. The most likely cells are microglia, which are often induced to express MHC class II antigens by viral infections of the CNS.[119,139] This response is partially dependent on mature T cells[139] but can also be induced to some degree by injury alone.[133] Microglia may not need to replicate virus to present viral antigens, since they are probably capable of taking up viral antigen released by other cells and processing it for presentation to and stimulation of CD4 T cells. Astrocytes and endothelial cells have also been reported to express class II antigens during viral infections of the CNS[119] and theoretically could also present viral antigen locally.

Since T cells must recognize antigen in the context of MHC antigens on cells, they are ideally suited for effecting virus elimination from tissue. Although CD4 T cells reacting with class II–expressing antigen-presenting cells appear to be important for initiating and amplifying the inflammatory response to most CNS viruses, they are not necessarily associated with virus clearance.[130,134] If a virus-infected cell also expresses MHC class I antigen, then it can serve as a target for cytotoxic CD8 T

lymphocytes. Antigens recognized by cytotoxic T lymphocytes are often synthesized early during viral replication, providing the opportunity for an infected cell to be recognized and killed prior to the production of more infectious virus. CD8 T cells are essential for elimination of certain coronaviruses (e.g., JHM virus)[134] and arenaviruses (e.g., lymphocytic choriomeningitis virus)[2] from the CNS. In addition, CD8 T cells are also responsible for mediating the fatal immunopathologic CNS disease lymphocytic choriomeningitis[2] and contribute to the development of late corona and Theiler's virus-induced demyelinating disease.[88,120,146]

Antibody

Antibody found in the CSF in the absence of infection comes from the blood. In the presence of an intact blood-brain barrier, antibody is present in CSF at approximately 0.5% to 1% of the concentration in blood. If the blood-brain barrier is not intact, then the CSF-to-serum antibody ratio must be corrected for this fact. Correction is based on the concentration of albumin relative to IgG in both the serum and the CSF (the IgG index).[34,45] Increased amounts of antibody in CSF suggest CNS infection with the agent against which the antibody is directed.

B cells, the producers of antibody, enter the blood, and thus have access to the brain, during two stages of maturation: when they leave the bone marrow before antigen stimulation (IgM$^+$ IgD$^+$ B cells), and when they leave the spleen after antigen stimulation (IgM$^+$, IgG$^+$, or IgA$^+$ B cells).[21,108] Selective homing of subsets of circulating B lymphocytes to certain types of lymphoid organs, inflamed joints, and skin, dependent on selective adhesion to specific endothelial cells, has been identified.[20,76] Selective homing to other organs, such as the brain, may also occur, but less specific mechanisms of B-cell entry into infected tissue are probably important as well. For in-

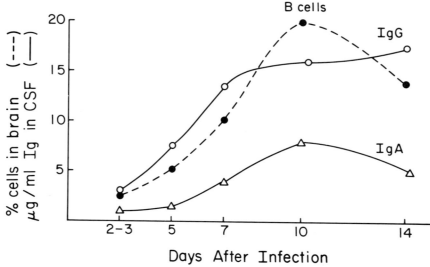

Figure 2–2. Correlation of the appearance of B cells in the brain parenchyma with the appearance of immunoglobulin (Ig) in the CSF during viral encephalitis. (From Griffin DE, Moench TR, Hess JL, and Johnson RT: Identification of the inflammatory cells in the central nervous system during acute viral encephalitis. In Lowenthal A and Raus J [eds]. Cellular and Humoral Immunological Components of Cerebrospinal Fluid in Multiple Sclerosis. Plenum Publishing Corporation, New York, 1987, p 364, with permission.)

stance, T cells present early in the inflammatory response may release factors that are chemotactic for B cells,[112] that make endothelial cells more adherent for B lymphocytes,[11,22,94,116] or that modify the tight junctions of the blood-brain barrier to allow passage of inflammatory cells of all types into the brain parenchyma.[6,95]

Local production of virus-specific antibody has been documented to occur during the recovery phase of many CNS viral infections.* Appearance of antiviral antibody in the CSF correlates with the appearance of B cells in the brain[55] (Fig. 2–2). This observation suggests that B cells are differentiating and producing immunoglobulin locally in the brain parenchyma. This immunoglobulin then moves with other components of interstitial fluid to appear in the CSF. The earliest B cells to enter the perivascular space are relatively immature and express IgM or IgM/IgD on the cell surface, as do essentially all the B cells in

blood.[138] It is not known what proportion of these IgM-expressing cells are antigen-specific, but local synthesis of virus-specific IgM has been described during a number of CNS viral infections.[38] It also is not known whether some of these immature B cells are induced to mature by the lymphokine-producing CD4 T cells present in the local inflammatory reaction, or if all remain IgM+.

As IgG- and IgA-expressing B cells enter the circulation, after undergoing antigen stimulation and isotype switching in the spleen, more and more of the B cells entering the evolving parenchymal inflammatory response are IgG+ or IgA+.[35,36,138] It is not known what proportion of these B cells produce virus-specific antibody, but local synthesis of significant amounts of virus-specific IgG and IgA has been documented in many types of viral encephalitis.† Local antibody production is likely to be important for neutralizing

*References 24, 38, 48, 51, 72, 83, 117, 142, 143.

†References 24, 48, 51, 72, 83, 117, 124, 142, 143.

infectious virus present in interstitial fluid and CSF. Furthermore, in alphavirus- and enterovirus-induced encephalitis, antibody also appears to be important for virus clearance from tissue by as-yet-undefined mechanisms.[70,86a,148]

IMMUNOLOGICALLY MEDIATED ENCEPHALOMYELITIS

A number of immunizations and infectious diseases are occasionally complicated by autoimmune diseases of the nervous system. These diseases typically are inflammatory, are demyelinating, occur within a few days to weeks of the inducing illness, and follow a monophasic course.[52] Experimental diseases with similar clinical and pathologic pictures can be produced in animals by inoculation of myelin constituents. The pathologic changes observed in the CNS of patients dying with postinfectious encephalomyelitis, perivenular mononuclear cell inflammation and demyelination, are similar to those seen in brains of animals with experimental autoimmune encephalomyelitis (EAE) and patients dying of the complications of neural tissue–derived (Semple) rabies vaccine.[91,118,141] The similarity of the pathology, the acute onset, and the monophasic clinical course have led to the hypothesis that all these diseases have an autoimmune etiology.[52,79]

Post–Rabies Vaccine Encephalomyelitis

Soon after Pasteur's introduction of postexposure rabies immunization with dessicated spinal cord from rabies virus–infected rabbits, neuroparalytic complications were recognized.[7] Semple rabies vaccine, still in use in many parts of the world, is a phenol-inactivated version of the early neural-tissue vaccines and is usually prepared from the brains of sheep or goats. In 1932, Hurst[73] postulated that the neuropara-

lytic disorders complicating rabies immunization were due to an immune reaction to the nervous system tissue in the vaccine. Subsequent attempts to produce a similar disease in animals were eventually successful,[118] resulting in the extensively studied animal model of autoimmune disease, EAE. To avoid these neurologic complications, tissue culture–produced vaccines, which elicit very few neurologic complications, have replaced neural tissue–produced vaccines in many countries.

The reported rates of neuroparalytic complications with Semple vaccine vary, but are approximately 1:400.[67] The first symptoms are usually fever, headache, and myalgias occurring 6 to 14 days after the initiation of the daily injections. Development of neurologic complications does not correlate with development of local inflammation at injection sites.[67] Objective neurologic signs typically occur within a week of the onset of the prodrome (Fig. 2–3) and include meningismus, altered consciousness, paralysis, sensory deficits, and movement disorders.[5,67,136] CSF examination at the time of presentation shows a moderate pleocytosis and increased protein (Table 2–5). Myelin basic protein (MBP) is present in the CSF in patients with encephalitis or myelitis, indicating myelin damage, but not in patients with meningitis or Guillain-Barré syndrome. The computed tomography scan may show white-matter lesions similar to those seen in multiple sclerosis.[67]

In most patients the disease follows a monophasic course, but occasionally it is progressive or relapsing.[66] The mortality rate is approximately 10%.[5,67,136] In general, patients with paralysis associated with a Guillain-Barré syndrome–type picture have greater morbidity and mortality than patients with CNS symptoms.[67]

Disease is postulated to be due to an autoimmune response to the injected neural tissue in the vaccine. Comparison of the antibody response of patients having clear neurologic complications with the antibody response to individ-

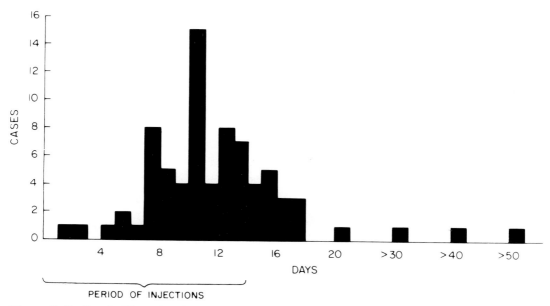

Figure 2–3. Onset of Semple rabies vaccine–induced encephalomyelitis after initiation of immunization. (From Griffin DE, Hemachudha T, and Johnson RT: Postinfectious and postvaccinal encephalomyelitis. In Gilden DH and Lipton HL [eds]: Clinical and Molecular Aspects of Neurotropic Virus Infection. Kluwer Academic Publishers, Boston, 1989, p 506, with permission.)

uals with minor complications (headache, myalgias, and so forth) or no complications has shown elevated levels of antibody to CNS myelin in those with major complications.[65] Assays for antibody to specific myelin antigens have shown that patients with major complications have high levels of serum and CSF antibody to MBP, the primary encephalitogen in EAE,[37] whereas patients without neurologic complications do not have such antibody (Table 2–6).[65] Most of the MBP antibody is directed against the C-terminal portion of the protein.[140] T-cell responses to MBP

are also demonstrable in most patients studied.[67] Many Semple vaccine–immunized individuals with and without neurologic complications have antibody to cerebroside and various gangliosides. Immune responses to these myelin components are more frequent in those with neurologic complications (Table 2–6) and may serve to enhance the demyelination associated with the response to MBP.[65]

The mechanism of demyelination and the relative roles of T cells and antibody in targeting myelin for immunologic attack are not known. T cells are

Table 2–5 CSF ABNORMALITIES IN PATIENTS WITH NEUROLOGIC COMPLICATIONS AFTER SEMPLE RABIES VACCINE AND AFTER MEASLES

Complications	Cells/mm³	Protein, mg/dL	MBP (+/Total)
Semple rabies vaccine			
Meningitis	221 ± 58	76 ± 12	0/13
Encephalitis	82 ± 30	73 ± 6	11/23
Measles			
Postinfectious encephalitis	71 ± 29	66 ± 15	6/10

Source: Griffin DE: Postinfectious and postvaccinal disorders of the central nervous system. Immunol Allergy Clinics N Am 8:241, 1988, with permission.

Table 2–6 PERCENTAGES OF PATIENTS RECEIVING SEMPLE RABIES VACCINE WHO DEVELOPED ELEVATED LEVELS OF ANTIBODY TO VARIOUS NEURAL ANTIGENS

| Neural Antigen | Neurologic Complications | | |
	Major, %	Minor, %	None (d14*), %
Myelin basic protein	75	0	0
Myelin-associated glycoprotein	0	0	0
Cerebroside	92	68	64
Ganglioside			
$\quad$GM1	85	55	53
$\quad$GD$_{1a}$	78	27	20
$\quad$GD$_{1b}$	44	0	7
$\quad$GT$_{1b}$	37	5	20

*Studied 14 days after beginning immunization.
Source: Adapted from Griffin DE: Postinfectious and postvaccinal disorders of the central nervous system. Immunol Allergy Clinics N Am 8:239, 1988, with permission.

clearly important for the induction of inflammation in EAE,[10,115] but full development of the demyelinating lesions also requires the presence of antibody[149] and macrophages[18] in addition to T lymphocytes. The nature of the antigen-presenting cells is not clear, but it is possible that MHC antigens are induced on CNS cells by systemic production of lymphokines. Genetic susceptibility to disease induction probably accounts, at least in part, for the relatively infrequent appearance of disease. Both MHC-linked and non–MHC-linked factors may well be important, as they are in EAE,[62,105] but have not yet been defined.

Postinfectious Encephalomyelitis

Neuroparalytic disease induced by a variety of infectious processes resembles encephalomyelitis induced by Semple rabies vaccine both clinically and pathologically. The incidence of disease after different infections varies greatly but is most frequent after measles (1 in 1000 cases) (Table 2–7). With measles, the incidence tends to increase with age.[79,99] The onset is usually abrupt, with a recurrence of fever and altered level of consciousness, frequently associated with seizures and multifocal neurologic signs. In measles the disease most often occurs within 4 to 8 days after the onset of rash (Fig. 2–4) and has a monophasic course. Mortality is approximately 10% to 20%, but most surviving patients have neurologic sequelae.[4,80,100]

The CSF usually shows a mild mononuclear cell pleocytosis, protein elevation, and presence of MBP (see Table 2–5) but may be completely normal.[80] The electroencephalogram is usually ab-

Table 2–7 INCIDENCE AND COMPLICATION RATES OF POSTINFECTIOUS ENCEPHALOMYELITIS AFTER DIFFERENT VIRAL INFECTIONS

Virus	Case Rate	Mortality	Sequelae
Measles	1:1000	20%	>50%
Vaccinia	1:63–1:300,000	10%	Rare
Mumps	1:6000	20%	30%
Varicella	<1:10,000	5%	10%
Rubella	<1:20,000	20%	Very rare

Source: Adapted from Johnson RT, Griffin DE, and Gendelman HE,[80] p 181.

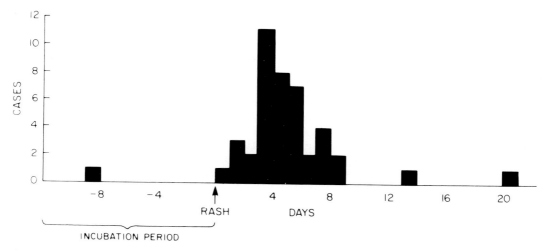

Figure 2–4. Onset of encephalomyelitis in relation to the incubation period and rash of measles. (From Griffin DE, Hemachudha T, and Johnson RT: Postinfectious and postvaccinal encephalomyelitis. In Gilden DH and Lipton HL [eds]: Clinical and Molecular Aspects of Neurotropic Virus Infection. Kluwer Academic Publishers, Boston, 1989, p 513, with permission.)

normal, with nonspecific diffuse slowing. When the neurologic disease occurs in association with an exanthema, the diagnosis is relatively straightforward, but when it follows other precipitating events, such as nonspecific respiratory illness, the diagnosis is more difficult.

There is little evidence of direct viral infection of the brain during postinfectious encephalomyelitis after measles. Virus has rarely been recovered from the brain,[79] viral antigen is not detectable by immunocytochemical staining,[47] viral nucleic acid is not detectable

by hybridization,[102] and there is no evidence of intrathecally synthesized antibody[81] or interferon[85] in the CSF. These features, along with the pathology, distinguish postinfectious encephalomyelitis from encephalitis due to direct virus infection of the CNS (see Tables 2–4 and 2–8).[77]

Neurologic abnormalities in the form of abnormal electroencephalograms and CSF pleocytosis are common even in uncomplicated measles,[49,61,111,114] however, raising the possibility that virus invasion of the CNS is common during measles but is rapidly cleared

Table 2–8 KEY FEATURES OF ACUTE VIRAL ENCEPHALITIS AND POSTINFECTIOUS ENCEPHALOMYELITIS

	Acute Viral Encephalitis	Postinfectious Encephalomyelitis
VIRUS IN CNS		
Culture	+ +	−
Antigen	+ +	−
Nucleic acid	+ +	−
Interferon α	+ +	−
HISTOPATHOLOGY		
Inflammation	+ + +	+ +
Demyelination	− to + +	+ + +
Neuronal damage	− to + +	−

and leads to CNS disease in only a few individuals. CNS tissue obtained at autopsy from children dying early during measles is also negative for viral antigen or nucleic acid at times when it is easily demonstrable elsewhere,[102] however, so there is little to suggest frequent infection of the CNS during measles. Alternatively, the CSF pleocytosis may be related to the systemic immune activation that occurs during measles.[57,58] Treatment of lymphocytes with IL-2 causes them to adhere to endothelial cells,[25a] and in vivo administration of IL-2 is associated with CNS toxicity[92b] thought to be due to alterations of capillary permeability.[121a] Similarly, treatment of patients with antibody to CD3, which activates T cells, is associated with acute aseptic meningitis.[22a] These observations suggest that systemic immune activation may lead to increased lymphocyte trafficking to the brain independent of the presence of virus in the CNS.

The pattern of demyelination suggests an immunologically mediated process. The loss of the myelin proteins MBP and myelin-associated glycoprotein is concordant, as it is in EAE, rather than discordant, as it is in viral infection of myelin-forming cells.[47] MBP is frequently present in the CSF (see Table 2–5).[80] Furthermore, many studies have documented an immune response to myelin proteins in patients with encephalomyelitis after a variety of infections,[9,59,80,90] and in many instances this response has been specific for MBP.[80] Soluble mononuclear cell products are found in CSF and show a pattern different from that observed during acute viral encephalitis (see Table 2–4). Levels of IFN-γ and soluble IL-2 receptor are low, while levels of neopterin and soluble CD8 are high.[15,40,57,58,84] These data suggest that the type of cellular immune response occurring within the CNS during postinfectious encephalomyelitis is distinct from that occurring during acute viral infection.[77]

The mechanism by which an auto-immune response to myelin proteins is induced during systemic infection has not been satisfactorily explained. There is well-documented immune dysregulation during measles* and other viral infections,[14,57,109,128] which may allow the proliferation of autoreactive T or B lymphocytes that are normally under restrictive control. A similar demyelinating pathology was found in a patient who died of encephalomyelitis after IL-2 treatment.[144a] It is also possible that many infectious agents contain antigens that cross-react with MBP or other myelin constituents. Some similarities have been identified in the sequences of MBP and viral proteins.[43,75] The biologic importance of "molecular mimicry" for measles virus, the agent most often associated with postinfectious encephalomyelitis, has not yet been established. Since the antigenic makeup of the virus (presumably including any portions cross-reacting with MBP) is relatively stable and the immune dysregulation, leading to emergence of autoreactive cells, is common, the relatively infrequent occurrence of postmeasles encephalomyelitis is likely to be host-related. No link to particular MHC genes has been identified,[1,86] but other genetic elements such as the availability of compatible T-cell–receptor variable regions, or histamine response genes, important for susceptibility to EAE,[1,89] have not been examined. It is likely that multiple factors ultimately will be found to contribute to the development of this postinfectious demyelinating disease.

SUMMARY

Immune responses in the CNS are probably initiated in peripheral lymphoid tissue. T cells activated in the periphery then enter the CNS by traversing the capillary endothelium. If the T cell encounters antigen in the CNS in

---

*References 53, 57, 58, 71, 129, 137, 145b.

the context of the appropriate MHC antigen, then effector activity in the form of lymphokine production or target cell lysis will be triggered. Locally produced lymphokines will amplify the inflammatory response by inducing endothelial changes; attracting B cells, monocytes, and other T cells from the blood; and stimulating cellular proliferation, differentiation, and increased MHC antigen expression in the local site.

During immunologically mediated encephalomyelitis, CNS myelin is the target antigen, and immunologic attack results in perivascular zones of demyelination. In both rabies vaccine–induced encephalomyelitis and postmeasles encephalomyelitis, the disease is monophasic, and myelin basic protein is an important target antigen within myelin. Host factors probably contribute significantly to susceptibility to these diseases.

ACKNOWLEDGMENTS

Work from the author's laboratory was supported by research grants from the National Multiple Sclerosis Society, the G. Harold and Leila Y. Mathers Charitable Foundation, and the National Institutes of Health (AI23047 and NS29234).

REFERENCES

1. Acha-Orbea H, Mitchell DJ, Limmermann L, et al: Limited heterogeneity of T cell receptors from lymphocytes mediating autoimmune encephalomyelitis allows specific immune intervention. Cell 54:263–272, 1988.

2. Allan JE and Doherty PC: Immune T cells can protect or induce fatal neurological disease in murine lymphocytic choriomeningitis. Cell Immunol 90:401–407, 1985.

3. Allan JE and Doherty PC: Natural killer cells contribute to inflammation but do not appear to be essential for the induction of clinical lymphocytic choriomeningitis. Scand J Immunol 24:153–162, 1986.

4. Appelbaum E, Dolgopol VB, and Dolgin J: Measles encephalitis. Am J Dis Child 77:25–48, 1949.

5. Appelbaum E, Greenberg M, and Nelson J: Neurological complications following antirabies vaccination. JAMA 151:188–191, 1953.

6. Askenase PW and Van Loveren H: Delayed-type hypersensitivity: Activation of mast cells by antigen-specific T cells factors initiates the cascade of cellular interactions. Immunol Today 4:259–264, 1983.

7. Bareggi C: Su cinque casi di rabbia paralitica (del laboratorio) nell'uomo. Gazz Med Lombarda 48:217–219, 1889.

8. Baringer JR and Griffin JF: Experimental herpes simplex encephalitis: Early neuropathologic changes. J Neuropathol Exp Neurol 29:89–104, 1970.

9. Behan PO, Geschwind N, Lamarche JB, Lisak RP, and Kies MW: Delayed hypersensitivity to encephalitogenic protein in disseminated encephalomyelitis. Lancet 2:1009–1012, 1968.

10. Ben-Nun A and Cohen IR: Experimental autoimmune encephalomyelitis (EAE) mediated by T cell lines: Process of selection of lines and characterization of the cells. J Immunol 129:303–308, 1982.

11. Bevilacqua MP, Stengelin S, Gimbrone MA Jr, and Seed B: Endothelial-leukocyte adhesion molecule 1. An inducible receptor for neutrophils related to complement regulatory proteins and lectins. Science 243:1160–1165, 1989.

12. Bierer BE and Burakoff ST: T cell adhesion molecules. FASEB J 2:2584–2590, 1988.

13. Bjerknes M, Cheng H, and Ottaway CA: Dynamics of lymphocyte-endothelial interactions in vivo. Science 232:402–405, 1986.

14. Bloomfield AL and Mateer JG:

Changes in skin sensitiveness to tuberculin during epidemic influenza. American Review of Tuberculosis 3:166–168, 1919.

15. Boutin B, Matsuguchi L, Lebon P, Ponsot G, Arthuis M, and Nelson D-L: Soluble IL-2 receptors in acute and subacute encephalitis. Ann Neurol 22:658–661, 1987.

16. Bradbury MWB, Cserr H, and Westrop RJ: Drainage of cerebral interstitial fluid into deep cervical lymph of the rabbit. Am J Physiol 240:F329–F336, 1981.

17. Brew BJ, Bhalla RB, Fleisher M, et al: Cerebrospinal fluid β2 microglobulin in patients infected with human immunodeficiency virus. Neurology 39:830–834, 1989.

18. Brosnan CF, Bornstein MB, and Bloom BR: The effects of macrophage depletion in the clinical and pathologic expression of experimental allergic encephalomyelitis. J Immunol 126:614–620, 1981.

19. Broudy VC, Kaushansky K, Harlan JM, and Adamson JW: Interleukin 1 stimulates human endothelial cells to produce granulocyte-macrophage colony-stimulating factor and granulocyte colony-stimulating factor. J Immunol 139:464–468, 1987.

19a. Burk PA, Hirschfeld S, Shirayoshi Y, et al: Developmental and tissue-specific expression of nuclear proteins that bind the regulatory element of the major histocompatibility complex class I gene. J Exp Med 169:1309–1321, 1989.

20. Butcher EC: The regulation of lymphocyte traffic. Curr Top Microbiol Immunol 128:85–122, 1986.

21. Cannon DC and Wissler RW: Migration of spleen cells into the blood stream following antigen stimulation of the rat. Nature 207:654–656, 1965.

22. Cavender DE, Haskard DD, Joseph D, and Ziff M: Interleukin-1 increases the binding of human B and T lymphocytes to endothelial cell monolayers. J Immunol 136:203–207, 1986.

22a. Centers for Disease Control: Aseptic meningitis among kidney transplant recipients receiving a newly marketed murine monoclonal antibody preparation. MMWR 35:551–552, 1986.

23. Ceredig R, Allan JE, Tabi Z, Lynch F, and Doherty PC: Phenotypic analysis of the inflammatory exudate in murine lymphocytic choriomeningitis. J Exp Med 165:1539–1551, 1987.

24. Cutler RWP, Merler E, and Hammerstad JP: Production of antibody by the central nervous system in subacute sclerosing panencephalitis. Neurology 18:129–132, 1968.

25. Czlonkowska A, Korlak J, and Iwinska B: Subacute sclerosing panencephalitis and progressive multiple sclerosis: T cell subsets in blood and CSF. Neurology 36:992–993, 1986.

25a. Damel NK, Doyle LV, Bender JR, and Bradley EC: Interleukin-2-activated human lymphocytes exhibit enhanced adhesion to normal vascular endothelial cells and cause their lysis. J Immunol 138:1779–1785, 1987.

26. Dixon JE, Allen JE, and Doherty PC: The acute inflammatory process in murine lymphocytic choriomeningitis is dependent on Lyt-2+ immune T cells. Cell Immunol 197:8–14, 1987.

27. Doherty PC: T cells and viral infections. Br Med Bull 41:7–14, 1985.

28. Doherty PC and Allan JE: Role of the major histocompatibility complex in targeting effector T cells into a site of virus replication. Eur J Immunol 16:1237–1242, 1986.

29. Doherty PC, Allan JE, and Ceredig R: Contributions of host and donor T cells to the inflammatory process in murine lymphocytic choriomeningitis. Cell Immunol 116:475–481, 1988.

30. Doherty PC, Allan JE, Dixon JE, Tabi Z, and Ceredig R: Characteristics of the CSF inflammatory exudate in murine lymphocytic choriomeningitis. In Lowenthal A and Raus J (eds): Cellular and Humoral Components of Cerebrospinal Fluid in Mul-

tiple Sclerosis. Plenum, London, 1987, pp 351–360.

31. Doherty PC, Ceredig R, and Allan JE: Immunogenetic analysis of cellular interactions governing the recruitment of T lymphocytes and monocytes in lymphocytic choriomeningitis virus-induced immunopathology. Clin Immunol Immunopathol 47:19–26, 1988.

32. Doherty PC and Korngold R: Characteristics of poxvirus-induced meningitis: Virus-specific and non-specific cytotoxic effectors in the inflammatory exudate. Scand J Immunol 17:1–7, 1983.

33. Dustin ML, Rothlein R, Bhan AK, Dinarello CA, and Springer TA: Induction by IL-1 and interferon, tissue distribution, biochemistry and function of a natural adherence molecule (ICAM-1). J Immunol 137:245–254, 1986.

34. Eichkoff K and Heipertz R: Discrimination of elevated immunoglobulin concentrations in CSF due to inflammatory reaction of the central nervous system and blood-brain-barrier dysfunction. Acta Neurol Scand 56:475–482, 1977.

35. Esiri MM: Poliomyelitis: Immunoglobulin-containing cells in the central nervous system in acute and convalescent phases of the human disease. Clin Exp Immunol 40:42–48, 1980.

36. Esiri MM, Oppenheimer DR, Brownell B, and Haire M: Distribution of measles antigen and immunoglobulin-containing cells in the CNS in subacute sclerosing panencephalitis (SSPE) and atypical measles encephalitis. J Neurol Sci 53:29–43, 1982.

37. Eylar EH, Salk J, Beveridge GC, and Brown LV: Experimental allergic encephalomyelitis: An encephalitogenic basic protein from bovine myelin. Arch Biochem Biophys 132:34–48, 1969.

38. Felgenhauer K and Schadlich H-J: The compartmental IgM and IgA response within the central nervous system. J Neurol Sci 77:125–135, 1987.

39. Fierz W, Endler B, Reske K, Wekerle H, and Fontana A: Astrocytes as antigen-presenting cells. I. Induction of Ia antigen expression on astrocytes by T cells via immune interferon and its effect on antigen presentation. J Immunol 134:3785–3793, 1985.

39a. Figdor CG, van Kooy KY, and Keizer GD: On the mode of action of LFA-1. Immunol Today 11:277–280, 1990.

40. Fredrikson S, Eneroth P, and Link H: Intrathecal production of neopterin in aseptic meningo-encephalitis and multiple sclerosis. Clin Exp Immunol 67:76–81, 1987.

41. Fredrikson S, Karsson-Parra A, Olsson T, and Lin H: HLA-DR antigen expression of T cells from cerebrospinal fluid in multiple sclerosis and aseptic meningo-encephalitis. Clin Exp Immunol 68:298–304, 1987.

42. Frohman EM, van den Noorts, and Gupta S: Astrocytes and intracerebral immune responses. J Clin Immunol 9:1–9, 1989.

43. Fujinami RS and Oldstone MBA: Amino acid homology between the encephalitogenic site of myelin basic protein and virus: Mechanism for autoimmunity. Science 230:1043–1045, 1985.

44. Gallo P, Frei K, Rordorf C, Lazdins J, Tavolato B, and Fontana A: Human immunodeficiency virus type 1 (HIV-1) infection of the central nervous system: An evaluation of cytokines in cerebrospinal fluid. J Neuroimmunol 23:109–116, 1989.

45. Ganrot K and Laurell C-B: Measurement of IgG and albumin content of cerebrospinal fluid and its interpretation. Clin Chem 20:571–573, 1974.

46. Geczy CL: The role of lymphokines in delayed-type hypersensitivity reactions. Springer Semin Immunopathol 7:321–346, 1984.

47. Gendelman H, Wolinsky JS, Johnson RT, Pressman NJ, Pezeshkpour GH, and Boisset GF: Measles encephalitis: Lack of evidence of viral invasion of the central nervous system and quantitative study of the na-

ture of demyelination. Ann Neurol 15:353–360, 1984.

48. Gessain A, Caudie C, Gout O, et al: Intrathecal synthesis of antibodies to human T lymphotropic virus type-1 and the presence of IgG oligoclonal bands in the cerebrospinal fluid of patients with endemic tropical spastic paraparesis. J Infect Dis 157:1226–1234, 1988.

49. Gibbs FA, Gibbs EL, Carpenter PR, and Spies HW: Electroencephalographic abnormality in "uncomplicated" childhood disease. JAMA 171:1050–1055, 1959.

50. Gowans JL and Knight EJ: The route of recirculation of lymphocytes in the rat. Proc R Soc Lond [Biol] 159:257–286, 1964.

51. Griffin DE: Immunoglobulins in the cerebrospinal fluid: Changes during acute viral encephalitis in mice. J Immunol 126:27–31, 1981.

52. Griffin DE: Monophasic autoimmune inflammatory diseases of the CNS and PNS. In Waksman BH (ed): Immunologic Mechanisms in Neurologic and Psychiatric Disease. Raven Press, New York, 1990, pp 91–104.

53. Griffin DE, Cooper SJ, Hirsch RL, et al: Changes in plasma IgE levels during complicated and uncomplicated measles virus infections. J Allergy Clin Immunol 76:206–213, 1985.

54. Griffin DE and Hess JL: Cells with natural killer activity in the cerebrospinal fluid of normal mice and athymic nude mice with acute Sindbis virus encephalitis. J Immunol 136:1841–1845, 1986.

55. Griffin DE, Hess JL, and Moench TR: Immune responses in the central nervous system. Toxicol Pathol 15:294–302, 1987.

56. Griffin DE and Mendoza Q: Identification of the mononuclear cells in the brains of mast cell deficient (W/W^v) and normal mice during Sindbis virus induced encephalitis. Cell Immunol 97:454–459, 1986.

57. Griffin DE, Ward BJ, Jauregui E, Johnson RT, and Vaisberg A: Immune activation during measles. N Engl J Med 320:1667–1672, 1989.

58. Griffin DE, Ward BJ, Jauregui E, Johnson RT, and Vaisberg A: Immune activation during measles: Interferon-γ and neopterin in plasma and cerebrospinal fluid in complicated and uncomplicated disease. J Infect Dis 161:449–453, 1990.

58a. Griffin DE, Ward BJ, Jauregui E, Johnson RT, and Vaisberg A: Immune activation during measles: β_2-microglobulin in plasma and cerebrospinal fluid in complicated and uncomplicated disease. J Infect Dis 166:1170–1173, 1992.

59. Hafler DA, Benjamin DS, Burks J, and Weiner HL: Myelin basic protein and proteolipid protein reactivity of brain and cerebrospinal fluid-derived T cell clones in multiple sclerosis and postinfectious encephalomyelitis. J Immunol 139:68–72, 1987.

60. Hamaoka T and Ono S: Regulation of B cell differentiation. Annu Rev Immunol 4:167–204, 1986.

61. Hanninen P, Arstila P, Lang H, Salmi A, and Panelius M: Involvement of the central nervous system in acute, uncomplicated measles virus infection. J Clin Microbiol 11:610–613, 1980.

62. Happ MP, Wettstein P, Dietzschold B, and Heber-Katz E: Genetic control of the development of experimental allergic encephalomyelitis in rats. J Immunol 141:1489–1494, 1988.

63. Harling-Berg C, Cserr HF, and Knopf PM: The role of cervical lymph nodes in the immune response to human serum albumin microinfused into rat CSF. J Neuroimmunol 25:185–193, 1989.

64. Hay JB, Cahill RNP, and Trnka Z: The kinetics of antigen-reactive cells during lymphocyte recruitment. Cell Immunol 10:145–153, 1974.

64a. Hedlund G, Sandberg-Wollheim M, and Sjogren HO: Increased proportion of CD4+ CDw29+ CD45R– UCHL-1+ lymphocytes in the cerebrospinal fluid of both multiple sclerosis patients and healthy individuals. Cell Immunol 118:406–412, 1989.

65. Hemachudha T, Griffin DE, Giffels JJ, Johnson RT, Moser AB, and Phanuphak P: Myelin basic protein as an encephalitogen in encephalomyelitis and polyneuritis following rabies vaccination. N Engl J Med 316:369–374, 1987.

66. Hemachudha T, Griffin DE, Johnson RT, and Giffels JJ: Studies of immune response in patients with chronic encephalitis induced by post-exposure rabies immunization. Neurology 38:42–44, 1988.

67. Hemachudha T, Phanuphak P, Johnson RT, Griffin DE, Ratanavonqsiri J, and Siriprasomsup W: Neurological complications of Semple type rabies vaccine: Clinical and immunological studies. Neurology 37:550–556, 1987.

68. Hemler ME: Adhesive protein receptors on hematopoietic cells. Immunol Today 9:109–113, 1988.

69. Hickey WF and Kimura H: Perivascular microglial cells of the CNS are bone marrow-derived and present antigen in vivo. Science 239:290–292, 1988.

70. Hirsch RL, Griffin DE, and Johnson RT: Interactions between immune cells and antibody in protection from fatal Sindbis virus encephalitis. Infect Immun 23:320–324, 1979.

71. Hirsch RL, Griffin DE, Cooper SJ, et al: Cellular immune responses during complicated and uncomplicated measles virus infections of man. Clin Immunol Immunopathol 31:1–12, 1984.

71a. Holzmann B, McIntyre BW, and Weissman IL: Identification of a murine Peyer's patch-specific lymphocyte homing receptor as an integrin molecule with an α chain homologous to human VLA-4α. Cell 56:37–46, 1989.

71b. Houssiau FA, Bukasa K, Sindic CJM, van Damme J, and van Snick J: Elevated levels of the 26K human hybridoma growth factor (interleukin 6) in cerebrospinal fluid of patients with acute infection of the central nervous system. Clin Exp Immunol 71:320–323, 1988.

72. Hovi T, Stenvik M, and Kinnunen E: Diagnosis of poliomyelitis by demonstration of intrathecal synthesis of neutralizing antibodies. J Infect Dis 153:988–999, 1986.

73. Hurst EW: The effects of the injection of normal brain emulsion into rabbits, with special reference in the aetiology of the paralytic accidents of antirabic treatment. J Hygiene 32:3–44, 1932.

74. Hurwitz JL, Korngold R, and Doherty PC: Specific and non-specific T cell recruitment in viral meningitis: Possible implications for autoimmunity. Cell Immunol 76:397–401, 1983.

75. Jahnke U, Fischer EH, and Alvord EC Jr: Sequence homology between certain viral proteins and proteins related to encephalomyelitis and neuritis. Science 229:282–284, 1985.

76. Jalkanen S, Steere AC, Fox RI, and Butcher EC: A distinct endothelial cell recognition system that controls lymphocyte traffic into inflamed synovium. Science 233:556–558, 1986.

77. Johnson RT: The pathogenesis of acute viral encephalitis and postinfectious encephalomyelitis. J Infect Dis 155:359–364, 1987.

78. Johnson RT, Burke DS, Elwell M, et al: Japanese encephalitis: Immunocytochemical studies of viral antigen and inflammatory cells in fatal cases. Ann Neurol 18:567–573, 1985.

79. Johnson RT, Griffin DE, and Gendelman HE: Postinfectious encephalomyelitis. Semin Neurol 5:180–190, 1985.

80. Johnson RT, Griffin DE, Hirsch RL, et al: Measles encephalomyelitis—clinical and immunologic studies. N Engl J Med 310:137–141, 1984.

81. Johnson RT, Intralawan P, and Puapanwatton S: Japanese encephalitis: Identification of inflammatory cells in cerebrospinal fluid. Ann Neurol 20:691–695, 1986.

82. Johnston GI, Cook RG, and McEver RP: Cloning of GMP-140, a granule

membrane protein of platelets and endothelium: Sequence similarity to proteins involved in cell adhesion and inflammation. Cell 56:1033–1044, 1989.

83. Koskiniemi M, Vaheri A, and Taskinen E: Cerebrospinal fluid alterations in herpes simplex virus encephalitis. Rev Infect Dis 6:608–618, 1984.

84. Lebon P, Boutin B, Dulac O, Ponsot G, and Arthus M: Interferon γ in acute and subacute encephalitis. Br Med J 296:9–11, 1988.

85. Lebon P, Ponsot G, Aicardi J, Goutieres F, and Arthuis M: Early intrathecal synthesis of interferon in herpes encephalitis. Biomedicine 31:267–271, 1979.

86. Lebon P, Ponsot G, Gony J, and Hors J: HLA antigens in acute measles encephalitis. Tissue Antigens 27:75–77, 1986.

86a. Levine B, Hardwick JM, Trapp BD, Crawford TO, Bollinger RC, and Griffin DE: Antibody-mediated clearance of alphavirus infection from neurons. Science 254:856–860, 1991.

87. Liew FY: Regulation of delayed-type hypersensitivity to pathogens and alloantigens. Immunol Today 3:18–23, 1982.

88. Lindsley MD and Rodriguez M: Characterization of the inflammatory response in the central nervous system of mice susceptible or resistant to demyelination by Theiler's virus. J Immunol 142:2677–2682, 1989.

89. Linthicum DS and Frelinger JA: Acute autoimmune encephalomyelitis in mice. II. Susceptibility is controlled by the combination of H-2 and histamine sensitization genes. J Exp Med 155:31–40, 1982.

90. Lisak RP and Zweiman B: In vitro cell-mediated immunity of cerebrospinal fluid lymphocytes to myelin basic protein in primary demyelinating diseases. N Engl J Med 297:850–853, 1977.

91. Litvak AM, Sands IJ, and Gibel H: Encephalitis complicating measles: Report of fifty-six cases with followup studies in thirty-two. Am J Dis Child 65:265–295, 1943.

92. Locksley RM, Heinzel FP, Shepard HM, et al: Tumor necrosis factors α and β differ in their capacities to generate interleukin 1 release from human endothelial cells. J Immunol 139:1891–1895, 1987.

92a. Long EO and Jacobson S: Pathways of viral antigen processing and presentation to CTL: Defined by the mode of virus entry? Immunol Today 10:45–48, 1989.

92b. Lotze MT, Matory YL, Rayner AA, Ettinghausen SE, Seipp CA, and Rosenberg SA: Clinical effects and toxicity of IL-2 in patients with cancer. Cancer 58:2764–2772, 1986.

93. Lynch F, Chaudhri G, Allan JE, Doherty PC, and Ceredig R: Expression of Pgp-1 (or Ly24) by subpopulations of mouse thymocytes and activated peripheral T lymphocytes. Eur J Immunol 17:137–140, 1987.

94. Makgoba MW, Sanders ME, Luce GEG, et al: ICAM-1 a ligand for LFA-dependent adhesion of B, T and myeloid cells. Nature 331:86–88, 1988.

95. Martin S, Maruta K, Burkart V, Gillis S, and Kolb H: IL-1 and IFN-γ increase vascular permeability. Immunology 64:301–305, 1988.

95a. Matsui M, Mori KJ, and Saida T: Cellular immunoregulatory mechanisms in the central nervous system: Characterization of non-inflammatory and inflammatory cerebrospinal fluid lymphocytes. Ann Neurol 27:647–651, 1990.

96. McArthur JC, Sipos E, Cornblath DR, et al: Identification of mononuclear cells in CSF of patients with HIV infection. Neurology 39:66–70, 1989.

97. McCarron RM, Spatz M, Kempski O, Hogan RN, Muehl L, and McFarlin DE: Interaction between myelin basic protein-sensitized T lymphocytes and murine cerebral vascular endothelial cells. J Immunol 137:3428–3435, 1986.

98. Merrill JE: Macroglia: Neural cells

responsive to lymphokines and growth factors. Immunol Today 8:146–150, 1987.

99. Miller DL: Frequency of complications of measles, 1963. Br Med J 2:75–78, 1964.

100. Miller HG and Stanton JB: Neurological sequelae of prophylactic inoculation. Q J Med 89:1–27, 1954.

101. Moench TR and Griffin DE: Immunocytochemical identification and quantitation of mononuclear cells in cerebrospinal fluid, meninges, and brain during acute viral encephalitis. J Exp Med 159:77–88, 1984.

102. Moench TR, Griffin DE, Obriecht CR, Vaisberg AJ, and Johnson RT: Acute measles in patients with and without neurological involvement: Distribution of measles virus antigen and RNA. J Infect Dis 158:433–442, 1988.

103. Mokhtarian F and Griffin DE: Role of mast cells in virus-induced CNS inflammation in the mouse. Cell Immunol 86:491–500, 1984.

104. Mokhtarian F, Griffin DE, and Hirsch RL: Production of mononuclear chemotactic factors during Sindbis virus infection of mice. Infect Immun 35:965–973, 1982.

105. Montgomery IN and Rauch HC: Experimental allergic encephalomyelitis (EAE) in mice: Primary control of EAE susceptibility is outside the H-2 complex. J Immunol 128:421–425, 1982.

106. Morishima T and Hayashi K: Meningeal exudate cells in vaccinia meningitis of mice: Role of local T cells. Infect Immun 20:752–759, 1978.

107. Naparstek Y, Ben-Nun A, Holoshitz J, et al: T lymphocyte lines producing or vaccinating against autoimmune encephalomyelitis (EAE). Functional activation induces peanut agglutinin receptors and accumulation in the brain and thymus of line cells. Eur J Immunol 13:418–423, 1983.

107a. Naparstek Y, Cohen IR, Fuks Z, and Vlodavsky I: Activated T lymphocytes produce a matrix-degrading heparan sulphate endoglycosidase. Nature 310:241–244, 1984.

108. Nieuwenhuis P: B-cell differentiation in vivo. Immunol Today 1:104–110, 1981.

109. Niwa Y, Sakane T, Kanoh T, Shichijo S, Wiederhold MD, and Yokoyama MM: Transient autoantibodies with elevated complement levels in common viral diseases. J Clin Lab Immunol 13:183–188, 1984.

110. Oehmichen M, Gruninger H, Wietholter H, and Gencic M: Lymphatic efflux of intracerebrally injected cells. Acta Neuropathol 45:61–65, 1979.

111. Ojala A: On changes in the cerebrospinal fluid during measles. Annales Medicinae Internae Fenniae 36:321–331, 1947.

112. Oppenheim JJ: Lymphokines. In Oppenheim JJ, Rosenstreich DL, and Potter M (eds): Cellular Functions in Immunity and Inflammation. Elsevier, New York, 1981, pp 259–282.

113. Osborn L: Leukocyte adhesion to endothelium in inflammation. Cell 62:3–6, 1990.

113a. Osborn L, Hession C, Tizard R, et al: Direct expression cloning of vascular cell adhesion molecule 1, a cytokine-induced endothelial protein that binds to lymphocytes. Cell 59:1203–1211, 1989.

114. Pampiglione G: Prodromal phase of measles: Some neurophysiological studies. Br Med J 2:1296–1300, 1960.

115. Paterson PY: Transfer of allergic encephalomyelitis in rats by means of lymph node cells. J Exp Med 111:119–135, 1960.

116. Pober JS, Gimbrone MA Jr, Lapierre LA, et al: Overlapping patterns of activation of human endothelial cells by interleukin-1, tumor necrosis factor, and immune interferon. J Immunol 137:1893–1896, 1986.

117. Resnick L, Di Marzo-Veronese F, Schupbach J, et al: Intra-blood-brain-barrier synthesis of HTLV-III-specific IgG in patients with neurologic symptoms associated with

AIDS or AIDS-related complex. N Engl J Med 313:1498–1504, 1985.

117a. Risau W, Engelhardt B, and Wekerle H: Immune function of the blood-brain barrier: Incomplete presentation of protein (auto-) antigens by rat brain microvascular endothelium *in vitro*. J Cell Biol 110:1757–1766, 1990.

118. Rivers TM and Schwentker FF: Encephalomyelitis accompanied by myelin destruction experimentally produced in monkeys. J Exp Med 61:689–702, 1935.

119. Rodriguez M, Price ML, and Howie EA: Immune response gene products (Ia antigens) on glial and endothelial cells in virus-induced demyelination. J Immunol 138:3438–3442, 1987.

120. Rodriguez M and Sriram S: Successful therapy of Theiler's virus-induced demyelination (DA strain) with monoclonal anti-Lyt-2 antibody. J Immunol 140:2950–2955, 1988.

121. Rosen H, Milon G, and Gordon S: Antibody to the murine type 3 complement receptor inhibits T lymphocyte-dependent recruitment of myelomonocytic cells *in vivo*. J Exp Med 169:535–548, 1987.

121a. Rosenstein M, Ettinghausen SE, and Rosenberg SA: Extravasation of intravascular fluid mediated by the systemic administration of recombinant IL2. J Immunol 137:1735–1742, 1986.

122. Savion N, Vlodavsky I, and Fuks Z: Interaction of T lymphocytes and macrophages with cultured vascular endothelial cells: Attachment, invasion and subsequent degradation of the subendothelial extracellular matrix. J Cell Physiol 118:169–178, 1984.

123. Schwartz RH: T-lymphocyte recognition of antigen in association with gene products of the major histocompatibility complex. Annu Rev Immunol 3:237–261, 1985.

124. Sindic CJM, Delacroix DL, Vaerman JP, Laterre EC, and Masson PL: Study of IgA in the cerebrospinal fluid of neurological patients with special reference to size, subclass and local production. J Neuroimmunol 7:65–75, 1984.

125. Sobel RA, Blanchette BW, Bhan AK, and Colvin RB: The immunopathology of experimental allergic encephalomyelitis. II. Endothelial cell Ia increases prior to inflammatory cell infiltration. J Immunol 132:2402–2407, 1984.

126. Sprent J: Circulating T and B lymphocytes of the mouse. I. Migratory properties. Cell Immunol 7:10–39, 1973.

127. Springer TA: Adhesion receptors of the immune system. Nature 346:425–434, 1990.

128. Starr S and Berkovich S: The depression of tuberculin reactivity during chickenpox. Pediatrics 33:769–772, 1964.

129. Starr S and Berkovich S: Effects of measles, gamma globulin-modified measles and vaccine measles on the tuberculin test. N Engl J Med 270:386–391, 1964.

129a. St. John T, Meyer J, Idzerda R, and Gallatin WM: Expression of CD44 confers a new adhesive phenotype on transfected cells. Cell 650:45–52, 1990.

130. Stohlman SA, Matsushima GK, Casteel N, and Weiner LP: *In vivo* effects of coronavirus-specific T cell clones: DTH inducer cells prevent a lethal infection but do not inhibit virus replication. J Immunol 136:3052–3056, 1986.

131. Stohlman SA, Sussman MA, Matsushima GK, Shubin RA, and Erlich SS: Delayed-type hypersensitivity response in the central nervous system during JHM virus infection requires viral specificity for protection. J Neuroimmunol 19:255–268, 1988.

132. Streit WJ, Graeber MB, and Kreutzberg GW: Functional plasticity of microglia: A review. Glia 1:301–307, 1988.

133. Streit WJ, Graeber MB, and Kreutzberg GW: Peripheral nerve lesion produces increased levels of major histocompatibility complex antigens

in the central nervous system. J Neuroimmunol 21:117–123, 1989.

134. Sussman MA, Shubin RA, Kyuwa S, and Stohlman SA: T cell-mediated clearance of mouse hepatitis virus strain JHM from the central nervous system. J Virol 63:3051–3056, 1989.

135. Suzumura A, Lavi E, Weiss SR, and Silberberg DH: Coronavirus infection induces H-1 antigen on oligodendrocytes and astrocytes. Science 232:991–993, 1986.

136. Swamy HS, Shankar SK, Chandra PS, Aroor SR, Krishna AS, and Perumal VG: Neurological complications due to beta-propiolactone (BPL)-inactivated antirabies vaccination. J Neurol Sci 63:111–128, 1984.

137. Tamashiro VG, Perez HH, and Griffin DE: Prospective study of the magnitude and duration of changes in tuberculin reactivity during complicated and uncomplicated measles. Pediatr Infect Dis J 6:451–454, 1987.

137a. Tedder TT, Penta AC, Levin HB, and Freedman AS: Expression of the human leukocyte adhesion molecule, LAM1: Identity with the TQ1 and Leu8 differentiation antigens. J Immunol 144:532–540, 1990.

138. Tyor WR, Moench TR, and Griffin DE: Characterization of the local and systemic B cell response of normal and athymic nude mice with Sindbis virus encephalitis. J Neuroimmunol 24:207–215, 1989.

139. Tyor WR, Stoll G, and Griffin DE: The characterization of local and systemic Ia expression during Sindbis virus encephalitis in normal and athymic nude mice. J Neuropathol Exp Neurol 49:22–30, 1990.

140. Ubol S, Hemachudha T, Whitaker JN, and Griffin DE: Antibody to peptides of human myelin basic protein in postrabies vaccine encephalomyelitis sera. J Neuroimmunol 26:107–111, 1990.

141. Uchimura I and Shiraki H: A contribution to the classification and the pathogenesis of demyelinating encephalomyelitis: With special reference to the central nervous system lesion caused by preventive inoculation against rabies. J Neuropathol Exp Neurol 16:139–203, 1957.

142. Vandvik B, Nielsen RE, Vartdal R, and Norrby E: Mumps meningitis: Specific and non-specific antibody responses in the central nervous system. Acta Neurol Scand 65:468–487, 1982.

143. Vartdal F, Vandvik B, and Norrby E: Intrathecal synthesis of virus-specific oligoclonal IgG, IgA and IgM antibodies in a case of varicella zoster meningoencephalitis. J Neurol Sci 57:121–132, 1982.

144. Vass K, Lassman H, Wekerle H, and Wisniewski HM: The distribution of Ia antigen in the lesions of rat acute experimental allergic encephalomyelitis. Acta Neuropathol 70:149–160, 1986.

144a. Vecht CJ, Keohane C, Menon RS, Henzen-Logmans SC, Punt CJA, and Stoter G: Acute fatal leukoencephalopathy after interleukin-2 therapy. N Engl J Med 323:1146–1147, 1990.

145. Vitetta ES and Capra JD: The protein of the murine 17th chromosome, genetics and structure. Adv Immunol 26:147–193, 1978.

145a. Walz G, Aruffo A, Kolanus W, Bevilacqua M, and Seed B: Recognition by ELAM-1 of the sialyl-Le^x determinant on myeloid and tumor cells. Science 250:1132–1135, 1990.

145b. Ward BJ, Johnson RT, Vaisberg A, Jauregui E, and Griffin DE: Cytokine production *in vitro* and the lymphoproliferative defect of natural measles virus infection. Clin Immunol Immunopathol 61:236–248, 1991.

146. Watanabe R, Wege H, and ter Meulen V: Adoptive transfer of EAE-like lesions from rats with coronavirus-induced demyelinating encephalomyelitis. Nature 305:150–153, 1983.

147. Wekerle H, Linington C, Lassmann H, and Meyerman R: Cellular immune reactivity within the CNS. Trends Neurosci 9:271–277, 1986.

148. Welsh CJR, Tonks P, Nash AS, and

Blakemore WF: The effect of L3T4 T cell depletion on the pathogenesis of Theiler's murine encephalomyelitis virus infection in CBA mice. J Gen Virol 68:1659–1667, 1987.

149. Willenborg DO, Sjollema P, and Danta G: Immunoglobulin deficient rats as donors and recipients of effector cells of allergic encephalomyelitis. J Neuroimmunol 11:93–103, 1986.

150. Williams KA, Hart DN, Fabre JW, and Morris PJ: Distribution and quantitation of HLA-ABC and DR (Ia) antigens on human kidney and other tissues. Transplantation 29:274–279, 1980.

151. Wong GHW, Bartlett PF, Clark-Lewis I, McKinnon-Breschkin JL, and Schrader JW: Interferon-γ induces the expression of H-2 and Ia antigens on brain cells. J Neuroimmunol 7:255–278, 1985.

Chapter 3

HIV AND HTLV INFECTIONS OF THE NERVOUS SYSTEM

Robert M. Levy, M.D., Ph.D., and Joseph R. Berger, M.D.

HIV-1
HIV-2
HTLV-I
HTLV-II

Retroviruses, a family of viruses widely distributed among vertebrate species, have been generally associated with oncogenesis. Indeed, retroviruses were first described in 1908 as a cause of sarcoma in chickens. Forty years later, Ludwik Gross identified a mammalian retrovirus that produced leukemia. Knowledge of their ability to cause neurologic disease has been significantly advanced as a result of the acquired immunodeficiency syndrome (AIDS) epidemic. Retroviruses are unique in that they contain ribonucleic acid (RNA)–dependent deoxyribonucleic acid (DNA) polymerase (reverse transcriptase), an enzyme that enables this RNA virus to produce DNA. The viral DNA may then be incorporated into the genome of the host cell. In addition to reverse transcriptase, other features of retroviruses that allow their recognition are their morphology and the structure of their RNA viral genomes. This family of viruses is divided into three subfamilies: lentivirus ("lente" = slow), oncovirus ("onco" = tumor), and spumivirus ("spuma" = foam).

In humans, the lentivirus subfamily is represented by the human immunodeficiency virus (HIV), types 1 and 2 (HIV-1 and HIV-2). Characteristics of the lentiviruses include latency of infection; a predilection for infection of mononuclear cells, particularly macrophages; an inability to transmit infection easily; exhibition of cell lysis in culture; and a high rate of chronic encephalopathy in the host animals. The prototypical lentivirus, visna, was first discovered in the 1930s in sheep brought to Iceland from Germany. These sheep developed a lymphocytic pneumonitis and a demyelinating disorder of the central nervous system (CNS). To date, all other lentiviruses have been demonstrated to be capable of causing neurologic disease.[62] Examples of these viruses include not only HIV and visna, but also caprine arthritis encephalopathy virus (CAEV), bovine visna, feline immunodeficiency virus, and simian immunodeficiency virus (SIV).

Human T-cell lymphotropic virus type I (HTLV-I) is a member of the largest retrovirus subfamily, the oncoviruses. HTLV-I was the first retrovirus infection described in humans and is capable of causing T-cell leukemia and lymphomas. Neurologic complications resulting from HTLV-I are not as common as those observed with HIV-1 and are only beginning to be characterized. In fact, the discovery of the neurologic complications of HTLV-I occurred serendipitously as a result of seroepidemiologic surveys of various populations.[39] The best characterized neurologic complication is a chronic, progressive myelopathy, which will be discussed later.

HIV-1

As of December 31, 1991, there had been 206,392 AIDS cases and 133,232 AIDS deaths in the United States.[27] By that time, it was estimated that as many as 2 million Americans would be infected with HIV-1. Although the name of this disease (AIDS) suggests that the immune system is the major target of HIV-1 infection, the nervous system is profoundly affected by this disease process, and neurologic complications represent a major source of AIDS-related morbidity and mortality. Although neurologic complications of HIV-1 infection have been reported since the beginning of the AIDS epidemic,[21,122] only recently have the breadth and frequency of these manifestations become apparent.[74,76] Neurologic illness can arise not only from opportunistic infections and neoplasms, but also from primary HIV-1 infection of the nervous system.[57,90,116] In light of this observation, the Centers for Dis-

Table 3–1 CDC CLASSIFICATION SYSTEM FOR HIV-1 INFECTION

Group I	Acute infection
Group II	Asymptomatic infection
Group III	Persistent generalized lymphadenopathy
Group IV	Other disease
Subgroup A	Constitutional disease
Subgroup B	Neurologic disease
Subgroup C	Secondary infectious diseases
Category C-1	Specified secondary infectious diseases listed in the CDC surveillance definition for AIDS
Category C-2	Other specified secondary infectious diseases
Subgroup D	Secondary cancers
Subgroup E	Other conditions

ease Control (CDC) has included HIV-1–related neurologic disease as a subcategory in the diagnosis of AIDS (Table 3–1).

Incidence and Epidemiology of HIV-1–Related CNS Disease

Of all AIDS patients, 40% to 60% will develop significant neurologic signs or symptoms during their lifetime. Of these AIDS patients with neurologic illness, one third present with these complaints as their initial manifestation of AIDS. Thus, approximately 10% to 20% of all AIDS patients first present with symptoms of neurologic illness.[13,70,74,76] The incidence of AIDS-related neuropathology is much higher in autopsy series, which demonstrate that 75% of AIDS patients have central nervous system pathology on postmortem evaluation.[97,129] Recent epidemiologic studies have confirmed that patients from different risk groups and geographic locations are at varying risk for contracting AIDS-related neurologic illness.[77] Toxoplasmosis occurs most frequently in Florida, in part reflecting the large number of Haitian AIDS patients in the community. In general, Haitian AIDS patients are more frequently reported to have neurologic complications than are patients in other risk groups. The subtropical climate in Florida may also contribute to the overall frequency of toxoplasmosis in AIDS patients residing in that state. Cryptococcal meningitis is reported most frequently in New Jersey and appears to be related to the higher percentage of AIDS patients in that state who are black or intravenous drug users.

Signs and Symptoms of HIV-1–Related Neurologic Disease

AIDS-related syndromes of the nervous system are many and varied, reflecting the breadth of primary and opportunistic diseases that can affect the patient with AIDS (Table 3–2). A specific diagnosis based on the clinical examination of the neurologically symptomatic AIDS patient may be virtually impossible because of the overlap in clinical presentations. Similarly, radiographic and serologic studies, though suggestive, may not allow for definitive diagnosis. The clinical signs and symptoms of AIDS-related CNS disease may arise as a result of diffuse or focal involvement of the brain or the development of increased intracranial pressure as a result of hydrocephalus. The symptoms include virtually all those related to nervous system dysfunction. The overall frequency with which many of

Table 3–2 HIV-1–RELATED CNS DISEASES

PRIMARY VIRAL (HIV-1) SYNDROMES
HIV-1 encephalopathy
Atypical aseptic meningitis
Vacuolar myelopathy

OPPORTUNISTIC VIRAL ILLNESSES
Cytomegalovirus
Herpes simplex virus, types 1 and 2
Varicella zoster virus
Papovavirus (progressive multifocal
    leukoencephalopathy)
Adenovirus type 2

NONVIRAL INFECTIONS
Toxoplasma gondii
Cryptococcus neoformans
Candida albicans
Aspergillus fumigatus
Coccidioides immitis
Mucormycosis
Rhizopus sp.
Acremonium alabamensis
Histoplasma capsulatum
Mycobacterium hominis tuberculosis
Mycobacterium avium intracellulare
Listeria monocytogenes
Nocardia asteroides

NEOPLASMS
Primary CNS lymphoma
Metastatic systemic lymphoma
Metastatic Kaposi's sarcoma

CEREBROVASCULAR COMPLICATIONS
Infarction
Hemorrhage
Vasculitis

**COMPLICATIONS OF SYSTEMIC AIDS
THERAPY**

Table 3–3 NEUROLOGIC SIGNS AND SYMPTOMS IN PATIENTS WITH AIDS

Signs and Symptoms	% of AIDS Patients with Neurologic Disease
Dementia	68
Headaches	55
Disordered gait	18
Focal weakness	18
Seizures	17
Aphasia	12
Incontinence	10
Cranial neuropathy	9
Hemisensory loss	8
Visual disturbance	8
Pain	1

Source: Adapted from Levy RM and Bredesen DE,[74] p 32, with permission.

the more common signs and symptoms are present in AIDS patients with neurologic illness are listed in Table 3–3. The most common disorders of cognition or of consciousness are evident in 68% of symptomatic patients with neurologic disease. Any neurologic symptom or sign may result from HIV-1 infection.

Phases of HIV-1 Infection of the Nervous System

At or about the time of seroconversion to HIV-1, most patients will develop abnormalities of the cerebrospinal fluid (CSF). A small number of patients will develop symptoms referable to this early infection, including headaches, encephalitis, meningitis,[26,33] myelopathy,[38] and plexitis.[25] The illness is usually monophasic, and symptoms usually resolve within weeks. Early asymptomatic infection of the CNS, however, appears to be the rule; several investigators have documented the presence of elevated protein, inflammatory cells, intra–blood-brain-barrier synthesis of immunoglobulins, and viral antigen in the CSF of asymptomatic HIV-1 patients. The acute meningitis that occurs in a minority of individuals at the time of HIV-1 seroconversion is clinically indistinguishable from other forms of aseptic meningitis and typically resolves within 10 days.[59]

A chronic, recurring meningitis can also develop around the time of sero-conversion but usually occurs in the setting of AIDS or AIDS-related complex (ARC). The chronic meningitis is characterized by headaches and CSF abnormalities without signs of meningeal irritation.[43] HIV-1 is often readily isolated from the CSF during these episodes. Late in the course of HIV-1 infection, patients may develop HIV-1–associated encephalopathy (AIDS dementia complex), HIV-1–associated myelopathy (vacuolar myelopathy), and neurologic problems secondary to opportunistic processes. Despite the frequency with which HIV-1 may be cultured from the CSF in early HIV-1 infection (in excess of 60% in some laboratories) and the frequent presence of evidence of chronic leptomeningeal inflammation, HIV encephalopathy does not usually develop until later stages of HIV infection, at a time when immunologic disturbances are prominent. Price and coworkers[108] posit that the "late" appearance of the encephalopathy indicates that HIV-1 is relatively nonpathogenic for the brain in the absence of immunosuppression.

CNS Complications of HIV-1 Infection

PRIMARY HIV-1
ENCEPHALOPATHY

Pathogenesis. Probably the most common CNS illness associated with AIDS is also one that is unique to this syndrome. This illness has been called subacute encephalitis, HIV-1 encephalopathy, AIDS dementia complex, and more recently, HIV-1–associated cognitive/motor disorder. Initial studies by Shaw and coworkers[121] using in situ hybridization techniques demonstrated the presence of HIV-1 in the brain of demented AIDS patients. The intra–blood-brain-barrier synthesis of anti–HIV-1 immunoglobulin G (IgG) in pa-

tients with AIDS and mental status changes was also detected,[116] and several investigators isolated HIV-1 from the CSF and neural tissues of patients with HIV-1–related neurologic symptoms.[57,72,73] Sharer and coworkers[118] demonstrated HIV-1 related to multinucleated giant cells in patients with HIV-1 encephalopathy, and more recently, Koenig and coworkers[68] as well as other investigators[114] demonstrated HIV-1 within brain macrophages in demented AIDS patients. Thus, the syndrome of HIV-1–related dementia appears to result at least in part from the primary infection of the brain by HIV-1. The cells containing the majority of the virus appear to be of macrophage origin. Recovery of HIV-1 from the CSF and intrathecal synthesis of anti–HIV-1 immunoglobulin has been detected in all stages of infection, however, and need not be associated with clinically evident neurologic disease.[115]

Compelling evidence suggests that a "neurotropic" strain of HIV-1 exists that is distinct from peripheral blood isolates of HIV-1. These strains can be distinguished by their growth characteristics, modulation of CD4 antigen on infected cell surfaces, and sensitivity to serum neutralizing antibody.[29] The evolution of peripheral blood HIV-1 into a brain-specific variant has been suggested by Epstein and colleagues.[43] Some studies suggest that brain and blood viral isolates can be distinguished by restriction enzyme sensitivity.[71] Wolinsky and colleagues have posited that changes in the V3 loop sequences of HIV-1 are associated with its neurotropic characteristics.[134]

The mechanism by which HIV-1 results in CNS dysfunction remains unanswered, although several mechanisms have been postulated.[11] First, the virus may be *neurotropic,* that is, have a propensity to infect glial cells and perhaps even neurons as detected by in situ hybridization, immunocytochemistry, and electron microscopy.[52,114,119,124] Both productive and nonproductive infections of human CNS cell lines have been demonstrated.[11] HIV-1 could directly induce brain cell dysfunction or death as a result of the infection, as suggested by the reported loss of cortical neurons.[44] Second, the virus may infect CNS endothelial cells and astrocytes, resulting in an *alteration of the blood-brain barrier.* Third, viral proteins of HIV-1 may be *directly toxic for cells of the CNS.* The envelope protein gp120 has been demonstrated to be toxic to neurons.[22] Some regions of the envelope protein may compete with neurotransmitters, e.g., vasoactive intestinal peptide.[104,105] This peptide can prevent neuronal cell killing by gp120.[22] Other viral proteins may also be neurotoxic.[49,113,117] The calcium channel blocker nimodipine can successfully block the toxic effect of gp120 in brain tissue culture, according to Lipton.[82] Fourth, *toxic cellular products,* including cytokines released by microglia and macrophages within the brain, may be elaborated as a result of HIV-1 infection. Quinolinic acid, an excitotoxin derived from tryptophan metabolism, correlates with degree of neurologic impairment.[56] Fifth, an *autoimmune response* may be induced. Sixth, *infectious cofactors,* such as cytomegalovirus (CMV), JC virus, and mycoplasma, may be important for the expression of neurologic disease. Last, *metabolic and nutritional factors* may be altered.

Clinical Manifestations. HIV-1–related dementia may be the presenting or sole manifestation of HIV-1 infection,[101] or it may occur in the setting of other HIV-1–related illnesses. Virtually all patients with this syndrome initially present with cognitive impairment that often, though not invariably, develops into a progressive, fatal dementia. It usually appears initially as a confusional state that may be accompanied by fevers or mild metabolic derangement. Less commonly, patients demonstrate weakness, altered personality, transient dysarthrias, seizures, or movement disorders.[98,99] The clinical description of this syndrome appears in Table 3–4.[107] The deficits associated with HIV-1 dementia meet the *Diag-*

Table 3–4 CLINICAL FEATURES OF THE AIDS DEMENTIA COMPLEX

SYMPTOMS
Cognitive: Poor concentration, forgetfulness, slowness
Motor: Loss of balance, clumsiness, leg weakness
Behavioral: Apathy, reduced spontaneity, social withdrawal

SIGNS
Mental status: Inattention, psychomotor slowing, impairment of complex processing; global dementia, mutism, organic psychosis
Motor findings: Impaired rapid movements, ataxia, tremor, hypertonia, paraparesis, incontinence, myoclonus

NEUROPSYCHOLOGIC TEST PROFILE
Impaired sequential-alternation problem solving and complex sequencing
Slowed verbal fluency and fine motor control

OVERALL CHARACTER
Subcortical dementia with diffuse cognitive deficit, psychomotor slowing, motor impairment, behavioral abnormalities

Source: Price RW, Sidtis JJ, Bradford AN, et al: The AIDS dementia complex. In Rosenblum ML, Levy RM, and Bredesen DE (eds): AIDS and the Nervous System. Raven Press, New York, 1988, p 204, with permission.

nostic and Statistical Manual of Mental Disorders (DMS-III) (Diagnostic Interview Schedule—Version IIIA) clinical diagnostic criteria for dementia.

On neuropsychologic testing, patients perform poorly on tests that measure performance under time contraints, problem solving, visual scanning, perceptual and visual motor integration, learning, memory, and alternation between two or more performance rules or sets.[127] The overall character of the disease is a dementia characterized by a diffuse cognitive deficit, psychomotor slowing, motor impairment, and behavioral abnormality. These deficits have been referred to as a "subcortical dementia"[107] and share common features with the dementias accompanying Parkinson's disease, Huntington's disease, and normal pressure hydrocephalus.

Incidence. The true incidence of HIV-1–related dementia has not been established. Point prevalence data on AIDS patients from a number of studies indicate that the prevalence ranges between 8% and 16%.[76,122] In a selected, autopsy-based series of patients referred to neurologists, this figure was as high as 66%.[107]

Although the presence of neurologic and neuropsychiatric illness in patients with AIDS has been recognized from the beginning of the AIDS epidemic, the occurrence of cognitive dysfunction in patients with ARC and possibly in asymptomatic HIV-1–infected individuals or those with persistent generalized lymphadenopathy has been only recently addressed.[48,61] While there is some evidence to the contrary, the available data strongly tend to support the hypothesis that cognitive deficits do not occur with any significantly increased frequency in HIV-1–seropositive people who are otherwise asymptomatic as compared with seronegative controls. It is, however, premature to make absolute conclusions based upon the available data. In fact, the clinical experience of many physicians is that a few otherwise asymptomatic HIV-1–infected individuals do exhibit and complain of cognitive dysfunction, although such patients are rare and the cause may not be HIV-1 infection per se but rather the associated stress and anxiety associated with its recent diagnosis.

ATYPICAL ASEPTIC MENINGITIS

Several patients in high-risk groups have been observed to develop an atypical aseptic meningitis that is characterized by chronicity and recurrence. Affected patients often have CSF pleocytosis and occasionally evidence of elevated intracranial pressure. Recent studies have demonstrated that HIV-1 can be cultured from the CSF of these patients; thus this syndrome may be better named acute, remitting HIV-1 meningitis. Common clinical features include headache, fever, and meningeal signs.

Two forms of meningitis have been described with HIV-1 infection.[59]

Shortly after infection, an acute meningitis may occur, characterized by headache, meningismus, photophobia, occasional global encephalopathy, and, more rarely, focal findings and seizures. CSF findings include a mononuclear pleocytosis, increased protein, and normal to low glucose.[59] HIV-1 may be cultured from the CSF at this time. Systemic features that may be observed at the time of acute HIV-1 infection include fever, lymphadenopathy, oropharyngitis, a maculopapular rash, and hepatosplenomegaly.[33]

The second form of meningeal inflammation is a chronic meningitis. Headache and CSF abnormalities (typically less striking than those observed in the acute form) are noted.[59] HIV-1 is recoverable from the CSF. In this meningitis, long periods of relative quiescence may be punctuated by periods of intense, unremitting headache. Generally, the CSF is persistently abnormal, despite the relative absence of symptoms at various times. Indeed, 60% of 459 CSF examinations in asymptomatic HIV-1–infected individuals (Reed stage 1 or 2) demonstrated at least one abnormal finding.[84]

SPINAL VACUOLAR MYELOPATHY

Vacuolar myelopathy appears to be a third unique AIDS-related CNS disease. Evidence of this disease is noted in about one quarter of AIDS patients at autopsy.[106] This process consists of a diffuse degeneration of the spinal cord that is most severe in the lateral and posterior areas of the thoracic spinal cord. Pathologically, this syndrome closely resembles the degeneration of the spinal cord seen with vitamin B_{12} deficiency, raising the question as to whether there is a nutritional cofactor to HIV-1 infection causing this disease. Certainly many AIDS patients suffer from malnutrition and malabsorption syndromes, but assays of vitamin B_{12} have failed to reveal any association with this illness.

This myelopathy is frequently overlooked clinically and discovered at the time of autopsy. The most common symptoms, leg weakness and incontinence, are often attributed to the patient's general state of debilitation. Neurologic examination often reveals spastic paraparesis, hyperreflexia, spastic-ataxic gait, and impaired distal sensory perception, particularly for vibration and position sense. Although HIV-1 can be cultured from the spinal cord and demonstrated in the spinal cord by in situ hybridization in some patients, the role of this virus in the etiopathology of this illness remains uncertain.

Not all myelopathies occurring in association with HIV-1 are spinal vacuolar myelopathy; other causes, some of which are treatable, need to be considered in the differential diagnosis of the HIV-1–infected patient presenting with a spinal cord syndrome. An acute myelopathy of uncertain pathogenesis has been described to occur at the time of HIV seroconversion.[38] Other myelopathies occurring in association with HIV infection include those due to *Herpes simplex* type 2,[23] CMV,[128] presumed *Herpes zoster*,[87] and HTLV-I.[15,88] Myelopathy may also be the consequence of tumors that occur with increased frequency in HIV infection, such as lymphomas,[64] plasmacytomas,[122] or gliomas.[133] Epidural abscesses may result from fungal, bacterial, or mycobacterial[40] infection. Mycobacterial meningomyelitis with an intramedullary granuloma has been reported.[136] Furthermore, a remitting and relapsing myelopathy has also been observed in several patients with a demyelinating disorder associated with HIV infection, which resembles multiple sclerosis.[16] Lastly, one of us (JRB) has observed syphilitic meningomyelitis in three patients with HIV-1 infection.

OPPORTUNISTIC VIRAL INFECTION

Progressive Multifocal Leukoencephalopathy. Progressive multifocal leukoencephalopathy (PML) is an unusual infectious CNS demyelinating disease caused by the JC papovavirus. This illness typically occurs in individuals with impaired cell-mediated immunity. Affected patients present with dementia, blindness, aphasia, hemiparesis, unsteadiness, ataxia, and other focal deficits, which slowly progress until death.[10] The characteristic computed tomography (CT) finding is that of low-density, non–contrast-enhancing, white matter lesions without significant mass effect. Magnetic resonance imaging (MRI) is more sensitive in detecting these lesions. On occasion, these lesions may enhance in contrast studies. CSF abnormalities are nonspecific, and the diagnosis can be firmly established only by brain biopsy. Pathologic findings reveal focal loss of myelin with axon sparing; bizarre astrocytes and enlarged oligodendrocytes containing eosinophilic intranuclear inclusions surround these areas of demyelination. PML has been reported in up to 4% of AIDS patients.[12] No effective therapy exists. The average survival after diagnosis of PML is 4 months,[12] although unexpectedly long survival and neurologic recovery have been observed in a rare individual.[14]

Herpesviruses. In AIDS patients, infection with CMV, herpes simplex viruses type 1 and 2 (HSV-1 and HSV-2), and varicella zoster virus (HVZ) is a significant source of central neurologic disease. Meningitis, encephalitis, myelitis, and radiculoneuritis caused by HSV-1, HSV-2, CMV, and HVZ, either alone or in combination, have been reported in patients with AIDS. In fact, infection with more than one opportunistic viral pathogen is now a well-recognized entity. Early studies of the neurologic complication of AIDS, such as that of Snider and coworkers,[122] suggested that CMV infection may have been the cause of the subacute encephalopathy observed in 18 of their 50 patients. Subsequent studies detected CMV in the brains of many patients with encephalitis by the use of immunoperoxidase staining techniques, radioactive probes, electron microscopy, and culture of nervous tissue and CSF. Pathologic examination of brains with CMV infection reveals microglial nodules and intranuclear CMV "owl's eye" inclusions that predominate in the subcortical gray matter.[96] The contribution of concomitant CMV infection to HIV encephalopathy is under active investigation.

While viruses other than papovaviruses or herpesviruses are potential opportunistic CNS pathogens in patients with AIDS, very few such cases have been reported. Opportunistic CNS viral infections are associated with a poor prognosis and an average survival of less than 4 months. Despite the availability of acyclovir for the treatment of herpesvirus infections and the development of dihydroxypropoxymethyl guanine (DHPG, ganciclovir), an antiviral agent useful in the treatment of CMV retinitis, therapy for opportunistic viral encephalitides has been largely ineffective. Recently, strains of herpesviruses have been identified that are resistant to these antiviral agents.

NONVIRAL INFECTIONS

Toxoplasma gondii. Toxoplasmosis, an infection caused by the protozoan *Toxoplasma gondii,* is one of the most common infections of animals and humans (see Chap. 11). In immunocompetent individuals, infection with *T. gondii* is asymptomatic in all but 5% of cases, in which a mononucleosis-like syndrome characterized by fever, lymphadenopathy, splenomegaly, and hepatitis may arise.[18] After the acute infection, the parasite assumes a latent form as tissue cysts containing bradyzoites. In the vast majority of patients with HIV-1 infection and active toxoplasmosis, the latter represents a reactivation of latent infection. In some communities (France, the Caribbean basin, south Florida), seroepidemiologic surveys reveal that the majority of the population is latently infected with toxoplasmosis. CNS infection with *T. gondii* produces acute focal or diffuse encephalitis with necrosis and signs of inflammation associated with both intracellular and extracellular organisms. Toxoplasmosis abscesses and large areas of infarction and necrosis resulting from thrombosis of blood vessels may produce CNS mass lesions. The lack of cell-mediated immunity may result in a persistent infection with severe lesions.

The incidence of cerebral toxoplasmosis ranges between 2% and 13% depending upon patient risk group and geographic location. Several series reporting AIDS-related CNS toxoplasmosis have appeared; all pointed to the increased risk of toxoplasmosis in the Haitian AIDS patient; to the common clinical findings of lethargy, intellectual slowness, seizures, and weakness; and to the frequency of bilateral, ring-enhancing basal ganglia lesions on CT scans.[28,53,66,74,79,83,110] CSF findings in patients with cerebral toxoplasmosis are nonspecific, with most showing elevation of protein (50 to 200 mg/dL) and one third exhibiting a mononuclear pleocytosis (<100 cell/mm^3). Rarely, mild hypoglycorrhachia is noted. Serologic studies are not particularly helpful in establishing the diagnosis, although IgG antibody directed against *T. gondii* in the blood is typically present before the onset of the illness and at the time of presentation.[100] CSF antibody studies may be negative, although some investigators[135] have suggested measuring local CSF antitoxoplasma IgG antibody production to support the diagnosis. Early aggressive diagnosis and therapy with antibiotics generally results in a dramatic clinical and radiographic response. Most patients respond to antibiotic therapy with pyrimethamine (50 to 100 mg to start and 25 mg/day thereafter) and sulfadiazine (6 to 8 g in four divided doses daily). Side effects are seen in up to 50% of AIDS patients on this regimen, with rash from the sulfadiazine and thrombocytopenia from pyrimethamine being the most common. In patients with confirmed toxoplasma encephalitis not responding to this regimen, or in those incapable of tolerating these antibiotics, trials with other antibiotics such as clindamycin may be of value. The possibility of another coexisting pathologic process needs to be considered.[45] Survival of 1 year or more is not uncommon, but the risk of recurrent toxoplasmosis exceeds 30%, so continued antibiotic therapy is necessary for secondary prophylaxis.

Cryptococcus neoformans. Epidemiologic data suggest that approximately 5% of all patients with AIDS will develop infection with the common soil fungus *Cryptococcus neoformans*. At particular risk are AIDS patients from New Jersey and those who are black or intravenous drug users; these factors may increase the risk of contracting cryptococcal meningitis to as high as 10%. Patients most frequently present with a short history of decreasing mental status, headache, and signs of meningeal irritation. Cranial CT scans are usually normal, although patients occasionally have cryptococcal mass lesions of the CNS. The diagnosis of cryptococcosis is made by CSF analysis with cryptococcal cultures, cryptococcal antigen titers, or direct staining with India ink. CSF analysis frequently reveals normal leukocyte count, protein, and glucose concentrations, but CSF cryptococcal antigen and a culture for cryptococci are almost always positive. Pathologically, cryptococcal meningitis results in a granulomatous meningitis with additional granulomas and cysts forming within the cerebral cortex and deeper brain structures. One feature unique to AIDS-related cryptococcal infection of the CNS is the frequency of intraparenchymal cryptococcal lesions. Although quite rare in immunocompetent patients, cryptococcomas are found in 10% of AIDS patients with cryptococcal meningitis.

Despite treatment with amphotericin B (0.6 to 1.0 mg/kg per day) for 6 weeks with or without the addition of flucytosine (see Chap. 12), the mortality rate of CNS cryptococcal infection in immunocompetent hosts is 40%, and it is at least that high in patients with AIDS.

Standard antibiotic therapy with amphotericin B (with or without flucytosine) tends to be quite effective for AIDS patients with newly acquired cryptococcal meningitis, but they often require chronic suppressive therapy after treatment of the acute disease. Recurrent cryptococcal meningitis is a significant problem, and mean survival after initial diagnosis has been only 2 to 3 months. Therefore, as with other opportunistic infections of the CNS in the HIV-1–infected patient, continued antibiotic prophylaxis is recommended after the initial treatment has been completed. Prophylactic regimens suggested include intravenous amphotericin B (100 mg/wk)[109] or oral fluconazole (50 to 200 mg/day).[126]

Other Fungal Infections. *Candida albicans* infection, usually associated with diabetes, leukemia, lymphoma, and intravenous drug abuse, has been reported in patients with AIDS. The combination of surgical abscess excision followed by amphotericin B appears to be the only effective therapy. Infections with the mold *Aspergillus fumigatus* have been reported in patients with AIDS and may present as meningitis, encephalitis, or abscess. CNS infection with *Coccidioides immitis* can result in a rapidly progressive, fulminant meningitis in the patient with AIDS. Treatment involves the long-term administration of intrathecal amphotericin B; frequently this requires the placement of a reservoir for intrathecal antibiotic therapy. Cases of AIDS-related CNS infection also have been reported with *Rhizopus* sp., *Acremonium alabamensis*, *Histoplasma capsulatum*, and mucormycosis.[111]

Mycobacterial Infections. Although infection with atypical mycobacterium is common in the HIV-1–infected individual, mycobacterial infection of the CNS is almost always the result of *Mycobacterium tuberculosis*. The clinical features and pathology of *M. tuberculosis* meningitis have been well described;[1,19] mycobacterial infection can result in meningitis, encephalitis, or brain abscess formation. Several series of patients with AIDS and *M. tuberculosis* infections of the central nervous system have been reported.[24,64,100,125] These patients were either intravenous drug abusers or Haitians, consistent with the endemic nature of tuberculosis in the Caribbean basin. Two thirds of AIDS patients with CNS *M. tuberculosis* infections present with CNS mass lesions, while one third present with signs and symptoms of meningitis only.

Although *M. avium* complex (MAC) infection is extremely common in the AIDS patient population, the CNS is rarely affected. In contrast to CNS *M. tuberculosis* infection, there does not appear to be a Haitian predilection for AIDS-related CNS MAC infection. Most patients have disseminated systemic MAC infection prior to their neurologic presentation with diffuse encephalitis. Meningitis, facial nerve palsy, and peripheral neuropathy have also been reported in association with MAC infection of the CNS. Survival after contracting CNS MAC infection is very short. Results with both standard tuberculosis chemotherapeutic agents and experimental regimens have been uniformly poor.[55]

Bacterial Infections. Reports of AIDS-related CNS complications from common bacterial pathogens have been conspicuously absent from the literature. None of the patients in the series presented by Snider and colleagues[122] or that of Levy's group[75] had bacterial infections of the CNS. Interestingly, an increased incidence of syphilis has been reported in patients with AIDS.[65] CNS infection with opportunistic bacterial pathogens has occasionally been reported. *Listeria monocytogenes*, the most common cause of bacterial meningitis in other types of immunocompromised patients, has rarely been the cause of AIDS-related neurologic disease, causing meningitis, diffuse encephalopathy, or focal neurologic deficit. Patients with *Listeria* infection may develop intraparenchymal mass lesions, but antibiotic therapy may re-

sult in complete resolution of the disease. *Nocardia asteroides* infection of the CNS usually accompanies pulmonary infection in immunosuppressed patients; CNS infection in the AIDS patient population is extremely rare.

NEOPLASMS

Primary CNS Lymphoma. Primary malignant lymphomas are rare tumors, representing less than 1.5% of primary brain tumors. The risk of developing primary CNS lymphoma in the general population has been estimated at 0.0001%. In immunosuppressed, non-AIDS patients, such as renal and cardiac transplant recipients, this risk increases to 0.2%, whereas in AIDS patients, the risk is about 2%. The annual incidence of primary CNS lymphoma in the United States prior to the AIDS epidemic was approximately 225 cases; projections suggested that more than 1800 cases of AIDS-related primary CNS lymphoma would occur in 1991. Thus, CNS lymphoma is becoming a disease predominantly affecting the AIDS patient population.

AIDS patients with CNS lymphoma typically present with the subacute onset of altered mental status, headaches, and, less commonly, focal weakness.[123] The diagnosis of primary CNS lymphoma is usually made by brain biopsy. Until recently, such patients have tended to survive for less than 2 months, with death related to progression of CNS disease. Recent experience with a protocol for the aggressive early treatment of these patients with radiation therapy suggests that these tumors are radiation sensitive and that such therapy may have a significant positive, although transient, effect on survival.[7]

Metastatic Neoplasms. Systemic lymphoma most frequently affects the CNS by invasion of the meningeal coverings of the brain, resulting in meningitis or cranial neuropathies. Additional neurologic manifestations include spinal cord or brachial plexus compression by metastatic tumor, or intracerebral hemorrhage within metastatic lesions. Although transient improvement has been noted following therapy, most patients succumb rapidly from metastatic systemic lymphomas.

Although Kaposi's sarcoma has been a primary feature of AIDS, CNS presentation of this neoplasm has been remarkably rare. Patients have presented with CNS mass lesions and seizures, focal neurologic deficits, or alterations in mental status. Although the CNS tumors are radiation sensitive, patients have died of their diffuse metastatic Kaposi's sarcoma.

CEREBROVASCULAR COMPLICATIONS

The frequency with which cerebrovascular complications have been reported with HIV infections varies considerably. In predominantly clinical studies, the incidence ranges from 0.5% to 7%,[13,42,64,76,87] whereas the incidence is even higher in autopsy series, in which estimates of stroke have varied from 11% to 34%.[5,95,120,132] Clearly the incidence of stroke in AIDS patients exceeds that in the general population of young adults, estimated at 10 to 25 cases per 100,000.[63,89] While multifocal ischemic infarction is the most common of these problems,[9] patients have also been seen with hemorrhagic infarction, hemorrhage into tumors, transient ischemic episodes, and both subdural and epidural hematomas. The etiology of ischemic cerebral infarction is quite variable and includes cardiac emboli, cerebral vasculitis resulting from HIV-1 or opportunistic infections (herpes zoster, cryptococcosis, syphilis, and so forth), other potential causes known to be associated with HIV-1 infection (lupus anticoagulant,[125] hyperviscosity[85]) and unknown factors.

COMPLICATIONS RESULTING FROM SYSTEMIC AIDS THERAPY

Neurologic symptoms arising as complications of AIDS therapy may be observed. A surprisingly common complication has been the appearance of extrapyramidal motor symptoms, particularly parkinsonism, with the use of low doses of the antiemetic metoclopramide (Reglan) and other dopamine receptor blockers.[58] This complication is often noted in individuals with frank dementia or previously unrecognized disturbances of cognitive function, suggesting that HIV-1 encephalopathy may contribute to the pathogenesis of this complication. Antiviral therapy may produce startle myoclonus, dysphasia, lethargy, delirium, and confusion. An acute myelopathy has occurred following the use of intrathecal chemotherapy for AIDS-related lymphoma.[6]

MULTIPLE CNS PATHOLOGIC PROCESSES

The evaluation and treatment of the AIDS patient with neurologic illness may be difficult, since many routine diagnostic tests, including clinical, serologic, and radiologic evaluations, can be unreliable and insensitive in this patient population. The evaluation of these patients has been further complicated by the presence of multiple intracranial pathologic processes in many patients with AIDS. In one series, nearly 30% of carefully evaluated, neurologically symptomatic AIDS patients had more than one disease process identified at some time during their lives.[56] These processes may occur both sequentially and simultaneously and have been identified both within the same lesion and within spatially separated lesions.

Peripheral Nervous System Complications of HIV-1 Infection

Abnormalities in patients with HIV infection have been described at every level of the peripheral nervous system.[35,76,81,92-94] Excluding neuropathies related to therapy (vincristine and di-

**Table 3–5 PERIPHERAL NEUROPATHIC SYNDROMES
IN HIV-INFECTED PATIENTS**

	Distal Symmetric Peripheral Neuropathy	Inflammatory Demyelinating Polyradiculo-neuropathy	Mononeuropathy Multiplex	Progressive Polyradiculopathy
Patients	Mostly AIDS	Mostly non-AIDS	Mostly non-AIDS	Mostly AIDS
Symptoms	Sensory > motor	Motor ≫ sensory	Motor and sensory	Motor > sensory
Symmetry	Yes	Yes	No	With progression
Cranial neuropathy	Rare	Common	Very common	Late, if at all
Urinary retention	No	No	No	Yes
Chronicity	Chronic	Acute to chronic	Usually subacute	Usually subacute
CSF	Usually normal	Mononuclear pleocytosis, increased gamma globulin	Mononuclear pleocytosis, increased gamma globulin	Hypoglycorrhachia, mononuclear and polymorphonuclear pleocytosis

Source: Adapted from Aminoff MJ. Neurology and General Medicine. Churchill Livingstone; New York, 1989, p 674, with permission.

deoxycytidine), neuropathies related to the nutritional disturbances that attend HIV-1 infection, and zoster radiculitis, nearly every patient has one of four readily distinguishable syndromes: distal symmetric peripheral neuropathy, inflammatory demyelinating polyradiculoneuropathy, mononeuropathy multiplex, or progressive polyradiculopathy (Table 3–5).

DISTAL SYMMETRIC PERIPHERAL NEUROPATHY

This is the most common syndrome of peripheral neuropathy observed in patients with HIV-1 infection. Symptoms and signs, which are often mild and chronically progressive, include hypesthesia, paresthesia, sensory ataxia, weakness, and hypoactive deep tendon reflexes. Pain is infrequent and seldom debilitating. Sensory function is usually affected more than motor, and dysautonomia may occur,[36,91] although such complaints have rarely been recorded.

Electrophysiologic findings are compatible with an axonal process.[92] The CSF is usually normal unless other processes such as toxoplasmosis coexist.[92] Nerve biopsy may be normal or may show axonal loss with absent or mini-

mal inflammation and demyelination. Some investigators believe that azidothymidine shows promise in treatment,[130] but treatment is largely symptomatic. Amitryptyline, phenytoin, carbamazepine, and topical capsaicin are often useful for the discomfort, and ankle-foot orthoses can be used for footdrop. Plasmapheresis is ineffective.[93]

INFLAMMATORY DEMYELINATING POLYRADICULONEUROPATHY

In HIV-1–infected patients, inflammatory demyelinating polyradiculoneuropathy may be acute, subacute, or chronic.[35,81,94] In contrast to distal symmetric peripheral neuropathy, this syndrome usually occurs in seropositive patients without AIDS. It usually produces more severe motor than sensory symptoms. Weakness is often most prominent distally, but there is usually definite proximal weakness as well. Muscle stretch reflexes are usually absent or markedly hypoactive throughout. Sensory symptoms are usually mild and distal, involving large-fiber modalities out of proportion to small-fiber modalities. In contrast to Guillain-Barré syndrome, autonomic symptoms are usually absent.

In contrast to typical Guillain-Barré syndrome, in which an albuminocytologic dissociation is observed, the CSF in these patients usually reflects inflammation, with elevation of both protein concentration and cell count.[81] Electromyography, nerve conduction studies, and biopsy results suggest that this syndrome in HIV-infected patients is predominantly (but usually not purely) demyelinating in nature.

Treatment with plasmapheresis is very successful when demyelination predominates over axonal loss.[93] Prednisone is often ineffective,[81] and there is at least theoretical concern about its ability to further compromise cellular immune function, although some argue that such effects are actually desirable in these patients.[54] In the patient who has persistent or progressive demyelinative peripheral neuropathy unresponsive to plasmapheresis, a trial of prednisone should be attempted. Spontaneous improvement also may occur.[10,35]

MONONEUROPATHY MULTIPLEX

As in mononeuropathy multiplex from other causes, such as diabetes mellitus or polyarteritis nodosa, the hallmark of mononeuropathy multiplex associated with HIV infection is the rapid development of sensory or motor loss (or both) in the distribution of one or more peripheral nerves, nerve roots, nerve trunks, or cranial nerves.[34,35] It is less common than inflammatory demyelinating polyradiculoneuropathy.

The CSF findings are nonspecific, typically reflecting inflammatory changes, with a mononuclear pleocytosis and oligoclonal bands.[81] Electromyography and nerve conduction studies usually show changes suggesting combined axonal loss and demyelination. Sural nerve biopsy may be normal or may show axonal degeneration, segmental demyelination, endoneurial edema, and inflammatory cells in the endoneurium and epineurium.[81] Vas-culitis is rarely seen. Plasmapheresis may lead to improvement.[81,92]

ETIOLOGIC CONSIDERATIONS REGARDING PERIPHERAL NERVE PATHOLOGY

The cause of these syndromes is unknown. HIV-1 has been cultured from nerve in at least one case,[57] but in situ hybridization studies in cases of inflammatory demyelinating polyradiculoneuropathy have been uniformly negative.[35] No evidence has been obtained for involvement of viruses other than HIV in these three syndromes.

Miller and coworkers[92] noted circulating antibodies to normal sural nerve in all 30 tested patients with AIDS or ARC and peripheral neuropathy (including patients with each of the three types of neuropathy), but in only 1 of 10 patients with AIDS or ARC but without peripheral neuropathy, and in only 3 of 20 seronegative patients with peripheral neuropathy. Seven of these patients with AIDS or ARC and peripheral neuropathy had sural nerve biopsies, all of which disclosed perineurial immunoglobulin M (IgM) deposits. The antigen(s) against which these antibodies are directed is unknown. It is noteworthy that in HIV-1–related immune thrombocytopenia, antibodies cross-reactive for a platelet surface membrane protein and HSV have been reported;[125] perhaps a similar phenomenon occurs in HIV-related peripheral neuropathies.

A third etiologic consideration involves neuroleukin, a lymphokine and neurotrophic factor that affects both the CNS and the peripheral nervous system.[50,51] An HIV-1 envelope glycoprotein, gp120, has a region of homology to neuroleukin (phosphohexose isomerase), and Gurney and colleagues[51] have found that gp120 is a competitive antagonist of neuroleukin's effects in tissue culture. Thus, conceivably, either gp120 or cross-reactive antibodies could cause a reduction in binding of neuroleukin to target neurons, resulting in neuronal death.

PROGRESSIVE POLYRADICULOPATHY

Progressive polyradiculopathy, a distinctive clinical syndrome that may manifest as a radiculopathy or a radiculomyelopathy, usually occurs in patients with AIDS.[41,92] It usually begins with leg weakness, often asymmetric, and progresses cephalad over several weeks. Sensory loss is less prominent but also spreads rostrally. Urinary retention is typical.

The CSF characteristically shows hypoglycorrhachia in addition to pleocytosis and elevated protein concentration. CMV or HSV may be cultured from the CSF. Polymorphonuclear cells often predominate in the CSF with CMV polyradiculopathy. Nerve conduction studies are usually normal initially, but later the size of compound muscle action potentials is reduced. The electromyogram shows a reduced recruitment pattern early and abnormal spontaneous activity later.[41,92] Pathologic and virologic results implicate CMV as the etiologic agent in this syndrome; in some cases, HSV may be involved.[128] In one treated case of progressive polyradiculopathy with HIV-1 infection, no benefit was noted from acyclovir, plasmapheresis, or DHPG, despite a concomitant arrest in CMV retinitis.[92] The prognosis is very poor. HIV-1–infected patients without AIDS may develop a transient, usually mild, sacral myeloradiculitis,[20,69] sometimes in association with perianal herpetic rashes. Similarly, individuals without HIV-1 infection may have transient myeloradiculitis with primary HSV-1 infection. Thus it is possible that progressive polyradiculopathy represents the more severe end of a spectrum of radicular involvement by viruses of the herpes family in patients with HIV-1 infection.

OTHER CAUSES OF PERIPHERAL NERVOUS SYSTEM DYSFUNCTION

Herpes zoster radiculitis is common in HIV-1–infected patients and may be associated with radicular sensory symptoms, motor symptoms (especially when radiculomyelitis occurs), cranial neuropathies, or postherpetic neuralgia. The diagnosis is usually straightforward because of the characteristic dermatomal rash.

Because of the association of herpes zoster infections with HIV-1,[32] young patients with herpes zoster infections, patients with complicated or disseminated herpes zoster, and patients with herpes zoster who are in groups associated with risk for HIV-1 infection should undergo serologic testing for HIV-1. After the development of shingles, there is a higher incidence in HIV-1–infected patients of neurologic complications such as stroke, cranial neuropathy, or myelopathy. It has therefore been suggested that all such patients receive acyclovir.[47]

Rare patients with transient brachial plexopathy of unknown cause (in one case due to Kaposi's sarcoma) have been observed.[92] Likewise, rare instances of cauda equina syndrome and lumbar radiculopathy may be seen.[37]

CRANIAL NEUROPATHIES

The pattern of cranial neuropathies may suggest an intra-axial or extra-axial process, or both. Of course, in patients with AIDS, the presence of multiple pathologic processes may make this distinction difficult. The differential diagnosis of intra-axial processes is similar to that for CNS dysfunction (see later). Among the common causes of HIV-1–related extra-axial cranial neuropathy are mononeuropathy multiplex and inflammatory demyelinating polyradiculoneuropathy. The fifth and seventh cranial nerves are the most frequently involved, followed by the third, fourth, and sixth nerves. These cranial neuropathies may be totally or partially reversible. As a point of differential diagnosis, it should be recalled that the first symptoms of mononeuropathy multiplex and inflammatory demyelinating polyradiculoneuropathy rarely appear after the diagnosis of AIDS.

Cryptococcal meningitis may produce either pattern, as may viruses of the herpes family and other infections. Herpes zoster (varicella zoster) virus is more often associated with an extra-axial pattern, whereas the reverse is true with herpes simplex and CMV. The upper division of the trigeminal nerve is the cranial nerve most often affected by HZV, but other cranial nerves, such as the nerves to the extraocular muscles, may be involved.

Meningeal lymphomatosis or focal (e.g., skull base) metastatic lymphoma may also cause cranial neuropathy, as may primary CNS lymphoma, which usually produces an intra-axial pattern, and aseptic meningitis, which especially affects the fifth, seventh, and eighth nerves. Other infections such as tuberculous meningitis or meningovascular syphilis may occasionally be responsible for cranial neuropathy in patients with HIV-1 infection.

Diagnosis of AIDS-Related CNS Illness

As with other neurologic illnesses, the first diagnostic steps are obtaining a history and physical examination. Because primary neurologic HIV-1 infection may produce subtle dementia before other signs of systemic or neurologic illness, careful cognitive assessment is critical. Radiologic and CSF examinations are then the mainstays of the diagnosis of AIDS-related nervous system illness. Examination of CSF may provide a definitive diagnosis in several AIDS-related neurologic diseases, including HIV-1 or other viral infections and cryptococcal meningitis. Tests for cryptococcal meningitis are very sensitive in patients with AIDS; cryptococcal antigen, culture, and India ink staining are positive in over 90% of cases. Although the presence of a positive toxoplasma titer is not a reliable indicator of active toxoplasma infection, a negative IgG titer may be of negative predictive value. Tests for HIV-1 infection (e.g., antibody, P24 core

antigen, or culture) indicate only exposure to the AIDS virus and not active disease. Quantitative measurement of HIV-1 antigen may better reflect active neurologic illness in these patients.

CT brain scans are still the most widely used radiologic examination in AIDS patients with neurologic signs or symptoms. Diffuse cerebral atrophy alone, probably a result of CNS HIV-1 infection, is seen in roughly 35% of scans, and focal cerebral lesions are noted in another 25%. The presence of diffuse cerebral atrophy is of some prognostic value: Patients with this CT finding are three times more likely than patients with normal CT scans to manifest neurologic progression and to demonstrate subsequent CNS histopathology.[80] In patients without focal CT abnormalities, HIV-1 encephalopathy and cryptococcal meningitis are by far the most frequent and second most frequent diagnoses, respectively (Fig. 3–1). Patients with focal abnormalities on CT scans most commonly have toxoplasmosis (50% to 70%), but primary CNS lymphoma (10% to 25%) and PML (10% to 22%) are not infrequent diagnoses. Patients with low-density lesions that demonstrate little or no enhancement after the administration of iodinated contrast material tend to have PML or primary CNS lymphoma. Restriction of these lesions to the white matter suggests the diagnosis of PML, whereas the presence of mass effect suggests lymphoma. The demonstration of ring-enhancing lesions, especially within the basal ganglia, suggests the diagnosis of toxoplasmosis (Fig. 3–2). Unfortunately, many ring-enhancing lesions are proven to be primary CNS lymphomas (Fig. 3–3), and many toxoplasma brain abscesses do not enhance. Thus, CT scans alone cannot provide a definitive diagnosis in AIDS-related CNS disease.

MRI is more sensitive than CT for the detection of intracranial pathology in the patient with AIDS and neurologic symptoms.[80,112] MRI also more accurately reflects the extent and distribution of histologically verified CNS dis-

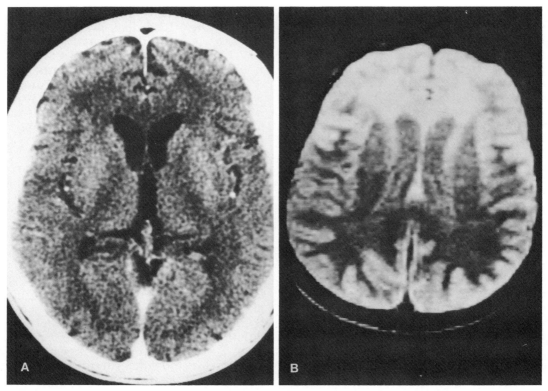

Figure 3–1. CT (*A*) and MRI (*B*) of a patient with HIV encephalitis. The CT scan reveals only diffuse cerebral atrophy. The MRI reveals bifrontal increases in signal intensity of the white matter; this finding correlated with the patient's bifrontal leukoencephalitis, noted on biopsy and autopsy.

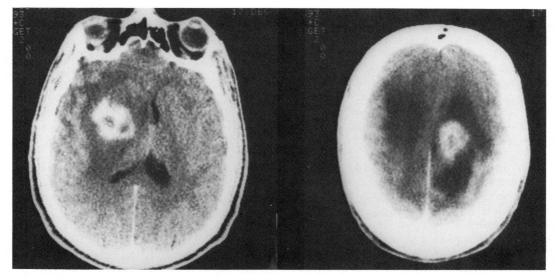

Figure 3–2. CT scan of a patient with toxoplasmosis. Note the bilateral deep ring-enhancing lesions that are characteristic (but not diagnostic) of this disease.

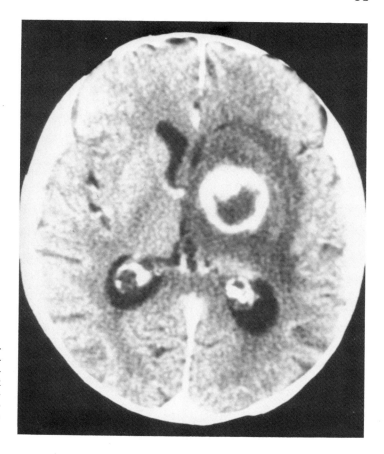

Figure 3–3. CT scan of a patient with primary CNS lymphoma. Note the contrast enhancement and mass effect that can make the radiologic differential diagnosis between lymphoma and toxoplasmosis extremely difficult.

ease. This increased sensitivity and accuracy has been demonstrated to have a significant impact on the evaluation and therapy of patients with AIDS-related CNS illness, including indication for and direction of brain biopsy, and alterations in both chemotherapeutic and radiation therapy protocols.[78] The MRI often demonstrates multiple bilateral intracranial abnormalities in patients with toxoplasmosis; a single lesion on MRI should suggest the possibility of an illness other than toxoplasmosis.

Algorithms for the Evaluation of the Patient with AIDS and Neurologic Symptoms

The evaluation and treatment of the AIDS patient with central neurologic ill-

ness is a difficult challenge. Figure 3–4 shows an algorithm to assist in the evaluation of the neurologically symptomatic AIDS patient. Close attention must be paid to subtle neurologic complaints, and careful neurologic examination is warranted in all AIDS patients. Once the patient complains of neurologic dysfunction or a neurologic abnormality is identified on examination, a careful work-up is indicated.

For patients with evidence of peripheral nervous system dysfunction, neurologic examination is usually followed by electromyography and nerve conduction studies. Occasionally, nerve biopsy may be necessary to establish a diagnosis. Inflammatory peripheral neuropathies (those with predominant demyelinative rather than axonopathic features) may respond to plasmapheresis. For the other peripheral neurologic

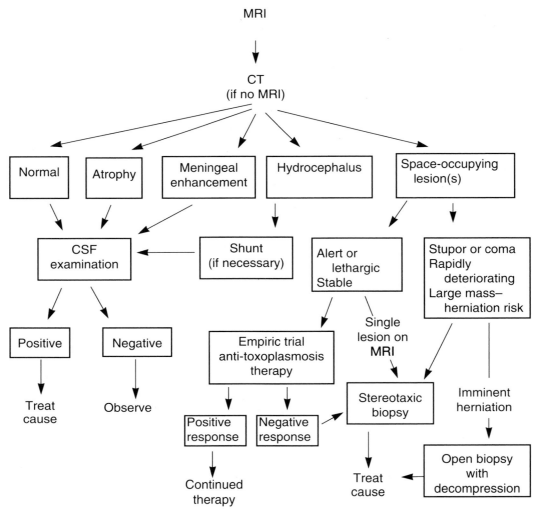

Figure 3–4. Algorithm for the evaluation of the patient with AIDS and signs of CNS disease. See text for details. (Adapted from Berger JR and Levy RM: Neurological emergencies associated with human immunodeficiency virus infection. In Weiner WJ [ed]: Emergent and Urgent Neurology. JB Lippincott, Philadelphia, 1992, pp 402, 405, with permission.)

diseases, the only treatments are symptomatic.

The current recommendation for the initial evaluation of the patient with central neurologic symptoms is MRI. If this is not readily available, then CT brain scanning should be performed. If the neuroradiologic study is normal or reveals diffuse cerebral atrophy only, then CSF examination should be performed. In addition to routine chemistries, cytology, and cultures, CSF examination should include viral cultures. Treatment should be initiated based upon these findings. If no diagnosis is made, then careful, regular clinical and radiologic follow-up is indicated.

Patients with focal mass lesions on MRI are divided into two groups: those who are stable (alert or lethargic) and those who are deteriorating. In stable patients, a trial of empiric therapy for toxoplasmosis with pyrimethamine and sulfadiazine is initiated. If there is clear radiologic and clinical response after 2 to 3 weeks of therapy, maximal antibiotic therapy is continued for life (although in some centers, a reduced dosage maintenance regimen for life is given after 6 weeks of full-dose therapy). If the patient fails to respond, then stereotaxic biopsy is indicated. In patients who are neurologically unstable, stereotaxic biopsy should be performed directly. Open craniotomy is reserved only for those patients with large mass lesions who are at risk of herniation and require emergent decompression, or individuals in whom stereotaxic biopsy proved to be nondiagnostic. In our experience, craniotomy is rarely necessary.

Specific diagnosis is thus made on the basis of CSF findings, response to empiric therapy, or biopsy. These patients must then be followed with great diligence to evaluate the response to therapy. The high incidence of multiple intracranial disease in patients with AIDS has profound implications for the diagnosis and treatment of intracranial lesions in this patient population. The reported frequency of cerebral toxoplasmosis[87] has led some authors to suggest that empiric therapy alone is sufficient for the treatment of AIDS patients with CNS mass lesions. Our experience suggests, however, that antibiotic therapy alone may ignore a potentially treatable disease in over half of neurologically symptomatic AIDS patients. In addition, even after a diagnosis has been reached by biopsy or response to empiric therapy, repeat clinical, CSF, and radiologic studies are indicated at regular intervals during therapy or whenever a patient deteriorates while receiving treatment even after the diagnosis is confirmed by biopsy. If new lesions appear, or if the response to therapy of other lesions differs from that of the biopsied lesion, the possibility of a second intracranial process must be considered. Repeat biopsy may be indicated and may reveal additional treatable disease. While such a diagnostic and therapeutic program requires extreme care and diligence, it is only with such an approach that we may optimally treat the patient with AIDS-related neurologic illness.

Impact of AIDS on the Practice of the Clinical Neurosciences

In light of the number of cases of AIDS in the United States, its dramatic increase, and the frequency of HIV-1–related neurologic illness, the impact of this epidemic on the practice of the clinical neurosciences promises to be profound. To estimate the impact of AIDS upon the practice of neurology and neurosurgery, we have combined projections of future AIDS cases by the CDC with our own neuroepidemiologic data. Recent CDC projections estimate that there will be 270,000 cumulative cases of AIDS in the United States, with 145,000 living AIDS patients, including 74,000 newly diagnosed AIDS cases. The cumulative number of neurologically symptomatic AIDS patients will rise to nearly 100,000, of which 54,000 will be alive during the calendar year 1992. Deaths from AIDS, virtually equal to the number of deaths from brain tumors in 1986, surpassed head injury as a cause of death in 1991.

The number of neurologically symptomatic AIDS patients relative to the number of patients in the United States with other neurologic illnesses is striking (Table 3–6). In 1986, neurologically symptomatic AIDS patients were intermediate in frequency between those with trigeminal neuralgia and those with multiple sclerosis. Currently, the number of neurologically symptomatic AIDS patients is nearly half the number of all patients with epilepsy and exceeds those with Parkinson's disease.

These figures take into account only those patients with AIDS (as defined by the CDC prior to 1983) and neurologic dysfunction; they may underestimate extremely the impact of AIDS on the practice of the clinical neurosciences. The large number of patients infected with HIV-1 but without signs of systemic illness creates a unique problem.

**Table 3–6 HIV-1–RELATED CNS DISEASE RELATIVE TO THE
ANNUAL INCIDENCE OF OTHER COMMON NEUROLOGIC DISEASES**

Neurologic Disease	Yearly Incidence in United States	
Stroke	337,500	
Epilepsy	112,500	Neurologic AIDS (1991)
Parkinson's disease	45,000	
Meningitis	33,750	
Cerebral palsy	20,250	
Tic douloureux	9,000	Neurologic AIDS (1986)
Multiple sclerosis	6,750	
Guillain-Barré syndrome	4,500	
Muscular dystrophy	1,575	
Huntington's disease	900	
Myasthenia gravis	900	

Source: Adapted from Rosenblum ML, Levy RM, and Bredesen DE: Overview of
AIDS and the nervous system. In Rosenblum ML, Levy RM, and Bredesen DE (eds):
AIDS and the Nervous System. Raven Press, New York, 1988, p 11, with permission.

CDC predictions suggest that 1.5 million people were infected wth the virus by 1986. Currently, 15 million Americans may be infected with HIV-1. As a significant number will develop primary HIV-1–related neurologic disease in the absence of other HIV-1–related illnesses, the potential number of HIV-1–related neurologically symptomatic patients may involve millions of individuals.

The possible impact of AIDS on the practice of neurosurgery can be predicted knowing the incidence of CNS space-occupying lesions in this patient population, defining the indications for biopsy of these lesions, and projecting into the future using the CDC projections. Our current indications for brain biopsy include the presence of intracranial space-occupying lesions that do not respond to empiric treatment for toxoplasmosis in patients with AIDS and the presence of intracranial space-occupying lesions in patients not yet known to have AIDS. This accounts for 6.8% of our patients with AIDS. Using these relatively conservative indications for biopsy, there were over 1000 potentially indicated biopsies in 1986; by 1992, there will be approximately 7000. The number of biopsies performed for AIDS-related CNS space-occupying lesions could, therefore, approximate the yearly incidence of malignant astrocytomas in the United States (Table 3–7). The number of biopsy procedures for AIDS-related primary CNS lymphomas is approaching the number of meningiomas in the United States.

The impact upon the practice of psychiatry is more difficult to ascertain. Most if not all patients with AIDS will experience appropriate and significant problems in coping with a fatal illness. Many of them will seek psychiatric assistance. In addition, as many as 75% of AIDS patients will demonstrate some degree of dementia,[108] frequently requiring psychiatric assessment and therapy. Finally, the potential impact of possible cognitive dysfunction in HIV-1–infected, non-AIDS patients is tremendous. The distinction among and differential weighting of biologic, psychologic, and social factors in this increasingly vast patient population will pose a major diagnostic task for neuropsychiatrists. Widely divergent therapeutic approaches exist for both organic and psychosocial HIV-1–related illness. Only through careful neurologic, psychiatric, and cognitive assessment can the complex needs of patients with AIDS be best addressed.

HIV-2

In 1986, a virus that was related to but distinct from the well-characterized

Table 3-7 PROJECTED NUMBER OF BRAIN BIOPSIES RELATIVE TO THE ANNUAL INCIDENCE OF PRIMARY BRAIN TUMORS IN THE UNITED STATES

Tumor	Yearly Incidence in United States
	—————————AIDS Brain Biopsies (1991)
Malignant astrocytoma	6000
Meningioma	2250
Astrocytoma	1500
Pituitary tumor	1500————————AIDS Brain Biopsies (1986)
Neurinoma/fibroma	750
Medulloblastoma	600
Congenital tumors	600
Ependymoma	300
Lymphoma	225

Source: Adapted from Rosenblum ML, Levy RM, and Bredesen DE: Overview of AIDS and the nervous system. In Rosenblum ML, Levy RM, and Bredesen DE (eds): AIDS and the Nervous System. Raven Press, New York, 1988, p 10, with permission.

AIDS virus was located in patients from West Africa.[30,31] This virus has been designated as HIV type 2 (HIV-2) and differs antigenically from standard HIV isolates, particularly in the envelope glycoprotein, which more closely resembles that of SIV.[31]

Individuals infected with HIV-2 may be asymptomatic or exhibit laboratory and clinical features of immunodeficiency identical to those caused by HIV-1.[31] The incubation period is estimated to be 11 to 19 years, substantially longer than that of HIV-1 infection.[4] Not unexpectedly, encephalopathy,[8,31,67] spastic paraplegia,[67] and peripheral neuropathy[67] may occur as a consequence of HIV-2 infection. Furthermore, the neurologic illness may be the presenting manifestation of the infection.[8,67]

Neurologic illness also may occur as a result of the immunodeficiency that attends HIV-2 infection, in addition to those illnesses that occur as a direct consequence of the viral infection. Two HIV-2–infected patients with toxoplasma encephalitis[24] and another with brain lymphoma[31] have been described.

HTLV-I

The neurologic manifestations of human T-cell lymphotropic virus type I (HTLV-I) were discovered serendipi-

tously. Of patients in the French West Indies suffering from a form of chronic myelopathy referred to as tropical spastic paraparesis (TSP), 68% to 80% were found to have antibodies directed to HTLV-I.[46,60,131] The evidence linking this chronic myelopathy with HTLV-I infection is quite convincing and includes (1) adult T-cell leukemia cells in the serum and CSF of patients with the disorder, (2) anti–HTLV-1 antibody titers that are highly positive in the serum and the CSF, (3) low incidence of anti–HTLV-1 antibody demonstrated.[102] In Japan, the myelopathy is referred to as HTLV-I–associated myelopathy (HAM).[102] Reports linking HTLV-I infection with multiple sclerosis, motor neuron disease, and polymyositis await further confirmation.

Clinically, the initial manifestations of the illness are leg weakness and lumbar and dorsal backache with or without painful legs or lower-limb arthralgia.[131] Although a single limb may be involved at the onset, generally signs are bilateral. The patients often comment on paresthesias of the distal lower extremities, and mild bladder dysfunction is occasionally observed.[131] Concordant with the chief effect of HTLV-I on the thoracic spinal cord, physical examination reveals spastic paraparesis or paraplegia, mild sensory loss of the lower extremities with vibratory and position sense generally more affected than other modalities, and an indistinct upper sensory level. CSF examination shows an elevated protein and lymphocytic pleocytosis in approximately 50% and an elevated gammaglobulin in approximately 66%.[131] The course of the illness is typically one of slow progression over months, although a rapidly progressive myelopathy may be noted.[131]

Pathologically examined cases have been few. Consistent findings have included a predominance of the abnormalities at the thoracic level; loss of myelin and axons chiefly in the lateral columns, but also in anterior and posterior columns; perivascular and parenchymal lymphocytic infiltration; the presence of foamy macrophages; the proliferation of astrocytes; and fibrillary gliosis.[2] Vacuolar changes may also be observed.[2]

Treatment is directed against the presumed autoimmune pathogenesis of the disorder. Treatment with corticosteroids[103] and plasmapheresis[86] has been reported. Trials with azidothymidine and other therapeutic modalities in the treatment of TSP and HAM are currently being conducted.

HTLV-II

The role, if any, of HTLV-II in the causation of neurologic disease is uncertain and under investigation. One patient dually infected with HIV-1 and HTLV-II developed a reversible myelopathy clinically indistinguishable from tropical spastic paraparesis.[17]

SUMMARY

HIV-1 is associated with a broad spectrum of neurologic diseases capable of affecting any part of the neuraxis. These neurologic diseases can be classified into those believed to be the direct result of the HIV-1 infection and those that occur as an indirect consequence of HIV-1 infection. The latter include opportunistic infection of the CNS due to immunosuppression, cerebrovascular diseases, primary and secondary CNS malignancies, and toxic/metabolic disorders that occur with AIDS. To date, the only other retrovirus that unequivocally causes neurologic illness in humans is HTLV-I, which results in a progressive myelopathy.[46,102,103]

REFERENCES

1. Adams RD and Victor M: Principles of Neurology, Ed 2. McGraw-Hill, New York, 1981, pp 475–506.
2. Akizuki S, Yoshida S, Seoguchi M, et al: The Neuropathy of Human T-Lymphotropic Virus Type-I-Associated Myelopathy. Roman GC, Vernant J-C, and Osame M (eds): HTLV-1 and the Nervous System. Alan R. Liss, New York, 1989, pp 253–260.
3. Aminoff MJ (ed): Neurology and General Medicine. Churchill Livingstone, New York, 1989, p 674.
4. Ancelle R, Bletry O, Baglin AG, Brun-Vezinet F, Rey MA, and Godeau P: Long incubation period for HIV-2 infection. Lancet 1:688–689, 1987.
5. Anders KH, Guerra W, Tomiyasu U, et al: The neuropathology of AIDS. UCLA experience and review. Am J Pathol 124:537–558, 1986.
6. Bates S, McKeever P, Masur H, et al: Myelopathy following intrathecal chemotherapy in a patient with extensive Burkitt's lymphoma and altered immune status. Am J Med 78:697–702, 1985.
7. Baumgartner JE, Rachlin JR, Beckstead JH, et al: Primary central nervous system lymphomas: Natural history and response to radiation therapy in 55 patients with acquired immunodeficiency syndrome. J Neurosurg 73:206–211, 1990.
8. Belec L, Martin PM, Georges-Courbot MC, et al: Dementia as the primary manifestation of HIV-2 infection in a Central African patient. Trans R Soc Trop Med Hyg 83:844–846, 1989.
9. Berger JR, Harris JO, Gregorios J, and Norenberg M: Cerebrovascular dis-

ease in AIDS: A case control study. AIDS 4:239–244, 1990.

10. Berger JR, Difini JA, Swercdloff MA, and Ayyar DR: HIV seropositivity in Guillain-Barré syndrome. Letter to the editor. Ann Neurol 22:393–394, 1987.

11. Berger JR and Levy JA: The human immunodeficiency virus type 1—the virus and its role in neurologic disease. Semin Neurol 12:1–9, 1992.

12. Berger JR, Kaszovitz B, Post MJD, and Dickinson G: Progressive multifocal leukoencephalopathy associated with human immunodeficiency virus infection: A review of the literature with a report of 16 cases. Ann Intern Med 107:78–87, 1987.

13. Berger JR, Moskowitz L, Fischl M, and Kelley RE: Neurologic disease as the presenting manifestation of acquired immunodeficiency syndrome. South Med J 80:683–686, 1987.

14. Berger JR and Mucke L: Prolonged survival and partial recovery in AIDS-associated progressive multifocal leukoencephalopathy. Neurology 38:1060–1065, 1988.

15. Berger JR, Raffanti S, Svenningsson A, McCarthy M, Snodgrass S, and Resnick L: The role of HTLV-I in HIV-I neurologic disease. Neurology 41:197–201, 1991.

16. Berger JR, Sheremata WA, Resnick L, Atherton S, Fletcher MA, and Norenberg M: Multiple sclerosis-like illness occurring with human immunodeficiency virus infection. Neurology 39:324–328, 1989.

17. Berger JR, Svenningsson A, Raffanti S, and Resnick L: Tropical spastic paraparesis-like illness occurring in a patient dually infected with HIV-1 and HTLV-II. Neurology 41:85–87, 1991.

18. Bia FJ and Barry M: Parasitic infections of the central nervous system. Neurol Clin 4:171–206, 1986.

19. Bishburg E, Sunderam G, Reichman LB, and Kapila R: Central nervous system tuberculosis with the acquired immunodeficiency syndrome and its related complex. Ann Intern Med 105:210–213, 1986.

20. Bredesen DE, Levy RM, and Rosen- blum ML: Clinical manifestations of HIV infection: Neurologic aspects. In Cohen PT, Sande MA, and Volberding P (eds): San Francisco General Hospital AIDS Knowledgebase (computer database). Mass Med Soc, Waltham, MA, 1988.

21. Bredesen DE and Messing R: Neurological syndromes heralding the acquired immune deficiency syndrome (abstr). Ann Neurol 14:141, 1983.

22. Brenneman DE, Westbrook GL, Fitzgerald SP, et al: Neuronal cell killing by the envelope protein of HIV and its prevention by vasoactive intestinal peptide. Nature 335:639–642, 1988.

23. Britton CB, Mesa-Tejada R, Fenoglio CM, Hays AP, Garvey GG, and Miller JR: A new complication of AIDS therapy: Thoracic myelitis caused by herpes simplex virus. Neurology 35:1071–1074, 1985.

24. Brun-Vezinet F, Katlama C, Roulot D, et al: Lymphadenopathy-associated virus type 2 in AIDS and AIDS-related complex. Lancet 1:128–132, 1987.

25. Calabrese LH, Proffitt MR, Levin KH, Yen-Lieberman B, and Starkey C: Acute infection with human immunodeficiency virus (HIV) associated with acute brachial neuritis and exanthematous rash. Ann Intern Med 107:849–851, 1987.

26. Carne CA, Smith A, Elkington SG, et al: Acute encephalopathy coincident with seroconversion for anti–HTLV-III. Lancet 2:1206–1208, 1985.

27. Centers for Disease Control: The second 100,000 cases of acquired immunodeficiency syndrome—United States. MMWR 41:28–29, 1991.

28. Chan JC, Moskowitz LB, Olivella J, Hensley GT, Greenman RL, and Hoffman TA: Toxoplasma encephalitis in recent Haitian entrants. South Med J 76:1211–1215, 1983.

29. Cheng-Mayer C and Levy JA: Distinct biologic and serologic properties of HIV isolates from the brain. Ann Neurol (Suppl) 23:S58–S61, 1987.

30. Clavel F, Guetard D, Brun-Vezinet F, et al: Isolation of a new human retrovirus from West African patients with AIDS. Science 233:343–346, 1986.

31. Clavel F, Mansinho K, Chamaret S, et al: Human immunodeficiency virus type 2 infection associated with AIDS in West Africa. N Engl J Med 316:1180–1185, 1986.

32. Cole EL, Meisler DM, Calabrese LH, et al: Herpes zoster ophthalmicus and acquired immune deficiency syndrome. Arch Ophthalmol 102:1027–1029, 1984.

33. Cooper DA, Maclean P, Finlayson R, et al: Acute AIDS retrovirus infection. Lancet 1:537–540, 1985.

34. Cornblath DR, McArthur JC, and Griffin JW: The spectrum of peripheral neuropathies in HTLV-III infection (abstr). Muscle Nerve 9:76, 1986.

35. Cornblath DR, McArthur JC, Kennedy PG, et al: Inflammatory demyelinating peripheral neuropathies associated with human T-cell lymphotropic virus type III infection. Ann Neurol 21:32–40, 1987.

36. Craddock C, Bull R, and Pasvol G: Cardiorespiratory arrest and autonomic neuropathy in AIDS. Lancet 2:16, 1987.

37. Crawfurd EJP, Baird PRE, and Clark AL: Cauda equina and lumbar nerve root compression in patients with AIDS. J Bone Joint Surg [Br] 69:36–37, 1987.

38. Denning DW, Anderson J, Rudge P, and Smith H: Acute myelopathy associated with primary infection with human immunodeficiency virus. Br Med J 294:143–144, 1987.

39. deThe G: HTLV-1 and chronic progressive encephalomyelopathies: An immunolovirological perspective. In Roman GC, Vernant J-C, and Osame M: (eds): HTLV-1 and the Nervous System. Alan R. Liss, New York, 1989, pp 3–8.

40. Doll DC, Yarbro JW, Philips K, and Klott C: Mycobacterial spinal cord abscess with an ascending polyneuropathy (letter). Ann Intern Med 106:333–334, 1987.

41. Eidelberg D, Sotrel A, Vogel H, et al: Progressive polyradiculopathy in acquired immune deficiency syndrome. Neurology 36:912, 1986.

42. Engstrom JW, Lowenstein DH, and Bredesen DE: Cerebral infarctions and transient neurological deficits associated with AIDS. Am J Med 86:528–532, 1989.

43. Epstein LG, Kinken C, Blumberg VM, et al: HIV-1 V3 domain variation in brain and spleen of children with AIDS: Tissue specific evolution within host-determined quasispecies. Virology 180:583–590, 1991.

44. Everall IP, Luthert PJ, and Lantos PL: Neuronal loss in the frontal cortex in HIV infection. Lancet 337:1119–1121, 1991.

45. Fischl MA, Pitchenik AE, and Spira TJ: Tuberculosis brain abscess and toxoplasma encephalitis in a patient with the acquired immunodeficiency syndrome. JAMA 253:3428–3430, 1985.

46. Gessian A, Barin F, Vernant JC, et al: Antibodies to human T-lymphotropic virus type I patients with tropical spastic paraparesis. Lancet 2:407–411, 1985.

47. Graham SH, Bredesen DE: Neurologic complication of herpes zoster in patients with HIV infection. Neurology (in press).

48. Grant I, Atkinson JH, Hesselink JR, et al: Evidence for early central nervous system involvement in the acquired immunodeficiency syndrome (AIDS) and other human immunodeficiency virus (HIV) infections. Ann Intern Med 107:828–836, 1987.

49. Giulian D, Vaca K, and Noonan CA: Secretion of neurotoxins by mononuclear phagocytes infected with HIV-1. Science 250:1593–1596, 1990.

50. Gurney ME, Apatoff BR, Spear GT, et al: Neuroleukin: A lymphokine product of lectin-stimulated T-cells. Science 234:574–581, 1986.

51. Gurney ME, Heinrich SP, Lee MR, and Yin HS: Molecular cloning and expression of neuroleukin, a neurotrophic factor for spinal and sensory neurons. Science 234:566–574, 1986.

52. Gyorkey F, Melnick JL, and Gyorkey P: HIV in brain biopsies of patients with AIDS and progressive encephalopathy. J Infect Dis 155:870–876, 1987.

53. Handler M, Ho KV, Whelan M, and Budzilovich G: Intracerebral toxoplasmosis in patients with acquired immune deficiency syndrome. J Neurosurg 59:994–1001, 1983.

54. Hausen A, Fuchs D, Reibnegger G, et al: Immunosuppressants in the treatment of patients with AIDS. Lancet 2:214, 1987.

55. Hawkins C, Gold JM, Whimbey E, et al: *Mycobacterium avium* complex infections in patient with acquired immunodeficiency syndrome. Ann Intern Med 105:184–188, 1986.

56. Heyes MP, Brew BJ, Martin A, et al: Quinolinic acid in cerebrospinal fluid and serum in HIV-1 infection: Relationship to clinical and neurological status. Ann Neurol 29:202–209, 1991.

57. Ho DD, Rota TR, Schooley RT, et al: Isolation of HTLV-III from cerebrospinal fluid and neural tissues of patients with neurologic syndromes related to the acquired immunodeficiency syndrome. N Engl J Med 313:1493–1497, 1985.

58. Hollander H, Bolden J, Mendelson T, and Cortland D: Extrapyramidal symptoms in AIDS patients given low-dose metoclopramide or chlorpramazine (letter). Lancet 2:1186, 1985.

59. Hollander H and Stringari S: Human immunodeficiency virus-associated meningitis. Am J Med 83:813–816, 1987.

60. Iwasaki Y: Pathology of chronic myelopathy associated with HTLV-1 infection (HAM/TSP). J Neurol Sci 96:103–123, 1990.

61. Janssen RS, Saykin AJ, Kaplan JE, et al: Neurological complications of human immunodeficiency virus infection in patients with lymphadenopathy syndrome. Ann Neurol 23(1):49–55, 1988.

62. Johnson RT, McArthur JC, and Narayan O: The neurology of human immunodeficiency virus infections. FASEB J 2:2970–2981, 1988.

63. Joint Committee for Stroke Facilities: I: Epidemiology for stroke facilities planning. Stroke 3:359–371, 1972.

64. Jordan BD, Navia BA, Petito C, Cho E-S, and Price RW: Neurological syndromes complicating AIDS. Front Radiat Ther Oncol 19:82–87, 1985.

65. Katz D and Berger JR. Neurosyphilis in AIDS. Arch Neurol 46:895–901, 1989.

66. Kelly WM and Brant-Zawadzki M: Acquired immunodeficiency syndrome: Neuroradiologic findings. Radiology 149:485–491, 1983.

67. Klemm E, Schneweis KE, Horn R, Tackmann W, Schulze G, and Schneider J: HIV-II infection with initial neurological manifestation. J Neurol 235:304–307, 1988.

68. Koenig S, Gendelman HE, Orenstein JM, et al: Detection of AIDS virus in macrophages in brain tissue from AIDS patients with encephalopathy. Science 233:1089–1093, 1986.

69. Komar J, Szalay M, and Dalos M: Acute retention of urine due to isolated sacral myeloradiculitis. J Neurol 228:215, 1982.

70. Koppel BS, Wormser GP, Tuchma AJ, Maayan S, Hewlett D Jr, and Daras M: Central nervous system involvement in patients with acquired immune deficiency syndrome (AIDS). Acta Neurol Scand 71:337–351, 1985.

71. Koyanagi Y, Miles S, Mitsuyasu TY, Merrill JE, Vinters HV, and Chen ISY: Dual infection of the central nervous system by AIDS viruses with distinct cellular tropisms. Science 236:819–822, 1987.

72. Kumar M, Resnick L, Lowenstein DA, Berger J, and Eisdorfer C: Brain-reactive antibodies and the AIDS dementia complex. J Acquir Immune Defic Syndr 2:469–471, 1989.

73. Levy JA, Shimabukuro J, Hollander H, Mills J, and Kaminsky L: Isolation of AIDS associated retroviruses from cerebrospinal fluid and brain of patients with neurological symptoms. Lancet 2:586–588, 1985.

74. Levy RM and Bredesen DE: Central nervous system dysfunction in acquired immunodeficiency syndrome. In Rosenblum ML, Levy RM, and Bredesen DE (eds): AIDS and the Nervous System. Raven Press, New York, 1988, pp 29–63.

75. Levy RM and Bredesen DE: Central nervous system dysfunction in acquired immunodeficiency syndrome. J Acquir Immune Defic Syndr 1:41–61, 1988.
76. Levy RM, Bredesen DE, and Rosenblum ML: Neurological manifestations of the acquired immunodeficiency syndrome (AIDS): Experience at UCSF and review of the literature. J Neurosurg 62:475–495, 1985.
77. Levy RM, Janssen RS, Bush RJ, et al: Neuroepidemiology of acquired immunodeficiency syndrome. J Acquir Immune Defic Syndr 1:31–40, 1988.
78. Levy RM, Mills C, Posin J, Moore S, Rosenblum M, and Bredesen D: The superiority of MR to CT in the detection of intracranial pathology in the acquired immunodeficiency syndrome (AIDS). Second International Conference on AIDS, Paris, France, 1986.
79. Levy RM, Pons VG, and Rosenblum ML: Central nervous system mass lesions in the acquired immunodeficiency syndrome (AIDS). J Neurosurg 61:9–16, 1984.
80. Levy RM, Rosenblum S, and Perrett LV: Neuroradiological findings in the acquired immunodeficiency syndrome (AIDS): A review of 200 cases. AJNR 7:833–839, 1986.
81. Lipkin WI, Parry G, Kiprov DD, and Abrams D: Inflammatory neuropathy in homosexual men with lymphadenopathy. Neurology 35:1479–1483, 1985.
82. Lipton SA: Calcium channel antagonists and human immunodeficiency virus coat protein-mediated neuronal injury. Ann Neurol 30:110–114, 1991.
83. Luft BJ, Conley F, and Remington JS: Outbreak of central-nervous-system toxoplasmosis in Western Europe and North America. Lancet 1:781–783, 1983.
84. Marshall DW, Brey RL, Cahill WT, Houk RW, Zajak RA, and Boswell RN: Spectrum of cerebrospinal fluid findings in various stages of human immunodeficiency virus infection. Arch Neurol 45:954–958, 1988.
85. Martin CM, Matlow AG, Chew E, Sutton D, and Pruzanski W: Hyperviscosity syndrome in a patient with acquired immunodeficiency syndrome. Arch Intern Med 149:1435–1436, 1989.
86. Matsuo H, Nakamura T, Tsujihata M, et al: Plasmapheresis (plasma-modulation) in patients with HTLV-1-associated myelopathy. In Roman GC, Vernant J-C, and Osame M (eds): HTLV-1 and the Nervous System. Alan R. Liss, New York, 1989, pp 343–349.
87. McArthur JC: Neurologic manifestations of AIDS. Medicine (Baltimore) 66(6):407–437, 1987.
88. McArthur JC, Griffin JW, Cornblath DR, and Farzadegan H: Progressive HTLV-1-associated myeloneuropathy in a patient with HIV-1 (abstract). Neurology (Suppl 1) 39:419, 1989.
89. Mettinger KL, Soderstrom CE, and Allander E: Epidemiology of acute cerebrovascular disease before the age of 55 in the Stockholm County, 1973–1977: I. Incidence and mortality rates. Stroke 15:795–801, 1984.
90. Meyenhofer MF, Epstein LG, Cho E-K, and Sharer LR: Ultrastructural morphology and intracellular production of human immunodeficiency virus (HIV) in brain. J Neuropathol Exp Neurol 46:474–484, 1987.
91. Miller RF and Semple SJG: Autonomic neuropathy in AIDS (letter). Lancet 2:343, 1987.
92. Miller RG, Kiprov DD, Parry G, and Bredesen DE: Peripheral nervous system dysfunction in acquired immunodeficiency syndrome. In Rosenblum ML, Levy RM, and Bredesen DE (eds): AIDS and the Nervous System. Raven Press, New York, 1988, p 65.
93. Miller RG, Parry GJ, Lang W, et al: AIDS-related inflammatory polyradiculopathy: Prediction of response to plasma exchange with electrophysiologic testing (abstr). Muscle Nerve 8:626, 1985.
94. Mishra BB, Sommers W, Koski CK, and Greenstein JI: Acute inflammatory demyelinating polyneuropathy in the acquired immune deficiency syn-

drome (abstr). Ann Neurol 18:131, 1985.

95. Mizusawa H, Hirano A, Llena JF, and Shintaku M: Cerebrovascular lesions in acquired immune deficiency syndrome (AIDS). Acta Neuropathol 76:451–457, 1988.

96. Morgello S, Cho E-S, Nielsen S, et al: Cytomegalovirus encephalitis in patients with acquired immunodeficiency syndrome: An autopsy study of 30 cases and a review of the literature. Hum Pathol 18:289–297, 1987.

97. Moskowitz LB, Hensley GT, Chan JC, Gregorios J, and Conley FK: The neuropathology of acquired immune deficiency syndrome. Arch Pathol Lab Med 108:867–872, 1984.

98. Navia BA, Cho E-S, Petito CK, et al: The AIDS dementia complex: II. Neuropathology. Ann Neurol 19:525–535, 1986.

99. Navia BA, Jordan BD, and Price RW: The AIDS dementia complex: I. Clinical features. Ann Neurol 19:517–524, 1986.

100. Navia BA, Petito CK, Gold JW, et al: Cerebral toxoplasmosis complicating the acquired immune deficiency syndrome: Clinical and neuropathological findings in 27 patients. Ann Neurol 19:224–238, 1986.

101. Navia BA and Price RW: The acquired immunodeficiency dementia complex as the presenting or sole manifestation of human immunodeficiency virus infection. Arch Neurol 44:65–69, 1987.

102. Osame M, Matsumoto M, Usuku K, et al: Chronic progressive myelopathy associated with elevated antibodies to human T-lymphotropic virus type I and adult T-cell leukemialike cells. Ann Neurol 21:117–122, 1987.

103. Osame M, Usuku K, Izumo S, et al: HTLV-1 associated myelopathy, a new clinical entity. Lancet 1:1031–1032, 1986.

104. Pert CB, Hill JM, Ruff MR, et al: Octapeptides deduced from the neuropeptide receptor-like pattern of antigen T4 in brain potently inhibit human immunodeficiency virus receptor binding and T cell infectivity. Proc

Natl Acad Sci USA 23:9254–9258, 1986.

105. Pert CB, Smith CC, Ruff MR, and Hill JM: AIDS and its dementia as a neuropeptide disorder: Role of VIP receptor blockade by human immunodeficiency virus envelope. Ann Neurol (Suppl) 23:S71–S73, 1988.

106. Petito CK, Navia BA, Eun-Sook C, Jordan BD, George DC, and Price RW: Vacuolar myelopathy pathologically resembling subacute combined degeneration in patients with the acquired immunodeficiency syndrome. N Engl J Med 312:874–879, 1985.

107. Price RW, Brew B, Sidtis J, Rosenblum M, Scheck AC, and Clearly P: The brain in AIDS: Central nervous system HIV-1 infection and AIDS dementia complex. Science 239:586–591, 1988.

108. Price RW, Sidtis JJ, Bradford AN, et al: The AIDS dementia complex. In Rosenblum ML, Levy RM, and Bredesen DE (eds): AIDS and the Nervous System. Raven Press, New York, 1988, pp 203–219.

109. Pons VG, Jacobs RA, and Hollander H: Nonviral infections of the central nervous system in patients with acquired immunodeficiency syndrome. In Rosenblum ML, Levy RM, and Bredesen DE (eds): AIDS and the Nervous System. Raven Press, New York, 1988, pp 263–382.

110. Post MJD, Hensley GT, Sheldon JJ, et al: CNS disease in AIDS: A CT-MR pathologic correlation. Radiology 153:55–56, 1984.

111. Post MJD, Dursunoglu SJ, Hensley GT, Chan JC, Moskowitz LB, and Hoffman TA: Cranial CT in acquired immunodeficiency syndrome: Spectrum of diseases and optimal contrast enhancement technique. AJNR 145:929–940, 1985.

112. Post JD, Sheldon JJ, Hensley GT, et al: Central nervous system disease in acquired immunodeficiency syndrome: Prospective correlation using CT, MR imaging, and pathologic studies. Radiology 158:141–148, 1986.

113. Pulliam L, Herndier BG, Tang NM, and McGrath MS: Human immunodefi-

ciency virus infected macrophages produce soluble factors that cause histological and neurochemical alteration in cultured human brains. J Clin Invest 87:503–512, 1991.

114. Pumarola-Sune T, Navia BA, Cordon-Cardo C, Cho E-S, and Price RW: HIV antigen in the brains of patients with AIDS dementia complex. Ann Neurol 21:490–496, 1987.

115. Resnick L, Berger JR, Shapshak P, and Tourtellotte WW: Early penetration of the blood-brain-barrier by HIV. Neurology 38:9–14, 1988.

116. Resnick L, DiMarzo-Veronese F, Schupbach J, et al: Intra-blood-brain-barrier synthesis of HRLC-III-specific IgG in patients with neurologic symptoms associated with AIDS or AIDS-related complex. N Engl J Med 313:1498–1504, 1985.

117. Sabatier JM, Vives E, Mabrouk K, et al: Evidence for neurotoxic activity of tat from human immunodeficiency virus type 1. J Virol 65:961–967, 1991.

118. Sharer LR, Cho ES, and Epstein LG: Multinucleated giant cells and HTLV-III in AIDS encephalopathy. Hum Pathol 16:760, 1985.

119. Sharer LR, Epstein LG, Cho ES, and Petito C: Pathological features of AIDS encephalopathy in children: Evidence of LAV/HIV infection of brain. Hum Pathol 17:271–284, 1986.

120. Sharer LR and Kapila R: Neuropathologic observations in acquired immune deficiency syndrome (AIDS). Acta Neuropathol (Berl) 66:188–198, 1985.

121. Shaw GM, Harper ME, Hahn BH, et al: HTLV-III infection in brains of children and adults with AIDS encephalopathy. Science 227:177–182, 1985.

122. Snider WD, Simpson DM, Nielsen S, Gold JWM, Metroka CE, and Posner JB: Neurological complications of acquired immune deficiency syndrome: Analysis of 50 patients. Ann Neurol 14:403–418, 1983.

123. So YT, Beckstead JH, and Davis RL: Primary central nervous system lymphoma in acquired immune deficiency syndrome. A clinical and pathologic study. Ann Neurol 20:566–572, 1986.

124. Stoler MH, Eskin TA, Benn S, Angerer RC, and Angerer LM: Human T-cell lymphotropic virus type III infection of the CNS. JAMA 256:2360–2364, 1986.

125. Stricker RB, Abrams DI, Corash L, and Shuman MA: Target platelet antigen in homosexual men with immune thrombocytopenia. N Engl J Med 313:1375–1380, 1985.

126. Sugar AM and Saunders C: Oral fluconazole as suppressive therapy of disseminated cryptococcosis in patients with acquired immunodeficiency syndrome. Am J Med 85:481–489, 1988.

127. Tross S, Price RW, Navia B, et al: Neuropsychological characteristics of the AIDS dementia complex: A preliminary report. AIDS 2:81–88, 1988.

128. Tucker T, Dix RD, Katzen C, Davis RL, and Schmidley JW: Cytomegalovirus and herpes simplex virus ascending myelitis in a patient with acquired immune deficiency syndrome. Ann Neurol 18:74–79, 1985.

129. Urmacher C and Nielsen S: The histopathology of the acquired immune deficiency syndrome. Pathol Annu 20:197–220, 1985.

130. Yarchoan R, Brouwers P, Spitzer AR, et al: Response of human-immunodeficiency-virus-associated neurological disease to 3′-azido-3′-deoxythymidine. Lancet 1:132, 1987.

131. Vernant JC, Maurs L, Gessain A, et al: Endemic tropical spastic paraparesis associated with human T-lymphotropic virus type I. A clinical and seroepidemiological study of 25 cases. Ann Neurol 21:123–130, 1987.

132. Vinters HV, Tomiyasu U, and Anders KH: Neuropathologic complications of infection with the human immunodeficiency virus. Prog AIDS Pathol 1:101–130, 1989.

133. Weill O, Finaud M, Bille F, et al: Gliome malin medullaire: Une nouvelle complication de l'infection par le HIV? (letter) Presse Med 16:1977, 1987.

134. Wolinsky S: Personal communication, June 1991.

135. Wong B, Gold JWM, Brown AE, et al: Central nervous system toxoplasmosis in homosexual men and parenteral drug abusers. Ann Intern Med 100:36–42, 1984.

136. Woolsey RM, Chambers TJ, Chung HK, and McGarry JD: Mycobacterial meningomyelitis associated with human immunodeficiency virus infection. Arch Neurol 45:691–693, 1988.

Chapter 4

HERPESVIRUS INFECTIONS OF THE CENTRAL NERVOUS SYSTEM

Donald H. Gilden, M.D.

HERPES SIMPLEX VIRUS TYPE 1
(HSV-1) ENCEPHALITIS
HERPES SIMPLEX VIRUS TYPE 2
(HSV-2)
VARICELLA-ZOSTER VIRUS (VZV)
CYTOMEGALOVIRUS (CMV)
EPSTEIN-BARR VIRUS (EBV)
HUMAN HERPESVIRUS 6 (HHV-6)

Herpesviruses are large, double-stranded deoxyribonucleic acid (DNA) viruses that share characteristics of cytopathology in vitro, replicative cycles, and the capacity to become latent.[46,84,85] More than 80 animal species harbor herpesviruses. There are six known human herpesviruses: herpes simplex virus (HSV) types 1 and 2, varicella-zoster virus (VZV), cytomegalovirus (CMV), Epstein-Barr virus (EBV), and human herpesvirus 6 (HHV-6). Reactivation from the latent state is an important cause of morbidity and mortality from these viruses. Furthermore, whereas HSV-1 and EBV encephalitis occur in immunocompetent individuals, HSV-2, VZV, and CMV encephalitis are complications of the immunocompromised patient. These and other important clinical features are summarized at the end of this chapter.

HERPES SIMPLEX VIRUS TYPE 1 (HSV-1) ENCEPHALITIS

Clinical Features

The symptoms and signs of HSV encephalitis are a consequence of virus replication and accompanying inflammation in the cerebrum. The predilection of HSV to propagate in the medial temporal lobe and orbital surface of the frontal lobe produces the characteristic clinical picture.[45] Patients develop fever, headache, irritability, and lethargy as well as confusion, seizures (major motor, complex partial, focal, and even absence attacks), aphasia (when the dominant temporal lobe is involved), and focal motor or sensory deficit. Furthermore, extensive hemorrhagic necrosis and temporal lobe edema may progress to uncal herniation, producing symptoms and signs indistinguishable from herniation due to tumor.[4] Because HSV becomes latent and periodically reactivates to produce recurrent herpes labialis, there is the misconception that HSV encephalitis is usually protracted or chronic. Although survivors of HSV encephalitis may have a permanent seizure disorder, mental changes, aphasia, or motor deficit, the onset of neurologic disease is, as in other viral encephalitides, usually acute or subacute, and early treatment is crucial to a favorable outcome. As discussed later, the mortality in untreated cases was 60% to 70% before the use of acyclovir.[112]

Laboratory Tests

Of all the viral encephalitides, HSV encephalitis is most amenable to diagnosis by laboratory tests. Cerebrospinal fluid (CSF) examination, electroencephalography (EEG), brain imaging, and biopsy all have a role in diagnosis and should be performed as soon as HSV encephalitis is suspected.

CEREBROSPINAL FLUID EXAMINATION

The CSF is usually abnormal in patients with HSV encephalitis. CSF opening pressure may be normal or may be very high if there is brain swell-

ing and impending temporal lobe herniation. The examination is usually performed in the first few days of illness, before significant brain swelling has occurred, so that concern over potential herniation after lumbar puncture in HSV encephalitis is lessened; furthermore, EEG and imaging studies may demonstrate features highly suggestive of HSV encephalitis, often obviating subsequent lumbar punctures. Approximately 90% of patients have CSF pleocytosis, although its absence does not rule out HSV encephalitis.[115] Cells in CSF range from 4 to 755/mm³, and more than 100 to 200 cells may be present weeks after the onset of disease.[69] The predominant cell type is mononuclear. In contrast to other viral encephalitides, HSV encephalitis may be characterized by red blood cells (RBC) in the CSF and xanthochromia, presumably reflecting the hemorrhagic nature of brain lesions. Instead of attributing the presence of RBCs in CSF to a "bloody tap," the astute clinician may use their occurrence to support the

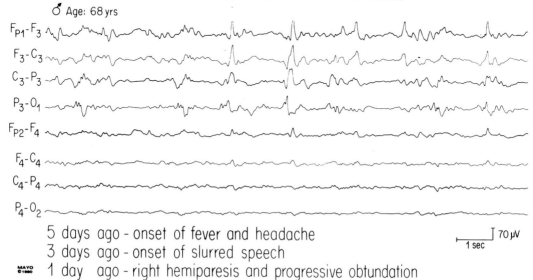

Figure 4–1. HSV encephalitis. EEG shows focal left hemispheric periodic sharp waves. (Reproduced with permission from Electroencephalography, 2nd Edition, edited by Ernst Niedermeyer and F. H. Lopes da Silva, 1987, Urban & Schwarzenberg, Baltimore-Munich.)

presumptive diagnosis of HSV encephalitis.

The CSF protein and immunoglobulin G (IgG) index are elevated in the majority of cases.[107] Increased levels of antibody to HSV, suggestive of recent infection, may be found in serum and CSF, but because increased antibody titers usually are not detected until 2 or more weeks after the onset of disease,[65] their practical value lies more in retrospective presumptive diagnosis than in the identification of acute encephalitis. Rarely, hypoglycorrhachia occurs.

Although HSV often can be isolated from cerebral biopsy or even autopsy material, the isolation of HSV from CSF during acute disease is exceptional. The reason for this is not known.

ELECTROENCEPHALOGRAM

Early in the disease, the EEG shows background disorganization with generalized or focal slowing, predominantly over the involved temporal region.[111] Within days, widespread, periodic, stereotyped complexes of sharp and slow waves develop, usually at regular intervals of 2 to 3 seconds.[96] Periodic complexes are seen when either side of the brain is involved (Fig. 4–1). Although these features may be seen in other CNS disorders (tumor, abscess, syphilis, infarct), their presence in the clinical setting of fever and rapidly progressive neurologic disease provides strong presumptive evidence for HSV encephalitis.

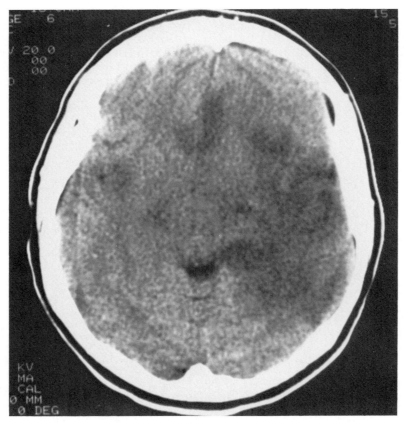

Figure 4–2. HSV encephalitis. CT scan of brain without contrast enhancement shows marked hypointensity in the left temporal lobe and areas of low absorption in the left frontal lobe and right temporal lobe. (Courtesy of Dr. Robert Grossman, Department of Radiology, The University of Pennsylvania School of Medicine, Philadelphia.)

IMAGING STUDIES

Computed tomography (CT) scanning shows hypodense lesions (Fig. 4–2) involving the medial temporal regions.[18] An important diagnostic clue is a sharp transition from the hypodense temporal lesion to the lateral basal ganglia.[120] Edema and mass effect occur in 80% of cases, and contrast enhancement (Fig. 4–3) is seen in more than 50%.[110]

Magnetic resonance imaging (MRI) reveals a decrease in T_1 and increase in T_2 signal (Fig. 4–4), and the signal abnormality includes a larger area of brain than is usually seen by CT scanning. In contrast to CT scanning, MRI of the temporal lobes is not subject to artifact from the petrous and sphenoid bones, which often obscures the temporal fossa.[103] A comparison of CT and MRI in four cases of HSV encephalitis showed that temporal lobe inflammation was obvious on MRI days before CT showed any changes.[91]

PATHOLOGIC AND VIROLOGIC STUDIES

A specific diagnosis of HSV encephalitis can be made by combined pathologic and virologic examination of tissue obtained by biopsy or at autopsy.

Pathologic changes are characterized by hemorrhagic necrotizing lesions and edema usually restricted to the medial temporal and orbital frontal region (Fig. 4–5; see color insert). Microscopically, inflammatory infiltrates are found in both meninges and cerebral paren-

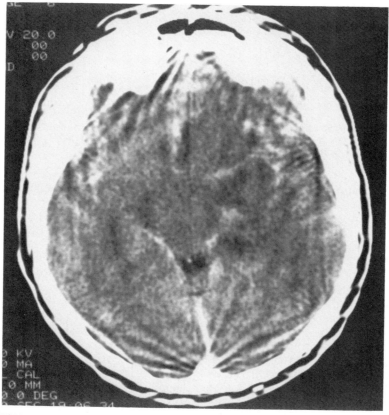

Figure 4–3. HSV encephalitis. Despite motion artifact, the CT brain scan performed with contrast medium shows enhancement in the left temporal lobe. (Courtesy of Dr. Robert Grossman, Department of Radiology, The University of Pennsylvania School of Medicine, Philadelphia.)

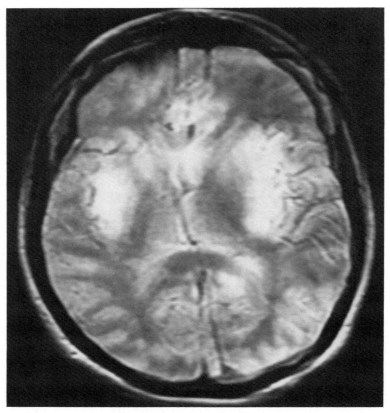

Figure 4–4. Superiority of brain MRI to CT scanning in diagnosis of HSV encephalitis. Compared with CT scans in Figures 4–2 and 4–3, this image produced by T_2-weighted MRI shows unequivocal involvement of both temporal lobes that does not extend beyond the insular cortex. Note also the involvement in the area of the cingulate gyrus. (Courtesy of Dr. Robert Grossman, Department of Radiology, The University of Pennsylvania School of Medicine, Philadelphia.)

chyma. The presence of Cowdry A intranuclear inclusions (Fig. 4–6; see color insert) is an important diagnostic feature for the neuropathologist. Although these inclusions may be found in encephalitis caused by any human herpesvirus, the Cowdry A inclusions in CMV encephalitis are usually larger and more "owl-eyed." Cowdry A inclusions also may be seen in subacute sclerosing panencephalitis (SSPE) produced by measles virus, but the clinical and radiologic features of SSPE are distinguished easily from those of HSV encephalitis.

Expression of HSV-specific proteins can be detected in infected brain by immunochemical staining. Immunofluo-rescent or immunoperoxidase staining can be applied either to brain biopsy impression smears (Fig. 4–7; see color insert) or to brain sections prepared from tissue (Fig. 4–8; see color insert) obtained by biopsy or at autopsy.

HSV can be isolated from infected brain by either of two techniques:

1. Explantation. In this procedure, brain tissue is finely minced and cells are allowed to attach to a petri dish or tissue culture flask. Within days to weeks, a cytopathic effect (CPE) characteristic for herpesviruses may develop. The virus isolate can then be typed using antisera specific for the different herpesviruses.

2. Cocultivation. In this case,

minced brain tissue is mixed (cocultivated) with indicator cells, usually fibroblasts or kidney cells, known to support HSV replication. Development of CPE in the indicator cell line is followed by typing of the specific herpesvirus.

The value of brain biopsy to corroborate the clinical diagnosis by pathologic and virologic analysis cannot be underestimated. Although biopsy is recommended to verify the diagnosis, it should not be performed unless expert neuropathologic and virologic studies can be applied to brain tissue. The effect of newer antiviral drugs can be determined only in biopsy-proven cases. Brain biopsies were essential to demonstrate lack of efficacy of the halogenated pyrimidines (idoxuridine [IUDR] and bromodeoxyuridine [BUDR]) and of cytosine arabinoside (Ara-C) in the treatment of HSV encephalitis. Finally, the argument that a specific diagnosis can be made by CSF antibody index must be weighed against the time elapsed before antibody develops in serum and CSF and testing is carried out. Polymerase chain reaction (PCR) technology has successfully detected HSV DNA in the CSF of patients with HSV encephalitis.[86] Use of PCR to expedite diagnosis could potentially obviate brain biopsy, although it is unlikely that an "HSV-DNA PCR-negative CSF" would definitely rule out HSV encephalitis.

Treatment with acyclovir 1 to 2 days before brain biopsy does not compromise the detection of pathologic changes of HSV encephalitis or the virologic detection of HSV antigen in diseased tissue. It is recommended that acyclovir treatment can and should be started immediately when the clinical features, CSF, EEG, and imaging studies suggest the diagnosis of HSV encephalitis; at the same time, brain biopsy can be scheduled within the next 1 to 2 days to substantiate the diagnosis. The incidence of complications with brain biopsy ranges from 0% to 3%,[113,114] and biopsy can miss diseased tissue.

Differential Diagnosis

The clinical features of HSV encephalitis can be mimicked by other viral and bacterial infections, cerebral abscess, tumor, and stroke. A focal area of decreased density and increased vascularity extending into subcortical areas is consistent with the cerebritis that heralds frank abscess formation[119] and helps to distinguish evolving abscess from HSV encephalitis. Ring-enhancing lesions characteristic of cerebral abscess are not seen in the first few days of illness. Glioma and infarct are not likely to be associated with fever or to be restricted to the medial temporal lobe on CT scan.

Treatment

Before acyclovir, the mortality in pathologically verified, untreated HSV encephalitis was approximately 60% to 70%. The use of acyclovir, 30 mg/kg per day for 10 days, has reduced the mortality to slightly under 30%.[112] Early treatment (before coma ensues) is associated with a more favorable outcome. Acyclovir appears to be safe. Mild hematologic, hepatic, and renal function abnormalities have been reported, and relapses after acyclovir therapy have been documented.[11,50]

Steroids and osmotic agents also may be used to control brain swelling. The benefits of a short course of steroids in instances of cerebral edema and impending herniation outweigh the small risk of potentiating HSV infection. Lastly, anticonvulsants are used to treat seizures. There are no controlled studies on the prophylactic use of steroids or anticonvulsants in HSV encephalitis.

Atypical HSV-1 Encephalitis

A clinical report of two patients with subacute encephalopathy in which HSV was isolated from brain tissue suggests that chronic encephalitis may be due to HSV,[87] but neither case was pathologically verified. Of particular interest is the description of a patient with HSV encephalitis who, after treatment with adenine arabinoside, developed recurrent encephalitis that was characterized histologically by perivenous demyelination.[51] This was the first pathologically verified case of HSV-associated postinfectious encephalomyelitis.

Pathogenesis and Latency

SPREAD OF VIRUS

In most individuals, HSV is acquired by exposure of skin or mucous membranes of the eye or mouth to the virus. The virus replicates locally and spreads along peripheral axons to ganglia where latency is established. Virus also has been shown to travel along peripheral nerves by infection of Schwann cells[44] and along autonomic nerves to superior cervical ganglia.[76] Virus is protected from the immune system during transport. After experimental infection, virus spreads not only to ganglia but also to the CNS for up to 2 weeks after infection.[101] Retrograde transport of virus from peripheral sites to the CNS in experimentally infected animals occurs in less than 1 week. Similarly, after trigeminal rhizotomy in humans, HSV is transported anterograde from ganglia back to skin within a few days. After experimental infection of skin on the face, HSV has also been shown to spread via olfactory pathways.[22] Although olfactory bulb necrosis has been observed in some patients dying of herpes encephalitis, it is not a uniform finding. Thus, while the restriction of human HSV-1 encephalitis to the medial temporal lobe and the orbital surface of the frontal lobe could reflect virus transport via olfactory pathways through the cribriform plate of the ethmoid bone into the anterior fossa, an alternative, but not necessarily mutually exclusive, explanation is that localized

temporal and frontal lobe encephalitis develops from herpesvirus that has reactivated from trigeminal ganglia and has then spread along trigeminal afferent fibers that innervate the basal meninges of the anterior and middle fossa.[10] Support for such a notion is provided by the facts that many patients with HSV-1 encephalitis have a past history of recurrent cold sores and that HSV-1 is latent in trigeminal ganglia.

In certain circumstances, HSV spread also may be blood-borne. Viremia is often detected in immunocompromised patients. Furthermore, after intravenous inoculation of HSV in experimentally infected animals, viremia is thought to result in the establishment of latency in multiple ganglia, the adrenal gland, and the CNS.[7]

LATENCY

The human herpesviruses, in particular the EBV, HSV, and VZV, have served as models for the study of latency and reactivation. Operationally, latency is characterized by virus-cell interactions in which viral DNA is maintained in infected cells and lytic replication of viral DNA rarely occurs. Virions are not visualized by electron microscopy, but virus can be rescued by explantation of latently infected cells or by cocultivation of latently infected cells with indicator cells. Virus gene expression during latency remains to be determined.

The first suggestion that HSV-1 might be latent in trigeminal ganglia came from the observation that trigeminal neurectomy was followed by HSV labialis.[9] Other trauma, including skin exposure to sun, dry ice, and coal tar, as well as x-irradiation, steroids, and immunosuppressive drugs all lead to virus reactivation. HSV-1 can be isolated readily from trigeminal and other cranial nerve ganglionic explants of normal adults at autopsy.[109] The mechanism of virus reactivation in vivo and in vitro is unknown.

Nucleic acid hybridization studies have revealed important differences among the human herpesviruses in the cell targeted for latency and the extent of viral gene expression, suggesting that the mechanism by which each herpesvirus is reactivated may be unique. In latently infected ganglia of humans and experimentally infected animals (mice, rabbits, and guinea pigs), HSV-1 is found exclusively in neurons.[82,102] The HSV DNA molecule is composed of a unique long and a unique short region each bounded by inverted repeat sequences. Thus, four isomeric forms of the HSV genome are predicted, and all four have been found during latency.[21] Restriction endonuclease analysis of HSV DNA isolated from latently infected humans and mice indicates submolar concentrations of end fragments relative to internal virus DNA fragments;[21,81] these "endless" HSV DNA molecules are thought to be the result of the ends of the virus genome being joined in circles or linear concatemers. Based on banding patterns in cesium chloride gradients, latent HSV DNA appears to be extrachromosomal.[63]

However, latent HSV DNA isolated from latently infected mouse trigeminal ganglia also has been shown by restriction endonuclease analysis to contain additional sequences at the termini of the virus genome, indicating site-specific integration of the virus genome into the host chromosomes.[77] Furthermore, latent HSV DNA is protected from digestion by micrococcal nuclease, which implies an association of virus DNA with nucleosomal structures.[13] These latter findings are more consistent with a model in which HSV DNA is integrated into specific sites within the chromosomes of latently infected ganglia. About 0.01 to 0.1 copy of the virus genome is present per cell in latently infected ganglia.[21]

Replication of HSV-1 is not essential for the establishment of latency.[99] Although mutants lacking the HSV-1 thymidine kinase (TK) gene establish latency in mouse trigeminal ganglia,[25] the frequency of virus reactivation in explant cultures is greatly reduced. The ability of HSV-1 to become latent in murine trigeminal ganglia independent of virus replication includes virus mutants deficient in the HSV-1 ribonucleotide reductase gene and the immediate early gene ICP4.[48]

Transcription of latent HSV-1 DNA has been demonstrated in humans,[30,100] rabbits,[82] and mice[97,108] and appears to be restricted to a set of nonpolyadenylated transcripts present at 10^4 to 10^5 molecules per infected neuron. Three major latency-associated transcripts (LATs) (2.0, 1.5, and 1.45 kilobases) have the same 5' end but different 3' termini, which result from alternative splicing.[53,82,97] Although the LATs contain several open reading frames, at least one of which is transcribed in vitro,[14] they may not be translated in vivo. In situ hybridization analysis of latently infected ganglia indicates that LATs are predominantly nuclear, and direct PCR-aided sequencing reveals multiple termination codons.[60] These features and the observation that LATs are less detectable during lytic infection in cell culture make their function obscure.

Mutant HSV-1 constructs that do not express LAT transcripts can establish and maintain latency, although the rate of reactivation is impaired.[92,98] If the LAT promotor region is maintained in the mutant HSV-1 genome, however, reactivation from latency approaches wild-type frequencies.[3,59,66] Thus the proposed action of the major LATs resides in the region about the promotor and extreme 5' end of the transcripts, a region shown to contain a binding site for the cyclic adenosine monophosphate (cAMP)–response element.[59]

Finally, a model of HSV-1 latency in vitro has been established. Primary sympathetic neuronal cultures have been maintained for more than 1 month after inoculation with HSV-1 by propagating cells in the presence of nerve growth factor (NGF).[116,117] During latency, virus cannot be detected, but within 24 hours of NGF deprivation, viral antigen is detected readily in neurons. Viral transcription in these latently infected neuronal cells in culture is restricted to LATs and appears to contain a LAT-encoded polypeptide.[14] This model system currently is being exploited not only to analyze the physical state of viral nucleic acid during latency but also to determine the factors that affect HSV-1 reactivation.

HERPES SIMPLEX VIRUS TYPE 2 (HSV-2)

HSV-2 is the causative agent of genital herpes. Two (possibly three) distinct neurologic conditions result from HSV-2 infection.

Aseptic Meningitis

The primary neurologic complication of HSV-2 is aseptic meningitis. In fact, HSV-2 accounts for about 5% of all cases of aseptic meningitis in the United States. In contrast to other viral meningitides that have a seasonal predilection, HSV-2 meningitis occurs any time of year. The typical clinical picture is characterized by headache, fever, stiff neck, and a CSF with a marked lymphocytic pleocytosis. Meningitis often is preceded by pain in the genital or pelvic region, and the astute clinician who suspects HSV-2 meningitis will ask about recent pelvic inflammatory disease (PID)–type symptoms or about penile or scrotal pain. Part of the workup for suspected HSV-2 meningitis is a careful external genital examination and pelvic examination for vesicular lesions in the vaginal vault or cervix. Unlike HSV-1, which usually cannot be isolated from the CSF of patients with encephalitis, HSV-2 can frequently be isolated from the CSF of patients with HSV-2 meningitis by adding fresh CSF to human or monkey indicator cells in tissue culture. Because HSV-2 meningitis is self-limited, treatment with acyclovir is not necessary.

Encephalitis

HSV-2 encephalitis is a rare disease, occurring most often in the newborn and rarely in the immunocompromised adult. In both age groups, HSV-2 causes diffuse CNS infection, whereas HSV-1 has a predilection for the medial temporal and orbital surface of the frontal lobes. Nevertheless, seizures, alterations in state of consciousness, and focal neurologic deficit (the common clinical features seen in HSV-1 encephalitis) also are characteristic of HSV-2 encephalitis. Today, HSV-2 encephalitis develops most commonly in patients with the acquired immunodeficiency syndrome (AIDS), frequently in association with CNS infection by other opportunistic agents, such as CMV.[73] HSV-2 encephalitis should be treated with acyclovir, 15 to 30 mg/kg per day.

HSV Neuropathy (Zosteriform Eruptions)

There are numerous reports of dermatomal distribution pain and sensory loss in association with zosteriform eruption. The syndrome usually is characterized by a prodrome of diffuse neuralgia, often with malaise and fever, followed within a few days by vesicular eruption.[54] Most reports describe lesions on the face in one or more areas served by the trigeminal nerve. Zosteriform eruptions due to HSV have also been described on the trunk, extremities, and genitalia.[95] Not surprisingly, episodes of dermatomal neuralgic pain and zosteriform eruptions may recur; a particularly interesting report of recurrent sciatica associated with HSV has been described by Morris and Peters.[68]

Although the clinical entity of HSV neuropathy is now well documented, the type of HSV responsible for disease is not clear. Details of HSV isolation in the literature indicate only that HSV was isolated from vesicles during acute disease and typed with anti-HSV immune serum. Although clinicians attribute herpes lesions "above the neck" to reactivation of HSV-1 and "below the waist" to reactivation of HSV-2, only future serotyping with monospecific polyclonal or monoclonal antibodies will identify specifically whether herpes neuropathy is caused primarily by HSV-1 or HSV-2.

With regard to treatment, most accounts of patients with HSV neuropathy occurred before acyclovir was developed. Acyclovir may reduce the number of days that patients have pain and rash. Nevertheless, it is unlikely that antiviral therapy will eradicate either HSV-1 or HSV-2; rather, resolution of acute disease will be followed by a return of the herpesvirus to the latent state with potential for future reactivation.

VARICELLA-ZOSTER VIRUS (VZV)

VZV, a human herpesvirus, causes chickenpox (varicella) in childhood, becomes latent in dorsal root ganglia, and reactivates decades later to produce shingles (zoster) in adults. The incidence of herpes zoster in the United States is 131/100,000 per year; approximately 50% of individuals older than 80 years will have had zoster once. Zoster and its attendant complications (Fig. 4–9) are more common in the immunocompromised and elderly population. A continuing increase in the immunocompromised (especially AIDS) and aging populations (it is estimated that by the year 2000, 25% of the population will be over age 65) will result in greater zoster-associated morbidity and mortality.

Epidemiology

Herpes zoster (shingles) is characterized by pain and vesicular rash on an erythematous base in one to three dermatomes (localized zoster). Zoster is common; approximately 300,000 cases are seen annually. It is approximately 8 to 10 times more frequent after age 60 years than before (Table 4–1). Fewer than 10% of zoster cases recur. Although chickenpox (varicella) occurs primarily in the spring, zoster occurs any time. There is no sex predilection. Although zoster most often reflects reactivation of latent VZV from dorsal root ganglia,[40] there are reports of zoster cases clustered in time,[67,70,104] supporting the notion that zoster may occasionally be acquired by exogenous reinfection. Zoster is more frequent in immunocompromised patients.[26] Before the AIDS era, the greatest frequency of zoster in immunocompromised individuals was in bone marrow transplant recipients,[1] followed in frequency by its occurrence in leukemia patients, particularly those receiving radiotherapy.[35] Zoster frequently develops at the site of primary radiation therapy.[89] In this author's experience, long-term, low-dose steroid therapy is also

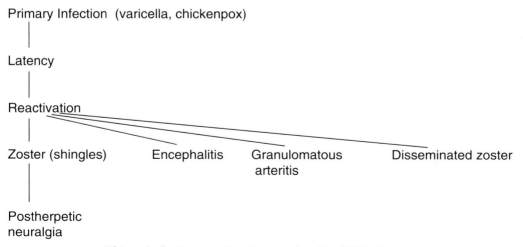

Figure 4–9. Primary disorders produced by VZV infection.

Table 4–1 ANNUAL INCIDENCE OF HERPES ZOSTER

Age	Cases, 1000/y
1–20	1.0
20–50	2.6
50–60	5.1
60–70	6.8
70–80	6.4
80–90	10.0

Source: Modified from Ragozzino MW, Melton LJ III, Kurland LT, Chu CP, Perry HO: Population-based study of herpes zoster and its sequelae. Medicine 61:310–316, 1982.

an important predisposing factor to zoster reactivation and to the serious complications of postherpetic neuralgia, disseminated zoster, and zoster encephalitis.

Clinical Features

The pain of zoster generally lasts 4 to 6 weeks, is severe, and is characterized by patients as "deep, burning and jabbing." Examination reveals both hypesthesia and hyperpathia in a dermatome distribution of mixed hypopigmentation and hyperpigmentation. Except for its longer duration, there does not appear to be any difference in the quality of pain with acute zoster or postherpetic neuralgia. When zoster occurs in cervical or lumbosacral dermatomes, muscle weakness may follow. The incidence of zoster paresis varies from as low as 0.5% to a high of 31%. Bladder and bowel dysfunction are often associated with sacral distribution zoster. The most complete study of clinical-pathologic correlations of herpes zoster was published nearly 100 years ago,[37] and clinicians are advised to review that paper before describing "new" zoster syndromes.

Zoster may involve any dermatome. The trunk, represented by 12 pairs of thoracic ganglia, is the most frequently involved site, but the face, supplied by the trigeminal nerve, is involved more often than any single thoracic dermatome. Trigeminal distribution zoster most frequently occurs in the ophthalmic branch (Fig. 4–10; see color insert).

Other abnormalities of the cranial nerves include peripheral facial weakness, often associated with vesicles in the ear (zoster oticus), the combination of which constitutes the Ramsay Hunt syndrome. Many cranial neuropathies occur weeks to months after cutaneous signs. One explanation offered for late-onset VZV-induced cranial neuropathy is that disease might be immune-mediated. Microinfarction of cranial nerves due to occlusion of the vasa vasorum is also possible. The blood supply of the cranial nerves is part of the carotid circulation.[56] Because trigeminal afferents innervate the large extracranial and intracranial blood vessels,[62] herpesvirus particles could spread along ganglionic afferent fibers to small vessels supplying cranial nerves. Such a mechanism has been proposed to explain the pathogenesis of VZV-induced granulomatous arteritis (see later discussion).

Treatment of Acute Infection

The treatment of acute zoster is controversial. Acyclovir administration during acute disease has not been proven to be efficacious, although it does reduce the duration of rash. Neither acute nor long-term pain (postherpetic neuralgia) appears to be affected (see later discussion). Because VZV has reduced in vitro sensitivity to acyclovir in comparison with HSV, a case can be made for treating acute zoster with higher doses of acyclovir and for a longer duration than is currently done, but neither the optimal dose nor time of treatment has been determined (see later discussion). Because postherpetic neuralgia occurs rarely in patients under age 50, there is currently no rationale for the use of antiviral agents in this age group. Furthermore, double-blind studies with antiviral agents are needed to determine their effectiveness in preventing postherpetic neuralgia in zoster patients over age 60. The use of glucocorticoids to prevent postherpetic neuralgia in the elderly has been advocated but not well studied. Their use in immunocompromised zoster patients is contraindicated. Whether glucocorticoids are effective in elderly immunocompetent individuals with zoster remains to be determined. Acute zoster pain should be controlled with analgesics, including codeine if necessary.

Complications of Zoster Infection

POSTHERPETIC NEURALGIA (PHN)

PHN, defined as pain persisting more than 4 to 6 weeks after zoster rash, is the most common complication of zoster. Age is the most important factor in predicting the development of PHN. The incidence of PHN is 46.9% in patients over age 60 years[83] but is 0 to 15% in patients under age 60, with most of these cases occurring in patients between ages 50 and 60 years. PHN is slightly more common in women than men and occurs more often after ophthalmic-distribution zoster in both sexes.

Treatment. The pain of PHN is initially managed with analgesic therapy. To avoid narcotics, the drugs carbamazepine, diphenylhydantoin, and amitriptyline are widely used. Best results are obtained by increasing the drug dose slowly to maximum subtoxic levels. Local applications of capsaicin (Zostrix) and Aspercreme are useful adjuncts when applied alternately throughout the day and before sleep. In most cases, medical treatment will obviate surgical nerve-root or ganglion block.

Recent studies suggest a possible link between PHN and VZV persistence.[106] These findings, together with a reduced sensitivity of VZV to acyclovir, provide a rationale for the use of high-dose acyclovir for more than 10 days to kill or reduce the persisting virus burden that triggers PHN. Studies are needed to determine whether acyclovir and/or glucocorticoid therapy initiated at the onset of zoster prevents PHN, and whether long-term, high-dose acyclovir is an effective treatment for PHN.

CNS DISEASE

CNS disease is the most alarming complication of zoster. Two conditions predominate: encephalitis and granulomatous arteritis.

Zoster Encephalitis. Encephalitis is the more common form of CNS involvement. CNS disease develops on a background of cancer, immunosuppression,[41] and AIDS. Neurologic disease is subacute, and death is common.

Clinical Manifestations. Zoster encephalitis presents with headache, fever, vomiting, and mental changes. Seizures may occur but are less frequent than with varicella encephalitis. Cranial nerve palsies affecting the third and seventh nerves are most frequent. An elevation of CSF pressure may be seen in frank zoster encephalitis, helping to distinguish it from the transient toxic encephalopathy seen in elderly people with zoster. A relaxed opening pressure should be recorded when spinal tap is performed. The CSF shows a mild pleocytosis (predominantly mononuclear), normal or mild elevation of CSF protein, and a normal CSF glucose. These findings do not significantly differ from zoster without encephalitis. There are two reports of hypoglycorrhachia in zoster meningoencephalitis.[79,118]

An accurate natural history of zoster encephalitis is not known, because earlier papers included patients both with and without an underlying immunodeficiency. Of the last five cases of zoster encephalitis at the University of Colorado Hospital, three were in AIDS patients; two occurred after long-term, low-dose glucocorticoids; and all five patients died.

Pathologic and Virologic Studies. Pathologic changes are characterized by perivenous encephalomalacia, focal hemorrhage and necrosis in both gray and white matter, and Cowdry A inclusions. Plaquelike demyelinative lesions at gray-white–matter junctions, originally described by Horton and colleagues,[41] are now a hallmark of disease in zoster encephalitis (Fig. 4–11). The

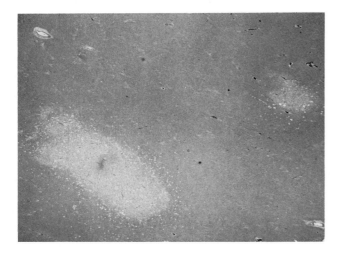

Figure 4-11. VZV encephalitis. Macroscopic section of brain showing characteristic large and small white-matter lesions. (Courtesy of Dr. B. K. DeMasters, Department of Pathology [Neuropathology], University of Colorado School of Medicine, Denver.)

differential diagnosis of multifocal white-matter lesions on CT or MRI scanning in patients with encephalitis, particularly those who are immunocompromised, should include VZV as a possible cause. The relationship of VZV to postinfectious encephalomyelitis remains to be determined.

A most recent complete study[29] shows that zoster encephalitis may be protracted for years and provides direct evidence of viral invasion of the CNS, as shown by the presence of Cowdry A inclusions and VZV antigen and DNA in glial cells.

Treatment. Treatment of zoster encephalitis includes acyclovir at a minimum of 30 mg/kg per day for 10 days. As already discussed, the reduced sensitivity of VZV to acyclovir compared with HSV suggests the use of higher doses for longer periods of time, particularly in severely immunocompromised patients.

Granulomatous Arteritis. This, the second form of VZV-induced CNS disease, is characterized by an acute focal deficit that develops weeks to months after contralateral trigeminal-distribution zoster. Stroke is the result of a necrotizing arteritis involving large and small cerebral arteries. In the comprehensive review by Hilt and associates,[38] most patients were over age 60 and there was no sex predilection. The mean onset of neurologic disease was 7

weeks after zoster; the longest interval was 6 months. Transient ischemic attacks and mental symptoms were common. Twenty-five percent of patients died. The majority of patients had CSF

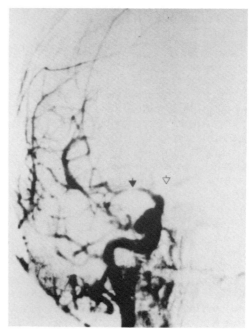

Figure 4-12. Angiogram in herpes zoster arteritis. Note severe narrowing of the A1 *(open arrow)* and M1 *(solid arrow)* segments, with less severe narrowing of the supraclinoid internal carotid artery. (From Fryer DG, Crane R, and Margolis MT: Angiographic changes in intracranial arteritis of ophthalmic herpes zoster. Ann Neurol 15:311, 1984, with permission.)

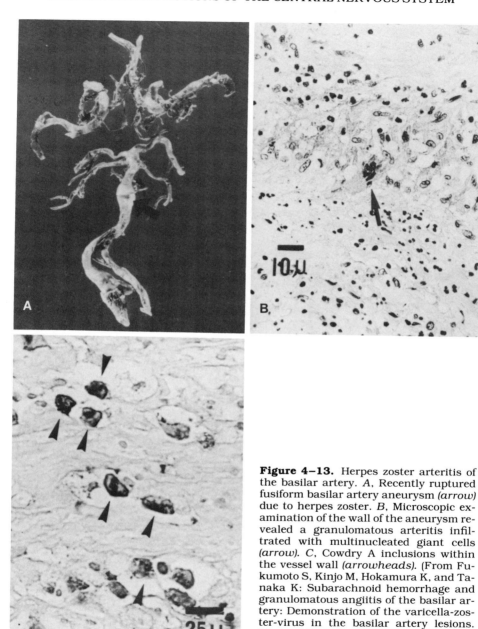

Figure 4–13. Herpes zoster arteritis of the basilar artery. *A*, Recently ruptured fusiform basilar artery aneurysm *(arrow)* due to herpes zoster. *B*, Microscopic examination of the wall of the aneurysm revealed a granulomatous arteritis infiltrated with multinucleated giant cells *(arrow)*. *C*, Cowdry A inclusions within the vessel wall *(arrowheads)*. (From Fukumoto S, Kinjo M, Hokamura K, and Tanaka K: Subarachnoid hemorrhage and granulomatous angiitis of the basilar artery: Demonstration of the varicella-zoster-virus in the basilar artery lesions. Stroke 17:1025–1026, 1986, with permission of the American Heart Association, Inc.)

pleocytosis (usually less than 100 cells, predominantly mononuclear), oligoclonal bands, and increased CSF IgG. Besides contralateral hemiplegia, ipsilateral central retinal artery occlusion[36] and posterior circulation involvement have been described. Angiographic examination revealed focal constriction and segmental narrowing primarily in middle cerebral, internal carotid, and anterior cerebral arteries (Fig. 4–12). Within diseased vessels, a necrotizing arteritis, primarily involving the intima and adventitia, is seen (Fig. 4–13). Multinucleated giant cells, VZV antigen, Cowdry A inclusions, and herpesvirus particles have been found. Pathologic examination revealed infarction in brain areas supplied by large cerebral arteries. Most zoster-associated granulomatous angiitis infarcts are pale,[55] but hemorrhagic infarction also occurs.[19]

Afferent trigeminal ganglionic fibers to both intracranial and extracranial blood vessels[62] provide an anatomic pathway for spread of virus. Because it is not clear whether the disease is exclusively viral or a viral-induced immunopathology, the proper definitive treatment is not known. Nevertheless, based on pathologic changes, a strong case can be made for using acyclovir to kill persistent virus and using glucocorticoids for their anti-inflammatory effect.

VZV Latency

No animal model for VZV latency is available, and VZV cannot be rescued from explants of thoracic ganglia.[75] Thus our knowledge of VZV latency is based on the application of nucleic acid hybridization techniques to human ganglia. Latent VZV DNA was first detected in trigeminal ganglia from humans without recent varicella or zoster by Southern blot analysis.[27] PCR studies revealed that VZV is latent in multiple ganglia of nearly all humans and that more than one region of the viral genome is present during latency.[61] These findings are consistent with the classic epidemiologic studies of Hope-Simpson,[40] in which the trigeminal and thoracic dermatomes were shown to be the most frequent sites of zoster.

Regarding the cell type in which VZV is latent, in situ hybridization initially detected VZV RNA,[42] and later both VZV DNA and RNA, in neurons of latently infected trigeminal[102] and thoracic[28] ganglia. Another report describes VZV RNA in satellite cells, but not in neurons.[8] The latter finding is of interest since viral integration would not be necessary for maintenance of VZV latency in dividing nonneuronal

cells, and virus would have to be shed periodically from these cells and simultaneously infect new satellite cells. On the other hand, if VZV is latent in nondividing neuronal cells, virus integration would be more likely. Further in situ hybridization studies designed to detect VZV transcripts and to analyze VZV configuration and integration in ganglia are needed to resolve these conflicting data. Finally, an attempt to develop a model of VZV infection in rats reports the presence of VZV exclusively in neurons.[64]

CYTOMEGALOVIRUS (CMV)

CMV produces neurologic disease primarily in infants as part of the clinical spectrum of congenital CMV infection. Although most congenital CMV infection is asymptomatic, many carriers develop sensorineural hearing loss and intellectual handicaps. Other neurologic complications of congenital infections include microcephaly, seizures, hypotonia, and spasticity. Lethargy and coma may follow a severe CMV meningoencephalitis.

In immunocompetent adults, the most common neurologic complication of CMV infection is Guillain-Barré syndrome. Two initial reports associated this syndrome with a "CMV mononucleosis,"[43,49] followed by a case study of a 35-year-old man who developed acute idiopathic polyneuritis; CMV was isolated from his blood buffy-coat cells, and CMV-IgM antibodies were detected in serum.[47] Further linkage of CMV with Guillain-Barré syndrome was the demonstration of a fourfold or greater alteration in complement-fixing antibody to CMV in 21 of 92 Guillain-Barré patients,[16] and the development of recurrent Guillain-Barré disease in a renal transplant patient after exposure to CMV by vaccination.[15] Serologic studies have also shown the onset of an acute brachial plexopathy in conjunction with recent CMV infection.[17]

CMV infection of the CNS in immunocompetent adults is rare. The clinical presentation is usually encephalitis, characterized by mental changes and pyramidal signs.[5] A case of self-limited encephalitis characterized by headache, right-sided sensory symptoms, and aphasia was presumed to be caused by CMV, based on high titer anti-CMV antibody (1:1024), which subsequently fell to 1:64; interestingly, encephalitic symptoms recurred 5 months later, when the anti-CMV titer was 1:8192.[80] The natural history of CMV encephalitis in immunocompetent individuals is not known, so a definitive treatment protocol has not been determined. Two patients with presumptive CMV encephalitis, based on the isolation of CMV from CSF and urine, were treated with vidarabine and responded well, however.[74]

In contrast to the rarity of CMV infection in the immunocompetent adult, CMV infections of the immunocompromised population, particularly AIDS patients, are common. CMV has now emerged as an important cause of encephalitis, myelitis, and polyradiculitis. The initial report of CMV encephalitis in renal transplant patients[90] was followed by the demonstration of CMV in the CNS of bone marrow transplant recipients.[71] As the AIDS era was beginning, an interesting report described CMV vasculitis and retinitis in a lymphoma patient receiving multiple cytotoxic and anti-inflammatory drugs.[52] Today CMV infection most commonly complicates AIDS; after human immunodeficiency virus (HIV), CMV is the most common infectious agent found in the brains of AIDS patients.[73] Complications include retinitis,[72] encephalitis,[57] progressive myelitis,[105] and polyradiculopathy. A distinct clinical syndrome of CMV encephalitis has been defined. The usual picture of CMV-associated subacute encephalopathy is that of progressive dementia, headache, focal or diffuse weakness, and seizures. In this regard, the clinician should consider CMV if the AIDS patient presents with diffuse or focal deficit. Focal disease has been attributed to CMV vasculitis or foci of demyelination. Characteristic owl-eyed cytomegalic inclusions and CMV-specific antigens have been found in the brain, spinal cord, and blood vessels of AIDS patients with subacute encephalopathy. Complicating the picture, however, is the additional presence of HIV or HSV-2,[105] so the attribution of specific symptoms and signs to CMV is difficult. CMV occasionally can be isolated from the CSF of AIDS patients.

Of particular interest is the occurrence in AIDS patients of a polyradiculopathy thought to be caused by CMV. Disease often begins insidiously as a cauda equina syndrome with distal weakness, paresthesias, incontinence, and sacral sensory loss. There is usually CSF pleocytosis (frequently characterized by a predominance of polymorphonuclear leukocytes), elevated protein, hypoglycorrhachia, and occasional isolation of CMV from CSF. Postmortem examination reveals inflammation, necrosis, and focal vasculitis of nerve roots, with typical CMV intranuclear and intracytoplasmic inclusions.[20]

EPSTEIN-BARR VIRUS (EBV)

EBV is the cause of infectious mononucleosis and also has been implicated as a cause of nasopharyngeal carcinoma and Burkitt's lymphoma. EBV is ubiquitous and affects most of the human population. Primary infection usually occurs in childhood or adolescence. By age 30, more than 90% of adults have antibody to EBV. Despite the prevalence of EBV infection, neurologic disease is rare. The most common presentation is meningoencephalitis,[31] often associated with acute cerebellar ataxia.[6] More serious meningoencephalopathy presenting with athetosis and chorea,[58] or with stupor and coma,[12,24] has been described. Two cases of ophthalmoplegic polyneuropathy have been associated with recent EBV infection.[88,94] Chiasmal neuritis may also complicate EBV infection.[78] Acute EBV mononucleosis may be followed by recurrent aseptic meningitis.[32] There are a few reports of myelopathy coincident with the onset of infectious mononucleosis.[33,34,93]

Finally, EBV DNA has been detected in CNS lymphoma tissue, both in immunocompetent[39] and immunocompromised[2] patients. A relationship between the detection of EBV sequences in CNS lymphomas and the induction or pathogenesis of disease remains to be determined, however.

HUMAN HERPESVIRUS 6 (HHV-6)

HHV-6 is the most recently recognized human herpesvirus. Serologic evidence indicates that HHV-6 is the cause of roseola infantum. HHV-6 appears to be lymphotropic but has not been associated with immunologic or neurologic disease. Most recently, a new human herpesvirus, designated RK, was isolated from CD4+ T cells of a healthy individual; analysis of the viral DNA by restriction enzyme analysis and blot hybridization yielded patterns different from HHV-6, suggesting that RK may be the prototype of a new seventh human herpesvirus.[23]

SUMMARY

The human herpesviruses are an important cause of neurologic disease. Figure 4–14 shows an algorithm for diagnosis and evaluation of acute encephalitis caused by the human herpesviruses. The two herpesviruses most commonly associated with morbidity and mortality are HSV-1 and VZV. Both produce encephalitis usually characterized by fever, mental status changes, seizures, and focal neurologic deficit. MRI reveals medial temporal lobe involvement in HSV-1 encephalitis and deep-seated white-matter lesions, primarily at gray-white–matter junctions, in VZV encephalitis. HSV-1 encephalitis develops in otherwise healthy individuals, whereas VZV encephalitis is seen after zoster in immunocompromised patients. Both viral encephalitides should be treated with acyclovir.

Other neurologic complications of VZV are postherpetic neuralgia (PHN) and granulomatous arteritis. PHN is defined as pain that persists for more than 4 to 6 weeks after zoster. Neither the mechanism by which PHN develops, nor its definitive treatment, is known. Granulomatous arteritis is usually characterized by acute hemiplegia that develops weeks to months after contralateral trigeminal-distribution zoster. Radiologic, pathologic, and virologic analyses demonstrate cerebral infarction, most often, but not exclusively, in the distribution of the middle cerebral artery, and the presence of multinucleated giant cells and VZV antigen and virions in affected blood vessels. Virus is presumably transported via trigeminal afferent fibers to large extracranial and intracranial arteries. Although the exact mechanism of disease is still unknown, the combination of an inflammatory response and the presence of virus in arteries justifies treatment of granulomatous arteritis with both glucocorticoids and acyclovir.

HSV-2 causes genital herpes. The most common neurologic complications in otherwise healthy adults are aseptic meningitis or painful zosteriform eruptions. Virus can be isolated from CSF or vesicles. The disease is self-limiting, and acyclovir treatment is not necessary. HSV-2 encephalitis occurs in newborns and immunocompromised individuals and should be treated with acyclovir.

CMV, with few exceptions, infects the adult nervous system only in immunocompromised individuals, especially those with AIDS. CNS disease is characterized by headache and diffuse mental changes or focal deficit. CMV may also cause polyradiculopathy with CSF pleocytosis, a predominance of polymorphonuclear leukocytes, and hypoglycorrhachia. Neurologic complica-

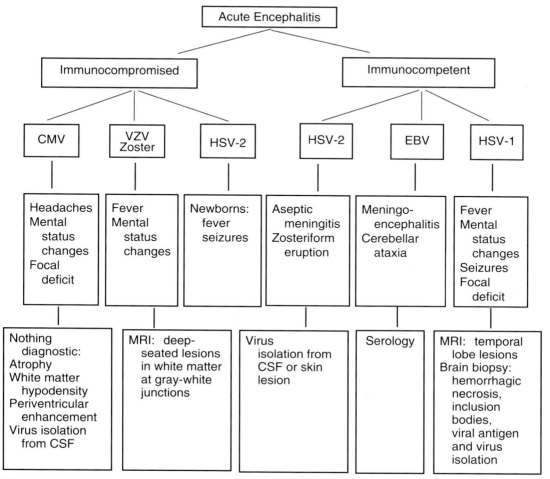

Figure 4–14. Algorithm for diagnosis and evaluation of acute encephalitis caused by the human herpesviruses.

tions of EBV infection are rare. Meningoencephalitis, often with cerebellar ataxia, is the most common presentation. HHV-6 has not been shown to cause neurologic disease.

ACKNOWLEDGMENTS

I wish to thank Marina Hoffman and Mary E. Devlin for editorial review, and Cathy Allen for preparation of this manuscript. This work was supported in part by Public Health Service Grants NS-07321, AG-06127, and AG-07347 from the NIH, and a grant from the Roy and Beatrice Backus Foundation.

REFERENCES

1. Artkinson K, Meyers JD, Rainer S, Ross LP, and Thomas ED: Varicella-zoster virus infection after marrow transplantation for aplastic anemia or leukemia. Transplantation 29:47–50, 1980.

2. Bashir RM, Harris NL, Hochberg FH, and Singer RM: Detection of Epstein-Barr virus in CNS lymphomas by in-situ hybridization. Neurology 39:813–817, 1989.

3. Block TM, Spivack JG, Steiner I, et al: A herpes simplex virus type 1 latency-associated transcript mutant reactivates with normal kinetics from latent

infection. J Virol 64:3417–3426, 1990.

4. Castleman B and McNeely BU: Case records of the Massachusetts General Hospital, Case 61-1964. N Engl J Med 271:1313–1320, 1964.

5. Chin W, Magoffin R, Frierson JG, and Lennette EH: Cytomegalovirus infection: A case with meningoencephalitis. JAMA 225:740–741, 1973.

6. Cleary TG, Henle W, and Pickering LK: Acute cerebellar ataxia associated with Epstein-Barr virus infection. JAMA 243:148–149, 1980.

7. Cook ML and Stevens JG: Latent herpetic infections following experimental viraemia. J Gen Virol 31:75–80, 1976.

8. Croen KD, Ostrove JM, Dragovic LJ, and Straus SE: Patterns of gene expression and sites of latency in human nerve ganglia are different for varicella-zoster and herpes simplex viruses. Proc Natl Acad Sci U S A 85:9773–9777, 1988.

9. Cushing H: The surgical aspects of major neuralgia of the trigeminal nerve: A report of 20 cases of operation on the Gasserion ganglion with anatomic and physiologic notes on the consequences of its removal. JAMA 44:773, 860, 920, 1002, 1088, 1905.

10. Davis LE and Johnson RT: An explanation for the localization of herpes simplex encephalitis? Ann Neurol 5:2–5, 1979.

11. Davis LE and McLaren LC: Relapsing herpes simplex encephalitis following antiviral therapy. Radiology 129:409–417, 1978.

12. Demey HE, Martin JJ, Leus RM, Moeremans CJ, and Bossaert LL: Coma as a presenting sign of Epstein-Barr encephalitis. Arch Intern Med 148:1459–1461, 1988.

13. Deshman SL and Fraser NW: During latency, herpes simplex virus type 1 DNA is associated with nucleosomes in a chromatin structure. J Virol 63:943–947, 1989.

14. Doerig C, Pizer LI, and Wilcox CL: An antigen encoded by the latency-associated transcript in neuronal cell cultures latently infected with herpes simplex virus type 1. J Virol 65:2724–2727, 1991.

15. Donaghy M, Gray JA, Squier W, et al: Recurrent Guillain-Barre syndrome after multiple exposures to cytomegalovirus. Am J Med 87:339–341, 1989.

16. Dowling P, Menonna J, and Cook S: Cytomegalovirus complement fixation antibody in Guillain-Barre syndrome. Neurology 27:1153–1156, 1977.

17. Duchowny M, Caplan L, and Siber G: Cytomegalovirus infection of the adult nervous system. Ann Neurol 5:458–461, 1979.

18. Dutt MK and Johnston IDA: Computed tomography and EEG in herpes simplex encephalitis. Arch Neurol 39:99, 1982.

19. Eible RJ: Intracerebral hemorrhage with herpes zoster ophthalmicus. Ann Neurol 14:591–592, 1983.

20. Eidelberg D, Sotrel A, Vogel H, Walker P, Kleefield J, and Crumpacker CS III: Progressive polyradiculopathy in acquired immune deficiency syndrome. Neurology 36:912–916, 1986.

21. Efstathiou SA, Minson AC, Field HJ, Anderson JR, and Wildy P: Detection of herpes simplex virus-specific DNA sequences in latently infected mice and in humans. J Virol 57:446–455, 1986.

22. Esiri MM and Tomlinson AH: Herpes simplex encephalitis: Immunohistological demonstration of spread of virus via olfactory and trigeminal pathways after infection of facial skin in mice. J Neurol Sci 64:213–217, 1984.

23. Frenkel N, Schirmer EC, Wyatt LS, et al: Isolation of a new herpesvirus from human CD4+ T cells (human herpesvirus 7/virus latency/T-cell activation). Proc Natl Acad Sci U S A 87:748–752, 1990.

24. Friedland R and Yahr MD: Meningoencephalopathy secondary to infectious mononucleosis: Unusual presentation with stupor and chorea. Arch Neurol 34:186–188, 1977.

25. Friedrich A, Kleim J-P, and Schnew-

eis KE: Detection of latent thymidine kinase-deficient herpes simplex virus in trigeminal ganglia of mice using the polymerase chain reaction. Arch Virol 113:107–113, 1990.

26. Gallagher JG and Merigan TC: Prolonged herpes-zoster infection associated with immunosuppressive therapy. Ann Intern Med 91:842–846, 1979.

27. Gilden DH, Vafai A, Shtram Y, Becker Y, Devlin M, and Wellish M: Varicella-zoster virus DNA in human sensory ganglia. Nature 306:478–480, 1983.

28. Gilden DH, Rosemann Y, Murray R, Devlin M, and Vafai A: Detection of varicella-zoster virus nucleic acid in neurons of normal human thoracic ganglia. Ann Neurol 22:377–380, 1987.

29. Gilden DH, Murray RS, Wellish M, Kleinschmidt-DeMasters BK, and Vafai A: Chronic progressive varicella-zoster virus encephalitis in an AIDS patient. Neurology 38:1150–1153, 1988.

30. Gordon YJ, Johnson B, Romanowski E, and Araullo-Cruz T: RNA complementary to herpes simplex virus type 1 ICPO gene demonstrated in neurons of human trigeminal ganglia. J Virol 62:1832–1853, 1988.

31. Gotlieb-Stematsky T and Arlazoroff A: Epstein-Barr virus. Handbook of Clinical Neurology 12:249–261, 1989.

32. Graman PS: Mollaret's meningitis associated with acute Epstein-Barr virus mononucleosis. Arch Neurol 44:1204–1205, 1987.

33. Grose C and Feorino PM: Epstein-Barr virus and transverse myelitis. Lancet 1:892, 1973.

34. Grose C, Henle W, Henle G, and Feorino PM: Primary Epstein-Barr-virus infections in acute neurologic diseases. N Engl J Med 292:392–395, 1975.

35. Guess HA, Broughton DD, Melton LJ, and Kurland LT: Epidemiology of herpes zoster in children and adolescents: A population-based study. Pediatrics 76:512–517, 1985.

36. Hall S, Carlin L, Roach SE, and McLean WT: Herpes zoster and central retinal artery occlusion. Ann Neurol 13:217–218, 1983.

37. Head H and Campbell AW: The pathology of herpes zoster and its bearing on sensory localization. Brain 23:353–523, 1900.

38. Hilt DC, Buchholz D, Krumholz A, and Weiss H: Herpes zoster ophthalmicus and delayed contralateral hemiparesis caused by cerebral angiitis: Diagnosis and management approaches. Ann Neurol 14:543–553, 1983.

39. Hochberg FH, Miller G, Schooley RT, Hirsch MS, Feorino P, and Henle W: Central-nervous-system lymphoma related to Epstein-Barr virus. N Engl J Med 309:745–748, 1983.

40. Hope-Simpson RE: The nature of herpes zoster: A long-term study and a new hypothesis. Proc R Soc Med 58:9–20, 1965.

41. Horton B, Price RW, and Jimenez D: Multifocal varicella-zoster virus leukoencephalitis temporally remote from herpes zoster. Ann Neurol 9:251–266, 1981.

42. Hyman RW, Ecker JR, and Tenser RB: Varicella-zoster virus RNA in human trigeminal ganglia. Lancet 2:814–816, 1983.

43. Ironside AG and Tobin JO: Cytomegalovirus infection in the adult. Lancet 2:615–616, 1967.

44. Johnson RT: The pathogenesis of herpes virus encephalitis. I. Virus pathways to the nervous system of suckling mice demonstrated by fluorescent antibody staining. J Exp Med 119:343–356, 1964.

45. Johnson RT: Viral Infections of the Nervous System. Raven Press, New York, 1982.

46. Joklik WK: The structure, components, and classification of viruses. In Joklik WK (ed): Principles of Animal Virology. Appleton-Century-Crofts, New York, 1980, pp 16–61.

47. Kabins S, Keller R, Peitchel RT, and Ali MA: Acute idiopathic polyneuritis caused by cytomegalovirus. Arch Intern Med 136:100–101, 1976.

48. Katz JP, Bodin ET, and Coen DM: Quantitative polymerase chain reaction analysis of herpes simplex virus DNA in ganglia of mice infected with replication-incompetent mutants. J Virol 64:4288–4295, 1990.

49. Klemola E, Kaarianen L, Von Essen R, Haltia K, Koivoniemi A, and Von Bondsdorff CH: Further studies on cytomegalovirus mononucleosis in previously healthy individuals. Acta Med Scand 182:311–322, 1967.

50. Knezevic W and Carrol WM: Relapse of herpes simplex encephalitis after acyclovir therapy. Aust N Z J Med 13:625–626, 1983.

51. Koenig H, Rabinowitz SG, Day E, and Miller V: Post-infectious encephalomyelitis after successful treatment of herpes simplex encephalitis with adenine arabinoside: Ultrasound observations. N Engl J Med 300:1089–1093, 1979.

52. Koeppen AH, Lansing LS, Peng S-K, and Smith RS: Central nervous system vasculitis in cytomegalovirus infection. J Neurol Sci 51:395–410, 1981.

53. Krause PR, Croen KD, Straus SE, and Ostrove JM: Detection and preliminary characterization of herpes simplex virus type 1 transcripts in latently infected human trigeminal ganglia. J Virol 62:4819–4823, 1988.

54. Krohel GB, Richardson JR, and Farrell DF: Herpes simplex neuropathy. Neurology 26:596–597, 1976.

55. Kuroiwa Y and Furukawa T: Hemispheric infarction after herpes zoster ophthalmicus: Computed tomography and angiography. Neurology 31:1030–1032, 1981.

56. Lapresle J and Lasjaunias P: Cranial nerve ischaemic arterial syndromes. A review. Brain 109:207–215, 1986.

57. Laskin OL, Stahl-Bayliss CM, and Morgello S: Concomitant herpes simplex virus type 1 and cytomegalovirus ventriculoencephalitis in acquired immunodeficiency syndrome. Arch Neurol 44:843–847, 1987.

58. Leavell R, Ray CG, Ferry PC, and Minnich LL: Unusual acute neurologic presentations with Epstein-Barr virus infection. Arch Neurol 43:186–188, 1986.

59. Leib DA, Nadeau KC, Rundle SA, and Schaffer PA: The promoter of the latency-associated transcripts of herpes simplex virus type 1 contains a functional cAMP-response element: Role of the latency-associated transcripts and cAMP in reactivation of viral latency. Proc Natl Acad Sci U S A 88:48–52, 1991.

60. Lynas C, Laycock KA, Cook SD, Hill TJ, Blyth WA, and Maitland NJ: Detection of herpes simplex virus type 1 gene expression in latently and productively infected mouse ganglia using the polymerase chain reaction. J Gen Virol 70:2345–2355, 1989.

61. Mahalingam R, Wellish M, Wolf W, et al: Latent varicella-zoster viral DNA in human trigeminal and thoracic ganglia. N Engl J Med 323:627–631, 1990.

62. Mayberg MR, Zervas NT, and Moskowitz MA: Trigeminal projections to supratentorial pial and dural blood vessels in cats demonstrated by horseradish peroxidase histochemistry. J Comp Neurol 223:46–56, 1984.

63. Mellerick DM and Fraser NW: Physical state of the latent herpes simplex virus genome in a mouse model system: Evidence suggesting an episomal state. Virology 158:265–275, 1987.

64. Merville-Louis M-P, Sadzot-Delvaux C, Delrée P, Moonen G, and Rentier B: Varicella-zoster virus infection of adult rat sensory neurons in vitro. J Virol 63:3155–3160, 1989.

65. Miller JK, Hesser F, and Tompkins VN: Herpes simplex encephalitis. Ann Intern Med 64:92–103, 1966.

66. Mitchell WJ, Lirette RP, and Fraser NW: Mapping of low abundance latency-associated RNA in the trigeminal ganglia of mice latently infected with herpes simplex virus type 1. J Gen Virol 71:125–132, 1990.

67. Morens DM, Bregman DJ, West CM, et al: An outbreak of varicella-zoster virus infection among cancer patients. Ann Intern Med 93:414–419, 1980.

68. Morris HH III and Peters BH: Recurrent sciatica associated with herpes simplex. Case report. J Neurosurg 41:97–99, 1974.

69. Olson LC, Buescher EL, Artenstein MS, and Parkman PD: Herpesvirus infections of the human central nervous system. N Engl J Med 277:1271–1277, 1967.

70. Palmer SR, Caul EO, Donald DE, Kwantes W, and Tillett W: An outbreak of shingles? Lancet 2:1108–1111, 1985.

71. Patchell RA, White CL III, Clark AW, Beschorner WE, and Santos GW: Neurologic complications of bone marrow transplantation. Neurology 35:300–306, 1985.

72. Pepose JS, Holland GN, Nestor MS, Cochran AJ, and Foos RY: Acquired immune deficiency syndrome: Pathogenic mechanisms of ocular disease. Ophthalmology 92:472–484, 1985.

73. Petito CK, Cho ES, Lehman W, Navis BA, and Price RW: Neuropathology of acquired immunodeficiency syndrome (AIDS): An autopsy review. J Neuropath Exp Neurol 45:635–646, 1986.

74. Phillips CA, Fanning WL, Gump DW, and Phillips CF: Cytomegalovirus encephalitis in immunologically normal adults: Successful treatment with vidarabine. JAMA 238:2299–2300, 1977.

75. Plotkin SA, Stein S, Snyder M, and Immesoette P: Attempts to recover varicella virus from ganglia. Ann Neurol 2:249, 1977.

76. Price RW, Walz MA, Wohlenberg C, and Notkins AB: Latent infection of sensory ganglia with herpes simplex virus: Efficacy of immunization. Science 188:938–940, 1975.

77. Puga A, Cantin EM, Wohlenberg C, Openshaw H, and Notkins AB: Different sizes of restriction endonuclease fragments from the terminal repetitions of the herpes simplex virus type 1 genome latent in trigeminal ganglia of mice. J Gen Virol 65:437–444, 1984.

78. Purvin V, Herr GJ, and De Myer W: Chiasmal neuritis as a complication of Epstein-Barr virus infection. Arch Neurol 45:458–460, 1988.

79. Reimer LG and Reller LB: CSF in herpes zoster meningoencephalitis. Arch Neurol 38:668, 1981.

80. Richert JR, Potolicchio S Jr, Garagusi VF, et al: Cytomegalovirus encephalitis associated with episodic neurologic deficits and OKT-8$^+$ pleocytosis. Neurology 37:149–152, 1987.

81. Rock DL and Fraser NW: Detection of HSV-1 genome in central nervous system of latently infected mice. Nature 302:523–525, 1983.

82. Rock DL, Nesburn AB, Ghiasi H, et al: Detection of latency-related viral RNAs in trigeminal ganglia of rabbits latently infected with herpes simplex virus type 1. J Virol 61:3820–3826, 1987.

83. Rogers RS and Tindall JP: Geriatric herpes zoster. J Am Geriatr Soc 19:495–503, 1971.

84. Roizman B: Provisional classification of herpesvirus. In de-The G, Henle W, and Rapp F (eds): Oncogenesis and Herpesviruses III. International Agency for Research on Cancer, Lyon, 1978, pp 1079–1082.

85. Roizman B, Carmichael LE, Deinhardt F, et al: Herpesviridae definition, provisional nomenclature, and taxonomy. Intervirology 16:201–217, 1981.

86. Rowley AH, Whitley RJ, Lakeman FD, and Wolinsky SM: Rapid detection of herpes-simplex-virus DNA in cerebrospinal fluid of patients with herpes simplex encephalitis. Lancet 335:440–441, 1990.

87. Sage JI, Weinstein MP, and Miller DC: Chronic encephalitis possibly due to herpes simplex virus: Two cases. Neurology 35:1470–1472, 1985.

88. Salazar A, Martinez H, and Sotelo J: Ophthalmoplegic polyneuropathy associated with infectious mononucleosus. Ann Neurol 13:219–220, 1983.

89. Schimpff S, Serpick A, Stoler B, et al: Varicella-zoster infection in patients with cancer. Ann Intern Med 76:241–254, 1972.

90. Schneck SA: Neuropathological features of human organ transplanta-

tion. I. Probable cytomegalovirus infection. J Neuropathol Exp Neurol 24:415–429, 1965.

91. Schroth G, Gawehn J, Thron A, Vallbracht A, and Voigt K: Early diagnosis of herpes simplex encephalitis by MRI. Neurology 37:179–183, 1987.

92. Sedarati F, Izumi KM, Wagner EK, and Stevens JG: Herpes simplex virus type 1 latency-associated transcription plays no role in establishment or maintenance of a latent infection in murine sensory neurons. J Virol 63:4455–4458, 1989.

93. Silverstein A, Steinberg G, and Nathanson M: Nervous system involvement in infectious mononucleosis. Arch Neurol 26:353–358, 1972.

94. Slavick HE and Shapiro RA: Fisher's syndrome associated with Epstein-Barr virus. Arch Neurol 38:134–135, 1981.

95. Slavin HB and Ferguson JJ Jr: Zoster-like eruptions caused by the virus of herpes simplex. Am J Med 8:456–467, 1950.

96. Smith JB, Westmoreland BF, Reagan TJ, and Sandok BA: A distinctive clinical EEG profile in herpes simplex encephalitis. Mayo Clin Proc 50:469–474, 1975.

97. Spivack JG and Fraser NW: Expression of herpes simplex virus type 1 latency-associated transcripts in the trigeminal ganglia of mice during acute infection and reactivation of latent infection. J Virol 62:1479–1485, 1988.

98. Steiner I, Spivack JG, Lirette RP, et al: Herpes simplex virus type 1 latency-associated transcripts are evidently not essential for latent infection. EMBO J 8:505–511, 1989.

99. Steiner I, Spivack JG, Deshmane SL, Ace CI, Preston CM, and Fraser NW: A herpes simplex virus type 1 mutant containing a nontransinducing Vmw65 protein establishes latent infection in vivo in the absence of viral replication and reactivates efficiently from explanted trigeminal ganglia. J Virol 64:1630–1638, 1990.

100. Stevens JG, Haarr L, Porter DD, Cook ML, and Wagner EK: Prominence of the herpes simplex virus latency-associated transcript in trigeminal ganglia from seropositive humans. J Infect Dis 158:177, 1988.

101. Stroop WG, Rock DL, and Fraser NW: Localization of herpes simplex virus in the trigeminal and olfactory systems of the mouse central nervous system during acute and latent infections by in situ hybridization. Lab Invest 51:27–38, 1984.

102. Tenser RB and Hyman RW: Latent herpesvirus infections of neurons in guinea pigs and humans. Yale J Biol Med 60:159–167, 1987.

103. ter Penning B: Inflammatory disease of the brain and spine. In Pomeranz SJ (ed): Craniospinal Magnetic Resonance Imaging. WB Saunders, Philadelphia, 1989, p 436.

104. Thomas M and Robertson WJ: Dermal transmission of virus as a cause of shingles. Lancet 2:1349–1350, 1971.

105. Tucker T, Dix RD, Katzen C, Davis RL, and Schmidley JW: Cytomegalovirus and herpes simplex virus ascending myelitis in a patient with acquired immune deficiency syndrome. Ann Neurol 18:74–79, 1985.

106. Vafai A, Wellish M, and Gilden DH: Expression of varicella-zoster virus in blood mononuclear cells of patients with postherpetic neuralgia. Proc Natl Acad Sci U S A 85:2767–2770, 1988.

107. Vandvik B, Skoldenberg B, Forsgren M, Stiernstedt G, Jeansson S, and Norrby E: Long-term persistence of intrathecal virus-specific antibody responses after herpes simplex virus encephalitis. J Neurol 231:307–312, 1985.

108. Wagner EK, Devi-Rao G, Feldman LT, et al: Physical characterization of the herpes simplex virus latency-associated transcript in neurons. J Virol 62:1194–1202, 1988.

109. Warren KG, Devlin M, Gilden DH, et al: Herpes simplex virus latency in patients with multiple sclerosis, lymphoma and normal humans. In De-The G, Henle W, and Rapp R (eds): Oncogenesis and Herpesvirus III, Part

2: Cell-virus Interactions, Host Response to Herpesvirus Infection and Associated Tumors, Role of Co-factors. International Agency for Research on Cancer, Lyon, 1978, vol 24, pp 765–768.

110. Weisberg L and Nice C: Herpes simplex encephalitis. Cerebral Computed Tomography: A Text Atlas. 3:295–297, 1989.

111. Westmoreland BF: The EEG in cerebral inflammatory processes. In Niedermeyer E and Lopes da Silva FH (eds): Electroencephalography, ed 2. Urban & Schwarzenberg, Baltimore-Munich, 1987, p 261.

112. Whitley RJ, Alford CA, Hirsch MS, et al: Vidarabine versus acyclovir therapy in herpes simplex encephalitis. N Engl J Med 314:144–149, 1986.

113. Whitley RJ, Soong SJ, Dolin R, Galasso GJ, Ch'ien LT, and Alford CA: Adenine arabinoside therapy of biopsy-proved herpes simplex encephalitis: National Institute of Allergy and Infectious Diseases Collaborative Antiviral Study. N Engl J Med 297:289–294, 1977.

114. Whitley RJ, Soong SJ, Hirsch MS, et al: Herpes simplex encephalitis: Vidarabine therapy and diagnostic problems. N Engl J Med 304:313–318, 1981.

115. Whitley RJ, Soong SJ, Linneman C Jr, Liu C, Pazin G, and Alford CA: Herpes simplex encephalitis. Clinical assessment. JAMA 247:317–320, 1982.

116. Wilcox CL and Johnson EM Jr: Nerve growth factor deprivation results in the reactivation of latent herpes simplex virus in vitro. J Virol 61:2311–2315, 1987.

117. Wilcox CL and Johnson EM Jr: Characterization of nerve growth factor-dependent herpes simplex virus latency in neurons in vitro. J Virol 62:393–399, 1988.

118. Wolf SM: Decreased cerebrospinal fluid glucose level in herpes zoster meningitis. Arch Neurol 30:109, 1974.

119. Zimmerman RA, Bilaniuk LT, Shipkin PM, Gilden DH, and Murtagh F: Evolution of cerebral abscess: Correlation of clinical features with computed tomography. Neurology 27:14–19, 1977.

120. Zimmerman RD, Russell EJ, and Leeds NE: CT in the early diagnosis of herpes simplex encephalitis. Am J Radiol 134:61–66, 1980.

EDITORS' COMMENTARY:

Brain Biopsy for the Diagnosis of Herpes Simplex Encephalitis

The management of cases involving suspected herpes simplex encephalitis (HSE) continues to pose a number of clinical dilemmas. Many studies have confirmed that prompt initiation of therapy is essential to minimize morbidity and mortality and maximize the probability of survival without substantial disability.[15] One of the most difficult problems remains whether to subject patients to brain biopsy to confirm the diagnosis before beginning antiviral therapy. Although the use of brain biopsy before beginning antiviral therapy has been advocated by many[7,8] and is supported by a recent decision-analysis study from the National Institute of Allergy and Infectious Diseases (NIAID) Antiviral Study Group (NIAID-ASG),[14] these recommendations are not universally supported,[5,6] run counter to actual practice at most institutions, and seem to fail the intuitive logic of the "What would you do for your mother?" test.

Supporters of the biopsy approach argue that brain biopsy is a reasonably safe procedure[11] that often leads to the discovery of previously unsuspected and treatable illnesses.[16] Opponents of biopsy argue that acyclovir is safe and unlikely to have adverse effects.[1,5,6] Each of these propositions needs to be analyzed independently.

Recent estimates suggest that the mortality rate associated with brain biopsy is approximately 0.2%,[14] with serious complications occurring in less than 1% to 2% of patients. These values are certainly reasonable estimates when brain biopsy is performed in a large hospital or teaching institution but might be substantially higher in community or local hospitals with less extensive neurosurgical experience. An increase in the rate of serious complications occurring as a result of biopsy to 5% to 10% makes biopsy an untenable diagnostic procedure.[3] Rates this high have been reported in some published series from reputable institutions.[1,9] Physicians should consult with their neurosurgical colleagues to determine how many brain biopsies are being performed at their institution and the expected local morbidity and mortality rates.

The second rationale for biopsy is that it may reveal previously unsuspected treatable illnesses. It was recently suggested that 40% of biopsy-negative patients (i.e., patients with no evidence of HSE) would have an alternative (non-HSE) diagnosis identified as a result of biopsy and that 40% of these diagnoses would be treatable illnesses.[14] In other words, 16% (about 1 in 6) of patients with brain biopsy results that are negative for HSE will instead have another treatable illness identified as a result of biopsy. It is important to recognize that these data were derived from studies performed before patients routinely had computed tomography (CT) studies or magnetic resonance imaging (MRI) studies, or both, included in their diagnostic evaluation. These estimates seem unrealistically high and do not reflect our current experiences. Previous NIAID-ASG reports have suggested a more reasonable incidence of 22% for non-HSE diseases, of which 40% were reportedly treatable,[16] providing an overall figure of 9% for the diagnosis of treatable non-HSE diseases. A recent study from Andersen and associates substantiates this lower incidence.[1] In this study, brain biopsy provided alternative diagnoses in 14% of patients (4 of 29) and diagnoses of treatable non-HSE diseases in 7% of patients.[1] These results seem much more in line with our own experience and suggest that in reviewing so-called decision-analysis studies,[3,4,14] one must carefully consider the studies' implicit assumptions before deciding to what degree to follow their recommendations.

Another important factor in the decision is the rate of serious complications resulting from acyclovir therapy. Serious adverse reactions to acyclovir are uncommon.[15] In the original collaborative trial of acyclovir versus vidarabine reatment in HSE, only 1 (3%) of 32 patients had an adverse clinical reaction to acyclovir therapy (erythema at the intravenous site).[15] Broader clinical experience with acyclovir suggest that serious complications (e.g., encephalopathy) occur in less than 2% of patients. Minor complications are more frequent and include phlebitis at the infusion site (9%); transient elevations in blood urea nitrogen (BUN) or creatinine, or both (5% to 10%); nausea or vomiting (7%); itching and hives (2%); and abnormalities in liver function tests (1%).

A final factor in the decision regarding biopsy is an estimate of the likelihood that a patient will actually have HSE (i.e., its prevalence). In a simplified sense, the more likely it is that a patient has HSE, the less necessary it is to consider biopsy. Ideally, biopsy should be reserved for the subset of patients who are unlikely to have HSE. In these patients, the risk of biopsy is outweighed by the proportionally greater chance that biopsy will provide an alternative treatable diagnosis. The high- and low-likelihood HSE patients must be accurately identified in a prospective fashion, using available clinical and laboratory resources. In the NIAID collaborative trials, the incidence of HSE in the population designated by experienced clinicians as having suspected HSE was approximately 35%. The probability that a patient has HSE is substantially enhanced if the patient has a cerebrospinal fluid (CSF) pleocytosis (≥ 5 cells/mm^3), is 30 years of age or older, and has focal findings on electroencephalography (EEG), CT, or MRI studies.[14]

We suggest that all patients over the age of 30 who have a CSF pleocytosis and focal findings on at least one diagnostic study should be given acyclovir without prior brain biopsy. Patients without a CSF pleocytosis are unlikely to have HSE ($\geq 95\%$ of documented HSE cases have a CSF pleocytosis) and should generally not receive acyclovir unless they have had a confirmatory biopsy. Patients with a CSF pleocytosis but no focal features on diagnostic study continue to be an ambiguous group. We currently treat these patients with acyclovir without obtaining a biopsy and reserve biopsy for those who fail to respond to therapy.

The debate about biopsy or no biopsy would quickly disappear if a safe, sensitive, and specific test could be developed that would allow diagnosis of HSE early after the onset of symptoms. A number of recent studies[2,10,12,13] suggest that polymerase chain reaction (PCR) amplification of herpes simplex virus DNA from the CSF may provide such a test. Although more detailed studies are required, early indications are that PCR is sensitive and specific[2,10,12,13] and that positive results may be reliably obtained within days after onset of the first neurologic symptoms.[2] If these results can be confirmed in large-scale studies, we may be able to reserve acyclovir therapy for patients with positive results of PCR amplification of herpes simplex virus DNA from the CSF.

References

1. Anderson NE, Willoughby EW, Synek BJL, Croxson MC, and Glasgow GL: Brain biopsy in the management of focal encephalitis. J Neurol Neurosurg Psychiatry 54:1001–1003, 1991.
2. Aurelius E, Johansson B, Skoldenberg B, Staland A, and Forsgren M: Rapid diagnosis of herpes simplex encephalitis by nested polymerase chain reaction assay of cerebrospinal fluid. Lancet 337:189–192 1991.
3. Barza M and Pauker SG: The decision to biopsy, treat, or wait in suspected herpes encephalitis. Ann Intern Med 92:641–649, 1980.
4. Braun P: The clinical management of suspected herpes viral encephalitis. Am J Med 69:895–902, 1980.
5. Caplan LR: Brain biopsy in herpes simplex encephalitis [letter]. N Engl J Med 303:700, 1980.
6. Fishman RA: No, brain biopsy need not be done in every patient suspected of having herpes simplex encephalitis. Arch Neurol 44:1291–1292, 1987.
7. Hanley DF, Johnson RT, and Whitley RJ: Yes, brain biopsy should be a prerequisite for herpes simplex encephalitis treatment. Arch Neurol 44:1289–1290, 1987.
8. Hirsch MS and Swartz MN: Brain biopsy in herpes simplex encephalitis [letter]. N Engl J Med 303:700–701, 1980.
9. Kaufman HH and Catalano LW: Diagnostic brain biopsy: A series of 50 cases and a review. Neurosurgery 4:129–136, 1979.
10. Klapper PE, Cleator GM, Dennett C, and Lewis AG: Diagnosis of herpes encephalitis via Southern blotting of cerebrospinal fluid DNA amplified by polymerase chain reaction. J Med Virol 32:261–264, 1990.
11. Morawetz RB, Whitley RJ, and Murphy DM: Experience with brain biopsy for suspected herpes encephalitis: A review of 40 consecutive cases. Neurosurgery 12:654–657, 1983.
12. Puchammer-Stockl E, Popow-Kraupp T, Heinz FX, Mandl CW, and Kunz C: Establishment of PCR for the early diagnosis of herpes simplex encephalitis. J Med Virol 32:77–82, 1990.
13. Rowley AH, Whitley RJ, Lakeman FD, and Wolinsky SM: Rapid detection of herpes-simplex-virus DNA in cerebrospinal fluid of patients with herpes simplex encephalitis. Lancet 335:440–441, 1990.
14. Soong S-J, Watson NE, Caddell GR, Alford CA Jr, Whitley RJ, and NIAID Collaborative Antiviral Study Group: Use of brain biopsy for diagnostic evaluation of patients with suspected herpes simplex encephalitis: A statistical model and its clinical implications. J Infect Dis 163:17–22, 1991.
15. Whitley RJ, Alford CA, Hirsch MS, et al: Vidarabine versus acyclovir therapy in herpes simplex encephalitis. N Engl J Med 314:144–149, 1986.
16. Whitley RJ, Cobbs CG, and Alford CA: Diseases that mimic herpes simplex encephalitis. Diagnosis, presentation, and outcome. JAMA 262:234–239, 1989.

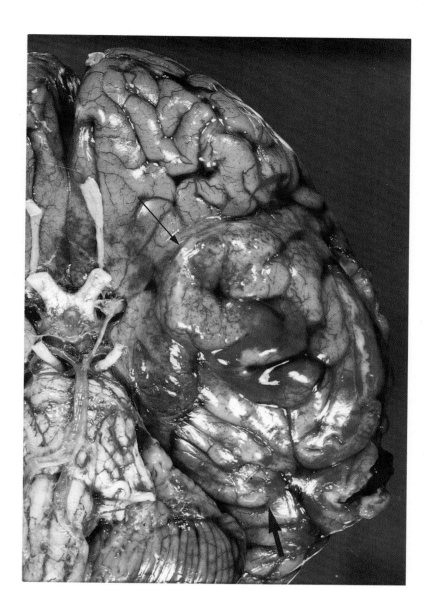

Figure 4–5. HSV encephalitis. At autopsy, the medial surface of the temporal lobe (*area between arrows*) shows petechial hemorrhage and congestion of small vessels. (Courtesy of Dr. J. Richard Baringer, Department of Neurology, University of Utah School of Medicine, Salt Lake City.)

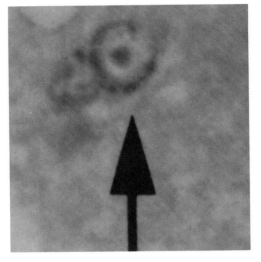

Figure 4-6

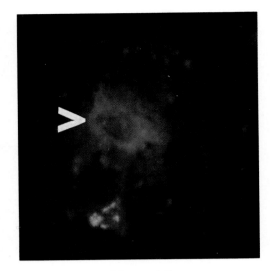

Figure 4-7

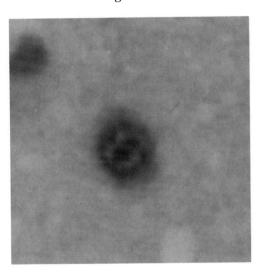

Figure 4-8

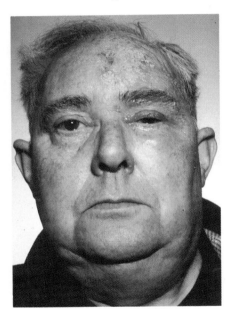

Figure 4-10

Figure 4–6. HSV encephalitis. Microscopic section shows a Cowdry A intranuclear inclusion body (*arrow*). (Original magnification x 880) (Courtesy of Dr. B. K. DeMasters, Department of Pathology [Neuropathology], University of Colorado School of Medicine, Denver.)

Figure 4–7. HSV encephalitis. Indirect immunofluorescence of brain biopsy impression smear with rabbit anti–HSV serum and goat anti–rabbit fluorescein isothiocyanate–conjugated immunoglobulin G. White arrow indicates characteristic apple-green fluorescence of an HSV-positive cell. (Original magnification x 880)

Figure 4–8. HSV encephalitis. Indirect immunoperoxidase stain of brain section with rabbit anti-HSV serum. Brown-staining cells contain HSV antigen. (Original magnification x 880)(Courtesy of Dr. B. K. DeMasters, Department of Pathology [Neuropathology], University of Colorado School of Medicine, Denver.)

Figure 4–10. Clinical ophthalmic distribution zoster. (From Blackwood W, Perkin GD, Rose FC, Shawdon HH: Slide Atlas of Neurology: Miscellaneous Disorders II. Presented by Sandoz Pharmaceuticals, Gower Medical Publishing, London, England, 1985, slide index no. 9.22, with permission.)

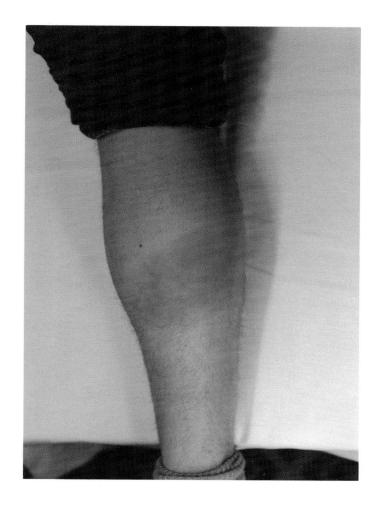

Figure 10–1. Erythema chronicum migrans.

Chapter 5

ENTEROVIRUS INFECTIONS OF THE CENTRAL NERVOUS SYSTEM

Howard L. Lipton, M.D., and Burk Jubelt, M.D.

CLASSIFICATION
PHYSICAL, BIOCHEMICAL, AND
  STRUCTURAL PROPERTIES
VIRUS REPLICATIVE CYCLE AND
  STRATEGY OF GENE EXPRESSION
PATHOGENESIS AND PATHOLOGY
NEUROVIRULENCE AND
  ATTENUATION
IMMUNITY
DISEASES
LABORATORY DIAGNOSIS
TREATMENT

The human enteroviruses, which include the polioviruses, coxsackieviruses, echoviruses, and the newer enteroviruses, were grouped together within the picornavirus family because they infect the human alimentary tract, their portal of entry to the host. Although central nervous system (CNS) involvement is a rare occurrence in enterovirus infections, these are the most frequent viruses recovered from the cerebrospinal fluid (CSF), probably because of the sheer frequency of such infections in the population.

Paralytic poliomyelitis (acute anterior poliomyelitis, infantile paralysis, Heine-Medin disease) was first depicted on the stele of Ruma from the 18th Egyptian dynasty (1580–1350 B.C.)[108] (Fig. 5–1). Poliomyelitis remained a sporadic and poorly defined disease until the occurrence of epidemics in the second half of the 19th century in Europe and North America. We now know that epidemic poliomyelitis is a modern disease, with outbreaks related to reduced "herd immunity" from improved hygiene, sanitation, and social conditions found in the more developed countries of the world. The development of the Salk killed-poliovirus vaccine in 1954–1955 and the Sabin live, attenuated oral poliovaccine in 1961 dramatically reduced the annual incidence of paralytic poliomyelitis in the United States from more than 20,000 cases in 1952 to fewer than 10 cases in the 1980s.[134] In 1948, the first nonpolio enteroviruses were isolated during an outbreak of poliomyelitis in the town of Coxsackie, New York. The virus was recovered from infant mice inoculated with suspensions made from the feces of children suffering from paralysis and was later designated a group A coxsackievirus after the place of discovery.[30] Subsequently, more than 70 additional human enteroviruses have been isolated in a variety of diseases.

Paralytic poliomyelitis is still a serious problem in underdeveloped areas of the world that lack adequate vaccination programs,[3,124] and the other enteroviruses remain a major cause of aseptic meningitis worldwide. Of the newly isolated enteroviruses, enterovirus 70

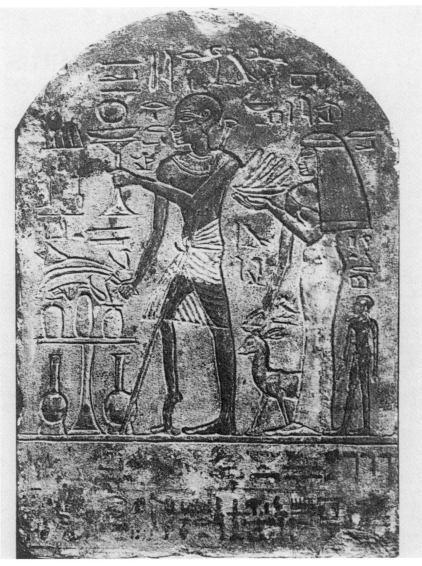

Figure 5–1. Egyptian stele, dating from the 18th dynasty (1580–1350 B.C.), now in the Carlsberg Glyptothek, Copenhagen, showing the typical wasting of a limb following poliomyelitis. (Reproduced courtesy of the National Foundation for Infantile Paralysis.)

has been the cause of epidemic acute hemorrhagic conjunctivitis in which lower-motor-neuron paralysis of the legs is a common complication.[139] Since its discovery, enterovirus 71 has been recognized as a prominent cause of aseptic meningitis and encephalitis.[21] Although poliomyelitis can now be prevented, there has been a renewed interest in the human polioviruses, since the development of modern molecular techniques has made poliovirus genetics particularly amenable to molecular pathogenetic studies of attenuation and virulence (vaccine versus wild-type strains).[71,103] The precise viral-coat amino acids that stimulate the production of neutralizing antibodies form the virion binding site that docks with the host cell receptor molecules and interact with antiviral agents are the target of refined crystallographic studies.[48,104,120,131] In addition, poliomyelitis infection provides the classic paradigm of selective neuronal vulnerability and provides an important experimental animal model system for studying the pathogenesis of neuronal infection.

CLASSIFICATION

The human enteroviruses comprise one group or genus of the family Picornaviridae. The word picornavirus was derived from *pico,* meaning "very small," and RNA, which denotes the type of nucleic acid found in the viral genome.[85] The other major groups of picornaviruses include the human rhinoviruses, hepatitis A virus, the aphthoviruses or foot-and-mouth–disease viruses, and the cardioviruses. The aphthoviruses were, in fact, the first animal viruses to be recognized. The human rhinoviruses are important etiologic agents of the common cold; hepatitis A virus, of infectious hepatitis; the aphthoviruses, of serious systemic illness in cloven-hooved animals; and the cardioviruses, which are known primarily to infect murine and other animal species, of aseptic meningitis in humans.[32,39]

The enteroviruses are distinguished by their common habitat, the alimentary tract, and by their similar physical and biochemical properties.[80] The human enteroviruses include 3 serotypes of polioviruses, 23 serotypes of group A and 6 serotypes of group B coxsackieviruses, 31 serotypes of echoviruses, and 5 serotypes of the newer enteroviruses (Table 5–1).[80] Originally, the various enterovirus groups were separated on the basis of the type of neurologic disease they caused (paralysis versus aseptic meningitis as well as systemic manifestations) and virologic properties (ability to kill newborn mice, growth in cell culture, and so forth). The nomenclature of the human enteroviruses has been changed, however, because many of the properties thought to be specific for the coxsackieviruses and echoviruses, especially mouse pathogenicity and replication in cell culture, in fact overlap. Because the original distinctions between these two groups have become obscured,[119] new enterovirus isolates are now being designated by number, such as enterovirus 68-72. The various enteroviruses are also distinguished serologically by the ability of specific antisera to neutralize the homologous or homotypic virus.[80]

PHYSICAL, BIOCHEMICAL, AND STRUCTURAL PROPERTIES

Although host range and tissue tropism are quite diverse, picornaviruses share many common properties and a unique strategy of gene expression. Picornavirions are isometric or spheroidal particles, 28 to 30 nm in diameter, and lack a lipid coat or envelope (Fig. 5–2). The virion consists of a protein shell or capsid (coat) surrounding an internal core of ribonucleic acid (RNA). The RNA accounts for 30% of the weight of the virion, and the protein coat, 70%. The virion coat consists of four structural proteins, originally

Table 5–1 CLASSIFICATION OF THE HUMAN ENTEROVIRUS GENUS IN THE FAMILY PICORNAVIRIDAE

Subgroups	No. of Serotypes	Member Species
Polioviruses	3	Human polioviruses 1–3
Coxsackieviruses		
Group A	23	Human coxsackieviruses A1–22, 24
Group B	6	Human coxsackieviruses B1–6
Echoviruses	31	Human echoviruses 1–9, 11–27, 29–33
Enteroviruses	5	Human enteroviruses 68–72

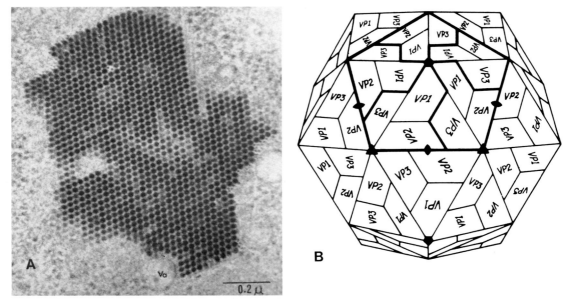

Figure 5–2. *A*, Electron micrograph of picornavirus crystals in the cytoplasm of an infected cell ×90,000. (From Dales et al,[29] p 386, with permission.) *B*, Schematic drawing of the external surface of a picornavirus, demonstrating the icosahedral symmetry. The basic protomeric unit consisting of VP1, VP2, and VP3 is thickly outlined; VP4 is buried beneath the surface. Five protomers make up one pentamer (also thickly outlined), and each virion consists of 12 pentamers. (Reprinted by permission from *Nature,* Vol 317, pp 145–153. Copyright © 1985 Macmillan Magazines Limited.)

numbered according to increasing electrophoretic mobility on sodium dodecyl sulfate (SDS)-polyacrylamide gels as virus protein (VP)1, VP2, VP3, and VP4 and now designated according to their position on the RNA genome.[125] A trace of a fifth protein, VP0, which undergoes cleavage to form VP2 and VP4 during virus assembly as the RNA is inserted into the coat, is present in the virion.[1] Recent x-ray diffraction studies of crystal picornaviruses have resolved the virion structure to an atomic level (2.9 Å).[48,120] Figure 5–2B shows the alignment of VP1, VP2, and VP3 chains in the protomer.

The genome of human enteroviruses consists of a single strand of RNA of positive or message-sense polarity, approximately 7400 nucleotides in size, with a molecular mass of 2.58×10^6 (polioviruses;[65,113,136] other enteroviruses cited in reference 63). A small protein, VPg, is covalently linked to the 5'end of the virion RNA, and a polyadenylated tail of variable length is present at the 3'end of the RNA.

Four neutralization antigenic sites have been mapped on the external loops of the major poliovirus proteins.[104] These sites have been identified by sequencing virus mutants that escape neutralization by monoclonal antibodies and then relating the mutated residues to the three-dimensional virus structure. Recent studies suggest that neutralization at the different poliovirus sites occurs by different mechanisms; these include induction of a conformational change that prevents uncoating and virion aggregation. In addition, the putative virus receptor attachment site has also been identified on poliovirus as a 25-Å-deep canyon circulating around each of the 12 pentamer vertices.[48] Site-specific mutations of residues lining a homologous crevice in human rhinovirus-14 (HRV-14) resulted in mutant viruses that exhibited altered binding affinities for host cells, thus providing strong evidence that the canyon is indeed involved in cell attachment.[22] Because the F(ab)₂ fragment of an antibody molecule has a diameter of approximately 35 Å, it would have difficulty reaching the canyon floor. Thus, it has been suggested that the residues in the canyon are not subjected to immune selection.[120]

VIRUS REPLICATIVE CYCLE AND STRATEGY OF GENE EXPRESSION

Viruses attach to a specific cellular receptor molecule as an initial step in the process of infection. In fact, attachment to a cellular receptor probably plays a major role in determining species and tissue tropism for all classes of viruses, including the human enteroviruses.[25] Enteroviruses do not have a common receptor; instead each group of enteroviruses probably attaches to its own specific receptor molecule. For example, the three poliovirus serotypes share a common receptor that differs from the receptor for the group A and B coxsackieviruses.[25,75] Remarkable progress has recently been made in identifying the human poliovirus receptor. Mendelsohn and colleagues[88] isolated complementary deoxyribonucleic acid (cDNA) clones encoding functional poliovirus receptors. The predicted amino acid sequence revealed that the poliovirus receptor is an integral membrane protein with the conserved amino acids and domain structure characteristic of members of the immunoglobulin superfamily. Interestingly, the HRV-14 receptor, intercellular adhesion molecule-1, which was also only recently identified, belongs to the immunoglobulin superfamily.[42,133,135] The natural function of the poliovirus receptor remains unknown. In contrast, little is known about the nature of the receptors for the other enteroviruses, although a plasma membrane protein of 50 kd has been isolated and identified as the coxsackievirus B3 receptor.[77]

After attachment, picornaviruses penetrate the cell by a poorly understood mechanism. This event is followed by uncoating and by release of the RNA into the cytoplasm. Picornaviruses then take over the synthetic machinery of the cell for replication and invariably inhibit host cell protein and nucleic acid synthesis (hepatitis A virus is an exception). Inhibition of host cell protein synthesis begins shortly after attachment, as early as ½ hour postinfection, and is essentially complete within several hours.[125] The mechanism of inhibition of host cell protein synthesis varies among the picornaviruses. For human poliovirus, the decline in protein synthesis is the result of inactivation of the complex of cap-binding proteins, collectively termed p220, by the poliovirus protein 2A.[68,74] Translation of poliovirus RNA is unaffected because the RNA does not possess a 5' cap structure and initiates translation via internal ribosome binding in the 5' noncoding region of the genome. Other picornaviruses, such as encephalomyocarditis virus (EMCV), shut off host cell protein synthesis by competition of viral RNA with cellular messenger RNA (mRNA), which is capped. A subsequent decline in cellular RNA synthesis is also seen in picornavirus-infected cells.

Picornavirus RNA is positive-sense and acts as its own mRNA. Since virus-encoded nonstructural proteins are not encapsidated in the virion and are required for replication, one of the first steps in this process is translation of the RNA genome.[125,130] A single large polyprotein of approximately 250 kd is synthesized from the viral RNA. This protein undergoes post-translational cleavage to form three primary products, which are then cleaved further to yield 11 viral polypeptides. These consist of the four coat proteins and a number of nonstructural proteins, some of which have defined functions, such as the viral protease that cleaves the polyprotein, and the viral RNA-dependent RNA polymerase.

Picornavirus RNA synthesis takes place in the cytoplasm on smooth membranes of the cell, in a structure called the replication complex. Virus RNA

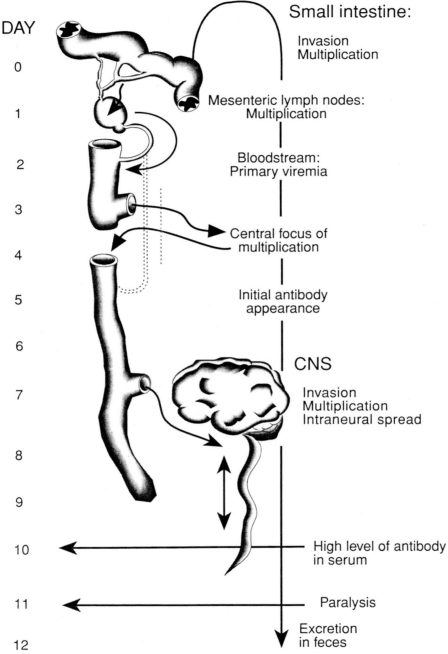

Figure 5–3. The pathogenesis of poliomyelitis. The virus enters by way of the alimentary tract, multiplies locally at the initial sites of virus attachment (eg, tonsils, Peyer's patches) or at the lymph nodes that drain these tissues, and is found in the throat and feces. Secondary virus spread occurs through the bloodstream to other susceptible tissues, namely other lymph nodes, brown fat, and the CNS. Within the CNS, the virus spreads along nerve fibers to susceptible cells such as motor neurons. If a high level of multiplication occurs, motor neurons are destroyed and paralysis develops. (From Melnick,[87] p 559, with permission.)

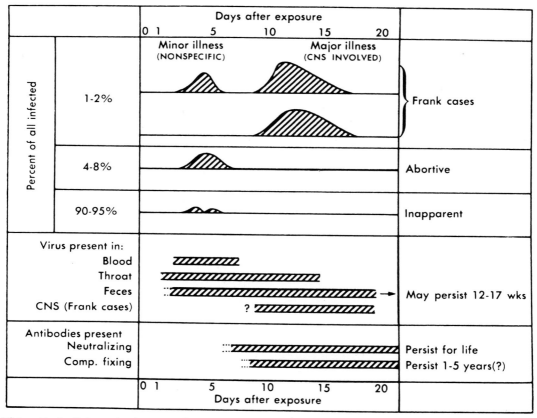

Figure 5–4. Schematic diagram of the clinical forms of poliomyelitis correlated with the times at which virus is present in various sites and the development of serum antibodies. (From Horstmann,[49] p 7, with permission.)

synthesis requires host cell factor(s) as well as the virus-encoded polymerase for generation of minus-strand RNAs from virion or plus-strand RNA.[70] Synthesis of new plus-strand RNAs then takes place in the replication complex, which consists of a minus-strand RNA and incomplete molecules of plus-strand RNA. Newly synthesized plus-strand RNAs are available for synthesis of more minus-strand RNAs, translation of the virus-encoded proteins, and packaging into virions.

PATHOGENESIS AND PATHOLOGY

CNS infection by polio and other enteroviruses is a rare consequence of enteric infection (Figs. 5–3 and 5–4). After fecal-hand-oral or, less commonly, oropharyngeal-oral transmission, enteroviruses replicate in cells of the oropharynx and intestines. Some coxsackieviruses and echoviruses occasionally spread by aerosols and enter through the respiratory tract, causing pharyngitis and, occasionally, bronchitis and pneumonia. The eye can also be the portal of entry for some enteroviruses.

The incubation period, or time from virus exposure until the onset of the disease, varies for the different enterovirus diseases. It is shortest for conjunctivitis (12 to 24 hours), upper respiratory infections (2 to 3 days), and gastroenteritis (2 to 3 days), and longer for systemic illness. The incubation period for systemic poliovirus manifested in minor illness is usually 1 to 5 days.

Extraneural Infection

In 90% to 95% of individuals exposed to poliovirus, the infection is subclinical or inapparent (see Fig. 5–4).[49,107] After replication in the oropharyngeal and intestinal mucosa, virus is excreted within 24 to 48 hours. Virus can be isolated from the oropharynx for several days and occasionally for 3 to 4 weeks, whereas excretion in the stool may last for 3 to 4 months.[49] After replication in the oropharynx and intestine, poliovirus may spread to the lymphatic tissues, tonsils, and lamina propria of the oropharynx and Peyer's patches of the ileum.[10] Virus may then spread to lymph nodes and the bloodstream (viremia). Primary viremia results in spread to nonneural target tissues, although CNS invasion may occur at this time. Nonneural target tissues include brown fat for the polioviruses, and muscle, skin, myocardium, pericardium, and pancreas for coxsackieviruses and echoviruses. After amplification of virus in nonneural tissues, a secondary viremia of greater magnitude then results in CNS invasion. The viremia occurs during the first week of infection and probably causes the minor illness (fever, headache, malaise) that is often accompanied by oropharyngeal and gastrointestinal symptoms (nausea, vomiting, abdominal discomfort, diarrhea). Minor illness only occurs in 5% to 10% of those infected.[49] At this point, poliovirus infection may be aborted or proceed to CNS invasion (see Fig. 5–4).

CNS Invasion

The precise route that poliovirus takes to the CNS remains unclear, but evidence suggests that viremia precedes CNS invasion.[95] Alternative pathways include direct spread of virus from the intestine along peripheral nerves,[126] or retrograde axonal transport of virus from neuromuscular junctions to the CNS.[7] The distal axon lacks a blood-brain barrier, and neurotropic strains of poliovirus can enter the CNS via retrograde transport after intramuscular inoculation.[58,94] The pantropic or viremic strains, however, which resemble wild-type poliovirus, preferentially spread by viremia to the CNS.[94,95] Immunization results in a neutralizing antibody response that prevents CNS invasion by curtailing viremia.[86,95] Although viremia is a prerequisite for CNS invasion in these instances, the possibility that viremia seeds the muscle and neuromuscular junction with virus, resulting in uptake by the terminal axon, cannot be excluded. Whereas polioviruses may replicate in skeletal muscle, coxsackieviruses and echoviruses clearly do replicate in muscle. Nonetheless, the weight of evidence favors poliovirus entering the neuraxis where the blood-brain barrier is defective, such as the area postrema.[9] The coxsackieviruses and echoviruses presumably enter the cerebrospinal fluid (CSF) through the choroid plexus.

Spread within the Central Nervous System

Although paralysis is the most dreaded complication of poliovirus infection, the ratio of paralytic to subclinical infections is low, ranging from 1:100 to 1:1000.[49,84] Polioviruses are believed to enter the CNS at one site[9] and then disseminate along nerve fiber pathways, probably by fast axonal transport, to other parts of the CNS.[10,59] Animal studies have demonstrated that the rate of fast axonal transport increases with age; thus, the increase in fast transport may explain why older children and adults are more prone to develop severe poliomyelitis.[59] Motor neurons, especially anterior horn cells, are susceptible to poliovirus, whereas glia, endothelium, and inflammatory cells appear to be spared (Fig. 5–5).[28,58] Results of in situ hybridization of polio RNA in neural lesions induced by poliovirus type 1 in monkeys demonstrated virus multiplication in motor neurons

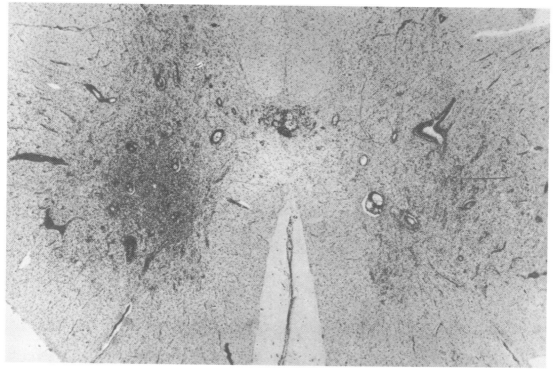

Figure 5–5. The lumbar spinal cord in acute poliomyelitis. Maximal pathology is localized to the anterior gray horn, where there is vascular congestion, motor neuron destruction, and perivascular and parenchymal inflammation, ×20. (From Bodian,[8] p 76, with permission.)

and in as-yet-unidentified small neural cells.[24] The destruction of anterior horn cells correlates with the clinical development of flaccid paralysis, but it is unclear whether the increased vulnerability of motor neurons is due to the presence and higher density of virus receptors on neurons, greater spread of virus along nerve fiber pathways, or other factors.

Intermediate and posterior horn neurons as well as bipolar neurons in the dorsal root ganglia may rarely be infected (Fig. 5–6). In the brain, large motor neurons in the precentral gyrus (Betz cells) and neurons in the thalamus and hypothalamus may be infected.[11] In the brainstem, motor nuclei (facial, hypoglossal, nucleus ambiguus), sensory nuclei (vestibular and trigeminal), and the reticular formation nuclei are involved. Infection within

these areas may result in brainstem encephalitis and respiratory insufficiency. The cerebellar vermis and roof nuclei may also be destroyed.[11]

Pathologic changes evolve rapidly after poliovirus infects a neuron (Fig. 5–7). Within several days, the Nissl bodies in the cytoplasm shrink and dissolve, leading to diffuse chromatolysis and loss of the basophilic staining reaction.[8] At this point, the infection may resolve and neurons may recover; alternatively, the infection may advance, leading to nuclear shrinkage with the appearance of eosinophilic type B inclusion bodies and ultimately cellular membrane disintegration. The inflammatory response consists of meningeal, perivascular, and parenchymal infiltrates. Polymorphonuclear cells may be seen early in the process, but the inflammatory cell response shifts primar-

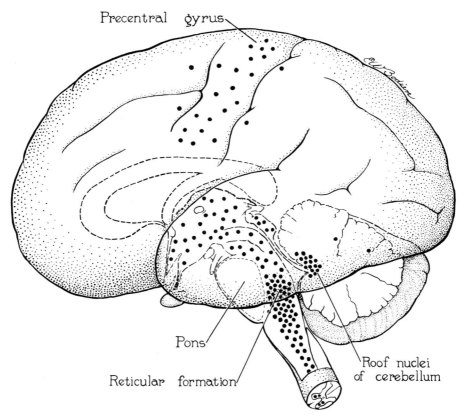

Figure 5–6. Lateral view of the brain and cervical spinal cord with schematic transparent projection of the midsagittal plane of the brainstem showing the usual distribution of lesions of poliomyelitis (indicated by *dots*). (From Bodian,[8] p 71, with permission.)

ily to mononuclear cells. Additional changes in the parenchyma include the proliferation of microglial cells and presence of neuronophagia (Fig. 5–8).

CNS involvement with some of the other enteroviruses, including enteroviruses 70 and 71, resembles that of poliovirus.[21,138] Coxsackieviruses and echoviruses probably are disseminated through the CSF and replicate in meningeal cells after entering through the choroid plexus. As mentioned, these viruses most frequently produce aseptic meningitis.

NEUROVIRULENCE AND ATTENUATION

Phenotypic markers intended to differentiate attenuated and wild-type polioviruses were in use by the late 1950s, but only recently have we begun to understand the molecular basis of poliovirus neurovirulence. Unsuccessful attempts were made to differentiate attenuated and wild-type strains by temperature sensitivity and by serology. Monkey neurovirulence is still required for licensing a poliovirus vaccine; attenuated polioviruses should demonstrate a reduced ability to induce paralysis and to spread within the monkey's CNS.[78]

Ribonuclease T1 oligonucleotide fingerprinting was the first technique that indicated genomic differences between attenuated and wild-type viruses.[99] Subsequently, Nomoto and coworkers[98] compared the complete nucleotide sequences for the poliovirus type 1 attenuated (vaccine) and wild-type strains.

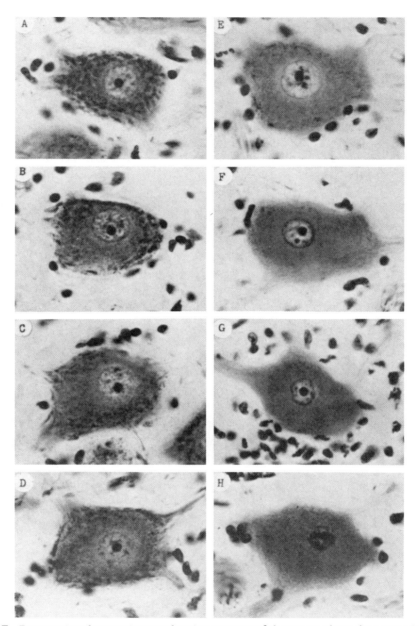

Figure 5–7. Progressive changes in spinal motor neurons of rhesus monkeys during acute poliomyelitis. *A*, Normal anterior horn cell. *B through D*, Early degenerative changes ×450. Note diffuse decrease in size of Nissl bodies (chromatolysis) and essentially normal nucleus. *E*, Severe chromatolysis with only a few small masses of Nissl substance at the cell periphery. Note clumping of chromatin in nucleus. *F*, Complete dissolution of Nissl bodies in cytoplasm. Nucleus is slightly shrunken and contains a small eosinophilic inclusion body. *G*, Cell similar to that in *F* with shrinkage of nucleus. *H*, Completely chromatolytic cell with severe, diffuse basophilia of cytoplasm and shrunken, distorted nucleus. (From Bodian,[8] p 164, with permission.)

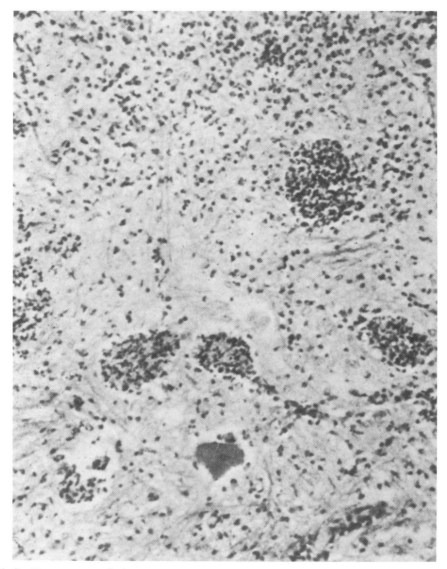

Figure 5–8. Microscopic inflammation. Anterior horn cells undergoing intense neuronophagia during acute poliomyelitis. Mononuclear inflammatory cells have also invaded the parenchyma. (From Price and Plum,[112] p 108, with permission.)

They identified 57 base substitutions and 21 amino acid changes. A cluster of amino acid changes were found in the coat proteins, especially in VP1. In contrast, only 10 nucleotide changes were identified between the poliovirus type 3 attenuated (vaccine) and wild-type strains, and there were only three amino acid substitutions (one each in VP1 and VP3 and one in protein 3B).[132]

A poliovirus type 3 revertant from the CNS of a child who died from vaccine-associated polio was then sequenced.[15] Seven nucleotide changes were found in the revertant virus, but only one change, nucleotide 472, a U—C, in the 5' noncoding region, was the same as that of the parental wild-type virus. Analysis of additional isolates from vaccine-related cases has confirmed that a

U—C mutation at position 472 correlates with reversion to neurovirulence.[35] Studies in which mice were inoculated with a mouse recombinant virus (type 3 vaccine 5' noncoding region and the remaining sequences from the Lansing type 2 strain) also showed that a U—C mutation at position 472 is associated with the virulence phenotype.[72] Several models have been proposed that suggest that mutations at this position change the predicted RNA secondary structure and reduce the efficiency of poliovirus translation.

Pathogenetic studies using recombinant poliovirus clones indicate that the sequences encoding the coat proteins influence host range and virulence.[71,103] La Monica and coworkers[73] found that monoclonal-antibody–selected variants of the Lansing strain of poliovirus type 2 had mutations in antigenic site 1 in VP1 as well as reduce neurovirulence in mice. Replacement of the residues of this site in poliovirus type 1 with the sequences from the Lansing strain of poliovirus type 2 showed that these residues are responsible for host range, i.e., mouse neurotropism in this instance.[79,92] Because the virion receptor attachment site abuts antigenic site 1, mutations in the latter are likely to alter poliovirus attachment to host cells and virulence.

Thus, two major areas in the viral RNA genome that influence poliovirus neurovirulence have been identified so far: sequences in the 5' noncoding region (particularly nucleotide 472), which affect the efficiency of viral translation; and sequences encoding the VP1 (1D) surface protein, which may relate to virion receptor activity.

Recombinant DNA technology is now being exploited to develop safer poliovirus vaccines. Inasmuch as most vaccine-related instances of paralysis are due to wild-type revertants of poliovirus type 3 (type 1 is remarkably stable), a hybrid virus combining the stability of the type 1 strain with the antigenic determinants of types 2 and 3 could be constructed. A chimeric Sabin type 1 strain containing an antigenic determinant of type 3 has been reported to induce neutralizing antibodies against both types 1 and 3.[14,92] Such a chimeric virus also had a more stable attenuated phenotype than did the type 3 parent.[67]

IMMUNITY

Natural infection or immunization with poliovirus leads to a brisk serotype-specific antibody response that is necessary for viral clearance. Immunoglobulin M (IgM)–neutralizing antibodies are detectable as early as 1 to 3 days, reach peak titers in 2 to 3 weeks, and then decline to undetectable levels by 3 months.[101] IgG-neutralizing antibodies increase slowly, reach peak titers in 2 to 3 months, and then decline over a period of several years. Thus, IgG-neutralizing antibodies can be detected for many years and provide life-long immunity.[118] Other types of antibodies that have been measured (for example, complement-fixing antibodies) do not persist for long periods of time. Some individuals who do not have detectable poliovirus antibodies resist reinfection because of an anamnestic response upon rechallenge with the live vaccines.[4]

High levels of neutralizing antibody depend on the occurrence of viremia.[9] Circulating antibodies are necessary to prevent hematogenous dissemination and neural invasion by poliovirus, and help to clear intestinal replication and prolonged shedding in the feces.[95] High levels of neutralizing antibody also protect monkeys and mice from intracerebral inoculation of poliovirus,[58,89] but the effect of circulating antibody on an established CNS infection is not clear. Evidence suggests that a local CNS antibody response to poliovirus is important in viral clearance.[90,102] Antibody responses in coxsackievirus and echovirus infections resemble those seen after poliovirus infections but have not been studied in detail (reviewed in Ref. 63).

The role of cell-mediated immunity in human enterovirus infections has not been well characterized. T-cell proliferative responses of low magnitude to poliovirus have been demonstrated in humans, presumably in previously exposed populations.[33] Studies in rodents have demonstrated virus-specific cellular immunity to coxsackievirus.[40] T-cell proliferative and delayed hypersensitivity responses to poliovirus in mice are mediated by CD4 T cells.[141]

DISEASES

The CNS is the organ system most commonly involved during the spread of human enterovirus infections from the alimentary tract. The neurologic syndromes that result are many, and each can be caused by a number of different types of enteroviruses. The syndromes associated with specific infecting viruses shown in Table 5–2 are only a guide for investigating clinical cases; some associations may have been overlooked, and new enterovirus isolates are continually being identified. Sys-

temic manifestations caused by the human enteroviruses are also diverse, and any single syndrome can be caused by multiple enterovirus serotypes.

Aseptic Meningitis

Aseptic meningitis is the most common neurologic syndrome due to enterovirus infection. In fact, enteroviruses are the most common causative agents of aseptic meningitis.[20,96] Earlier in the century, aseptic meningitis was thought primarily to be a form of nonparalytic poliomyelitis, but the majority of cases were probably caused by nonpolio enteroviruses. In 1976, the last year of surveillance reports from the Centers for Disease Control, enteroviruses were identified in 83% of the cases of viral meningitis in which a viral cause could be established.[16] Enterovirus meningitis is primarily caused by coxsackieviruses and echoviruses (see Table 5–2).[20,26,43]

Aseptic meningitis is characterized

Table 5–2 NEUROLOGIC SYNDROMES ASSOCIATED WITH THE HUMAN ENTEROVIRUSES

Syndrome	Virus Type
Aseptic viral meningitis	Polioviruses 1–3
	Coxsackieviruses A1–11, 14, 16–18, 22, 24
	Coxsackieviruses B1–6
	Echoviruses 1–7, 9, 11–25, 27, 30–33
	Enterovirus 71
Encephalitis	Polioviruses 1–3
	Coxsackieviruses A2, 4–9
	Coxsackieviruses B1–6
	Echoviruses 2–4, 6, 7, 9, 11, 14, 17–19, 25
	Enteroviruses 71, 72 (hepatitis A virus)
Lower-motor-neuron paralysis	Polioviruses 1–3
	Coxsackieviruses A2–4, 6–11, 14, 16, 21
	Coxsackieviruses 1–4, 6, 7, 9, 11, 13, 14, 16, 18–20, 30, 31
	Enteroviruses 70, 71
Acute cerebellar ataxia	Polioviruses 1, 3
	Coxsackieviruses A2, 4, 7, 9, B1–6
	Echoviruses 6, 9
	Enterovirus 71
Cranial nerve palsies	Polioviruses 1–3
	Coxsackieviruses A10, B5
	Echoviruses 4
	Enteroviruses 70
Chronic infections	Polioviruses 1–3 (vaccinelike strains)
	Coxsackieviruses A15, B3
	Echoviruses 2, 3, 5, 7, 9, 11, 15, 17–19, 22, 24, 25, 27, 29, 30, 33

by the acute onset of fever, headache, and meningeal signs; a CSF pleocytosis; sterile CSF bacteriologic cultures; and a benign course. Viruses are by far the most common cause of aseptic meningitis; hence the terms *viral* and *aseptic meningitis* are often used interchangeably. The meningeal inflammatory reaction is usually mononuclear in nature and presumably results from the replication of virus in meningeal and ependymal cells lining the CSF pathways.

Viral meningitis may begin as a nonspecific flulike illness with low-grade fever, pharyngitis, malaise, and photophobia. During enterovirus infections, involvement of other organ systems may coincide with meningitis; thus neurologic symptoms may be accompanied by rash, pleurodynia, or pericarditis. At other times, the onset of aseptic meningitis may be abrupt and heralded only by meningismus. Fever may range from 38° to 40°C, meningeal symptoms may vary from only subjective neck pain or stiffness to severe nuchal rigidity, and Kernig and Brudzinski signs may be elicited. Acute illness usually lasts for only a week, but malaise and fatigue may persist for a longer period.

The differential diagnosis of enterovirus meningitis includes other viruses as well as bacterial, fungal, and parasitic agents. Other viruses that frequently cause aseptic meningitis include the childhood agents of measles, mumps, varicella, and rubella, as well as herpes simplex virus, togaviruses, and bunyaviruses (arthropod-borne viruses), and lymphocytic choriomeningitis. It is impossible to differentiate among these viruses based on the clinical findings of aseptic meningitis alone, but differential diagnosis may be narrowed by the occurrence of specific nonneurologic manifestations, such as pleurodynia. On occasion, other infections may present as aseptic meningitis with a predominant mononuclear CSF pleocytosis. These conditions include subacute forms of bacterial infections (brucellosis, listeriosis, and mycoplasma), partially treated bacterial meningitis, parameningeal infections, leptospirosis, secondary syphilis, Lyme disease, tuberculosis, rickettsial infections (principally Rocky Mountain spotted fever), fungal meningitis (cryptococcosis, candidiasis, and coccidioidomycosis), and parasitic infections (cysticercosis and *Angiostrongylus* eosinophilic meningitis).[57,62] As many of these diseases progress, the CSF glucose level falls, directing the clinician to the correct causative category, since hypoglycorrhachia is rarely found in viral meningitis. The correct diagnosis may be made from appropriate bacterial and acid-fast organism stains and cultures. Noninfectious diseases, such as carcinomatous meningitis, collagen-vascular disorders, and sarcoidosis, should also be considered since they may present as aseptic meningitis.

Encephalitis

Human enteroviruses have accounted for almost one fourth of all cases of encephalitis of established cause in the years when there is increased seasonal activity of these viruses. On the other hand, the human enteroviruses are not a common cause of encephalitis except in infants. Enterovirus encephalitis is primarily due to infections with coxsackieviruses, echoviruses, and enterovirus 71. When poliovirus is the cause, the brainstem reticular activating system and cranial nerve motor nuclei are involved more often (bulbar polio) than the cerebral cortex. Apparently, hepatitis A virus (enterovirus 72) can also cause encephalitis, but hepatic encephalopathy is more frequently the cause of confusion during hepatitis A virus infections.[13,46]

Human enterovirus encephalitis is the result of direct virus invasion of the CNS and cytolytic destruction of neurons, in contrast to immune-mediated damage, which is the postulated mechanism of tissue damage in postinfectious encephalomyelitis. Patients may have symptoms and signs of aseptic meningitis, particularly fever, headache, and nuchal rigidity, in addition to signs of parenchymal involvement. The latter include alterations in consciousness or behavior, seizures, and focal deficits.[43] Mental status changes are usually only those of mild obtundation, although bizarre behavior and coma may be seen. The seizures usually are isolated and do not recur or progress to status epilepticus; focal deficits are also mild and transient in nature. Thus, human enterovirus encephalitis in older children and adults tends to be mild, with an excellent chance for full recovery. The fulminant encephalitis seen with neonatal coxsackievirus group B infections and chronic encephalitis seen in agammaglobulinemic patients are more serious disorders. Sells and colleagues[128] reported that enterovirus encephalitis in infants can produce subtle residual intellectual deficits.

Lower-Motor-Neuron Paralysis

Since the introduction of the polio vaccines over 30 years ago, the incidence of paralytic poliomyelitis has plummeted in the developed countries of the world. Only 154 cases of paralytic poliomyelitis were reported in the United States between 1975 and 1988, and the majority of cases were caused by the reversion to virulence of attenuated viruses in the live vaccines.[97,134] Nonetheless, poliomyelitis remains a serious health problem in the underdeveloped countries of the world.[3,124]

The term poliomyelitis is derived from the Greek words *polios* ("gray") and *myelon* ("marrow"). Thus, poliomyelitis is a virus infection of anterior horn motor neurons located in the spinal cord gray matter. In the 24 to 48 hours prior to the onset of paralysis, symptoms of fever, headache, nausea, vomiting, malaise, and sore throat constitute the minor illness (abortive or nonspecific poliomyelitis). Immediately or within 3 to 4 days after recovery, this stage may give way to the major illness.

The major illness encompasses all forms of CNS disease: nonparalytic polio or aseptic meningitis, polioencephalitis, bulbar polio, and paralytic poliomyelitis. Thus, aseptic meningitis may be seen prior to the onset of paralysis, as may polioencephalitis, which is characterized by tremulousness, agitation, obtundation, and upper-motor-neuron signs of hyperactive tendon reflexes, spasticity, and extensor plantar responses (Babinski sign). In addition, radicular pains, muscle aches and cramping, and fasciculations in an extremity may precede the onset of paralysis. At any of these stages, poliovirus may be neutralized and cleared by the reticuloendothelial system, aborting progression to paralysis.

PARALYTIC POLIOMYELITIS

Paralytic poliomyelitis, which occurs in spinal, bulbar, and bulbospinal forms, accounts at most for only 5% of clinically apparent and 0.1% to 2% of all poliovirus infections.[49,84] Spinal poliomyelitis occurs more frequently than the bulbar form. The lumbar region of the spinal cord is affected more often than the cervical segments. Characteristically, paralysis is flaccid, asymmetric, affects proximal more than distal muscles, and unpredictably skips muscle groups of an extremity (see Fig. 5-1). As paralysis progresses, tendon reflexes are lost, additional extremities become paralyzed, and the medulla may be involved causing an impairment in respiration. Extension of paralysis is unlikely after the fifth or sixth day. Spinal poliomyelitis can also produce autonomic dysfunction (hyperhidrosis or hypohidrosis and decreased skin temperature), urinary retention, and sensory symptoms, but very rarely, sensory signs.[111]

Bulbar poliomyelitis constitutes 10% to 15% of the paralytic cases and may involve any cranial nerve and/or the pontomedullary reticular formation. Bulbar polio without paralysis of the limbs is more common in children, whereas adults with bulbar involvement usually have limb paralysis. Cranial nerves that are commonly affected include the seventh, ninth, and tenth, resulting in facial weakness, dysphonia, and dysphagia. Less commonly, the fifth and twelfth cranial nerves are affected, in which case weakness of the mastication muscles and tongue is seen. Infrequently, diplopia due to extraocular muscle paresis has been reported. Involvement of the reticular formation produces irregularities of respiration and cardiovascular function (hypotension, hypertension, and cardiac arrhythmias).

A number of factors has been associated with increased risk of paralytic poliomyelitis. Adults are not only at greater risk than young children, but the paralysis is likely to be more severe in adults (reviewed in Ref. 63). Tonsillectomy has also been shown to be predisposing for bulbar poliomyelitis,[100] and antecedent intramuscular injections, trauma, and exercise predispose the involved extremity(s) to paralysis.[44] Rindge[115] found that pregnancy is associated with increased risk of paralytic polio.

PARALYSIS CAUSED BY NONPOLIO ENTEROVIRUSES

Although uncommon, paralysis caused by nonpolio enteroviruses has been reported. Of 52 recorded cases of paralysis caused by human enteroviruses in the United States from 1976 to 1979, 25 cases were caused by polioviruses, 18 by echoviruses, 7 by coxsackieviruses, and 2 by enterovirus 71.[17] Paralysis seen with coxsackievirus and echovirus infections is usually mild. In fact, the absence of a residual deficit 60 days after the onset of paralysis has been used as a criterion for differentiating nonpolio enterovirus paralysis from that due to the polioviruses.

Enterovirus 70 has caused epidemics of acute hemorrhagic conjunctivitis (AHC) in many parts of the world. AHC epidemics began in Asia and Africa and have spread to Latin America and the United States.[106] It has been estimated that the neurologic involvement seen principally in adults occurs in 1:10,000 to 1:15,000 cases of AHC.[138,139] Typically, paralysis begins several days to weeks following AHC. Neurologic involvement often begins with backache and radicular pains several days before the onset of flaccid paralysis of the lower limbs; paralysis tends to be asymmetric and to affect more proximal muscles. Because of early reports of the frequent occurrence of radicular pains and paresthesias, the disorder was thought to be a radiculomyelitis.[51] There has been little objective evidence of radicular sensory abnormalities, however, and during more recent epidemics, radicular symptoms have been less common.[64,139] Approximately one half of patients with leg paralysis develop proximal arm weakness. Isolated cranial nerve palsies, particularly facial weakness, vertigo, pyramidal tract signs, and urinary incontinence, are other manifestations of enterovirus 70 infection. Paralysis following AHC has not been reported in the Americas.[106]

Enterovirus 71 infection has a variable clinical picture. Enterovirus 71 was first isolated in California in 1969 in association with hand-foot-and-mouth disease and aseptic meningitis.[127] In Bulgaria, enterovirus 71 caused a severe outbreak of poliolike paralysis; although aseptic meningitis was the most common CNS manifestation, different forms of paralysis were seen, including fatal bulbar paralysis.[21] In an enterovirus 71 epidemic in Hungary in 1979, encephalitis was almost as common as meningitis, and paralysis occurred infrequently.[93] During a limited outbreak of enterovirus 71 infection in New York State, two individuals were reported to have mild paralysis.[19]

DIFFERENTIAL DIAGNOSIS

The differential diagnosis of paralysis should include those enteroviruses listed in Table 5–2 as causing paralysis. In addition, several other viruses have occasionally caused flaccid paralysis, including rabies and herpes zoster virus. Guillain-Barré syndrome, botulism, toxic neuropathies, acute intermittent porphyria, acute transverse myelitis, and acute spinal cord compression from epidural abscess should also be considered.[41]

Acute Cerebellar Ataxia

Whereas this syndrome is more commonly associated with other viruses, several of the human enteroviruses have been reported to cause acute cerebellar ataxia in children (see Table 5–2) (reviewed in Ref. 61). In addition, enterovirus 71 has been reported to be associated with cerebellitis in Japan.[53]

Cranial Nerve Palsies

Enterovirus 70 has caused cranial nerve palsies in as many as one half of patients with neurologic sequelae in epidemics of AHC.[64,139] Isolated cranial nerve palsies have occurred in as many as a quarter of these patients, although the incidence was much lower in some epidemics.[64,139] The seventh nerve is affected most frequently, followed by involvement of the motor division of the fifth nerve, and, less commonly, the other cranial nerves. Isolated seventh nerve palsy after poliovirus, coxsackievirus, and echovirus infections has been reported (reviewed in Ref. 63).

Uncommon Neurologic Complications

Human enterovirus infections have been implicated in the pathogenesis of several other neurologic disorders, but the causal relationship has not always been clear. Coxsackievirus A9 has been isolated from the CSF of two patients with acute infantile hemiplegia.[18,117] Kuban and colleagues[69] reported the isolation of coxsackievirus B3 from two children with the opsoclonus-myoclonus syndrome. The isolate in one case

was from the CSF and in the other, from the stool, but there was serologic confirmation in the latter instance. Coxsackievirus B2 encephalitis has resulted in parkinsonism in two patients.[12,140] Hemichorea as a manifestation of focal encephalitis was reported in a case of serologically confirmed echovirus infection.[109] Transverse myelitis appears to have been caused by poliovirus in one instance,[37] echoviruses in two cases,[6,55] and hepatitis A virus (enterovirus 72) in one case.[137] Guillain-Barré syndrome has been associated with coxsackieviruses A2, 5, 6, and 9, B1 and 5, and with echoviruses 6, 7, 9, and 22.[38,41,43,105]

Chronic (Persistent) Enterovirus Infections

Although uncommon, chronic human enterovirus infections typically occur in patients with profound immunodeficiencies, not in individuals with normal immune function. The viruses that cause these infections are characterized by low virulence and reduced invasiveness, and include the poliovirus vaccine strains,[143,144] echoviruses,[82] and, less often, coxsackieviruses.[23,82] Children with hypogammaglobulinemia or agammaglobulinemia and normal cellular immunity are at greatest risk. Poliovirus infections have been seen in patients with combined immunodeficiency, however, and in one patient with cellular immune deficiency.[114,143]

The clinical picture is that of a slowly progressive neurologic disease that lasts for months to years. In the poliovirus cases, several months usually elapse between vaccination and onset of disease. Affected individuals may present with lower-motor-neuron paralysis or progressive intellectual and cerebral dysfunction with delayed paralysis.[31,114] In persistent echovirus infections, the brain is preferentially involved, and patients develop headaches, mental status or behavioral changes, seizures, pyramidal tract involvement, and tremors.[82] One half of patients also develop dermatomyositis, presumably from virus invasion of muscle, but echovirus has been isolated from muscle in only two instances.[2,83] Intense mononuclear cell infiltrates are found in the meninges and perivascular sites; microglial proliferation, microglial nodule formation, and neuronophagia are seen in the CNS despite humoral immunodeficiency. CSF examination also reveals a mononuclear pleocytosis.

Echoviruses but not poliovirus have been isolated from CSF, whereas both viruses can be isolated from feces because of chronic intestinal infection.[31,142] Recently, Rotbart and co-workers[123] detected echovirus 11 in the CSF of a 12-year-old boy with X-linked agammaglobulinemia and chronic meningoencephalitis by polymerase chain reaction (PCR) (see later discussion) despite negative routine virus cultures and negative nucleic acid hybridization studies. Most patients do not survive even when treated intravenously or intrathecally with specific antiviral antibodies.[34,36,45,56,83]

Postpolio Syndrome and Postpoliomyelitis Progressive Muscle Atrophy

Postpolio syndrome (PPS) is a well-described condition, principally of weakness, that develops many years after a bout of paralytic poliomyelitis.[60] PPS includes systemic symptoms, musculoskeletal complaints, and neurologic manifestations. Fatigue, pain, and weakness are the most common symptoms. When the combination of weakness and atrophy is present, the disorder is referred to as postpoliomyelitis progressive muscular atrophy (PPMA).[27] The insidious onset of weakness begins 30 to 40 years after paralysis in patients who have been clinically stable.[60,91] In general, the new weakness develops and progresses slowly in muscles that were previously affected by polio. Neither electromyographic nor muscle biopsy evidence of ongoing de-

nervation is able to distinguish between the stable postpolio patients and those developing weakness. Extensive virologic search has provided limited evidence of chronic poliovirus infection in PPMA,[60] although inflammatory changes have been found postmortem in the spinal cord, suggesting either an infectious or immune-mediated basis of this enigmatic disorder.[110] Another hypothesis of the cause has invoked overwork or excessive metabolic demand on motor units that remain after the initial bout of polio and that have reinnervated denervated fibers. The excessive metabolic demand from the increased motor unit territory results in loss of the reinnervating terminal sprouts or the motor neuron itself. This theory is supported by the observation that the association of more widespread and severe paralysis and greater functional recovery is a risk factor for development of PPMA.[66]

LABORATORY DIAGNOSIS

General laboratory tests are uninformative, and the CSF parameters, although abnormal, are no different than those seen with other CNS virus infections. The CSF cell count is increased, and typically an initial polymorphonuclear leukocyte response shifts to a predominantly mononuclear leukocyte one within 8 to 48 hours. Thus, it may be important to repeat lumbar puncture to exclude bacterial infection. Pleocytosis often reaches several hundred cells per mm^3, and occasionally several thousand cells, but declines precipitously within 2 weeks. Initially, CSF protein content is normal or mildly elevated, rising to 100 to 300 mg/dL over several weeks and possibly remaining elevated for months. Only rarely has hypoglycorrhachia been reported.[76] In patients with encephalitis, the electroencephalogram often reveals nonspecific mild to moderate slow wave activity that may be generalized or slightly asymmetric. Computed tomography and angiography are almost always normal since the infections are mild, but magnetic resonance imaging of the brain and spinal cord would be expected to show the areas of damage and surrounding edema.

Virus isolation, serologic tests, or both will reveal a specific human enterovirus etiology. Polioviruses, coxsackieviruses, echoviruses, and enterovirus 71 can be isolated from the oropharynx for several weeks and from the stool for several months after infection.[49] Several stool specimens should be tested because excretion may be intermittent. Enterovirus 70 is difficult to isolate except from the eye during conjunctivitis. Coxsackieviruses and echoviruses can be isolated from CSF in about one half of the cases; polioviruses and enteroviruses 70 and 71 are almost never recovered from the CSF.[26,53,138]

Because asymptomatic human enterovirus infections of the gastrointestinal tract are common, especially during the summer months, it is essential to determine the relevance of stool isolation by serology. Serologic testing for the group A coxsackieviruses and echoviruses is impractical because of the larger number of serotypes, but serology is helpful in diagnosing infections with poliovirus, group B coxsackieviruses, and enteroviruses 70 and 71. A fourfold or greater rise in serum antibody titer between acute- and convalescent-phase samples is considered diagnostic of acute infection. Therefore, acute- and convalescent-phase serum samples should be obtained, and the earlier in the infection that the acute-phase serum sample is drawn, the more likely a fourfold rise in titer will be detected. The convalescent-phase serum should be obtained at least 2 weeks, and preferably 4 weeks, after the acute-phase specimen has been drawn. Recently, an increased serum:CSF antibody ratio has been shown to be diagnostic of CNS infections for a number of viruses, including the human enteroviruses. The normal serum:CSF ratio is approximately 150:1.[50]

Recently, the PCR, a powerful method for amplifying nucleic acid sequences, has been used diagnostically to identify CNS infections by human enteroviruses in infants and children.[121] Since nucleotide sequences in the 5' noncoding region of the human enteroviruses are highly conserved, it has been possible to design a single set of oligonucleotide primers that will amplify all enteroviruses.[52,122] PCR is rapid and highly sensitive in detecting low levels of a virus genome, and it is possible to amplify less than 1 plaque-forming unit of an enterovirus from unconcentrated CSF (an equivalent of 1 to 10 fg of RNA or 10 RNA molecules). PCR is likely to be in common use in diagnostic laboratories in the near future.

TREATMENT

Treatment of enterovirus infections includes supportive care for the affected individual and prevention for others. Some degree of supportive care is needed for all patients with CNS enterovirus infections, but it is of paramount importance for those with encephalitis and paralytic disease. These patients require adequate fluids and electrolytes and support for cardiovascular and autonomic abnormalities and respiratory failure.[112] Encephalitic patients may also require anticonvulsants for seizures and sedation for delirium. Paralytic disease in the acute stage should be treated with bed rest, analgesics, hot packs for muscle pains, and appropriate positioning, such as splints to prevent contractures, foot boards to prevent foot drop, and frequent turning to prevent decubiti. Physical therapy is usually deferred until the convalescent stage except for nonvigorous range-of-motion exercise to prevent contractures. During convalescence, active physical therapy can be instituted. Bracing and other orthoses may be required. Orthopedic surgical intervention, if needed, should be postponed for 1 to 2 years, when recovery is maximal.[54]

The mainstay of prevention for poliomyelitis is vaccination. Both the inactivated poliomyelitis vaccine (Salk) and the live oral polio vaccine (Sabin) have dramatically reduced the incidence of poliomyelitis.[108,134] The advantages and disadvantages of the two vaccines have recently been reviewed.[5] In brief, the killed vaccine does not cause paralysis, but a very high level of vaccination in the population is required to prevent the spread of virulent viruses. Also, relatively short-term immunity with the Salk vaccine necessitates frequent revaccination. In contrast, the live vaccine, although more effective at producing long-term immunity, has the added risk of causing paralysis as the result of revertants' restoring the virulent phenotype. Still, the spread of live vaccine strains has eliminated virulent strains from the population in some countries and also has resulted in herd immunity with only an intermediate level of vaccination. The use of live oral vaccine appears to be most practical in the United States;[47] most developed countries, with the exceptions of the Scandinavian countries and Holland, use it.[5] A more potent inactivated poliovirus vaccine is now in use[116,129] and strategies for safer live oral polio vaccines are being investigated.[14,67] Vaccination is not available for other enterovirus infections.

No specific antiviral therapy is currently available for enterovirus infections, although the experimental agents arildone and its derivative, disoxaril, have been used successfully in treating acute poliovirus paralysis in mice[81] and in clearing persistent poliovirus infection in mice.[63] Analogs of these agents hold promise for an effective treatment of poliovirus and other enterovirus infections.

SUMMARY

The human enteroviruses, which include the polioviruses, coxsackieviruses, echoviruses, and some newly isolated enteroviruses, enter the body through the alimentary tract and usually do not affect the CNS. Because they are so widespread among the popula-

tion, however, they represent a major source of CNS infection. The virus initially spreads from the alimentary tract to the lymph nodes and bloodstream, then to various nonneural target tissues, producing a minor illness that may precede invasion of the CNS.

The systemic manifestations of infection and resulting neurologic syndromes vary, and each may be caused by any of a number of different enteroviruses. Enteroviruses are the most common cause of aseptic meningitis and may also cause encephalitis (especially in infants), lower-motor-neuron paralysis, and occasionally other syndromes. Polymerase chain reaction testing is expected to facilitate the future diagnosis of CNS enterovirus infections.

Treatment consists of supportive care, which is especially important for those with encephalitis or paralytic disease. Vaccination has been effective in preventing poliomyelitis, but no effective vaccine is available for other enterovirus infections.

REFERENCES

1. Arnold E, Luo M, Vriend G, et al: Implications of the picornavirus capsid structure for polyprotein processing. Proc Natl Acad Sci U S A 84:21–25, 1987.
2. Asherson GL and Webster ABD: Sex-linked hypogammaglobulinemia. In Asherson GL and Webster ABD (eds): Diagnosis and Treatment of Immunodeficiency Diseases. Blackwell, Oxford, 1980, pp 7–36.
3. Assaad F and Ljungars-Esteves F: World overview of poliomyelitis: Regional patterns and trends. Rev Infect Dis 6:S302–S307, 1984.
4. Bass JW, Halstead SB, Fischer GW, Podgore JK, and Wiebe RA: Oral poliovaccine-effect of booster vaccination 1 to 14 years after primary series. JAMA 239:2252–2255, 1978.
5. Beale AJ: Polio vaccines: Time for a change in immunisation policy? Lancet 335:839–842, 1990.

6. Bell EJ and Russell SJ: Acute transverse myelopathy and ECHO-2 virus infection. Lancet 2:1226–1227, 1963.

7. Blinzinger K and Anzil AP: Neural route of infection in viral diseases of the central nervous system. Lancet 2:1374–1375, 1974.

8. Bodian D: Poliomyelitis: Pathologic anatomy. In Poliomyelitis: Papers and Discussions Presented at the First International Poliomyelitis Conference. Lippincott, Philadelphia, 1949, pp 62–84.

9. Bodian D: Viremia in experimental poliomyelitis. I. General aspects of infection after intravascular inoculation with strains of high and low invasiveness. Am J Hyg 60:339–357, 1954.

10. Bodian D: Emerging concepts of poliomyelitis infection. Science 122:105–108, 1955.

11. Bodian D: Poliomyelitis. In Minckler J (ed): Pathology of the Nervous System. McGraw-Hill, New York, 1972, pp 2323–2394.

12. Bojinov S, Mitov G, and Nivov N: Attempted virologic and serologic verification of contemporary acute parkinsonism encephalitis. Nevrol Psikhiatr Nevrokhir 13:369–378, 1974.

13. Bromberg K, Newhall DN, and Peter G: Hepatitis A and meningoencephalitis. JAMA 247:815, 1982.

14. Burke KL, Dunn G, Ferguson M, Minor PD, and Almond JW: Antigen chimaeras of poliovirus as potential new vaccines. Nature 332:81–82, 1988.

15. Cann ALJ, Stanway G, Hughes PJ, et al: Reversion to neurovirulence of the live-attenuated Sabin type 3 oral poliovirus vaccine. Nucleic Acids Res 12:7787–7792, 1984.

16. Centers for Disease Control: Aseptic meningitis surveillance. Annual summary, 1976. 1979.

17. Centers for Disease Control: Enterovirus surveillance report, 1970–1979. US Dept of Health and Human Services, Atlanta, 1981.

18. Chalhub EG, Devivo DC, Siegel BA, Gado MH, and Feigin RD: Coxsackie A9 focal encephalitis associated with acute infantile hemiplegia and porencephaly. Neurology 27:574–579, US Dept of Health and Human Services, Atlanta, 1977.

19. Chonmaitree T, Menegus MA, Schervish-Swierkosz EM, and Schwalenstocker E: Enterovirus 71 infection: Report of an outbreak with two cases of paralysis and a review of the literature. Pediatrics 67:489–493, 1981.

20. Chonmaitree T, Menegus MA, and Powell KR: The clinical relevance of "CSF viral culture." A two year experience with aseptic meningitis in Rochester, N.Y. JAMA 247:1843–1847, 1982.

21. Chumakov M, Voroshilova M, Shindarov L, et al: Enterovirus 71 isolated from cases of epidemic poliomyelitis-like disease in Bulgaria. Arch Virol 60:329–340, 1979.

22. Colonno RJ, Condra JH, Mizutani S, Callahan PL, Davies ME, and Murcko MA: Evidence for the direct involvement of the rhinovirus canyon in receptor binding. Science 85:5449–5453, 1988.

23. Cooper JB, Pratt WP, English BK, and Shearer WT: Coxsackievirus B3 producing fatal meningoencephalitis in a patient with X-linked agammaglobulinemia. Am J Dis Child 137:82–83, 1983.

24. Couderc T, Christodoulou C, Kopecka H, et al: Molecular pathogenesis of neural lesions induced by poliovirus type 1. J Gen Virol 70:2907–2918, 1989.

25. Crowell RL and Landau BJ: Receptors in the initiation of picornavirus infections. In Fraenkel-Conrat H, and Wagner RR (eds): Comprehensive Virology. Plenum, New York, 1983, vol 18, pp. 1–42.

26. Dagan R, Jenista JA, and Menegus MA: Association of clinical presentation, laboratory findings, and virus serotypes with the presence of meningitis in hospitalized infants with enterovirus infection. J Pediatr 113:975–978, 1988.

27. Dalakas MC, Eldre G, Hallett M, et al: A long term follow up study of patients with post-poliomyelitis neuromuscu-

lar symptoms. N Engl J Med 314:959–963, 1986.

28. Dal Canto MC, Barbano RL, and Jubelt B: Ultrastructural immunohistochemical localization of poliovirus during virulent infection of mice. J Neuropathol Exp Neurol 45:613–617, 1986.

29. Dales S, Eggers HJ, Tamm I, and Palade GE: Electron microscopic study of the formation of poliovirus. Virology 26:379–389, 1965.

30. Dalldorf G and Sickles GM: An identified, filterable agent isolated from the feces of children with paralysis. Science 108:61–62, 1948.

31. Davis LE, Bodian D, Price D, Butler I, and Vickers J: Chronic progressive poliomyelitis secondary to vaccination of an immunodeficient child. N Engl J Med 297:241–245, 1977.

32. Dick GWA, Haddow AJ, Best AM, and Smith-Burn KC: Mengo encephalomyelitis: A hitherto unknown virus affecting man. Lancet 2:286–295, 1948.

33. Elves MW, Roath S, and Israels MC: The response of lymphocytes to antigen challenge in vitro. Lancet 1:806–807, 1963.

34. Erlendsson K, Swartz T, and Dwyer JM: Successful reversal of echovirus encephalitis in X-linked hypogammaglobulinemia by intraventricular administration of immunoglobulin. N Engl J Med 312:351–353, 1985.

35. Evans DMA, Dunn G, Minor PD, et al: Increased neurovirulence associated with a single nucleotide change in a noncoding region of the Sabin type 3 poliovaccine genome. Nature 314:548–550, 1985.

36. Farmer K, MacArthur BA, DeZoete JA, and Croxson MC: A case of agammaglobulinemia complicated by meningoencephalitis due to echo virus 27. Aust Paediatr J 20:229–231, 1984.

37. Foley KM and Beresford RH: Acute poliomyelitis beginning as transverse myelopathy. Arch Neurol 30:182–183, 1974.

38. Forbes SJ, Brumlik J, and Harding HB: Acute ascending polyradiculo-

myelitis associated with ECHO 9 virus. Dis Nerv Syst 28:537–540, 1967.

39. Gajdusek CC: Review article: Encephalomyocarditis virus infection in childhood. Pediatrics 16:902–906, 1955.

40. Gauntt CJ, Paque RE, Trousdale MD, et al: Temperature-sensitive mutant of coxsackievirus B3 establishes resistance in neonatal mice that protects them during adolescence against coxsackievirus B3-induced myocarditis. Infect Immun 39:851–864, 1983.

41. Gear JH: Nonpolio causes of polio-like paralytic syndromes. Rev Infect Dis 6:S379–S384, 1984.

42. Greve JM, Davis G, Meyer AM, et al: The major human rhinovirus receptor is ICAM-1. Cell 56:839–847, 1989.

43. Grist NR, Bell EJ, and Asaad F: Enteroviruses in human disease. Prog Med Virol 24:114–187, 1978.

44. Guyer B, Bisong AAE, Gould J, Brigaud M, and Aymard M: Injections and paralytic poliomyelitis in tropical Africa. Bull World Health Organ 58:285–291, 1980.

45. Hadfield MG, Seidlin M, Houff SA, Adair CF, Markowitz SM, and Strauss E: Echovirus meningomyeloencephalitis with administration of intrathecal immunoglobulin. J Neuropathol Exp Neurol 44:520–529, 1985.

46. Hammond GW, MacDougall BK, Plummer F, and Sekla LH: Encephalitis during the prodromal stage of acute hepatitis A. Can Med Assoc J 126:269–270, 1982.

47. Hinman AR, Koplan JP, Orenstein WA, Brink EW, and Kowane BM: Live or inactivated poliomyelitis vaccine; an analysis of benefits and risks. Am J Public Health 78:291–295, 1988.

48. Hogle JM, Cho M, and Filman DJ: Three-dimensional structure of poliovirus at 2.9 A resolution. Science 229:1358–1365, 1985.

49. Horstmann DM: Epidemiology of poliomyelitis and allied diseases—1963. Yale J Biol Med 36:5–26, 1963.

50. Hovi TM, Stenvik M, and Kinnunen E: Diagnosis of poliomyelitis by demonstration of intrathecal synthesis of

neutralizing antibodies. J Infect Dis 153:998–999, 1986.

51. Hung TP, Sung SM, Liang HC, Landsborough D, and Green IJ: Radiculomyelitis following acute haemorrhagic conjunctivitis. Brain 99:771–790, 1976.

52. Hypia T, Auvinen P, and Maaronen M: Polymerase chain reaction for human picornaviruses. J Gen Virol 70:3261–3268, 1989.

53. Ishimaur Y, Nakano S, Yamaoka K, and Takami S: Outbreaks of hand, foot and mouth disease by enterovirus 71: High incidence of complicating disorders of central nervous system. Arch Dis Child 55:583–588, 1980.

54. James JIP: Poliomyelitis: Essentials of Surgical Management. Edward Arnold Ltd, London, 1987.

55. Johnson DA and Eger AW: Myelitis associated with an echovirus. JAMA 201:143–144, 1967.

56. Johnson PR Jr, Edward KM, and Wright PF: Failure of intraventricular gamma globulin to eradicate echovirus encephalitis in patients with X-linked agammaglobulinemia. N Engl J Med 313:1546–1547, 1985.

57. Johnson RT: Viral Infections of the Nervous System. Raven Press, New York, 1982.

58. Jubelt B, Gallez-Hawkins G, Narayan O, and Johnson RT: Pathogenesis of human poliovirus infection in mice. I. Clinical and pathological studies. J Neuropathol Exp Neurol 39:138–148, 1980.

59. Jubelt B, Narayan O, and Johnson RT: Pathogenesis of human poliovirus infection in mice. II. Age dependency of paralysis. J Neuropathol Exp Neurol 39:149–159, 1980.

60. Jubelt B and Cashman NR: Neurological manifestations of post-polio syndrome. Crit Rev Neurobiol 3:199–200, 1987.

61. Jubelt B and Lipton HL: Enterovirus infections. In Vinken PJ, Bruyn GW, and Klawans HL (eds): Handbook of Clinical Neurology. Elsevier Science Publishers, Amsterdam, vol 12, Viral Diseases, 1989, pp 307–347.

62. Jubelt B and Miller JR: Viral infections. In Rowland LP (ed): Merritt's Textbook of Neurology. Lea & Febiger, Philadelphia, 1989, pp 96–136.

63. Jubelt B, Wilson AK, Guidiner PL, Ropka SL, and McKinly MA: Clearance of a persistent human enterovirus infection of the mouse central nervous system by the antiviral agent disoxaril. J Infect Dis 159:866–871, 1989.

64. Katiyar BC, Misra S, Singh RB, et al: Adult polio-like syndrome following enterovirus 70 conjunctivitis (natural history of the disease). Acta Neurol Scand 67:263–274, 1983.

65. Kitamura N, Semler B, Rothbert PG, et al: Primary structure, gene organization and polypeptide expression of poliovirus RNA. Nature 291:547–553, 1981.

66. Klingman NJ, Chul H, Corgiat M, and Perry J: Functional recovery: A major risk factor for the development of post-poliomyelitis muscular atrophy. Arch Neurol 45:645–647, 1988.

67. Kohara M, Abe S, Komatsu T, Tago K, Arita M, and Nomoto A: A recombinant virus between the Sabin 1 and Sabin 3 vaccine strains of poliovirus as a possible candidate for a new type 3 poliovirus live vaccine strain. J Virol 62:2828–2835, 1988.

68. Krausslich HG, Nicklin MJ, Toyoda H, Etichson D, and Wimmer E: Poliovirus proteinase 2A induces cleavage of eucaryotic initiation factor 4F polypeptide p220. J Virol 61:2711–2718, 1987.

69. Kuban KC, Ephros MA, Freeman RL, Laffell LB, and Bresnan MJ: Syndrome of opsoclonus-myoclonus causes by coxsackie B3 infection. Ann Neurol 13:69–71, 1983.

70. Kuhn RJ and Wimmer E: The replication of picornaviruses. In Rowlands DJ, Mayo MA, and Mahy BWJ (eds): The Molecular Biology of Positive Strand RNA Viruses. Academic Press, New York, 1987, pp 17–51.

71. La Monica N, Meriam C, and Racaniello VR: Mapping of sequences required for mouse neurovirulence of poliovirus type 2 Lansing. J Virol 56:515–525, 1986.

72. La Monica N, Almond JW, and Racaniello VR: A mouse model for poliovirus neurovirulence identifies mutations that attenuate the virus for humans. J Virol 61:2917–2920, 1987.

73. La Monica N, Kupsky WJ, and Racaniello VR: Reduced mouse neurovirulence of poliovirus type 2 Lansing antigenic variants selected with monoclonal antibodies. Virology 61:429–437, 1987.

74. Lloyd RE, Grubman MJ, and Ehrenfeld E: Relationship of p220 cleavage during poliovirus infection to 2A proteinase sequencing. J Virol 62:4216–4223, 1988.

75. Lonberg-Holm K, Crowell RL, and Philipson L: Unrelated animal viruses share receptors. Nature 259:679–716, 1976.

76. Malcolm BS, Eiden JJ, and Hendley JO: ECHO virus type 9 meningitis simulating tuberculous meningitis. Pediatrics 65:725–726, 1980.

77. Mapoles JE, Krah DL, and Crowell RL: Purification of HeLa cell receptor protein for group B coxsackieviruses. J Virol 55:560–566, 1985.

78. Marsden SA, Boulger SR, Macgrath DI, Reeve P, Schild GC, and Taff LF: Monkey neurovirulence of live, attenuated (Sabin) type I and type II poliovirus vaccines. J Biol Stand 8:303–309, 1980.

79. Martin A, Wychowski C, Couderc T, Crainic R, Hogle J, and Girard M: Engineering a poliovirus type 2 antigenic site on a type 1 capsid results in a chimaeric virus which is neurovirulent for mice. EMBO J 7:2839–2847, 1988.

80. Matthews REF: Classification and nomenclature of viruses. Intervirology 17:1–200, 1982.

81. McKinley MT, Miralles JV, Brisson CJ, and Pancic F: Prevention of human poliovirus-induced paralysis and death in mice by the novel antiviral agent arildone. Antimicrob Agents Chemother 22:1022–1025, 1982.

82. McKinney RE, Katz SL, and Wilfert CM: Chronic enteroviral meningoenchephalitis in agammaglobulinemic patients. Rev Infect Dis 9:334–356, 1987.

83. Mease PJ, Ochs HD, and Wedgewood RJ: Successful treatment of echovirus meningoencephalitis and myositis-fascitis with intravenous immune globulin therapy in a patient with X-linked agammaglobulinemia. N Engl J Med 304:1278–1281, 1981.

84. Melnick JL and Ledinko N: Development of neutralizing antibodies against the three types of poliomyelitis virus during an epidemic period: The ratio of inapparent infections to clinical poliomyelitis. Am J Hyg 58:207–222, 1953.

85. Melnick JL, Cockburn WC, Dalldorf G, et al: Picornavirus group. Virology 19:114–116, 1963.

86. Melnick JL, Proctor RO, Ocampo AR, Diwan AR, and Ben-Porath E: Free and bound virus in serum after administration of oral poliovirus vaccine. Am J Epidemiol 84:329–342, 1966.

87. Melnick JL: Enteroviruses: Polioviruses, coxsackieviruses, and new enteroviruses. In Fields BN (ed): Virology. Raven Press, New York, 1990, pp 549–605.

88. Mendelsohn CL, Wimmer E, and Racaniello VR: Cellular receptor for poliovirus: Molecular cloning nucleotide sequence, and expression of a new member of the immunoglobulin superfamily. Cell 56:855–865, 1989.

89. Morgan I: Level of serum antibody associated with intracerebral immunity in monkeys vaccinated with Lansing poliomyelitis virus. J Immunol 62:301–310, 1949.

90. Morgan IM: The role of antibody in experimental poliomyelitis. III. Distribution of antibody in and out of the central nervous system in paralyzed monkeys. American Journal of Hygiene 45:390–400, 1947.

91. Mulder DW, Rosenbaum RA, and Layton DD Jr: Late progression of poliomyelitis or forme fruste amyotrophic lateral sclerosis. Mayo Clin Proc 47:756–761, 1972.

92. Murray MG, Bradley J, Yang XF, Wimmer E, Moss EG, and Racaniello

VR: Poliovirus host range is determined by a short amino acid sequence in neutralization antigenic site 1. Science 241:213–215, 1988.

93. Nagy G, Takatsy S, Kukan E, Mihaly I, and Domok I: Virological diagnosis of enterovirus type 71 infections: Experiences gained during an epidemic of acute CNS diseases in Hungary in 1978. Arch Virol 71:217–227, 1982.

94. Nathanson N and Bodian D: Experimental poliomyelitis following intramuscular virus injection. I. The effect of neural block of a neurotropic and pantropic strain. Bull Johns Hopkins Hosp 108:308–319, 1961.

95. Nathanson N and Bodian D: Experimental poliomyelitis following intramuscular virus injection. III. The effect of passive antibody. Bull Johns Hopkins Hosp 111:198–220, 1962.

96. Nicolosi A, Hauser WA, Beghi E, and Kurland LT: Epidemiology of the central nervous system infection in Olmsted County, Minnesota, 1950–1981. J Infect Dis 154:399–408, 1986.

97. Nokowane BM, Wassilak SGF, Orenstein WA, et al: Vaccine associated paralytic poliomyelitis: United States 1973 through 1984. JAMA 257:1335–1340, 1987.

98. Nomoto A, Omata T, Toyoda H, et al: Complete nucleotide sequence of the attenuated poliovirus Sabin 1 strain genome. Proc Natl Acad Sci U S A 79:5793–5797, 1982.

99. Nottay BK, Kew OM, Hatch MH, Heyward JT, and Obijeski JF: Molecular variation of type I vaccine-related and wild polioviruses during replication in human. Virology 108:405–423, 1981.

100. Ogra PL: Effect of tonsillectomy and adenoidectomy on nasopharyngeal antibody response to poliovirus. N Engl J Med 284:59–64, 1971.

101. Ogra PL, Karzon DT, Righthand F, and MacGillivray M: Immunoglobulin response in serum and secretions after immunization with live and inactive polio vaccine and natural infection. N Engl J Med 279:893–900, 1968.

102. Ogra PL, Ogra SS, and Al-Nakeed S: Local antibody response to experimental poliovirus infection in the central nervous system of rhesus monkeys. Infect Immun 8:931–937, 1973.

103. Omata T, Kohara M, Kuge S, et al: Genetic analysis of the attenuation phenotype of poliovirus type 1. Virology 58:248–358, 1986.

104. Page GS, Mosser AG, Hogle JM, Filman DJ, Rueckert RR, and Chow M: Three-dimensional structure of poliovirus serotype 1 neutralizing determinants. J Virol 62:1781–1794, 1988.

105. Parker W, Wilt JC, Dawson JW, and Stackiw W: Landry-Guillain-Barré syndrome—the isolation of an ECHO virus type 6. Can Med Assoc J 82:813–815, 1960.

106. Patriarca PA, Onorato IM, Seklar VE, et al: Acute hemorrhagic conjunctivitis: Investigation of a large-scale community outbreak in Dade County, FL. JAMA 249:1283–1289, 1983.

107. Paul JR: Epidemiology of poliomyelitis. In Poliomyelitis. WHO Monograph Series No 26, Geneva, 1955.

108. Paul JR: History of poliomyelitis. Yale University Press, New Haven, 1971.

109. Peters ACB, Vielvoyem GHM, Veerstag J, Bots GTAM, and Lindeman J: Echo 25 focal encephalitis and subacute hemichorea. Neurology 29:676–681, 1979.

110. Pezeshkpour GH and Dalakas MC: Long-term changes in the spinal cords of patients with old poliomyelitis: Signs of continuous disease activity. Arch Neurol 45:505–508, 1988.

111. Plum F: Sensory loss with poliomyelitis. Neurology 6:166–172, 1956.

112. Price RW and Plum F: Poliomyelitis. In Vinken PJ, Bruyn GW, and Klawans HL (eds): Handbook of Clinical Neurology, vol 34. Infections of the Nervous System. Part II. North-Holland Publishing, Amsterdam, 1978, pp 93–132.

113. Racaniello VR and Baltimore D: Molecular cloning of poliovirus cDNA and determination of the complete nucleotide sequence of the viral genome. Proc Natl Acad Sci U S A 78:4887–4891, 1981.

114. Riker JB, Brandt CD, Chandra R, Ar-

robio JO, and Nakano JH: Vaccine-associated poliomyelitis in a child with thymic abnormality. Pediatrics 48:923–929, 1971.

115. Rindge ME: Poliomyelitis in pregnancy: A report of 79 cases in Connecticut. N Engl J Med 256:281–285, 1957.

116. Robertson SE, Traverso HP, Drucker JA, et al: Clinical efficacy of a new, enhanced-potency, inactivated poliovirus vaccine. Lancet 1:897–899, 1988.

117. Rodden VJ, Cantor HE, O'Conner DM, Schmidt RR, and Cherry JD: Acute hemiplegia of childhood associated with Coxsackie A9 viral infection. J Pediatr 86:56–58, 1975.

118. Roebuck M and Chamberlain R: Prevalence of antibodies of poliovirus in 1978 among subjects aged 0-88 years. Br Med J 284:697–700, 1982.

119. Rosen L, Melnick JL, Schmidt NJ, and Wenner HA: Subclassification of enteroviruses and echovirus type 34. Arch Gesmte Virusforsch 30:89–92, 1970.

120. Rossmann MG, Arnold E, Erickson JW, et al: Structure of a human common cold virus and functional relationship to other picornavirus. Nature 317:145–153, 1985.

121. Rotbart HA: Enzymatic RNA amplification of the enteroviruses. J Clin Microbiol 28:438–442, 1990.

122. Rotbart HA: Diagnosis of enteroviral meningitis with the polymerase chain reaction. J Pediatr 117:85–89, 1990.

123. Rotbart HA, Kinsella JP, and Wasserman RL: Persistent enterovirus infection in culture-negative meningoencephalitis: Demonstration by enzymatic RNA amplification. J Infect Dis 161:787–791, 1990.

124. Rotti SB, Saypathy SK, and Mehta SP: Prevalence of paralytic poliomyelitis in Pondicherry, South India. J Epidemiol Community Health 36:279–281, 1982.

125. Rueckert RR: Picornaviruses and their replication. In Fields BN, Knipe DM, Chanock RM, et al: (eds): Virology. Raven Press, New York, 1990, pp 507–548.

126. Sabin AB: Pathogenesis of poliomyelitis. Reappraisal in the light of new data. Science 123:1151–1157, 1956.

127. Schmidt JJ, Lennette EH, and Ho HH: An apparently new enterovirus isolated from patients with disease of the central nervous system. J Infect Dis 129:304–309, 1974.

128. Sells CJ, Carpenter RL, and Ray CG: Sequelae of central nervous system enterovirus infections. N Engl J Med 293:1–4, 1975.

129. Slater PE, Orenstein WA, Morag A, et al: Poliomyelitis outbreak in Israel in 1988: A report with two commentaries. Lancet 335:1192–1198, 1990.

130. Sonenberg N and Pelletier J: Poliovirus translation: A paradigm for a novel initiation mechanism. BioEssays 11:128–132, 1989.

131. Smith TJ, Kremer MJ, Luo M, et al: The site of attachment in human rhinovirus 14 for antiviral agents that inhibit uncoating. Science 233:1286–1293, 1986.

132. Stanway G, Hughes PJ, Mountford RC, et al: Comparison of the complete nucleotide sequences of the genomes of the neurovirulent poliovirus P3/Leon/37 and its attenuated Sabin vaccine derivation P3/Leon 12ab. Proc Natl Acad Sci U S A 81:1539–1543, 1984.

133. Stauton DE, Merluzzi VJ, Rothlein R, Barton R, Martin SD, and Springer TA: A cell adhesion molecule, ICAM-1, is the major surface receptor for rhinoviruses. Cell 56:849–853, 1989.

134. Sutter RW, Brink EW, Cochi SL, et al: A new epidemiologic and laboratory classification system for paralytic poliomyelitis cases. Am J Public Health 79:495–498, 1989.

135. Tomassini JE, Graham D, DeWitt CM, Lineberger DW, Rodkey JA, and Colonno RJ: cDNA cloning reveals that the major group rhinovirus receptor on HeLa cells is intercellular adhesion molecule 1. Proc Natl Acad Sci U S A 86:4907–4911, 1989.

136. Toyoda H, Kohara M, Karaoka Y, et al: Complete nucleotide sequences of all three poliovirus serotype genomes. Implication for genetic relationship, gene function and antigenic deter-

minants. J Mol Biol 174:561–585, 1984.

137. Tyler KL, Gloss RA, and Cascino GD: Unusual viral causes of transverse myelitis: Hepatitis A virus and cytomegalovirus. Neurology 36:855–858, 1986.

138. Vejjajiva A: Hemorrhagic conjunctivitis with neurologic complications. In Vinken PJ, Bruyn GW, Klawans HL, and McKendall RR (eds): Handbook of Clinical Neurology, Viral Disease, vol 56. Elsevier North-Holland, Amsterdam, 1989, p. 349–354.

139. Wadia NH, Katrak SM, Misra VP, et al: Polio-like motor paralysis associated with acute hemorrhagic conjunctivitis in an outbreak in 1981 in Bombay, India: Clinical and serologic studies. J Infect Dis 147:660–668, 1983.

140. Walters JH: Postencephalitic Parkinson syndrome after meningoencephalitis due to Coxsackievirus group B, type 2. N Engl J Med 263:744–747, 1960.

141. Wang K, Sun L, Jubelt B, and Waltenbaugh C: Cell mediated immune responses to poliovirus. I. Conditions for induction, characterization of effector cells, and cross-reactivity between serotypes for delayed hypersensitivity and T cell proliferative responses. Cell Immunol 119:252–262, 1989.

142. Wilfert CM, Buckley RH, Mohanakumar T, et al: Persistent and fatal central nervous system ECHO virus infections in patients with agammaglobulinemia. N Engl J Med 296:1485–1489, 1977.

143. Wright PF, Hatch MH, Kasselberg AG, Lowry SP, Wadlington WB, and Karzon DT: Vaccine-associated poliomyelitis in a child with sex-linked agammaglobulinemia. J Pediatr 91:408–412, 1977.

144. Wyatt HV: Poliomyelitis in hypogammaglobulinemics. J Infect Dis 128:802–806, 1973.

Chapter 6

CHRONIC AND SLOW INFECTIONS OF THE CENTRAL NERVOUS SYSTEM

Leslie P. Weiner, M.D.

SUBACUTE SCLEROSING PANENCEPHALITIS
PROGRESSIVE MULTIFOCAL LEUKOENCEPHALOPATHY
SPONGIFORM ENCEPHALOPATHIES

Over the past 30 years, a number of chronic degenerative diseases of the nervous system have been found to be caused by unusual infections. These infections have long, asymptomatic incubation periods of months or years followed by the insidious onset of slowly progressive symptoms and signs of nervous system dysfunction. In 1954, Sigurdsson was the first to characterize several transmissible diseases of sheep as "slow infections."[128] Sigurdsson compared the long incubation periods and the prolonged and progressive course of these infections to a "slow motion picture of the chain of events occurring in the acute infection."

A number of these unusual infections can be defined as being caused by classic or conventional viruses and are termed "chronic viral infections." Other prolonged infections, however, appear to be caused by agents that lack the physical, biochemical, and genetic characteristics of classic viruses. These latter unconventional agents do not contain nucleic acid and have been termed *prions*.[111] Prions produce "slow infections" when transmitted to experimental animals.

Chronic and slow infections that occur in humans are listed in Table 6–1. The pathogenesis of chronic infections involves a variety of factors that include the nature of the invading organism and the host response. With some viruses, such as the rabies virus, the agent enters the host and replicates in peripheral tissues. After a long incubation period, it produces a subacute central nervous system (CNS) disease.[67] Other agents, such as the herpesviruses [herpes simplex virus (HSV), cytomegalovirus (CMV), Epstein-Barr virus (EBV), and varicella-zoster virus (VZV)], can produce either an acute infection with clinical symptoms or a subclinical infection without a recognizable clinical picture (see Chapter 4). EBV and CMV are known to produce syndromes of infectious mononucleosis, and VZV produces chickenpox, whereas HSV-1 during an acute infection may produce a nondescript, flulike illness. If the patient does not succumb to the initial infection, herpesviruses become latent in most subjects. In latent states, an infectious virus may not be present at all, but viral genetic information remains in the cell. This latent state can be activated and produce an acute or subacute disease (see Table 6–2).[77]

The CNS appears to be particularly

Table 6-1 HUMAN CHRONIC AND SLOW CNS INFECTIONS

Disease	Virus
CHRONIC INFECTIONS	
Subacute sclerosing panencephalitis (SSPE)	Measles
Measles inclusion body encephalitis (MIBE)	Measles
Progressive multifocal leukoencephalopathy (PML)	JCV (papovavirus)
Kozhernikov's epilepsy chronic tick-borne encephalitis	Tick-borne virus (flavivirus)
Progressive rubella panencephalitis (PRPE)	Rubella
Tropical spastic paraparesis/HTLV-1–associated myelopathy (TSP/HAM)	HTLV-1
AIDS dementia complex, myelopathy, peripheral neuropathy, myositis	HIV
Cytomegalovirus encephalitis	CMV
Varicella-zoster syndrome, shingles, myelopathy, cranial arteritis	VZV
Herpes simplex, encephalitis, myelitis, radiculopathy	HSV-1 and HSV-2
Adenovirus encephalitis	Adenovirus
Enterovirus encephalitis and myositis	Coxsackie, polio, and enterocytopathogenic human orphan (ECHO)
SLOW INFECTIONS	
Kuru	Prion
Creutzfeldt-Jakob disease (CJD)	Prion
Gerstmann-Sträussler-Scheinker syndrome (GSS)	Prion

susceptible to the establishment of chronic infections and is also the site of disease in slow infections. The basic biology of CNS cells clearly plays a major role in the establishment of chronic infection and the nature of the disease process. In a host with a normal immune response, the CNS is protected from invasion by most organisms, and infection is a rare complication of a systemic illness. Invasion by conventional viruses is usually inhibited by the host defenses and the blood-brain barrier (BBB). Viruses may, however, enter the brain either by infecting endothelial cells and diffusing through the cells within pinocytotic vesicles or, rarely, via retrograde axonal transport mechanisms within peripheral nerves. Once entry into the CNS has occurred, the BBB appears to protect viruses by shielding them from the host's immune defenses. Because there are no true lymphatics in the CNS, immune surveillance is at best limited, even with a normal immune response. The cells of the CNS also are unique in that most are highly differentiated and have an increased metabolic rate and little mitotic

activity. The intracellular volume is extensive and may also play a role in the sequestering and transporting of viruses within the CNS without immune system detection. These properties may contribute to either an altered replication cycle, producing a chronic defective infection, or to a failure in aborting replication, producing a chronic productive infection.

The virus-immune-response interaction is even more critical to the outcome of an infection. The establishment, activation, and eventual clinical manifestations of latent and persistent viral infections depend on the presence of a functioning immune response.[148] The normal immune response is designed to eliminate invading microorganisms. Under certain circumstances, however, it is presumed that viral replication modulates, rather than ceases. The result is the selection of pathogens with intrinsic mutagenicity. This immune selection or pressure appears to contribute inadvertently to the establishment of persistent measles virus in subacute sclerosing panencephalitis (SSPE), rubella virus in progressive rubella panencephalitis (PRPE), and human immunodeficency virus (HIV) and human T-cell lymphotrophic virus type I (HTLV-I) in diseases of the CNS associated with those viruses.

When the immune response malfunctions, an invading virus, which would ordinarily produce an acute, limited infection, has the "opportunity" to replicate and infect tissues it would not ordinarily penetrate. This is seen in a variety of inherited and acquired immunodeficiencies (see Table 6–6).[146] For example, an opportunistic infection with JCV, a human papovavirus, causes progressive multifocal leukoencephalopathy (PML) in individuals who are immunoincompetent. Table 6–2 lists possible mechanisms for the activation and establishment of chronic viral infections.

The pathogenesis of slow infections is even less clear than that of chronic viral infections. Although our understanding of prion diseases has advanced dramatically over the past several years, very little is known about how these agents produce transmissible spongiform encephalopathies (SE). In some cases, they are inherited as autosomal dominant diseases such as familial Creutzfeldt-Jakob disease (FCJD) or Gerstmann-Sträussler-Scheinker syndrome (GSS), but in most instances they occur as either spontaneous processes or, rarely, as the result of inadvertent inoculation of contaminated human tissue, as appears to have occurred with kuru in New Guinea[54] and from the use of contaminated human tissues for transplantation or the extraction of growth hormone.[19,110,151]

A number of chronic and slow viral infections have been defined, and the list will probably expand as the causes of new diseases and syndromes are discovered. This may be the case in the newly described fatal familial insomnia.[95] In this review, we discuss two chronic infections, subacute sclerosing panencephalitis (SSPE) and progressive multifocal leukoencephalopathy (PML), from the perspective of clinical manifestations and pathogenesis. Because a number of recent reviews have appeared on prions, this chapter will concentrate on the clinical picture of prion diseases and a few points related to the nature of these novel infectious agents.

Table 6–2 PUTATIVE MECHANISMS FOR ACTIVATION AND PERSISTENCE OF VIRUSES IN HUMAN NERVOUS SYSTEM

Virus	Activation	Persistence
LATENCY		
HCV	Trauma, fever, IS, ultraviolet light	IS
CMV	IS	IS
VZV	Aging, fever, IS	IS
CHRONIC INFECTION		
Measles		
MIBE		IS
SSPE		Defective virus
PML (JCV)	IS	IS
Adenoviruses		IS
Enteroviruses		IS
Rabies		Tropism and replication cycle
Rubella		Unknown
Tick-borne encephalitis		Unknown
HIV	(Latency) unknown	IS
HTLV-1	(Latency) unknown	IS

IS = Immunosuppresion (primary or secondary), including pregnancy, viral infection, or use of immunosuppressive agents.

SUBACUTE SCLEROSING PANENCEPHALITIS

Definition and Epidemiology

SSPE is a chronic measles infection of children and young adults that leads to severe neurologic dysfunction or death. Dawson originally described a degenerative process characterized by gray-matter disease with intracytoplasmic and intranuclear eosinophilic inclusions.[40] Van Bogeart described a similar clinical entity, but with demyelination and gliosis in the white matter.[141] It soon became apparent that these two entities were the same, and the name SSPE was suggested. The cause remained unknown until a series of observations led to the recognition that SSPE was caused by the measles virus.[16,32,37,51,69,108]

SSPE is a rare disease occurring worldwide, whose risk has been estimated at 8.5 SSPE cases per million cases of measles.[31] The risk after measles vaccination is only 0.7 per million vaccinations. The effectiveness of the vaccine is found in the falling incidence of SSPE in the United States since 1960, from 0.61 cases per million persons under 20 to approximately 0.06 cases in 1980.[31] The disease has occurred in infants less than 1 year old and in adults over 30 years, but most infected persons are between the ages of 5 and 15 years.[96] The occurrence of measles before the age of 18 months appears to increase the risk of SSPE.[96] In general, the average age of measles infection in patients with SSPE is 2.4 years, whereas their unaffected playmates had measles at age 4 years.[63]

Clinical Manifestations

The clinical course of SSPE can vary in duration from 6 weeks to 10 years. Long-term stabilization and even improvement have been reported in some patients,[35] but on the average patients survive about 3 years.

Although the clinical course varies,

Table 6–3 CLINICAL STAGES OF SUBACUTE SCLEROSING PANENCEPHALITIS

Stage 1	Mental and behavioral changes
	Irritability
	Lethargy
	Forgetfulness
	Indifference
	Withdrawal
	Drooling
	Speech changes
Stage 2	Myoclonic jerks and seizures
	Incoordination of trunk and limbs
	Choreoathetosis
	Tremors
	Dyskinetic movements
Stage 3	Decerebrate rigidity
	Exterior hypertonus
	Irregular respirations
	Coma
Stage 4	Loss of cortical functions
	Flexion posturing of limbs
	Pathologic laughter or crying
	Hypotonia
	Occasional limb myoclonus
	Startle response to noise
	Mutism

Source: Modified from Jabbour et al.[76]

SSPE can be divided into four phases (Table 6–3).[76] Stage 1 appears insidiously as a decline in school performance or a change in behavior. This stage may last for months. Most patients are diagnosed in stage 2, with the appearance of myoclonic jerks at a frequency of 5 to 10 per minute, which are synchronous with high-amplitude slow waves on the electroencephalogram (EEG) (Fig. 6–1). After several months, the patient progresses to stage 3 (see Table 6–3). In stage 4, the patient may appear to improve because of reduced myoclonic jerks and abnormal posturing, but most cortical function has been lost. Stabilization and occasional remission can occur at any stage but are most frequent in stages 2 and 3.

Diagnosis

SSPE can be diagnosed by clinical findings and positive serologic testing (Table 6–4). The cerebrospinal fluid (CSF) is often acellular, with a normal protein early in the illness. As the dis-

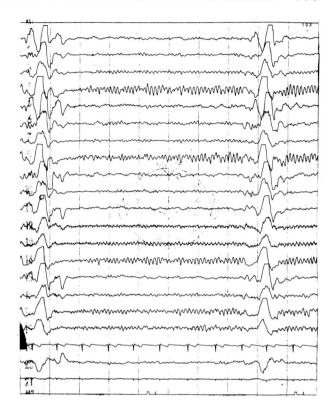

Figure 6–1. A typical EEG of SSPE, with long interburst intervals between periodic slow waves. (Courtesy of Dr. Elizabeth Horton, Children's Hospital, Los Angeles.)

ease progresses, the protein usually becomes elevated, the immunoglobulin G (IgG) level increases, and the electrophoretic pattern reveals oligoclonal bands. Of the IgG in the CSF, 50% to 80% is measles-specific.[142] Serum measles antibody concentrations are usually very high, but most critical to the diagnosis is the ratio of serum measles antibody to measles antibody in the CSF, an indicator that the antibody to measles is being synthesized intrathecally.[139]

The diagnosis is often confirmed by typical EEG abnormalities. Synchronous high-amplitude slow waves recur at intervals of 5 to 15 seconds, often synchronous with myoclonic jerks.[2] With progression, other EEG abnormalities appear, including diffuse slowing and other dysrhythmias.

Although computed tomography (CT) scans may be normal early in the course, low-density white-matter lesions develop as the disease progresses, and cortical and brainstem atrophy and

Table 6–4 LABORATORY AND RADIOGRAPHIC AIDS IN THE DIAGNOSIS OF SUBACUTE SCLEROSING PANENCEPHALITIS

Cerebrospinal fluid	Increased IgG synthesis
	Oligoclonal bands
	Measles antibody
Serum	Increased measles antibody
EEG	Abnormal with periodic high-amplitude slow waves
CT scan	Normal in stage 1
	Subsequently dilated ventricles, cortical atrophy, and low-density lesions
MRI	Subcortical and periventricular lesions

ventricular dilatation may be seen. Subcortical and periventricular white-matter lesions have also been reported on magnetic resonance imaging (MRI) scan.[136]

Pathology

The brain in SSPE shows inflammation and necrosis. The inflammatory response consists of lymphocytes and macrophage/microglial cells, both forming perivascular cuffs and diffusely infiltrating brain tissue. Lesions are found in both gray and white matter.[136] Neuronal loss may be widespread. Loss of myelin may be secondary to neuronal degeneration, or primary demyelination may follow oligodendroglial infection. There is generally a marked reactive astrogliosis. Intranuclear and intracytoplasmic inclusions can be found in astroglia, oligodendroglia, and neurons. In patients with predominantly gray-matter disease, most inclusions are in neurons.

Immunochemical staining shows that the inclusions contain measles antigen. Electron microscopic examination shows tubular structures consistent with paramyxovirus nucleocapsids.[68] Budding virions have not been found in SSPE brain specimens, consistent with the concept of a defective infection lacking viral assembly.

Pathogenesis

A fundamental question remains in the pathogenesis of SSPE: How does the measles virus persist within the CNS? Measles is an enveloped, negative-strand RNA virus. In acute measles infection, RNA-containing nucleocapsids align beneath the cell surface membrane. The RNA-nucleocapsid is surrounded by an envelope derived from the host cell membrane, into which viral glycoproteins are inserted. The assembled virus then buds through the cell membrane. In SSPE, nucleocapsids fail to align with the membrane and budding virions are not seen.

The transcriptional and translational components of the measles virus are listed in Table 6–5. All viral structural proteins have been found in varying amounts in the brains of SSPE patients.[98] Defective replication of measles virus is the major feature associated with persistence of virus. The defect in measles virus replication has been attributed to either restriction by cellular factors unique to CNS cells or defects in the structure or formation of measles gene products. A decrease in viral proteins, or the presence of defective viral proteins, may also explain viral persistence. Molecular studies of measles gene expression in brain tissue of SSPE patients has shown defects in matrix (M), hemagglutinin (H), and fusion (F) proteins.[4,5,24–29,62,127,135] When M has been decreased, it has been found to be a result of altered M gene transcription, prematurely terminated M protein translation, or production of an unstable M protein. The viral genetic defects were initially thought to be random mutations, but some strains isolated from different SSPE patients contained similar mutations.[4,28,30] Over 90% of the mutations were identical to the hypermutated nucleotides in measles inclusion-body encephalitis. This "biased hypermutation" is nonrandom and has host cell restriction.[28,152] It is not known why certain residues are more often affected by mutation than others.[30]

How these mutants are induced and then selected is unknown. It has been suggested that antiviral antibodies, which are present in high titer in infected individuals, may cause a decrease in the amount of available measles proteins and thereby disrupt viral assembly.[53] This process, referred to as antigenic modulation, has been demonstrated in vitro and in vivo in experimental systems.[53,120] In addition, monoclonal antibodies against viral glycoprotein H can induce subacute encephalitis in measles-infected mice. In

Table 6–5 TRANSCRIPTIONAL AND TRANSLATIONAL COMPONENTS OF MEASLES VIRUS IN SUBACUTE SCLEROSING PANENCEPHALITIS

Component	Function	Genomic RNA	mRNA	Protein
Nucleocapsid (NP)	Nucleocapsid	Normal	Normal	Normal
Phosphoprotein (P)	Nucleocapsid	Normal	Normal	Normal
Large protein (L)	Nucleocapsid	Normal	Normal	Normal
Matrix (M)	Nucleocapsid	Normal	Not always functional	Variable (diminished normal or absent)
Hemagglutinin (H)	Attachment	Reduced copies	Reduced	Variable
Fusion (F)	Fusing membrane	Reduced copies	Reduced	Variable

Source: Modified from Swoveland.[135]

the absence of antibody, the mice die of acute encephalitis.[120]

A second mechanism by which mutants may be induced relates to cellular factors that may be unique to CNS cells. When researchers analyzed measles virus in primary rat astroglial cultures, they found defective replication, with a reduced synthesis of viral envelope proteins and an expression gradient of viral messenger ribonucleic acids (mRNAs). These defects were not seen in nonneural cells.[125] Restriction in CNS cells appears to result from premature termination of transcription of viral mRNA.

In summary, persistent measles infection, once established, is characterized by continuous production of viral genomic mutations. Host factors, including antigenic modulation by antibody and CNS cell restriction, probably induce viral persistence. The host factors appear to act by attenuating the transcription of the measles genome so that viral proteins are not expressed on the cell surface. Subsequent replication cycles result in the accumulation of mutations that further compromise transcription and translation, resulting in SSPE. The mechanism of viral-induced cell death is unknown.

Treatment

The abolition of childhood measles infection by vaccination remains the best means to prevent SSPE. Treat-

ment of SSPE has been unsatisfactory. Intrathecal and intraventricular administration of interferon preparations has been reported to result in improvement.[22,65,73,107] Alpha interferon has been most effective, improving the clinical status in about half the patients. Since interferon crosses the BBB poorly, it should be administered intrathecally or intraventricularly. Definitive studies have not been carried out with newer recombinant preparations utilizing beta interferon.

Isoprinosine has also been reported to stabilize or improve SSPE in two thirds of patients,[47] but other studies have failed to show benefits.[59] Isoprinosine is most effective in slowly progressive, rather than rapidly advancing, disease.

PROGRESSIVE MULTIFOCAL LEUKOENCEPHALOPATHY

Definition and Epidemiology

Progressive multifocal leukoencephalopathy is a subacute demyelinating disease caused by the human papovavirus JCV. It is usually associated with an immunocompromised state, but on rare occasions PML has occurred in patients without obvious underlying disease.[49] Astrom and colleagues[3] first described PML as a complication of lymphoproliferative disorders. Virus was implicated following electron microscopic evidence of papovavirus-like particles in the nuclei of abnormal oligodendroglia.[154] JCV was isolated from the brain of a PML patient in 1971.[105] Although another viral isolate, SV40, was recovered from patients with PML, this finding has never been confirmed.[147]

PML is a rare disorder, but JCV is a common human infection, as evidenced by the widespread presence of antibody to JCV found in patients throughout the world.[21] The acquisition of JCV antibody occurs early in life; up to 60% of the population is positive by age 10.[21,104,137] Evidence suggests that JCV infection remains latent, only to be activated with immunoincompetent states (Table 6–6). Activation can also occur during pregnancy.[36] Antibody to JVC is usually IgG; only the rare patient shows IgM antibody,[104] strong evidence that JCV is not a primary infection in PML.

Although the virus has been isolated from urine, kidney, and peripheral-blood mononuclear cells in patients with PML,[34,61,70] there is no evidence of a non-CNS pathologic process. JCV has also been found in the brain of patients dying without clinical evidence of PML.[97]

PML has been associated with every form of immunoincompetence, but it was a rare disorder prior to the acquired immunodeficiency syndrome (AIDS) epidemic.[144] The autopsy incidence of PML in AIDS patients is reported to be 3% to 5%.[9,86,100]

Clinical Manifestations

Patients with PML develop progressive multifocal neurologic signs that typically result in death in 6 to 12 months, although some patients have survived up to 5 years.[49] In AIDS patients, the course can be more fulminant, with death occurring within 2 months from the onset of CNS signs and symptoms. The clinical manifestations are summarized in Table 6–7. Initially, the disease may be localized to one hemisphere. The occipital lobe is affected, most often producing visual deficits. Other common clinical manifestations include motor deficits such as monoparesis, hemiparesis, and quadriplegia, as well as dysarthria and dysphasia. Deficits in higher cerebral function are common and may be an early sign in AIDS-related PML. Intellectual impairment, finger agnosia, dyscalculia, right-left confusion, memory disturbances, and personality changes have been described.

Cerebellar ataxia may be more common in AIDS patients with PML than in

Table 6–6 IMMUNODEFICIENCY STATES

PRIMARY
Severe combined immunodeficiency
Thymic hypoplasia
Purine nucleoside phosphorylase deficiency
Ataxia telangiectasia
X-linked agammaglobulinemia
Selective IgA deficiency
IgG subclass deficiency
Wiskott-Aldrich syndrome
Varied immunodeficiency
　Predominantly immunoglobulin
　Predominantly T cell
　Phagocytic disorders
　Hyperimmunoglobulin E
　Complement deficiency

ACQUIRED
Malignancies and disorders of
　reticuloendothelium
　Gammopathies
　Hodgkin's disease
　Leukemia
　Aplastic anemia and agranulocytosis
Immunosuppressive and chemotherapeutic
　agents
　Radiation
　Corticosteroids
　Antimetabolites
　Cyclosporine
Infections
　Bacterial
　Parasitic
　Fungal
　Viral
Hereditary and metabolic disorders
　Diabetes mellitus
　Malnutrition
　Chromosome abnormalities (Down's
　　syndrome)
　Sickle cell disease
　Exudative enteropathy
Surgery and trauma
　Burns
　Splenectomy

Table 6–7 SIGNS AND SYMPTOMS OF PROGRESSIVE MULTIFOCAL LEUKOENCEPHALOPATHY

Signs and Symptoms at Onset	Percent of Cases
Mental deficits	36.1
Attention	
Memory	
Confusion	
Personality change	
Dementia	
Speech deficits	17.3
Dysarthria	
Dysphasia	
Visual deficits	34.7
Homonymous hemianopia	
Diplopia	
Cortical blindness	
Motor weakness	33.3
Monoparesis	
Hemiparesis	
Tone alterations	2.8
Bradykinesia	
Rigidity	
Incoordination	13.0
Ataxia	
Cerebellar dysarthria	
Miscellaneous	17.3
Headache	
Vertigo	
Seizures	
Coma	

Source: Modified from Brooks and Walker.[17]

those with other immunoincompetent disorders. Headache, vertigo, and seizures may be seen early and have to be differentiated from signs or symptoms caused by other opportunistic infections.

Diagnosis

PML should be suspected in immunoincompetent patients who present with CNS signs and symptoms. The CSF is usually normal but may have mild elevations of protein and myelin basic protein. An abnormal cellular response is rare. The EEG may show focal slowing, but this finding is not usually helpful. Serum antibody levels are useful if rising concentrations of anti-JCV are seen over time in the presence of progressive neurologic signs.

In the absence of inflammatory or neoplastic changes in the CSF, the presence in an immunoincompetent patient of multiple, nonenhancing lesions in the white matter, as seen by CT scan or MRI, is diagnostic. Typically, MRI shows numerous, clearly demarcated white-matter lesions in subcortical regions, pons, and cerebellum (Fig. 6–2). MRI may show similar lesions secondary to other viruses, parasites, or neoplasms, but these lesions usually enhance with contrast media, or they are accompanied by CSF changes. Some patients require brain biopsy for diagnosis, such as a patient with a single, space-occupying white-matter lesion with cerebral edema.[83,85] The biopsy may be taken by computer-assisted CT or MRI stereotaxis. If it is an open biopsy, it should be in a region with obvious radiographic evidence of a lesion. As well as looking for the classic pathologic changes of PML, which is described in the next section, the biopsy should be examined with JCV-specific probes. Large, abnormal oligodendroglia stained with anti-JCV monoclonal antibody will show antigen in inclusions and diffusely within the cytoplasm.[74,99] JCV mRNA can be demon-

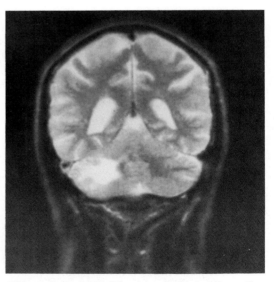

Figure 6–2. MRI of focal cerebellar white matter lesions in an AIDS patient with autopsy-proven PML.

strated within abnormal astrocytes and oligodendroglial cells by in situ hybridization methods utilizing a JCV-specific complementary deoxyribonucleic acid (cDNA) probe.[1]

It is likely that in the next few years, methods utilizing the polymerase chain reaction (PCR) to study CSF will become available for the demonstration of JCV and will greatly facilitate the diagnosis. Studies utilizing PCR in brain detect JCV in 83% of specimens studied.[138]

Pathology

Pathologic features of PML consist of focal areas of white-matter degeneration that are visible on gross sections of the brain. Microscopically, these are foci of demyelination (Fig. 6–3). Within the areas of demyelination are marked destruction of myelin with relative axon sparing, oligodendroglia loss, and astroglia proliferation. Areas of necrosis are sometimes seen, and lesions may extend into subcortical and cortical gray matter. The oligodendroglial cells have enlarged, swollen basophilic nuclei and may contain eosinophilic inclusions when stained by hematoxylin and eosin.[3,144] Astroglia are enlarged and often appear bizarre, with irregularly lobulated hyperchromatic nuclei.

Electron microscopic examination reveals large numbers of 25 to 45 nm papovavirus-like virions, either singly or in dense crystalline arrays in both the nuclei and cytoplasm of oligodendroglial cells. On rare occasions, virions can be seen in astroglia and in macrophages containing components of phagocytosed cells. Bizarre-appearing astrocytes usually do not contain virions.[154,155] Astroglia with characteristic morphologic changes of PML are more likely to contain viral DNA than are reactive astrocytes.

Pathogenesis

The pathogenesis of PML is not understood. As mentioned, antibody to JCV is widespread in human populations,[21] and most evidence suggests that JCV persists in some patients, although the possibility of a primary infection in PML has been suggested.[61,148] Until recently, JCV had not been detected in patients with other neurologic diseases or in the brains of normal peo-

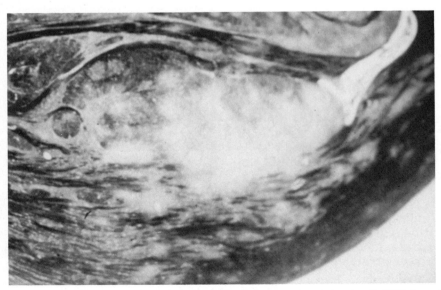

Figure 6–3. Focal pontine demyelination and confluent lesions in a patient with PML (Luxol fast blue, original magnification ×40).

ple,[34] but there is now evidence that JCV DNA and capsid protein can be found in the brain of some elderly patients without evidence of PML.[97] This report, if confirmed, would be important, but a previous study using PCR did not find evidence of JCV in normal brain.[138] The discrepancy could relate to the age of the patients.

JCV is a nonenveloped-DNA virus of the papovaviridae family that includes BKV, a virus not associated with CNS disease. These viruses have an icosohedral shape that measures between 37 and 39 nm in diameter. JCV genomes from different patients have marked variability when analyzed by restriction enzyme analysis, suggesting that subtypes may exist.[52,60,89,90] JCV can be found in other tissues, particularly the kidney, but in PML patients 1000 times fewer DNA copies have been found in these sites than in the brain.[61]

The molecular biology of JCV has been of great interest since its discovery and elucidation as a unique human papovavirus.[103,105,145] JCV has enhancer/promoter elements that have been cloned and sequenced.[78] These are short sequences of nucleotides that regulate viral gene expression. Studies of the enhancer/promoter region in transgenic mice have shed further light on the mechanisms of JCV-induced demyelination. JCV early-region genes that are under the control of the promoter/enhancer elements were injected into one-cell mouse embryos.[129] Some offspring showed a PML-like myelin abnormality in the CNS but not in the peripheral nervous system. The oligodendroglia showed bizarre nuclei, much like those seen in PML. These results suggest that the expression of JCV early-region genes in oligodendroglia may result in demyelination. One of the proteins encoded by early-region genes is the T antigen. When T antigen of JCV is expressed in oligodendroglia, transcription of the major structural proteins of CNS myelin is decreased.[140] The JCV T antigen has a region of amino acid sequence homology with myelin basic protein (MBP). The T antigen may

compete with MBP for phosphorylation,[32] and this competition may block the production of myelin and arrest the maturation of the oligodendroglia. The JCV T antigen has been found in the oligodendroglia of patients with PML but not with the major demyelinating disease, multiple sclerosis.[134]

The interaction of JCV and human immunodeficiency virus (HIV) infection has also been of interest from a molecular point of view because of the frequent association of PML with AIDS. In vitro studies suggest that HIV replication is increased in cells infected with both HIV and JCV.[57] The relevance of this observation is diminished, however, by a recent study that failed to detect cells containing both JCV and HIV antigens or mRNA, suggesting that dual infection may not occur in vivo.[143,150] Another possibility is that JCV infection and CNS demyelination act as a stimulus to bring HIV-infected macrophages into the brain. The influx of infected macrophages may in turn lead to the development of HIV encephalopathy.

Treatment

No treatment of PML has been shown to be effective. A few patients with minimal immunoincompetence have been reported to live longer, as have some patients treated with 1-β-D-arabino-furanosylcytosine (cytarabine).[7,10,88,130] One patient suffering from non-Hodgkin's lymphoma had a prolonged remission of PML after intrathecal cytarabine.[102] In our own experience, two AIDS patients with PML failed to improve with intrathecal cytarabine.

SPONGIFORM ENCEPHALOPATHIES

Definition and Epidemiology

Eight diseases can be characterized as spongiform encephalopathies (SEs) or prion diseases (Table 6–8).[112] Of the four human diseases, Creutzfeldt-

Table 6–8. SPONGIFORM ENCEPHALOPATHIES OF HUMANS AND ANIMALS

Disease	Natural Hosts
Creutzfeldt-Jakob disease (CJD)	Human
Gerstmann-Sträussler-Scheinker syndrome (GSS)	Human
Kuru	Human
Fatal familial insomnia	Human
Bovine spongiform encephalopathy	Cattle
Chronic wasting disease	American elk, mule deer
Scrapie	Sheep, goats
Transmissible mink encephalopathy	Mink

Jakob disease (CJD) is by far the most common of these rare processes and is discussed in some detail. Kuru was the first of these human diseases to be described. A number of excellent reviews have been written on the biologic and cultural aspects of this disease, found in the native population of the highlands of New Guinea.[54,56] GSS is considered to be a heterogeneous disorder with several subtypes. It resembles kuru in the distribution of lesions and the clinical picture of dementia and ataxia, but the illness is longer and the amyloid plaques differ.[92,93,117] As mentioned earlier, a new human prion disease, fatal familial insomnia, was recently described and awaits further study.[95]

CJD was first described by Creutzfeld and Jakob in the early 1920s.[38,75] The age of onset is usually in the fifth to seventh decade, although patients as young as 17 years old have been reported.[91] The epidemiology of CJD is not characteristic of an infectious disease.[18,19] The incidence is one new case per million, and it is slightly more prevalent in females.[91] Case clustering appears to be correlated with genetic predisposition, rather than with geography or environmental factors. The genetic predisposition is in the form of ethnic foci and a familial tendency, which is seen in 5% to 15% of cases.[92] In some families, CJD occurs as an autosomal dominant disorder.

Symptomatic patients have not been shown to spread the disorder. Direct inoculation is the only proven way to spread CJD from human to human. The proven cases of CJD transmission have all been iatrogenic, including corneal transplant, placement of deep EEG electrodes into the brain, infected surgical instruments used in brain surgery, and dura mater graft.[11,46,50,110,151] All of these were essentially equivalent to an intracerebral inoculation. The incubation period ranged from 16 to 28 months.

A more recent problem of transmission has been a growing number of CJD cases related to the use of growth hormone (GH) derived from human cadaver pituitary glands.[20,82,109] Patients were hypopituitary dwarfs treated with GH from pools of pituitary glands. The GH was administered by multiple injections per week over several years. The incubation period from the last dose to clinical disease ranged from 4 to 19 years. A recent review identified one batch of pituitary glands, processed in 1967, from which extracts were taken by each of five US patients with CJD.[19] This contaminated material was administered at some point between 1967 and 1970. Of two foreign cases of CJD after GH administration, one from New Zealand also received the same material as the US patients, but a patient from England had no obvious connection to the other cases.

Clinical Manifestations

Patients with CJD frequently have behavioral disturbances that are diagnosed as psychiatric disorders. After a brief interval of weeks to months, the patients progress to frank dementia characterized by memory loss, impaired judgment, sleep disturbances, and general intellectual decline. The loss of cognitive function is usually accompanied by myoclonic spasms and seizures. Fever or chills are not evident, and few give a history of systemic signs other than general malaise and occasional weight loss secondary to anorexia. Patients may present with either seizures or myoclonic jerks, both of which may appear at any time during the illness. Visual disturbances and cerebellar signs such as incoordination and gait difficulties are far less common.[117,122] Lower-motor-neuron disturbances with muscle wasting and fasciculations are rare,[122] and it is possible that the lower-motor-neuron form of the disease may not be transmissible.[124] Chimpanzees injected with CJD do develop widespread fasciculations.[58]

Most patients live 6 to 12 months after the beginning of signs and symptoms, although some have lived up to 5 years.

Diagnosis

The diagnosis of CJD is to be suspected in patients over 50 years of age presenting with dementia and myoclonic jerks. The general evaluation fails to reveal any systemic illness. The CSF is usually normal, and no specific lesion has been seen on CT scan or MRI, although it is common late in the course to see significant cortical atrophy with large ventricles secondary to loss of CNS tissue.

At some point in the illness, the EEG will be abnormal and very suggestive of CJD, in the setting of rapidly advancing dementia and myoclonic spasms. The EEG may show repetitive, high-voltage, triphasic and polyphasic sharp discharges. When stereotyped periodic bursts occur at 1- to 2-second intervals, the diagnosis is most likely CJD, although in some instances periodicity may be absent.[153]

Although no specific diagnostic test yet exists, abnormal CSF proteins have been reported that may be useful in the premortem diagnosis of CJD.[12,64]

Pathology

The pathologic picture of all the SEs, including CJD, shows vacuolation, loss of neurons, and astrogliosis. The spongiform changes, although variable in intensity, are most profound in the cerebral cortex, putamen, caudate nucleus, and thalamus in CJD.[84] The vacuoles are in the neuropil, primarily in the dendritic and axonal processes, and to a lesser extent in the neuronal soma.[91] Astroglia, and rarely oligodendroglia, may also show vacuolar degeneration. Amyloid plaques can be found in each of these disorders. Staining of these plaques with specific antiserum suggests that they consist of filamentous arrays of prion protein.[80] There is no evidence of an inflammatory response in the brain, spinal cord, or meninges, nor of lymphocytic infiltrates or perivascular cuffing.

Ultrastructural studies have never shown the presence of virions or virion-like material, although spheres, rods, fibrils, and tubules have been described.[8,84] The vacuoles appear to be surrounded by a membrane, within which are usually many membrane fragments.[8,84]

Pathogenesis

Evidence mounts that the causes of SEs are both infectious and genetic. This is a rapidly changing field (see recent reviews on prion proteins[133] and the molecular biology of prion diseases[115]). This section briefly reviews some of the current data and thoughts about these unique biologic processes.

It was first noted over 200 years ago that scrapie, the prototype SE (which occurs in sheep), is an inherited disease. Scrapie was transmitted by inoculation into sheep in 1936, confirming that it also was infectious.[39] A striking similarity between scrapie in sheep and kuru and CJD in humans was subsequently recognized.[48,55,56,58,81,113] The scrapie, kuru, and CJD agents resembled viruses in that they were transmissible and filterable, and strains appeared to vary in specificity, virulence, and pathogenicity. Initial studies of the kinetics of inactivation of the scrapie agent by ionizing radiation suggested that a nucleic acid genome was present,[121] but repeated subsequent attempts to demonstrate nonhost nucleic acid or nonhost protein have failed. The agent is resistant to nucleases, ultraviolet light, and reagents known to inactivate nucleic acids.[54]

As purification methods improved and the tools of molecular biology became available, a substantial body of evidence accumulated that transmissibility may depend on protein devoid of nucleic acid. In a series of elegant experiments, Prusiner and colleagues showed that partially purified material retained its transmissibility when treated with agents known to destroy nucleic acid but not when treated with proteolytic or denaturing chemicals.[13,14,111] Prusiner introduced the term "prion," defined as "small *pro*teinaceous *in*fectious particles which resist inactivation by procedures that modify nucleic acids."[111] The development of a more rapid bioassay for the scrapie agent led to the finding of a scrapie-associated protein PrP 27-30.[13,116] This polypeptide has a molecular weight of 27,000 to 30,000 d, and its heterogeneity appeared to be related to its sialic acid content.[15] It was realized that PrP mRNA was found in both normal and scrapie-infected brains.[6,33] The sequencing of the cellular gene[87,101] opened the way to the finding that PrP 27-30 was generated from a larger protein with a molecular weight of 33,000 to 35,000 d. There appeared to be a scrapie isoform of prion protein (PrP 33-35^{Sc}) and a cellular isoform (PrP 33-35^{C}). The PrP^C is completely degraded by proteinase K. The PrP^{Sc} is resistant to proteases, and treatment with proteinase K generates PrP 27-30.[94] PrP^C is solubi-

lized when treated with detergents, whereas PrP^{SC} polymerizes and forms amyloid rods.[118] This amyloid appears to be composed mainly of PrP 27-30 and PrP^{Sc} proteins, unlike amyloid from nonprion diseases.[41,116]

PrP^C and PrP^{Sc} are both glycosylated membrane proteins of host origin and have been mapped to homologous regions of mouse chromosome 2 and human chromosome 20.[131] The gene encoding PrP is tightly linked to genes known to determine scrapie incubation time.[23] Strains of mice that develop scrapie after long incubation periods differ in the composition of their PrP from strains with short incubation times.[149] Another gene controlling incubation time in experimental CJD has been found on mouse chromosome 17 within the D region of the H-2 complex.[79]

The function of PrP^C is still unclear, but the amino acid sequence suggests a transmembrane protein that spans the lipid bilayer twice[66] and is anchored to the cell surface by a glycosylphosphatidylinositol linkage that can be solubilized by ionic detergents or by phospholipase C.[132] A secretory form of the protein may also exist.

The intricate relationship between a host gene and transmissibility has been documented by the finding that GSS is linked to mutation in the PrP alleles, resulting in amino acid substitutions. The first example was a mutation in codon 102 of PrP, resulting in a substitution of leucine for proline.[71] This mutation was not found in normals, nor in other prion diseases. A number of other PrP mutations have been reported in cases of familial GSS,[45] but not all family members with the PrP mutation have developed GSS. This finding, and that related to the long and short incubation period in scrapie, suggests that amino acid substitutions may influence prion diseases.

Three fundamental questions can be asked about prion biology: (1) Do prions contain nucleic acid, and therefore are really viruses? (2) Is the prion the sole cause of SEs? and (3) Are these diseases infectious, genetic, or both?

No evidence to date suggests that a scrapie-specific nucleic acid is a component of the prion particle. Procedures that alter proteins invariably reduce prion infectivity, whereas treatments that degrade nucleic acids have no effect.[111,114] Thus it appears that prions are not likely to be viruses.

The perplexing problem of "scrapie strains" still remains to be explained, however. It has been suggested that if strains of scrapie exist, then an informational molecule must be part of the infectious agent.[42-44] This argument is based on the fact that even if the dose of the agent; route of injection; and age, sex, and strain of the host are kept constant, the incubation periods, vacuolation patterns, amyloid plaques, and clinical course may differ with a given strain of scrapie. Explanations given for strains of scrapie have included the possibilities that the inoculum may be impure or that the differences are due to mutations.[114] In the case of mutations, one would expect the differences to disappear with one or two passages when scrapie strains derived from different sources are passaged in the same mouse strain. In most instances this is the case, but differences between scrapie strains are sometimes seen in the same inbred host after repeated passages.

The evidence in support of the prion as the sole factor in SE has been convincingly reviewed by the Prusiner group.[119,126] Transgenic mice expressing the hamster and mouse prion protein genes have been produced.[119] Transgenic mice harboring a hamster PrP gene expressed cellular hamster PrP in their brains. When inoculated with hamster prions, such mice synthesized de novo hamster PrP. Transgenic mice inoculated with mouse prions produced mouse PrP. Thus, the prion inoculum dictated which prions were synthesized, even though the cells expressed both PrP genes. The neuropathologic distribution of disease was also characteristic of hamster if hamster PrP was inoculated into transgenic mice, whereas those inoculated with

mouse prions had the pattern found in nontransgenic mice inoculated with scrapie. A compelling argument was made that species specificity of scrapie prions resides in the primary structure of PrP, and the formation of infectious prions is the result of interaction between PrP^{Sc} in the inoculum and homologous PrP^C.

Transgenic mice expressing a mouse PrP gene with a codon 102 mutation similar to that found in GSS were also produced. These mice spontaneously develop a CNS degenerative disease that is clinically and neuropathologically indistinguishable from scrapie. Preliminary data suggest that brain material from these mice, when inoculated into normal mice, transmits scrapie. If these data hold true, these results would clearly establish that prions are the causative agent of scrapie and that no foreign nucleic acid is required for transmission of the disease.[72]

Nevertheless, questions remain about the pathogenesis of SE in both humans and animals. Human SE is undoubtedly transmissible, but it remains unclear whether these are truly "infectious" diseases. CJD is a sporadic worldwide illness with a consistent pattern and frequency, and a stable incidence of about one case per million. Clusters of human SE cases seem to reflect genetic, rather than infectious, factors. Familial CJD and GSS are inherited as autosomal dominant diseases with defined mutations in the prion gene, but most cases of CJD are sporadic and thus far have not been shown to be associated with mutations. It was recently reported that 40 out of 45 cases of sporadic CJD were homozygous at the amino acid residue 129, whereas 51% of the normal population are heterozygous at this site.[106] These data suggest that environmental prion infection may not cause most sporadic CJD cases.

It is still not clear how the inoculation of prion protein modifies an analogous protein and induces disease in the infected host. Evidence is sufficient to suggest that SE are indeed genetic dis-

Table 6–9 STERILIZATION PROCEDURES FOR TISSUES AND MATERIALS SUSPECTED OF HAVING PRION DISEASE

RECOMMENDED MINIMAL PROCEDURES
Steam autoclaving for 1 hour at 132°C
Immersion in 1 N sodium hydroxide for 1 hour at room temperature

NOT RECOMMENDED (Partially or completely ineffective procedures)
Steam autoclaving for less than 1 hour and/or at a lower temperature than 132°C
Immersion in sodium hydroxide for less than 1 hour and/or at a lower concentration than 1 N
Boiling, ultraviolet radiation, enthylene oxide sterilization, ethanol, formalin, β-proprioammonium compounds, Lysol, alcoholic iodine, acetone, potassium permanganate

Source: Modified from Rosenberg et al.[123]

eases, but it still must be determined whether these diseases have to be induced in their sporadic occurrence.

Treatment

There is no treatment for any of the SEs. The biohazard in the handling of contaminated fluids and tissues calls for certain precautions. Perhaps one of the most important aspects of preventing the inadvertent transmission of these diseases is the careful screening of patients whose organs are being considered for transplantation or grafting, and the thorough decontamination of all materials, particularly needles, bone, and other sharp objects, that have come in contact with patients diagnosed as having neurodegenerative processes. Table 6–9 describes current sterilization procedures.[123]

SUMMARY

Chronic and slow infections of the nervous system, although comparatively rare, continue to be perplexing clinical and biologic problems. SSPE is preventable by measles vaccination. PML, for the most part a complication of immunoincompetence, appears to be associated with HIV infection and may well be prevented with control or treatment of AIDS. The recent progress in our understanding of prion diseases could provide significant insights into the nature of other neurodegenerative diseases such as Alzheimer's disease, amyotrophic lateral sclerosis, and Parkinson's disease. All these processes serve as valuable models of the interaction between the host's genetic makeup, the biology of neuronal and glial elements, and invading agents, whether they be viruses or prions.

REFERENCES

1. Aksamit AJ, Mourrain P, and Sever JL: Progressive multifocal leukoencephalopathy: Investigation of three cases using in situ hybridization with JC virus biotinylated DNA probe. Ann Neurol 18:490–494, 1985.
2. Asher AM: Slow viral infections of the human nervous system. In Scheld WM, Whitley RJ, and Durack DT (eds): Infections of the Central Nervous System. Raven Press, New York, 1991, pp 145–166.
3. Astrom KE, Mancall EL, and Richardson EP Jr: Progressive multifocal leukoencephalopathy, a hitherto unrecognized complication of chronic lymphatic leukemia and Hodgkin's disease. Brain 81:93–111, 1958.
4. Ayata M, Hirano A, and Wong TC: Structural defect linked to non random mutations in the matrix of Biken strain subacute sclerosing panencephalitis virus defined by cDNA cloning and expression of chimeric genes. J Virol 63:1162–1173, 1989.
5. Baczko K, Liebert UG, Billeter M, Cattaneo R, Budka H, and ter Meulen V: Expression of defective measles virus

genes in brain tissues of patients with subacute sclerosing panencephalitis. J Virol 59:472–478, 1986.

6. Barry RA, Kent SBH, McKinley MP, et al: Scrapie and cellular prion proteins share polypeptide epitopes. J Infect Dis 153:848–854, 1986.

7. Bauer WR, Truel AP, and Johnson KP: Progressive multifocal leukoencephalopathy and cytarabine. JAMA 226:174–176, 1973.

8. Beck E, Daniel PM, Davey AJ, Gajdusek DC, and Gibbs CJ Jr: The pathogenesis of transmissible spongiform encephalopathy—an ultrastructural study. Brain 105:755–786, 1982.

9. Berger JR, Kaszovitz B, Donavan Post JM, and Dickinson G: Progressive multifocal leukoencephalopathy associated with human immunodeficiency virus infection. Ann Intern Med 107:78–87, 1987.

10. Berger JR and Mucke L: Prolonged survival and partial recovery in AIDS-associated progressive multifocal leukoencephalopathy. Neurology 38:1060–1065, 1988.

11. Bernoulli C, Siegfried J, Baumgartner G, et al: Danger of accidental person to person transmission of Creutzfeldt-Jakob disease by surgery. Lancet 1:478–479, 1977.

12. Blisard KS, Davis LE, Harrington MG, Lovell JK, Kornfeld M, and Berger ML: Pre-mortem diagnosis of Creutzfeldt-Jakob disease by detection of abnormal cerebrospinal fluid proteins. J Neurol Sci 99:75–81, 1990.

13. Bolton DC, McKinley MP, and Prusiner SB: Identification of protein that purifies with the scrapie prion. Science 218:1309–1311, 1982.

14. Bolton DC, McKinley MP, and Prusiner SB: Molecular characteristics of the major scrapie prion protein. Biochemistry 23:5898–5905, 1984.

15. Bolton DC, Meyer RK, and Prusiner SB: Scrapie PrP 27-30 is a sialoglycoprotein. J Virol 53:596–606, 1985.

16. Bouteille M, Fontaine C, Vedrenne C, and Delarue J: Sur un cas d'encephalite subaigue a inclusion. Etude anatomoclinique et ultrastructurale. Rev Neurol 118:454–458, 1965.

17. Brooks BR and Walker DL: Progressive multifocal leukoencephalopathy. Neurol Clin 2:299–313, 1984.

18. Brown P: An epidemiologic critique of Creutzfeldt-Jakob disease. Epidemiol Rev 2:113–135, 1980.

19. Brown P: The clinical neurology and epidemiology of Creutzfeldt-Jakob disease with special reference to iatrogenic cases. In Bock G and March J (eds): Novel Infectious Agents and the Central Nervous System. CIBA Foundation Symposium 135:3–23, 1988.

20. Brown P, Gajdusek DC, Gibbs CJ Jr, and Asher DM: Potential epidemic of Creutzfeldt-Jakob disease from human growth hormone therapy. N Engl J Med 313:728–731, 1985.

21. Brown P, Tsai T, and Gajdusek DC: Seroepidemiology of human papovaviruses. Am J Epidemiol 102:331–340, 1975.

22. Bye A, Balkwill F, and Wilson J: Use of interferon in the management of patients with subacute sclerosing panencephalitis. Dev Med Child Neurol 27:170–175, 1985.

23. Carlson GA, Kingsbury DT, Goodman PA, et al: Linkage of prion protein and scrapie incubation time genes. Cell 46:503–511, 1986.

24. Carter MJ, Willcocks MM, and ter Meulen V: Defective translation of measles virus matrix protein in a subacute sclerosing panencephalitis cell line. Nature 305:153–155, 1983.

25. Cattaneo R, Rebmann G, Baczko K, ter Meulen V, and Billeter MA: Altered ratios of measles virus transcripts in diseased human brains. Virology 160:523–526, 1987.

26. Cattaneo R, Rebmann G, Schmid A, Backzo K, ter Meulen V, and Billeter MA: Altered transcription of a defective measles virus genome derived from a diseased brain. EMBO J 6:681–688, 1987.

27. Cattaneo R, Schmid A, Billeter MA, Shepperd RD, and Udem SA: Multiple viral mutations rather than host factors cause defective measles virus gene expression in a subacute sclerosing panencephalitis cell line. J Virol 62:1488–1497, 1988.

28. Cattaneo R, Schmid A, Eschle D, Baczko K, ter Meulen V, and Billeter MA: Biased hypermutation and other genetic changes in defective measles viruses in human brain infections. Cell 55:255–265, 1988.

29. Cattaneo R, Schmid A, Rebmann G, et al: Accumulated measles virus mutations in a case of subacute sclerosing panencephalitis: Interrupted matrix protein reading frame transcription alteration. Virology 154:97–107, 1986.

30. Cattaneo R, Schmid A, Spielhofer P, et al: Mutated and hypermutated genes of persistent measles viruses which caused lethal human brain diseases. Virology 173:415–425, 1989.

31. Centers for Disease Control: Subacute sclerosing panencephalitis surveillance—United States. MMWR 31:585–588, 1982.

32. Chan K-FJ, Stoner GL, Hashim GA, and Huang K-P: Substrate specificity of rat brain calcium-activated and phospholipid-dependent protein kinase. Biochem Biophys Res Commun 134:1358, 1986.

33. Chesebro B, Race R, Wehrly K, et al: Identification of scrapie prion protein-specific mRNA in scrapie-infected and uninfected brain. Nature 315:331–333, 1985.

34. Chesters PM, Heritage J, and McCance DJ: Persistence of DNA sequences of BK viruses and JC virus in normal human tissues and in diseased tissues. J Infect Dis 147:676, 1983.

35. Cobb WA, Marshall J, and Scaravilli F: Long survival in subacute sclerosing panencephalitis in Italy: An epidemiological study. Acta Neurol Scand 73:160–167, 1984.

36. Coleman DV, Gardner SD, and Mullholland C: Human polyomavirus in pregnancy: A model for the study of defense mechanisms to virus reactivation. Clin Exp Immunol 53:289–296, 1983.

37. Connolly JH, Allen IV, Hurwitz LJ, and Miller JHD: Measles virus antibody and antigen in subacute sclerosing panencephalitis. Lancet 1:542–544, 1967.

38. Creutzfeldt HG: Uber eine eigenartige herdformige Erkrankung des Zentralnervensystems. Z Gesamte Neurol Psychiatry 57:1–18, 1920.

39. Cuille J and Chelle PL: Pathologie animal—la maladie dite tremblante du mouton: est-elle inoculable? CR Acad Sci [D] (Paris) 203:1552–1554, 1936.

40. Dawson JR: Cellular inclusions in cerebral lesions of lethargic encephalitis. Am J Pathol 9:7–15, 1933.

41. DeArmond SJ, McKinley MP, Barry RA, Braunfeld MB, McColloch JR, and Prusiner SB: Identification of prion amyloid filaments in scrapie-infected brain. Cell 41:221–235, 1985.

42. Dickinson AG, Bruce ME, Outram GW, and Limberlin RH: Scrapie strain differences: The implications of stability and mutation. In Tateishi J (ed): Proceedings of Workshop on Slow Transmissible Disease. Tokyo, Japanese Ministry of Health and Welfare, 1984, pp 105–118.

43. Dickinson AG, Fraser H, and Outram GW: Scrapie incubation time can exceed natural lifespan. Nature 256:732–733, 1981.

44. Dickinson AG and Leikle VM: Host-genotype and agent effects in scrapie incubation: Change in allelic interaction with different strains of agent. Mol Gen Genet 112:73–79, 1971.

45. Doh-ura K, Tateishi J, Kitamoto T, Sasaki H, and Sakaki Y: Creutzfeldt-Jakob disease patients with congophilic kuru plaques have the missense variant prion protein common to Gerstmann-Sträussler syndrome. Ann Neurol 27:121–126, 1990.

46. Duffy P, Wolf J, Collins G, Devoe A, Streeten B, and Cowen D: Possible person to person transmission of Greutzfeldt-Jakob disease. N Engl J Med 290:692–693, 1974.

47. Dyken PR, Swift A, and Durant RH: Long-term follow-up of patients with subacute sclerosing panencephalitis treated with inosiplex. Ann Neurol 11:359–364, 1982.

48. Eklund CM, Kennedy RC, and Hadlow

CHRONIC AND SLOW INFECTIONS OF THE CENTRAL NERVOUS SYSTEM   149

WJ: Pathogenesis of scrapie virus infection in the mouse. J Infect Dis 17:15–22, 1967.

49. Fermaglich J, Hardman JM, and Earle KM: Spontaneous progressive multifocal leukoencephalopathy. Neurology 20:479, 1970.

50. Foncin J, Gaches J, Cathala F, El Sharif E, and LeBeau J: Transmission iatrogene interhumaine possible de maladie de Creutzfeldt-Jakob avec atteinte des grains du cervelet. Rev Neurol 136:280, 1980.

51. Freeman JM, Magoffin RL, Lennette EH, and Herndon RM: Additional evidence of the relationship between subacute inclusion-body encephalitis and measles virus. Lancet 2:129–131, 1967.

52. Frisque RJ, Bream GL, and Cannella MT: Human polyomavirus JC virus genome. J Virol 51:458–469, 1984.

53. Fujinami RS and Oldstone MB: Alterations in expression of measles virus polypeptides by antibody. Molecular events in antibody-induced antigenic modulation. J Immunol 125:78–85, 1980.

54. Gajdusek DC: Unconventional viruses and the origin and disappearance of kuru. Science 197:943–960, 1977.

55. Gajdusek DC, Gibbs CJ Jr, and Alpers M: Experimental transmission of a kuru-like syndrome to chimpanzees. Nature 209:794–796, 1966.

56. Gajdusek DC and Zigas V: Degenerative disease of the central nervous system in New Guinea—the endemic occurrence of 'kuru' in the native population. N Engl J Med 257:974–978, 1957.

57. Gendelman HE, Phelps W, Feigenbaum L, et al: Transactivation of the human immunodeficiency virus long terminal repeat sequence by DNA viruses. Proc Natl Acad Sci U S A 83:9759–9763, 1986.

58. Gibbs CJ Jr, Gajdusek DC, Asher DM, Alpers MP, Beck E, and Mathews WB: Creutzfeldt-Jakob disease (spongiform encephalopathy): Transmission to the chimpanzee. Science 161:388–389, 1968.

59. Griffin DE: Therapy of viral infections of the central nervous system. Antiviral Res 15:1–10, 1991.

60. Grinnell BW, Padgett BL, and Walker DL: Comparison of infectious JC virus DNAs cloned from human brain. J Virol 45:299–308, 1983.

61. Grinnell BW, Padgett BL, and Walker DL: Distribution of non-integrated DNA from JC papovavirus in organs of patients with progressive multifocal leukoencephalopathy. J Infect Dis 147:669–675, 1983.

62. Hall WW and Choppin PW: Measles virus proteins in the brain tissue of patients with subacute sclerosing panencephalitis; absence of the M protein. N Engl J Med 304:1152–1155, 1981.

63. Halsey NA, Modlin JF, Jabbour JT, Dubey L, Eddins DL, and Ludwig DD: Risk factors in subacute sclerosing panencephalitis. A case control study. Am J Epidemiol 111:415–424, 1980.

64. Harrington MG, Merril CR, Asher DM, and Gajdusek DC: Abnormal proteins in the cerebrospinal fluid of patients with Creutzfeldt-Jakob disease. N Engl J Med 315:279–283, 1986.

65. Hatanaka T, Sigimoto T, and Yohnosuke K: Electroencephalographic changes during interferon therapy in a case of subacute sclerosing panencephalitis. Eur Neurol 29:6–9, 1990.

66. Hay B, Barry RA, Lieberburg I, Prusiner SB, and Lingappa VR: Biogenesis and transmembrane orientation of the cellular isoform of the scrapie prion protein. Mol Cel Biol 7:914–920, 1987.

67. Hemachudha T: Rabies. In McKendall RR (ed): Viral Disease. Handbook of Clinical Neurology, vol 56. Elsevier Science Publishers, Amsterdam, 1989, pp 383–404.

68. Herndon RM and Rubinstein LJ: Light and electron microscopy observations in the development of viral particles in the inclusions of Dawson's encephalitis (subacute sclerosing panencephalitis). Neurology 18:8–20, 1967.

69. Horta-Barbosa L, Fucillo DA, London WT, Jabbour JT, Zeman W, and Sever

JL: Isolation of measles virus from brain cell cultures of two patients with subacute sclerosing panencephalitis. Proc Soc Exp Biol Med 132:272–277, 1969.

70. Houff SA, Major EO, Katz DA, et al: Involvement of JC virus-infected mononuclear cells from the bone marrow and spleen in the pathogenesis of progressive multifocal leukoencephalopathy. N Engl J Med 318:301–305, 1988.

71. Hsiao KK, Baker HF, Crow TJ, et al: Linkage of prion protein missense variant to Gerstmann-Sträussler syndrome. Nature 338:342–345, 1989.

72. Hsiao KK: Scott M, Foster D, Groth DF, DeArmond SJ, and Prusiner SB: Spontaneous neurodegeneration in transgenic mice with mutant prion protein. Science 250:1587–1590, 1991.

73. Huttenlocher PR, Picchietti DL, and Roos RP: Intrathecal interferon in subacute sclerosing panencephalitis. Ann Neurol 19:303–305, 1986.

74. Itoyama Y, Webster H deF, Sternberger NH, et al: Distribution of papovavirus, myelin-associated glycoprotein, and myelin basic protein in progressive multifocal leuko-encephalopathy lesions. Ann Neurol 11:396–407, 1982.

75. Jakob A: Uber eigenartige erkrankungen des zentralnervensystems mit bemerkenswertem anatomischen befunde (spastische pseudosclerose-encephalomyelopathies mit disseminierten degenerationsherden). Preliminary communication. Dtsch Z Nervenheilkd 70:132–146, 1921.

76. Jabbour JT, Garcia JG, Lemmi H, Ragland J, Duenas DA, and Sever JL: Subacute sclerosing panencephalitis. A multidisciplinary study of eight cases. JAMA 207:2248–2254, 1969.

77. Johnson RT: Viral Infections of the Nervous System. Raven Press, New York, 1982.

78. Kenney S, Natarajan V, Strike D, Khoury G, and Salzman NP: JC virus-promoter active in human brain cells. Science 226:1337–1339, 1984.

79. Kingsbury DT, Kasper KC, Stites DP,

Watson JC, Hogan RN, and Prusiner SB: Genetic control of scrapie and Creutzfeldt-Jakob disease in mice. J Immunol 131:491–496, 1983.

80. Kitamoto R, Tateishi J, Tashima T, et al: Amyloid plaques in Creutzfeldt-Jakob disease stain with prion protein antibodies. Ann Neurol 20:204–208, 1986.

81. Klatzo I, Gajdusek DC, and Zigas V: Pathology of kuru. Lab Invest 8:799–847, 1959.

82. Koch TK, Berg BO, DeArmond SJ, and Gravina RF: Creutzfeldt-Jakob disease in a young adult with idiopathic hypopituitarism: Possible relation to the administration of cadaveric human growth hormone. N Engl J Med 313:731–733, 1985.

83. Krupp LB, Lipton RB, Swerdlow ML, Leeds NE, and Llena J: Progressive multifocal leukoencephalopathy. Clinical and radiographic features. Ann Neurol 17:344–349, 1985.

84. Lampert PW, Gajdusek DC, and Gibbs CJ Jr: Subacute spongiform virus encephalopathies—scrapie, kuru and Creutzfeldt-Jakob disease: A review. Am J Pathol 68:626–652, 1972.

85. Levy JD, Cottingham KL, Campbell RJ, et al: Progressive multifocal leukoencephalopathy and magnetic resonance imaging. Ann Neurol 19:399–401, 1986.

86. Levy RM, Bredesen DE, and Rosenblum ML: Neurological manifestations of the acquired immunodeficiency syndrome (AIDS). Experience at UCSF and review of the literature. J Neurosurg 62:475–495, 1985.

87. Locht CM, Chesbro B, Race R, and Keith JM: Molecular cloning and complete sequence of prion protein cDNA from mouse brain infected with scrapie agent. Proc Natl Acad Sci U S A 83:6372–6376, 1986.

88. Marriott PJ, O'Brien MD, MacKensie ICK, and Janota I: Progressive multifocal leukoencephalopathy: Remission with cytarabine. J Neurol Neurosurg Psychiatry 38:205–209, 1975.

89. Martin JD and Foster GC: Multiple JC virus genomes from one patient. J Gen Virol 65:1405–1411, 1984.

90. Martin JD, King DM, Slauch JM, and Frisque RJ: Differences in regulatory sequences of naturally occurring JC virus variants. J Virol 53:306–311, 1985.

91. Masters CL and Richardson EP Jr: Subacute spongiform encephalopathy Creutzfeldt-Jakob disease—the nature and progression of spongiform change. Brain 101:333–344, 1978.

92. Masters CL, Gajdusek DC, and Gibbs CJ Jr: Creutzfeldt-Jakob disease virus isolations from the Gerstmann-Sträussler syndrome. Brain 104:559–588, 1981.

93. Masters CL, Gajdusek DC, and Gibbs CJ Jr: The familial occurrence of Creutzfeldt-Jakob disease and Alzheimer's disease. Brain 104:535–558, 1981.

94. McKinley MP, Bolton DC, and Prusiner SB: A protease-resistant protein is a structural component of the scrapie prion. Cell 35:57–62, 1983.

95. Medori R, Tritschler H-J, LeBlanc A, et al: Fatal familial insomnia, a prion disease with a mutation at codon 178 of the prion protein gene. N Engl J Med 326:444–449, 1992.

96. Modlin JF, Halsey NA, Eddins DL, et al: Epidemiology of subacute sclerosing panencephalitis. J Pediatr 94:231–236, 1979.

97. Mori M, Kurata H, Tajima M, and Shimada H: JC virus detection in brain tissue from elderly patients by in situ hybridization. Ann Neurol 29:428–432, 1991.

98. Mountcastle WE and Choppin PW: A comparison of the polypeptides of four measles virus strains. Virology 78:463–474, 1977.

99. Narayan ON, Penny OJB, Johnson RT, Herndon RM, and Weiner LP: Etiology of progressive multifocal leukoencephalopathy. N Engl J Med 289:1278–1282, 1973.

100. Navia BA, Jordan BD, and Price RW: Central nervous system complications of immunosuppression. In Parsillo JE and Masier H (eds): The Critically Ill Immunosuppressed Patient. Aspen, Rockville, MD, 1987, pp 119–142.

101. Oesch B, Westaway DM, Walchli M, et al: A cellular gene encodes scrapie PrP 27-30 protein. Cell 40:735–746, 1985.

102. O'Ricordan T, Daly PA, Hutchinson M, Shatlock AG, and Gardner SD: Progressive multifocal leukoencephalopathy—remission with cytarabine. J Infect 20:51–54, 1990.

103. Padgett BL and Walker DL: New human papovaviruses. Prog Med Virol 22:1–35, 1976.

104. Padgett BL and Walker DL: Virologic and serologic studies of progressive multifocal leukoencephalopathy. In Sever JL and Madden DL (eds): Polyomaviruses and Human Neurological Diseases. Alan Liss, New York, 1983, pp 107–118.

105. Padgett BL, Walker DL, ZuRhein GM, Eckroade RJ, and Dessell BH: Cultivation of papova-like virus from human brain with progressive multifocal leukoencephalopathy. Lancet 1:1257–1260, 1971.

106. Palmer MS, Dryden AJ, Hughes JT, and Collinge J: Homozygous prion protein genotype predisposes to sporadic Creutzfeldt-Jakob disease. Nature 352:340–341, 1991.

107. Panitch HS, Gomez-Plascencia J, Norris FH, Cantell K, and Smith RA: Remission of subacute sclerosing panencephalitis in patients treated with intraventricular interferon. Neurology 36:563–566, 1986.

108. Payne FE, Baublis VV, and Itabashi HH: Isolation of measles virus from cell cultures of brain from a patient with subacute sclerosing panencephalitis. N Engl J Med 281:585–589, 1969.

109. Powell-Jackson J, Kennedy P, Whitcombe EM, Weller RO, Preece MA, and Newsom-Davis J: Creutzfeldt-Jakob disease after administration of human growth hormone. Lancet 2:244–246, 1985.

110. Prichard J, Thadani V, Kalb R, and Manuelidis E: Rapidly progressive dementia in a patient who received cadaveric dura mater graft. MMWR 36:49–55, 1987.

111. Prusiner SB: Novel proteinaceous in-

fectious particles cause scrapie. Science 216:136–144, 1982.

112. Prusiner SB: Prions and neurodegenerative disease. N Engl J Med 317:1571–1581, 1987.

113. Prusiner SB: Creutzfeldt-Jakob disease and scrapie prions. Alzheimer Disease and Associated Disorders 3:52–78, 1989.

114. Prusiner SB: Scrapie prions. Annu Rev Microbiol 43:345–374, 1989.

115. Prusiner SB: Molecular biology of prion diseases. Science 252:1515–1522, 1991.

116. Prusiner SB, Cochran SP, and Alpers MP: Transmission of scrapie in hamsters. J Infect Dis 152:971–978, 1985.

117. Prusiner SB, Hsiao KK, Bredesen DE, and DeArmond SJ: Prion disease. In McKendall RR (ed): Handbook of Clinical Neurology, vol 56. Elsevier Science Publishers, Amsterdam, 1989, pp 543–580.

118. Prusiner SB, McKinley MP, Bowman KA, et al: Scrapie prions aggregate to form amyloid-like birefringent rods. Cell 35:349–358, 1983.

119. Prusiner SB, Scott M, Foster D, et al: Transgenic mouse studies implicate interactions between homologous PrP isoforms in scrapie prion replication. Cell 63:673–686, 1990.

120. Rammohan KW, McFarland HF, and McFarlan DE: Induction of subacute murine measles encephalitis by monoclonal antibody to virus hemagglutinin. Nature 290:588–589, 1981.

121. Rohwer RG: Scraple infectious agent is virus-like in size and susceptibility to inactivation. Nature 308:658–662, 1984.

122. Roos R, Gajdusek DC, and Gibbs CJ Jr: The clinical characteristics of transmissible Creutzfeldt-Jakob disease. Brain 96:1–20, 1973.

123. Rosenberg RN, White CL, Brown P, et al: Precautions in handling tissues, fluids, and other contaminated materials from patients with documented or suspected Creutzfeldt-Jakob disease. Ann Neurol 19:75–77, 1986.

124. Salazar AM, Masters CL, Gajdusek DC, and Gibbs CJ Jr: Syndromes of amyotrophic lateral sclerosis and de-mentia: Relation to transmissible Creutzfeldt-Jakob disease. Ann Neurol 14:17–26, 1983.

125. Schneider-Schaulies S, Liebert UG, Baczko K, and ter Meulen V: Restricted expression of measles virus in primary rat astroglial cells. Virology 177:802–806, 1990.

126. Scott M, Foster D, Mirenda C, et al: Transgenic mice expressing hamster prion protein produce species-specific scrapie infectivity and amyloid plaques. Cell 59:847–857, 1989.

127. Sheppard RR, Raine CS, Bornstein MS, and Udem SA: Rapid degradation restricts measles virus matrix protein expression in a subacute sclerosing panencephalitis cell line. Proc Natl Acad Sci U S A 83:7913–7917, 1986.

128. Sigurdsson B: Rida, a chronic encephalitis of sheep, with general remarks on infections which develop slowly and some of their special characteristics. Br Vet J 110:341–354, 1954.

129. Small JA, Scangos GA, Cork L, Jay G, and Khoury G: The early region of human papovavirus JC induces dysmyelination in transgenic mice. Cell 46:13–18, 1986.

130. Smith CR, Sima AF, and Gentili F: Progressive multifocal leuko-encephalopathy: Failure of cytarabine therapy. Neurology 32:200–203, 1982.

131. Sparkes RS, Simon M, Cohn VH, et al: Assignment of the human and mouse prion protein genes to homologous chromosomes. Proc Natl Acad Sci U S A 83:7358–7362, 1986.

132. Stahl N, Borchelt DR, Hsiao KK, and Prusiner SB: Scrapie prion protein contains a phosphatidylinositol glycolipid. Cell 51:229–240, 1987.

133. Stahl N and Prusiner SB: Prions and prion protein. FASEB J 5:2799–2807, 1991.

134. Stoner GL, Ryschkewitsch CF, Walker DL, and Webster H deF: JC papovavirus large tumor (t)-antigen expression in brain tissue of acquired immunodeficiency syndrome (AIDS) and non AIDS patients with progressive multifocal leukoencephalopathy. Proc Natl Acad Sci U S A 83:2271, 1986.

135. Swoveland PT: Molecular events in

measles virus infection of the central nervous system. Int Rev Exp Pathol 32:255–275, 1991.

136. Swoveland PT and Johnson KP: Subacute sclerosing panencephalitis and other paramyxovirus infections. In McKendall RR (ed): Handbook of Clinical Neurology, vol 56. Elsevier Science Publishers, Amsterdam, 1989, pp 417–438.

137. Taguchi J, Kajioka J, and Miyamura T: Prevalence rate and age of acquisition of antibodies against JC virus and BK virus in human sera. Microbiol Immunol 26:1057–1064, 1982.

138. Telenti A, Aksamit AJ, Proper J, and Smith TF: Detection of JC virus DNA by polymerase chain reaction in patients with progressive multifocal leukoencephalopathy. J Infect Dis 162:858–861, 1990.

139. Tourtellotte WW, Ma BI, Brandes DB, Walsh MJ, and Potvin AR: Quantification of de novo central nervous system IgG measles antibody synthesis in SSPE. Ann Neurol 9:551–556, 1981.

140. Trapp BD, Small JA, Pulley M, Khoury G, and Scangos GA: Dysmyelination in transgenic mice containing JC virus early region. Ann Neurol 23:38–43, 1988.

141. Van Bogaert L: Une leuco-encephalité sclerosante subaigue. J Neurol Neurosurg Psychiatry 8:101–120, 1945.

142. Vandvik B and Norrby E: Oligoclonal IgG antibody response in the central nervous system to different measles virus antigens in subacute sclerosing panencephalitis. Proc Natl Acad Sci U S A 70:1060–1063, 1973.

143. Vazeux R, Cumont M, Girard PM, et al: Severe encephalitis resulting from coinfections with HIV and JC virus. Neurology 40:944–948, 1990.

144. Walker DL: Progressive multifocal leukoencephalopathy: An opportunistic infection of the central nervous system. In: Handbook of Clinical Neurology, vol 34. North-Holland, Amsterdam, 1978, pp.

145. Weiner LP: Role of viruses in brain disorders: An overview. In Jones E (ed): Molecular Biology of the Human Brain. Alan R Liss, New York, 1988, pp 149–164.

146. Weiner LP: Viruses in immunocompromised hosts. In McKendall RR (ed): Handbook of Clinical Neurology, vol 56. Elsevier Science Publishers, Amsterdam, 1989, pp 467–488.

147. Weiner LP, Herndon RM, Narayan ON, et al: Isolation of virus related to SV40 from patients with progressive multifocal leukoencephalopathy. N Engl J Med 286:385–390, 1972.

148. Weiner LP and Stohlman SA: Immunodeficiency and CNS disease. In Rose FC (ed): Clinical Neuroimmunology. Blackwell Scientific Publications, London, 1979, pp 53–89.

149. Westaway D, Goodman PA, Mirenda CA, McKinley MP, Carlson GA, and Prusiner SB: Distinct prion proteins in short and long scrapie incubation period mice. Cell 51:651–662, 1987.

150. Wiley CA and Nelson JA: Role of the human immunodeficiency virus and cytomegalovirus in AIDS encephalitis. Am J Pathol 133:73–81, 1988.

151. Will RG and Matthews WB: Evidence for case-to-case transmission of Creutzfeldt-Jakob disease. J Neurol Neurosurg Psychiatry 45:235–238, 1982.

152. Wong TC, Ayate M, Hirano A, Yoshikawa Y, Tsuruoka H, and Yamanouchi K: Generalized and localized biased hypermutation affecting the matrix gene of a measles virus strain that causes subacute sclerosing panencephalitis. J Virol 63:5464–5468, 1989.

153. Zochodne DW, Young GB, McLachlan RS, Gilbert JJ, Vinters JV, and Kaufmann CJE: Creutzfeldt-Jakob disease without periodic sharp wave complexes. Neurology 38:1056–1060, 1988.

154. ZuRhein GM: Polyoma-like virions in a human demyelinating disease. Acta Neuropathol 8:57, 1967.

155. ZuRhein GM: Association of papovavirions with human demyelinating disease (progressive multifocal leukoencephalopathy). Prog Med Virol 11:185–247, 1969.

Part II

BACTERIAL, FUNGAL, AND PARASITIC INFECTIONS

Chapter 7

FOCAL SUPPURATIVE INFECTIONS OF THE CENTRAL NERVOUS SYSTEM

Kenneth L. Tyler, M.D.,
Joseph B. Martin, M.D., Ph.D.,
and
W. Michael Scheld, M.D.

BRAIN ABSCESS
CEREBRAL SUBDURAL EMPYEMA
SPINAL SUBDURAL EMPYEMA AND
　EPIDURAL ABSCESS
INTRACRANIAL EPIDURAL ABSCESS

Focal suppurative infections of the central nervous system (CNS) are typically classified according to their anatomic location. Epidural empyemas are confined to the space between the dura and the overlying bones; subdural empyemas lie beneath the dura but outside the pia-arachnoid, and brain abscesses lie within the brain parenchyma itself. The clinical features of these infections depend in part on the location of the infection, and each type of infection has unique clinical, pathophysiologic, diagnostic, and therapeutic aspects, which are discussed below.

BRAIN ABSCESS

Epidemiology

The basic epidemiology of brain abscesses has been extensively re-

viewed.* In general, the frequency of brain abscesses is higher in men than women, although the difference has been small in some studies. The typical patient is a young adult (median age 30 to 40 years), although as many as 25% of brain abscesses occur in children younger than 15 years of age.[21,37,68] Very young children (younger than 2 years) rarely get brain abscesses unless there is an intercurrent meningitis. The age distribution of patients with abscesses arising from contiguous sites of intracranial infection reflects the prevalence of the underlying primary infection. For example, abscesses secondary to otitis media have bimodal age peaks, one during childhood and one in older adulthood (older than 40 years). Abscess associated with paranasal sinusitis[6,38] typically occurs in young adults (ages 10 to 30).

Pathogenesis

Brain abscesses may result from contiguous spread of infection from a pri-

---

*References 7, 11, 50, 58, 69, 71, 80, 90, 92.

157

mary site of suppuration ($\approx 50\%$), or infection may reach the brain through the bloodstream ($\approx 25\%$). In rare cases, such as following cranial trauma or neurosurgical procedures, microorganisms may be introduced directly into the brain.[64,79] Even after all these possibilities are considered, a significant proportion of cases ($\approx 25\%$) remain idiopathic in nature.[7,50,58,69]

The two major sources for direct spread of infection are from the middle-ear–mastoid region[5,49,70] and from the paranasal sinuses.[6,12,38] Otogenic abscesses more commonly seem to follow chronic rather than acute cases of otitis. Infection may spread from the middle ear through the tegmen tympani or from the mastoid through the tegmen mastoideum or may travel to the brain through the major venous sinuses. In adults, otogenic abscesses commonly occur in the temporal lobe, whereas in children the most frequently involved site is the cerebellum.[73] As a general corollary, when abscess occurs in either the cerebellum or temporal lobes, the possibility of mastoid or middle-ear infection should always be considered. In some series, nearly 90% of cerebellar abscesses are associated with mastoid or middle-ear infections.[73] Infection in the paranasal sinuses typically results in an abscess located in the frontal lobes, although sphenoid sinusitis is also associated with temporal lobe (and, more rarely, intrasellar) abscesses.

Another important, and often overlooked, primary site of suppuration is dental infection,[33] which may account for up to 10% of brain abscesses. Infection often takes the form of periapical abscesses, especially involving molar teeth.

Hematogenous spread of infection from a distant site to the CNS occurs in about 25% of cases of brain abscess. These abscesses frequently occur in the territory of the middle cerebral artery at the corticomedullary junction.[91] The presence of multiple abscesses suggests the possibility of hematogenous infection. Unfortunately the converse is not true, and solitary abscesses may arise from either blood-borne spread or direct extension of local infection.

The most common primary source of blood-borne infection is the lung. The initiating processes are diverse and include lung abscess, pneumonia, bronchiectasis, and empyema. Patients with pulmonary arteriovenous (AV) fistulas (Osler-Weber-Rendu syndrome)[25,61] are at increased risk. A specific association between pulmonary alveolar proteinosis and nocardial brain abscess has frequently been described.[89,91]

Patients with cardiac disease resulting in right-to-left shunting also have a higher than expected incidence of brain abscesses. The most common underlying cardiac pathologies include tetralogy of Fallot, ventricular septal defects, patent foramen ovale, and transpositions of the great vessels.[93] Surprisingly, bacterial endocarditis is not associated with brain abscess as frequently as might be expected.[43,62] In endocarditis, when abscesses do occur, they are typically small (< 1 cm). Although all types of endocarditis may be associated with abscess, *Staphylococcus aureus* endocarditis appears to pose the greatest threat. Less common sites of primary infection than cardiopulmonary sources include intra-abdominal and pelvic infections and osteomyelitis.

Organisms may also be directly introduced into the brain parenchyma by cranial trauma, penetrating head injuries, or neurosurgical procedures.[64,79,80] Improvements in neurosurgical techniques have greatly reduced the incidence of postoperative infections, and brain abscess now complicates less than 0.2% of procedures. Penetrating head wounds, particularly gunshot injuries and other forms of trauma producing retained bone, clearly predispose to subsequent abscess development.

Microbiology

Aerobic bacteria including *Staph. aureus*, streptococci, and coliform bacteria account for about two thirds of the organisms isolated from brain abscesses.[7,11,50,69,71,90] Aerobic and microaerophilic streptococci, predominantly of the *Streptococcus milleri* group (*Strep. anginosus, Strep. constellatus, Strep. intermedius,* etc.), account for nearly 50% of these aerobic isolates. *Staph. aureus* accounts for another 25% and should always be considered in cases that follow trauma or neurosurgical procedures. Gram-negative bacilli, often in mixed culture, account for the majority of the remaining aerobes; these include *Proteus* species, *Escherichia coli, Klebsiella* species, *Enterobacter* species, and *Pseudomonas aeruginosa.* Improved techniques for culture of anaerobic organisms has led to the recognition that they are also important etiologic agents, which account for at least one third of the organisms isolated from abscesses. The most frequently encountered organisms are *Bacteroides* species (including *B. fragilis*), *Fusobacterium* species, anaerobic streptococci, and *Clostridium* species. Anaerobic infection appears particularly important in abscesses associated with chronic otitis or pulmonary disease.

The location of an abscess may provide an important clue to the infectious cause. Abscesses in the frontal lobe often result from paranasal sinusitis or dental sepsis and are typically associated with streptococci (often in pure culture), *B. fragilis,* and Gram-negative bacilli. Chronic sinusitis often results in abscesses with mixed aerobic and anaerobic microorganisms.[6,38] Abscesses in the cerebellum and temporal lobes[73] may complicate otitis media and mastoiditis, which frequently result in polymicrobial infection with streptococci, *Bacteroides* species, and Gram-negative aerobic bacilli. Because acute otitis, in contrast to chronic otitis, is only rarely associated with abscess, the organisms responsible for acute infection (e.g., *Strep. pneumoniae, Haemophilus influenzae,* and *Moraxella (Branhamella) catarrhalis*) are only rarely responsible for otogenic abscesses. By contrast, the organisms encountered in chronic otitis, including streptococci, Gram-negative aerobes (e.g., *P. aeruginosa*), anaerobic cocci, and *Bacteroides* species, are commonly encountered in otogenic brain abscesses. Abscesses that follow neurosurgical procedures or trauma are often caused by *Staph. aureus* or clostridia species.

The microbial cause of brain abscesses is strikingly altered in immunocompromised patients,[1,34,67,90] including those with acquired immunodeficiency syndrome (AIDS).[44,47] In this group, *Toxoplasma gondii* and fungal infections (e.g., *Cryptococcus neoformans*), as well as infections with *Nocardia asteroides, Listeria monocytogenes,* and *Mycobacterium* species, are of paramount importance. The causative agents in neutropenic patients differ from those in patients with impaired cell-mediated immunity; in neutropenic patients, infection may result from aerobic Gram-negative bacteria, *Candida* species, *Aspergillus* species, and zygomycetes.

Pathology

The frequency with which different regions of the brain are involved with abscesses reflects the prominence of spread from contiguous primary sites of infection. The order of frequency is shown in Table 7–1.

Studies of experimentally induced abscesses suggest that infection

Table 7–1 REGIONS OF THE BRAIN AFFECTED BY ABSCESSES (IN DECREASING ORDER OF FREQUENCY)[59,89,90]

1. Frontal lobe
2. Frontoparietal lobes
3. Parietal lobes
4. Cerebellum
5. Occipital lobe
Rarely involved
    Basal ganglia[3,14,66]
    Thalamus
    Pituitary
    Brainstem

evolves through a series of four histopathologic stages.[9,89] The first stage (early cerebritis) is characterized by a necrotic central focus, striking edema, and a surrounding zone of prominent perivascular inflammatory response. In the second stage (late cerebritis), the necrotic zone becomes more discrete and is surrounded by a peripheral zone of fibroblasts and neovascularization. In the third stage, a distinct capsule begins to appear, with a well-developed layer of fibroblasts and associated persisting cerebritis and neovascularity. The final stages consist of completion and thickening of capsule formation. Capsule formation is frequently more complete on the cortical side of the abscess when compared to the ventricular side.[9,89] This may explain the propensity for abscesses to rupture medially into the ventricular system rather than laterally into the subarachnoid space. Capsule formation is often less extensive in abscesses resulting from hematogenous spread of infection,[89] compared to those arising from local infection. Maturity of the lesion(s) also depends on factors such as local oxygen concentration, the offending microorganism, and the host immune response.[89] Although these discrete stages cannot always be appreciated in natural infection in humans, they do seem to correlate well with specific patterns seen on computed tomography (CT) and magnetic resonance imaging (MRI) studies.[8]

Clinical Features

The signs and symptoms of brain abscess are produced by the primary infection (if present), the focal effects of the abscess and its particular localization within the brain parenchyma, and by the more generalized effects of increased intracranial pressure.[28,82,89-91] The clinical presentation may range from indolent to fulminant, although the majority of patients present with a subacute illness with symptoms that have been present for less than 2 weeks.

General signs and symptoms include fever, chills, and malaise. Fever is more commonly present in acute cases and may be minimal or absent in chronic ones. Fever appears to result predominantly from the primary infection (e.g., otitis or sinusitis) rather than from the abscess itself. Because fever is present in less than half the patients, its absence should never be used to exclude abscess as a diagnostic consideration.

Headache occurs in 50% to 70% of patients and may be either generalized or focal in location. Like fever, its absence does not preclude the diagnosis of abscess. Seizures occur in one third to one half of patients and may be either generalized or focal, although the former occur more frequently. Headache, nausea, vomiting, and papilledema appear to reflect increased intracranial pressure rather than particular focal locations of infection. Focal neurologic signs are present in the majority of cases. The most commonly encountered signs are hemiparesis, alterations in mental status, nuchal rigidity, papilledema, cranial nerve deficits, and visual field abnormalities. The appearance of particular signs and symptoms obviously depends on the location of the lesion. Frontal lobe abscesses may produce deterioration in memory function, attention, and other abnormalities of mental status. Grasp, snout, or suck responses may occur. Some patients have focal or generalized seizures that may be associated with contraversive head or eye movements. Abscesses in the temporal lobe may be associated with hemiparesis, superior quadrantanopsia, and aphasia (dominant lesions). Motor weakness may be subtle, if present, and can consist of only faciobrachial paresis. In cerebellar abscesses, suboccipital headache with radiation to the neck and interscapular region may be prominent. This may be associated with nystagmus, ataxia, dysmetria, and other signs of cerebellar dysfunction.

Diagnosis

Studies of the blood are rarely useful in the specific diagnosis of brain abscess.[38,90] Leukocytosis ($>$ 10,000 cells/mm^3) is present in about 50% of patients but rarely exceeds 20,000/mm^3.[89] The erythrocyte sedimentation rate (ESR) is elevated in 75% of cases (mean value 50 mm/h) and may provide a diagnostic clue to the presence of infection. Acute phase reactants, including serum C reactive protein, may also provide hints of the presence of infection. Although as many as 25% of abscesses arise from primary extracranial infections, less than 10% of blood cultures are positive.[11,68,69]

Although the cerebrospinal fluid (CSF) is often abnormal in patients with abscess, lumbar puncture should be avoided in cases of suspected abscess, owing to the danger of subsequent herniation.[11,69,71,89,91] Post–lumbar-puncture deterioration occurs in 20% to 33% of cases, typically within 24 to 48 hours. When CSF has been examined,[58,59,69] it typically shows a mild pleocytosis ($\approx$70% of cases) with either mononuclear or polymorphonuclear cell predominance, an elevated protein level, and a normal glucose level. Cell counts may be higher in cases of cerebritis and tend to fall in the presence of an encapsulated abscess. Cell counts are also higher when the abscess is located in proximity to either the subarachnoid space (e.g., near the cortical surface) or the ventricles. It is important to recognize that a CSF pleocytosis is absent in 10% to 20% of cases. Cultures and stains for microorganisms are negative in more than 90% of cases unless there is an associated meningitis, or ventricular rupture of the abscess has occurred.[11]

The introduction of CT and MRI has revolutionized the diagnostic and therapeutic approach to brain abscess. Older imaging procedures such as radionuclide brain scans and arteriography are now essentially obsolete as aids in the diagnosis of brain abscess and should be reserved for rare situations when CT and MRI are unavailable. CT is extremely useful in the evaluation of localized infections involving the sinuses, mastoid, and middle ear, and a scan should be obtained, along with a chest x-ray, in all patients with suspected brain abscess. CT scan will identify virtually all cases of abscess and provides valuable information about the extent of associated edema, midline shift, and hydrocephalus.[56] Abscesses typically appear as hypodense lesions surrounded by a uniform ring of enhancement following contrast administration. The zone of enhancement may in turn be surrounded by a hypodense peripheral region of edema. It is important to recognize that a similar CT appearance may be produced by tumors, granuloma, hematomas, or infarcts.[76] Ring enhancement may be absent in the early stages of abscess development (cerebritis) and may also be absent in up to one half of patients receiving steroid therapy.[76]

MRI (Fig. 7–1) appears to be at least as sensitive as CT in delineating brain abscesses[16] and is clearly more sensitive during the initial phases of abscess development (cerebritis). MRI also allows more optimal imaging of the posterior fossa and brainstem and a clearer delineation of the presence and extent of associated edema. The typical MRI appearance of a fully developed abscess is of a ring lesion with a T_1-weighted hyperintense and T_2-weighted hypointense capsule. With gadolinium administration the ring enhances on T_2-weighted images. When it is readily available, MRI should be considered the imaging procedure of choice in cases of suspected brain abscess.

Treatment

Optimal treatment of most patients with brain abscess consists of a combination of antimicrobial and neurosurgical therapy. Some patients may respond to antimicrobial therapy alone,[4] without the need for surgical intervention. In general, this approach should

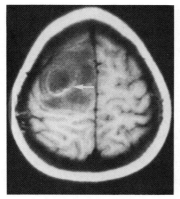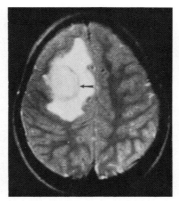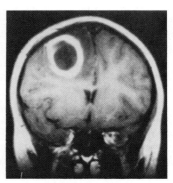

Figure 7–1. MRI appearance of brain abscess. *Left,* An axial T$_1$-weighted image shows a bright, hyperintense ring lesion *(arrow)* in the right frontal lobe with a hypointense central and surrounding area. *Center,* On a T$_2$-weighted axial image, the ring *(arrow)* is slightly hypointense and the central and surrounding regions are hyperintense. *Right,* A gadolinium-enhanced T$_1$-weighted coronal image demonstrates ring enhancement of the lesion. In both the T$_1$- and T$_2$-weighted images, the ring corresponds to the abscess capsule, the surrounding zone is edema in the brain parenchyma, and the central zone is necrotic debris within the abscess capsule. (From Smith RS and Arvin MC: Neuroradiology of intracranial infection. Reprinted with permission from Seminars in Neurology 12:248–262, 1992, Thieme Medical Publishers, Inc.)

be reserved for patients with multiple lesions, lesions that are surgically inaccessible, and cases of cerebritis. Patients treated in this fashion often require prolonged (longer than 2 months) courses of high-dose intravenous antimicrobial therapy and must be closely followed both clinically and with sequential imaging studies.

Recommended antibiotic regimens for the therapy of brain abscess reflect both the nature of the inciting microbial organisms and the necessity for good penetration of the abscess cavity. In typical cases, intravenous antibiotics are used for 4 to 6 weeks. This may be followed by several months of oral antibiotic treatment, although the efficacy of this type of supplemental therapy has never been clearly established. For many years the standard regimen for empiric therapy in immunocompetent adults with normal renal function was a combination of intravenous penicillin G (e.g., 2 to 4 million units every 2 to 4 hours) plus chloramphenicol (1.0 to 1.5 g every 6 hours). Penicillin remains a mainstay of therapy because of its excellent activity against the majority of organisms typically encountered in brain abscesses and the abundant

accumulated clinical experience supporting its efficacy. However, chloramphenicol has been largely supplanted by other agents (see below). When *Staph. aureus* infection is suspected, such as following trauma or neurosurgical procedures, a semisynthetic penicillin such as nafcillin or oxacillin (1.5 g every 4 hours intravenously) should be substituted for penicillin. Vancomycin[45] (1 g every 12 hours) may be used for patients who are allergic to penicillin or from whom methicillin-resistant staphylococci are isolated. Vancomycin dosage should be adjusted to keep peak serum concentrations at 20 to 40 mg/mL and trough concentrations at 5 to 10 mg/mL.

The use of chloramphenicol in conjunction with penicillin to provide enhanced activity against anaerobes such as *B. fragilis* has become less common.

In most centers, metronidazole (15 mg/kg loading dose followed by 7.5 mg/kg every 6 hours intravenously) has supplanted chloramphenicol[85] because it is more potent against many anaerobes, is bactericidal against *B. fragilis,* and attains good concentrations in both brain parenchyma and abscess cavities. Some studies suggest that metronidazole, when substituted for chloramphenicol, may lead to more rapid abscess healing and a lower mortality rate. The absorption of metronidazole after oral administration is excellent, with serum levels equivalent to those obtained with intravenous administration. As a result, oral dosing (e.g., 500 mg every 6 hours) may be used in place of intravenous therapy in certain situations, especially after clinical stabilization in preparation for outpatient administration.

Patients with otogenic abscesses frequently have Gram-negative bacilli isolated from their lesions. The combination of penicillin and metronidazole does not offer adequate coverage of these organisms, and in this setting a third-generation cephalosporin such as cefotaxime[75] (2 g every 4 hours) should be used, either in addition to the other agents or as a replacement for penicillin. Trimethoprim-sulfamethoxazole has also been used in this setting.

Although advocated by many neurosurgeons, few studies of the effects of instillation of antibiotics into the abscess cavity have been performed. In one small series, the group receiving local instillation of antibiotics did have a lower mortality rate.[42] Nonetheless, this practice should not be used routinely until further studies documenting efficacy are available.

As noted earlier, optimal therapy for brain abscess combines antimicrobial therapy with neurosurgical treatment. Controversy exists about whether aspiration alone or total excision of the brain abscess provides the best surgical approach.[18,65,66,77,78,90] Some studies have suggested that excision may be associated with a lower mortality rate, although this may reflect the fact that patients selected for excision are often in better medical condition than those undergoing aspiration.[77,78] Many surgeons advocate excision for lesions in the posterior fossa and for fungal abscesses.[89] Stereotaxic CT-guided aspiration of the abscess cavity can be performed with minimal morbidity and allows specimens to be obtained for definitive microbiologic and pathologic diagnosis. Aspiration is the procedure of choice for most patients with multiple abscesses and for inaccessible lesions such as those involving the brainstem.[18,66]

If the CT scan or MRI suggests the presence of cerebritis, rather than a fully encapsulated abscess, and the patient is neurologically stable, empiric antibiotic therapy should be started and the patient carefully followed until cerebritis resolves. If the patient remains stable and the abscess encapsulates, CT-guided aspiration is then desirable to facilitate a specific pathologic and microbiologic diagnosis. Although this delay may render operative cultures negative, aspiration during the cerebritis stage may be associated with an unacceptable risk of hemorrhage, especially in children.

If on initial CT scan or MRI the lesion appears to be already encapsulated, aspiration for diagnosis and drainage should be performed immediately in conjunction with empiric antimicrobial therapy. Therapy should then be adjusted as required when culture results become available. Neurologic deterioration or failure of the lesion to resolve on follow-up imaging studies is an indication for further surgery, often excision if feasible.

In addition to definitive antimicrobial and surgical therapy, patients with brain abscess are frequently treated with both anticonvulsants and corticosteroids. As noted, seizures occur acutely in one third to one half of patients. This frequency is probably high enough to justify prophylactic anticonvulsant therapy, although no specific data on this subject exist. The agents employed are the same as for seizures resulting from noninfectious causes. Once instituted, therapy should probably be continued for at least 6 to 12 months. At that point, if the patient has remained seizure-free, a gradual attempt to discontinue treatment can be considered. It should be recognized, however, that seizures occur as a late complication of brain abscess in up to 90% of patients in some series,[89] and seizure recurrence after discontinuation of early anticonvulsant therapy is common.

Steroids are often used in patients with brain abscess to reduce edema and help control intracranial pressure, although documentation of their utility is not available. Animal studies have not provided evidence of a clear beneficial effect.[89] Corticosteroids may reduce the entry of some antibiotics into the CNS and can also reduce abscess encapsulation by inhibiting collagenization and glial response. In addition, steroids may alter the appearance of brain abscess on CT scans by affecting the inflammatory response and the associated capsular enhancement. Nonetheless, steroids should probably be used (e.g., dexamethasone 0.15 mg/kg IV every 6 hours), in conjunction with hyperosmotic agents and hyperventilation, when increased intracranial pressure is present. Once definitive therapy, such as drainage or excision, allows reversion of intracranial pressure to normal, steroids should be tapered as rapidly as possible.

Prognosis

The mortality rate of brain abscess has declined sharply since the advent of CT. In most recent studies, the mortality rate is consistently below 10%. However, neurologic sequelae remain common and may occur in 30% to 55% of those with brain abscess. The late occurrence of seizures, reported in up to 90% of abscess survivors[89] in some series, remains particularly problematic.

CEREBRAL SUBDURAL EMPYEMA

Subdural empyema (SDE) can be defined as a collection of pus in the preformed space between the cranial dura and arachnoid membranes. More than 90% of cases occur supratentorially, as the tentorium cerebelli serves as an effective mechanical barrier to infraten-

torial spread of infection.[57] SDE accounts for approximately 10% to 20% of all purulent intracranial infections.[10,29,52] In the preantibiotic era, SDE was almost invariably fatal, but improvements in diagnosis and therapy have now reduced the mortality rate to less than 30%.

Epidemiology and Pathogenesis

SDE is primarily an infection of young adults, with a striking (70%) male predilection.[10,29,40,52] The majority of cases arise as a complication of paranasal sinusitis (50% to 70%),[12,29,35,39,84] with otitis media and mastoiditis now accounting for less than 20% of cases. In most cases, the frontal sinus is involved, with the SDE beginning near the frontal pole and extending posteriorly. Cases may also follow maxillary and sphenoid sinusitis. Otitis or mastoiditis may extend directly into the subdural space by direct erosion through the adjacent bone of the tegmen tympani or may spread indirectly by way of a progressive thrombophlebitis of the perforating veins. Otitis-induced subdural empyema is localized initially on or around the tentorium but may spread into the posterior fossa or laterally over the temporal lobe. Less common antecedents of SDE include head trauma or neurosurgical procedures, local osteomyelitis, and facial infections. Rarely, secondary infection of subdural hematomas, extension of an epidural abscess through a dural fistula, or septic cerebral thrombophlebitis can lead to SDE. Cases may also occur as a result of hematogenous spread of infection from a distant, extracranial primary site. Posterior fossa SDEs,[57] which account for less than 10% of all SDEs, may arise as a complication of septic labyrinthitis or petrous apicitis. In children, SDE may be due to secondary bacterial infection of an initially sterile subdural effusion or may be an unusual complication of meningitis.[36,88] In adults, SDE rarely arises following bacterial meningitis.[10,29] SDE can spread rapidly along the falx cerebri and over the cerebral hemispheres. Complicating septic cortical vein thrombophlebitis may lead to hemorrhagic cerebral infarction, brain edema, and fatal transtentorial herniation.

Microbiology

In distinction to the commonly polymicrobial cause of brain abscesses, SDE is typically due to a single microorganism. The major pathogens include aerobic and anaerobic streptococci (50%), staphylococci (20%), aerobic Gram-negative bacilli (5% to 10%), and other anaerobic bacteria (5%).[29,32,40,52,55] As with brain abscess, a clue to the cause may be obtained from the nature of the preceding primary infection. Otorhinogenic subdural empyemas are usually caused by streptococci (including members of the *Strep. milleri* group), whereas staphylococci and anaerobe infections are unusual. Infections resulting as a complication of neurosurgical procedures or indwelling foreign devices commonly involve staphylococci and/or aerobic Gram-negative bacilli. Subdural empyema rarely complicates meningitis, but cases due to *Strep. pneumoniae* or *Haemophilus influenzae* have been described.[35] Rare etiologic agents include *Salmonella* species, *Campylobacter fetus*, *Neisseria meningitidis*, *Pasteurella* species, *Candida albicans*, and actinomycetes.[10]

Clinical Features

The cardinal clinical features of SDE are due to (1) the signs and symptoms of the associated local infection, (2) increased intracranial pressure, and (3) focal neurologic dysfunction.[10,29,32,36,40,88] SDE may present as an acute, fulminant, progressive, life-threatening condition, but more commonly patients have a history of several days or even weeks of nonspecific illness followed by an abrupt deterioration. The most common symptoms and signs include fever, headache, nuchal rigidity, and focal neurologic deficits. Most patients (90%) appear acutely ill with fever in excess of 39°C. Headache, initially localized to the infected sinus or ear, is a prominent complaint (75%) and can become generalized as the infection progresses. There may be pain and tenderness over the brow, between the eyes, or in the area of the involved ear or sinus. Orbital swelling and mild proptosis may be a clue to obstruction of the orbital veins. Scalp swelling or cellulitis suggests the possibility of cranial osteomyelitis or an associated extradural empyema. Nausea and vomiting occur in one half to two thirds of cases and reflect associated increased intracranial pressure. Alterations in consciousness develop in approximately 50% to 75% of patients. These may range from mild sleepiness to obtundation or even coma. Focal neurologic findings appear within the first few days of illness and may progress rapidly. Contralateral hemiparesis and hemiplegia are the most common focal findings and eventually develop in almost all patients. These are usually associated with an extensor plantar (Babinski) response. Ocular palsies and paresis of conjugate gaze toward the side of the lesion (resulting in eyes deviated toward the side of the lesion) are common. Additional findings vary with the location of the SDE and may include dysphasia, homonymous hemianopsia, cerebellar signs, and pupillary abnormalities. The presence of bilateral Babinski responses or papilledema should suggest the possibility of transtentorial herniation or the presence of coexisting sinus thrombosis. More than half the patients with SDE will develop seizures, which may be focal or generalized. Focal motor or jacksonian seizures may precede the development of generalized seizures. Rare patients develop status epilepticus. Meningeal irritation (particularly meningismus) is found in 70% to 80% of patients, although Kernig's and/or

Brudzhinski's signs are less frequently noted. In the absence of treatment, neurologic deterioration occurs rapidly, with signs of increased intracranial pressure and cerebral herniation.

This classic clinical picture of SDE may not be seen in patients with SDE as a complication of cranial trauma or neurosurgical procedures or in patients receiving antimicrobial therapy.[10,23,29] Atypical presentations may also occur when SDE complicates a preexisting hematoma or results from spread of infection from an extracranial primary site.

Diagnosis

Studies of blood and CSF are of limited value in the evaluation of patients with suspected SDE.[29,32,40,88] Almost all patients will have a peripheral blood leukocytosis. CT, MRI, or plain films will often delineate a predisposing local infection such as sinusitis, otitis, or mastoiditis. Lumbar puncture is contraindicated because of the risk of cerebral herniation and rarely adds useful diagnostic information. When CSF has been examined, the findings are as shown in Table 7–2.

CT with contrast enhancement and MRI[29,32,86,94] are the diagnostic procedures of choice in patients with suspected SDE. The typical CT appearance

is of a crescentic or elliptically shaped hypodense zone overlying one or both cerebral hemispheres and situated immediately beneath the skull or adjacent to the falx cerebri. Associated mass effect and displacement of midline structures are common. The underlying brain parenchyma may show hyperintensity of the cortical gray matter and hypointensity of the underlying white matter. Following contrast administration, there may be enhancement at the boundary between the SDE and the cortex. Gyral enhancement, if present, should suggest the possibility of associated meningitis, cerebritis, or venous thrombosis.[29]

MRI appears to be more sensitive than CT in detecting SDE and provides better morphologic details (Fig. 7–2). MRI is of particular value in identifying SDE located in the posterior fossa, along the falx cerebri, or at the base of the brain. SDEs differ in signal intensity from both subdural hematomas and effusions.

Arteriography is now only infrequently used in the diagnosis of SDE. It may be of value in cases where the CT is negative and MRI is unavailable. The typical angiographic findings of SDE include displacement of vessels away from the inner skull table, which indicates the presence of an extra-axial avascular mass. Intrafalcial empyemas may produce a characteristic S-shaped distortion of the vessels of the anterior cerebral artery, with the proximal branches being displaced away from, and the distal branches toward, the side of the empyema.

Treatment

Subdural empyema is a fulminant, life-threatening emergency, and diagnostic and therapeutic studies should be performed as expeditiously as possible in all suspected cases. Empiric antimicrobial therapy is warranted prior to definitive surgical intervention. Commonly used empiric therapy in

Table 7–2 CSF FINDINGS IN PATIENTS WITH SUBDURAL EMPYEMA

Finding	% of Patients
Increased intracranial pressure	70
Elevated protein level (almost always < 200 mg/dL)	85
Normal glucose level	90
Pleocytosis (varying severity)	90
Cell count < 500/mm³	75
Lymphocytes predominating	30
Polymorphonuclear cells predominating	70
Negative Gram stain*	90–95
Negative cultures*	90–95

*Except in cases with coexistent bacterial meningitis.

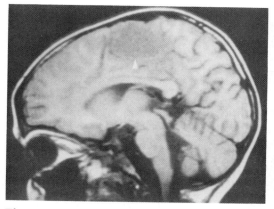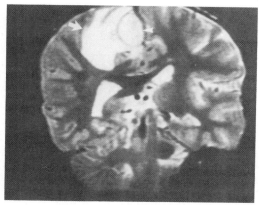

Figure 7–2. MRI appearance of cerebral subdural empyema. *Left,* A sagittal T_1-weighted image shows a slightly hypointense region *(arrowhead)* representing a collection of fluid along the right side of the falx cerebri. *Right,* The fluid collection is seen as a hyperintense lesion *(arrowhead)* with an adjacent hyperintense zone of edema *(arrow)* on a T_2-weighted coronal image. (From Smith RS and Arvin MC: Neuroradiology of intracranial infection. Reprinted with permission from Seminars in Neurology 12:248–262, 1992, Thieme Medical Publishers, Inc.)

adult patients with normal renal function includes a semisynthetic penicillin (e.g., nafcillin or oxacillin 1.5 g every 4 hours) and metronidazole (15 mg/kg loading dose followed by 7.5 mg/kg every 6 hours). Vancomycin (1 g every 12 hours) may be used in patients who are allergic to penicillin or when methicillin-resistant staphylococci are suspected. Although detailed clinical data are lacking, a third-generation cephalosporin (e.g., cefotaxime 2 g every 4 hours) in combination with metronidazole is used as alternative empiric therapy in many centers. Ceftazidime is useful in patients in which *P. aeruginosa* is a consideration (after neurosurgery or trauma, for instance), but may not adequately cover *Staphylococcus aureus.* Parenteral antibiotic therapy is generally maintained for 4 weeks following evacuation of the SDE. Longer periods of intravenous therapy and/or continuation as an oral regimen may be required if an associated osteomyelitis is present.

Optimal therapy for SDE includes a combination of surgical drainage and antimicrobial treatment.[29,40,55,82] Isolated reports of cure of SDE by antibiotics alone exist,[51] but this approach is not recommended except in exceptional circumstances. Surgical drainage may be achieved via craniotomy or through the placement of multiple burr holes.[20,29,53,55] In general, craniotomy is probably the procedure of choice.[20,53,55] Many neurosurgeons irrigate the empyema site with antibiotics at the time of surgery, but the utility of this practice has never been clearly demonstrated. Patients with coexisting sinusitis or otitis may need emergent surgical therapy for these conditions as well.

Steroids and hyperosmolar agents may be required to control intracranial pressure. Definitive surgery, by eliminating the presence of the inciting mass lesion, normally allows for rapid discontinuation of these adjunctive therapies. The frequency of focal and generalized seizures in patients with SDE is probably high enough to justify prophylactic anticonvulsant therapy.[40]

Prognosis

The overall mortality rate of subdural empyema averages 15% to 25%, with severe neurologic sequelae (chiefly disabling hemiparesis or aphasia) found in 5% to 25% of survivors. Chronic seizures develop in a significant number of patients.

SPINAL SUBDURAL EMPYEMA AND EPIDURAL ABSCESS

Epidemiology and Pathogenesis

Spinal epidural abscess (SEA) is second only to meningitis as a common suppurative infection of the spinal cord.* By contrast, spinal subdural empyema (SSE) is an extraordinarily rare condition, with less than 30 cases reported in the literature.[10,13,22,29,82] In the reported cases of SEA there has been a slight male predominance and an increased incidence in patients older than 50 years of age. There is no obvious age or sex predilection for SSE. Risk factors for both infections include alcoholism, cancer, intravenous drug abuse, diabetes mellitus, and preexisting degenerative joint disease.[10,15,31]

Most cases of SEA and SSE follow hematogenous dissemination of infection from a distant primary site.[15] Other causes of both SEA[10,15,17,26] and SSE[10,24,83] include direct extension of infection from a contiguous site, such as osteomyelitis or discitis, or direct inoculation of microorganisms following lumbar puncture or neurosurgical procedures.[10,19] SSE may also follow spread of infection through a sinus fistula, and SEA may complicate pelvic or intra-abdominal infections.[10]

Microbiology

Staph. aureus is the most commonly isolated organism in cases of SSE.[22] Other cases due to streptococci, Gram-negative bacilli, Staph. epidermidis, and polymicrobial flora have been reported.[10,29] Staph. aureus is also the most commonly encountered organism in SEA,[26] but many cases associated with streptococcus species, anaerobes, Gram-negative bacilli, and polymicrobial flora have been reported.

---

*References 2, 10, 15, 17, 19, 26, 30, 31, 54, 82.

Clinical Features

The distinction between SSE and SEA can rarely be made clinically, and the two conditions can coexist.[2,63] The signs and symptoms include fever, back pain, and spinal cord compression.[10,15,26,30,54,82] The pain is typically severe and localized. Most patients hold their spine rigid and report an increase in pain with movement. In contrast to the pain of SEA, that of SSE may not be increased by percussion or local pressure.[13,29] Fever is almost invariably present and may be associated with chills or rigors. Headache and meningeal signs are also common. Neurologic signs and symptoms typically develop acutely and may progress rapidly. The initial symptoms include bilateral leg weakness (paraparesis), sensory loss, and urinary incontinence. These reflect the propensity of SSE to involve the lumbar and thoracic spine, typically along the posterior aspect. Patients may present with a cord compression syndrome that is either spastic (hyperactive deep tendon reflexes and Babinski responses) or flaccid (hypoactive reflexes, absent Babinski responses) depending on the balance between upper- and lower-motor-neuron involvement.

Diagnosis

Routine laboratory tests in patients with SEA and SSE usually show a peripheral leukocytosis and an elevated ESR. All patients should have blood cultures because these may be positive. CSF examination should be deferred, because it may result in spread of infection into the subarachnoid, subdural, or epidural space, and should generally be limited to patients undergoing emergency myelography. The CSF findings are rarely diagnostic, usually revealing a polymorphonuclear pleocytosis, elevated protein level, and normal glucose level. An extremely high CSF protein level occurs in the presence of subarachnoid block. CSF Gram stains and cultures may be positive. MRI should be considered the diagnostic procedure of choice for both SEA and SSE,[15,17,27,46,60] although studies in SSE are limited to case reports because of the rarity of the infection. The classic finding in SEA is a localized T_2-hyperintense extradural lesion. Metrizamide spinal CT[41,46,81] is also of proven value in the diagnosis of both SEA and SSE. Myelography should be reserved for cases where MRI and CT are unavailable.

Treatment

Empiric treatment of SEA and SSE in adult patients with normal renal function consists of an anti-staphylococcal penicillin such as nafcillin (2 g every 4 hours) in combination with a third-generation cephalosporin (e.g., cefotoxamine 2 g every 4 hours). Metronidazole (15 mg/kg loading dose followed by 7.5 mg/kg every 6 hours) can be added to improve anaerobic coverage. Although favorable responses have been reported with antibiotic therapy alone,[10,15,27,46] optimal therapy of both SEA and SSE includes emergency laminectomy for drainage and culture of the infection. Antibiotic therapy should be adjusted based on results obtained at surgery and should be continued for at least 4 weeks.

INTRACRANIAL EPIDURAL ABSCESS

Epidural abscess (EA) is produced by suppurative infection in the epidural space, which is a potential space located between the dura mater and the overlying bone. The cause, pathogenesis, and microbiology of EA are similar to that of SDE. An associated primary focus of infection is commonly found in the paranasal sinuses, middle ear, or mastoids.[10,48] Although the exact incidence of EA is difficult to calculate, it appears to be about half as common as SDE in most series, making it the third most frequent form of focal intracranial

infection, after brain abscess and SDE.[10] EA does not appear to have distinctive age or sex predilections, unlike SDE.

Pathogenesis

EA primarily results from contiguous extension of localized cranial infections including sinusitis, mastoiditis, and scalp or orbital cellulitis. Cases may also result from direct introduction of microorganisms through skull fracture or neurosurgical procedure. Less commonly, EA arises as a complication of other focal intracranial infections such as SDE or septic thrombophlebitis.

Microbiology

The organisms responsible for EA are similar to those encountered in SDE. Aerobic and anaerobic streptococci predominate in infections complicating paranasal sinusitis, whereas *Staph. aureus* or *Staph. epidermidis* and aerobic Gram-negative bacilli are associated with penetrating injuries and neurosurgical procedures. Less commonly isolated organisms include *Salmonella* species, *Eikenella corrodens, Aspergillus* species, and Zygomycetes.

Clinical Features

Symptoms begin slowly, perhaps reflecting the gradual formation of the abscess in the restricted potential space between the dura and skull.[10,48,72,82] Most patients are febrile and complain of headache, but this may be absent or not prominent in some cases.[48] Focal neurologic signs or symptoms may also be mild or absent. Patients with associated SDE will often present with symptoms referable to the SDE rather than the EA. As the abscess enlarges, focal neurologic signs and symptoms may include obtundation, hemiparesis, and focal or generalized seizures. At this point the clinical differentiation between EA and SDE may be impossible. EA involving the petrous bone may result in facial pain and/or sensory loss and diplopia due to involvement of the fifth and sixth cranial nerves (Gradenigo's syndrome).

Diagnosis

CT and MRI are the diagnostic procedures of choice for the detection of EA.[10,87] The typical CT appearance (Fig. 7–3) is of a superficial, circumscribed hypointense area with a strongly contrast-enhancing rim. The rim enhancement may be thicker and more irregular in appearance than that associated with SDE. MRI appears to be superior to CT in the evaluation of EA.[87] The advantages of MRI include its improved capacity to identify small abscesses and to distinguish between SDE and EA. These results are due in part to the absence of bone artifact, which permits clearer visualization of the subosteal region.

Treatment

Optimal therapy for EA includes both surgical drainage and antimicrobial therapy. Empiric antimicrobial therapy[10,26,48,74,82] is directed against aerobic streptococci, staphylococci, and anaerobic bacteria. In adult patients with normal renal function, the combination of intravenous penicillin G (2 to 4 million units every 2 to 4 hours) and metronidazole (15 mg/kg loading dose followed by 7.5 mg/kg every 6 hours) is suitable for cases associated with sinusitis. In cases associated with trauma, cranial defects, or neurosurgical procedures, an anti-staphylococcal penicillin (e.g., nafcillin 1.5 g every 4 hours) should replace penicillin. In patients with otogenic EA or in whom the

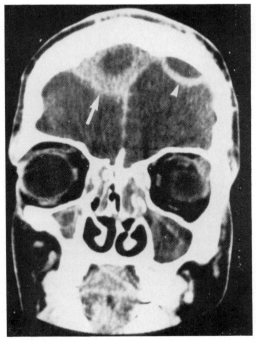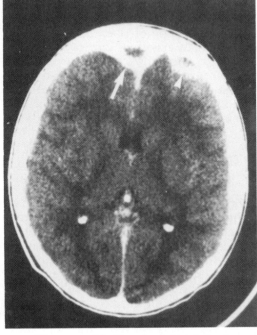

Figure 7–3. CT appearance of cerebral epidural abscess. The coronal *(left)* and axial *(right)* enhanced images show two epidural abscesses with associated dural enhancement *(arrows)*. Evidence of paranasal sinusitis can also be seen on the coronal image. (From Smith RS and Arvin MC: Neuroradiology of intracranial infection. Reprinted with permission from Seminars in Neurology 12:248–262, 1992, Thieme Medical Publishers, Inc.)

cause is unknown, a third-generation cephalosporin (e.g., cefotaxime 2 g every 4 hours) should be used in combination with metronidazole and penicillin or nafcillin. Vancomycin is a suitable alternative in penicillin-allergic patients or in patients found to harbor methicillin-resistant staphylococci. Parenteral antibiotic therapy is generally continued for 4 weeks after surgical drainage. Antibiotic therapy can be modified based on the organisms isolated from surgical cultures.

All patients should undergo surgical drainage of their EAs in addition to receiving antimicrobial therapy. Drainage may be attempted through burr holes, craniotomy, or craniectomy. As is the case for SDE, controversy exists as to which procedure is preferable.[10,23,26,74] The choice depends in part on the location and extent of the lesion and the presence or absence of associated cranial osteomyelitis.

SUMMARY

Focal suppurative infections of the CNS typically arise from either local spread of primary intracranial infections such as sinusitis or via hematogenous dissemination of microorganisms from a distant focus of infection. The clinical syndromes vary with the particular infection, but localized CNS infection should always be suspected in patients who present with focal neurologic symptoms and evidence of a primary infectious process or symptoms (e.g., fever, leukocytosis) suggesting the presence of such an infection. The diagnosis of brain abscess, subdural empyema, and epidural empyema has been revolutionized by the widespread availability of CT and MRI. Either CT or MRI should be performed emergently on all patients with suspected focal CNS infections. When both tests are readily available, MRI should generally be considered the diagnostic procedure of choice. Lumbar puncture should be avoided in patients suspected of harboring focal CNS infections, because of the danger of precipitating an abrupt clinical deterioration. Optimal therapy of focal CNS infections generally consists of a combination of appropriate antimicrobial therapy and prompt neurosurgical drainage.

REFERENCES

1. Armstrong D: Central nervous system infections in the immunocompromised host. Infection 12(Suppl 1):S58–S64, 1984.
2. Baker AS, Ojemann RG, Swartz MN, and Richardson EP Jr: Spinal epidural abscess. N Engl J Med 293:463–468, 1975.
3. Berger SA, Edberg SC, and David G: Infectious disease of the sella turcica. Rev Infect Dis 8:747–755, 1986.
4. Boom WH and Tuazon C: Successful treatment of multiple brain abscesses with antibiotics alone. Rev Infect Dis 7:189–199, 1985.
5. Bradley PJ, Manning K, and Shaw MD: Brain abscess secondary to otitis media. J Laryngol Otol 98:1185–1191, 1984.
6. Bradley PJ, Manning K, and Shaw MD: Brain abscess secondary to paranasal sinusitis. J Laryngol Otol 98:719–725, 1984.
7. Brewer NS, McCarty CS, and Wellman WE: Brain abscess: A review of recent experience. Ann Intern Med 82:571–576, 1975.
8. Britt RH and Enzmann DR: Clinical stages of human brain abscesses on serial CT scans after contrast infusion. Computerized tomographic, neuropathological, and clinical correlations. J Neurol Sci 59:972–989, 1983.
9. Britt RH, Enzmann DR, and Yeager A: Neuropathological and computerized tomographic findings in experimental brain abscess. J Neurol Sci 55:590–603, 1981.
10. Brock DG and Bleck TP: Extra-axial suppurations of the central nervous system. Semin Neurol 12:263–272, 1992.

11. Chun CH, Johnson JD, Hofstetter M, and Raff M: Brain abscess. A study of 45 consecutive cases. Medicine 65:415–431, 1986.

12. Clayman GL, Adams GL, Paugh DR, and Koopman CF Jr: Intracranial complications of paranasal sinusitis: A combined institutional review. Laryngoscope 101:234–239, 1991.

13. Dacey RG, Winn HR, Jane JA, and Butler AB: Spinal subdural empyema: Report of two cases. Neurosurgery 3:400–403, 1978.

14. Dake MD, McMurdo SK, Rosenblum ML, and Brant-Zawadzki M: Pyogenic abscess of the medulla oblongata. Neurosurgery 18:370–372, 1986.

15. Danner RL and Hartmann BJ: Update of spinal epidural abscess: 35 cases and review of the literature. Rev Infect Dis 9:265–274, 1987.

16. Davidson M and Steiner R: Magnetic resonance imaging in infections of the central nervous system. AJNR 6:499–504, 1985.

17. Del Curling O Jr, Gower DJ, and McWhorter JM: Changing concepts in spinal epidural abscess: Report of 29 cases. Neurosurgery 27:185–192, 1990.

18. Dyste G, Hitchon P, Memezes A, Van Gilder J, and Groene G: Stereotactic surgery in the treatment of multiple brain abscesses. J Neurol Sci 69:188–194, 1988.

19. Ericsson M, Algers G, and Schliamser SE: Spinal epidural abscess in adults: Review and report of iatrogenic cases. Scand J Infect Dis 22:249–257, 1990.

20. Feuerman T, Wackym PA, Gade G, and Dubrow T: Craniotomy improves outcome in subdural empyema. Surg Neurol 32:105–110, 1989.

21. Fischer E, McLennan J, and Suzuki Y: Cerebral abscess in children. Am J Dis Child 135:746–769, 1981.

22. Frasier RA, Ratzan K, Wolpert SM, and Weinstein L: Spinal subdural empyema. Arch Neurol 28:235–238, 1973.

23. Galbraith JG and Barr VW: Epidural abscess and subdural empyema. Adv Neurol 6:257–267, 1974.

24. Gelfand M, Bakhtian B, and Simmons B: Spinal sepsis due to *Streptococcus milleri:* Two cases and review. Rev Infect Dis 13:559–563, 1991.

25. Gelfand M, Stephens D, Howell E, Alford R, and Kaiser A: Brain abscess: Association with pulmonary arteriovenous fistula and hereditary hemorrhagic telangiectasia. Am J Med 85:718–720, 1988.

26. Gellin BG, Weingarten K, Gamache FW Jr, and Hartman BJ: Epidural abscess. In Scheld WM, Whitley RJ, and Durack DT (eds): Infections of the Central Nervous System. Raven Press, New York, 1991, pp 499–514.

27. Hanigan WC, Asner NG, and Elwood PW: Magnetic resonance imaging and nonoperative treatment of spinal epidural abscess. Surg Neurol 34:408–413, 1990.

28. Harrison MJ: The clinical presentation of intracranial abscess. Q J Med 51:461–468, 1982.

29. Helfgott DC, Weingarten K, and Hartman BJ: Subdural empyema. In Scheld WM, Whitley RJ, and Durack DT (eds): Infections of the Central Nervous System. Raven Press, New York, 1991, pp 487–498.

30. Heusner AP: Nontuberculous spinal epidural infections. N Engl J Med 239:845–854, 1984.

31. Hlavin ML, Kaminski HJ, Ross JS, and Ganz E: Spinal epidural abscess: A ten-year perspective. Neurosurgery 27:177–184, 1990.

32. Hodges J, Anslow P, and Gillett G: Subdural empyema—Continuing diagnostic problem in the CT scan era. Q J Med 59:387–393, 1986.

33. Hollin SA, Hayashi H, and Gross S: Intracranial abscesses of odontogenic origin. Oral Surgery 23:277–293, 1967.

34. Hooper DC, Pruitt AA, and Rubin RH: Central nervous system infections in the chronically immunocompromised. Medicine 61:166–188, 1982.

35. Hoyt DJ and Fischer SR: Otolaryngologic management of patients with subdural empyema. Laryngoscope 101:20–24, 1991.

36. Jacobson PL and Farmer TW: Subdural empyema complicating meningitis in infants: Improved prognosis. Neurology 31:190–193, 1981.

37. Jadavji T, Humphreys RP, and Prober CG: Brain abscesses in infants and children. Pediatr Infect Dis J 4:393–398, 1985.

38. Kaplan K: Brain abscess. Med Clin North Am 69:345–360, 1985.

39. Kaufman DM, Litman N, and Miller M: Sinusitis-induced subdural empyema. Neurology 33:123–132, 1983.

40. Kaufman DM, Miller MM, and Steigbigel NH: Subdural empyema: Analysis of 17 recent cases and review of the literature. Medicine 54:485–498, 1975.

41. Knudsen LL, Voldby B, and Stagaard M: Computed tomographic myelography in spinal subdural empyema. Neuroradiology 29:99, 1987.

42. Kourtopoulos H, Holm S, and West K: The management of intracranial abscesses: Comparative study between two materials with different rates of mortality. Acta Neurochir 56:127–128, 1981. (Cited in reference 89.)

43. Lerner PJ: Neurologic complications of infective endocarditis. Med Clin North Am 69:385–399, 1985.

44. Levy R, Bredesen D, and Rosenblum ML: Neurological manifestations of the acquired immunodeficiency syndrome (AIDS): Experience at UCSF and review of the literature. J Neurol Sci 62:475–495, 1985.

45. Levy R, Gutin P, Baskin D, and Pons VG: Vancomycin penetration of a brain abscess: Case report and review of the literature. Neurosurgery 18:633–636, 1986.

46. Leys D, Lesoin F, Viaud C, et al: Decreased morbidity from acute bacterial spinal epidural abscess using computed tomography and non-surgical treatment in selected patients. Ann Neurol 17:350–355, 1985.

47. MacArthur JC: Neurologic manifestations of AIDS. Medicine 66:407–437, 1987.

48. Maniglia AJ, Goodwin AJ, Arnold JE, and Ganz E: Intracranial abcesses secondary to nasal, sinus and orbital infections in adults and children. Arch Otolaryngol Head Neck Surg 115:1424–1429, 1989.

49. Mathews TJ and Marcus G: Otogenic intradural complications: A review of 37 patients. J Laryngol Otol 102:121–124, 1988.

50. Mathisen GE, Meyer RD, George W, Ditrin DM, and Finegold SM: Brain abscess and cerebritis. Rev Infect Dis 6(Suppl 1):S101–S106, 1984.

51. Mauser HW, Ravijst RA, Elderson A, Van Gijn J, and Tulleken C: Nonsurgical treatment of subdural empyema: Case report. J Neurol Sci 63:128–130, 1985.

52. Mauser HW and Tulleken CA: Subdural empyema: A review of 48 patients. Clin Neurol Neurosurg 86:255–263, 1984.

53. Mauser HW, Van Houwelingen H, and Tulleken CA: Factors affecting the outcome in subdural empyema. J Neurol Neurosurg Psychiatry 50:1136–1141, 1987.

54. McGee-Collett M and Johnson IH: Spinal epidural abscess: Presentation and treatment. Med J Aust 155:14–17, 1991.

55. Miller ES, Dias PS, and Uttley D: Management of subdural empyema: A series of 24 cases. J Neurol Neurosurg Psychiatry 50:1415–1418, 1987.

56. Miller ES, Psrilal SD, and Uttley D: CT scanning in the management of intracranial abscess: A review of 100 cases. Br J Neurosurg 2:439–446, 1988.

57. Morgan DW and Williams B: Posterior fossa subdural empyema. Brain 108:983–992, 1985.

58. Morgan H, Wood M, and Murphy F: Experience with 88 consecutive cases of brain abscess. J Neurol Sci 38:698–704, 1973.

59. Nielsen H, Glydensted C, and Harmsen A: Cerebral abscess: Etiology and pathogenesis, symptoms, diagnosis and treatment. Acta Neurol Scand 65:609–622, 1982.

60. Post MJ, Sze G, Quencer RM, et al: Gadolinium-enhanced MR in spinal infection. J Comput Assist Tomogr 14:721–729, 1990.

61. Press OW and Ramsey PG: Central nervous system infections associated with hereditary hemorrhagic telangiectasia. Am J Med 77:86–92, 1984.

62. Pruitt AA, Rubin RH, Karchmer AW, and Duncan GW: Neurologic complica-

tions of bacterial endocarditis. Medicine 57:329–343, 1978.

63. Ravicovitch MA and Spallone A: Spinal epidural abscess: Surgical and parasurgical management. Eur Neurol 21:347–357, 1982.

64. Rish BL, Ceveness WF, Dillon JD, Kistler JP, Mohr JP, and Weiss GH: Analysis of brain abscess after penetrating craniocerebral injuries in Vietnam. Neurosurgery 9:535–541, 1981.

65. Rosenblum ML, Manpalam TJ, and Pons VG: Controversies in the management of brain abscesses. Clin Neurosurg 33:603–632, 1986.

66. Rossitch E, Alexander E, Schiff S, and Ballard D: The use of computed tomography-guided stereotactic techniques in the treatment of brainstem abscesses. Clin Neurol Neurosurg 90:365–368, 1988.

67. Rubin RH and Hooper DC: Central nervous system infections in the compromised host. Med Clin North Am 69:281–296, 1985.

68. Saez-Llorens XJ, Umann MA, Odio CM, McCracken GH, and Nelson JD: Brain abscess in infants and children. Pediatr Infect Dis J 8:449–458, 1989.

69. Sampson DS and Clark K: A current review of brain abscess. Am J Med 54:201–210, 1973.

70. Samuel J, Fernandes C, and Steinberg J: Intracranial otogenic complications: A persisting problem. Laryngoscope 96:272–278, 1986.

71. Schliamser SE, Backman K, and Norrby SR: Intracranial abscess in adults: An analysis of 54 consecutive cases. Scand J Infect Dis 20:1–9, 1988.

72. Sharif HS and Ibrahim A: Intracranial epidural abscess. Br J Radiol 55:81–84, 1982.

73. Shaw MD and Russell JA: Cerebellar abscess—a review of 47 cases. J Neurol Neurosurg Psychiatry 38:429–435, 1975.

74. Silverberg AL and DiNubile MJ: Subdural empyema and cranial epidural abscess. Med Clin North Am 90:361–374, 1985.

75. Sjolin J, Eriksson N, Arneborn P, and Cars O: Penetration of cefotaxime and desacetylcefotaxime into brain abscesses in humans. Antimicrob Agents Chemother 35:2606–2610, 1991.

76. Solzman C and Tuazon C: Value of the ring enhancing sign in differentiating intracerebral hematomas and brain abscesses. Arch Intern Med 147:951–957, 1987.

77. Sterpanov S: Surgical treatment of brain abscess. Neurosurgery 22:724–730, 1988.

78. Taylor JC: The case for excision in the treatment of brain abscess. Br J Neurosurg 1:173–178, 1987.

79. Tenney JH: Bacterial infections of the central nervous system in neurosurgery. Neurol Clin 4:91–114, 1986.

80. Tenney JH, Vlahov D, Salcman M, et al: Wide variation in risk of wound infection following clean neurosurgery. J Neurosurg 62:243–247, 1985.

81. Theodotou B, Woosley RE, and Whaley RA: Spinal subdural empyema: Diagnosis by spinal computed tomography. Surg Neurol 21:610–612, 1984.

82. Tyler KL: Localized infections of the central nervous system. In Bayless TM, Bram MC, and Cherniak RM (eds): Current Therapy in Internal Medicine, Ed 2. BC Decker, Toronto, 1987, pp 231–240.

83. Verner EF and Musher DM: Spinal epidural abscess. Med Clin North Am 69:375–384, 1985.

84. Wackym PA, Canalis RF, and Feuerman T: Subdural empyema of otorhinological origin. J Laryngol Otol 104:118–122, 1990.

85. Warner J, Perkins R, and Cordero L: Metronidazole therapy of anaerobic bacteremia, meningitis, and brain abscess. Arch Intern Med 139:167–169, 1979.

86. Weingarten K, Zimmerman R, Becker R, Heier L, Haimes A, and Deck M: Subdural and epidural empyemas: MR imaging. AJNR 10:81–87, 1987.

87. Weingarten K, Zimmerman R, Becker RD, et al: Subdural and epidural empyemas: MR imaging. AJR 152:615–621, 1989.

88. Weisberg L: Subdural empyema: Clinical and computed tomographic corre-

lations. Arch Neurol 43:497–500, 1986.

89. Wispelwey B, Dacey RG Jr, and Scheld WM: Brain abscess. In Scheld WM, Whitley RM, and Durack DT (eds): Infections of the Central Nervous System. Raven Press, New York, 1991, pp 457–486.

90. Wispelwey B and Scheld WM: Brain abscess. Semin Neurol 12:273–278, 1992.

91. Wood M and Anderson M. Neurological Infections. WB Saunders, London, 1988, pp 249–380.

92. Yang SH: Brain abscess. A review of 400 cases. J Neurol Sci 55:794–799, 1981.

93. Yang SY: Brain abscess associated with congenital heart disease. Surg Neurol 31:129–132, 1989.

94. Zimmerman RD, Leeds NE, and Danziger A: Subdural empyema: CT findings. Radiology 150:417–422, 1984.

Chapter 8

BACTERIAL MENINGITIS

Joseph B. Martin, M.D., Ph.D.,
Kenneth L. Tyler, M.D., and
W. Michael Scheld, M.D.

DEFINITION

Bacterial meningitis is an inflammatory response to bacterial invasion of the meninges and cerebrospinal fluid (CSF). Infection of the subarachnoid space, which is contiguous with the brain and extends over the spinal cord, around the optic nerves, and into the ventricles, can rapidly disseminate and, when the pathogen is virulent, can lead to serious morbidity and mortality.

PATHOGENESIS

Bacterial meningitis occurs when pathogenic organisms overcome host defense mechanisms and reach the subarachnoid CSF. As reviewed by Quagliarello and Scheld, the "successful meningeal pathogen must sequentially colonize host mucosal epithelium, invade and survive in the intravascular space, cross the blood-brain barrier, and survive in the cerebrospinal fluid (CSF)."[14]

Most bacterial meningitides are hematogenous in origin. The first step in entry to the tissues surrounding the brain and spinal cord is believed to occur after nasopharyngeal mucosal colonization and invasion of pathogens (Table 8–1). This step requires overcoming the protection of immunoglobulin A (IgA) secreted by plasma cells in the mucus, avoidance of ciliary mechanisms of clearance, and transfer across the apical epithelium cell by first adhering to its nasal surface and then passing to the basal lateral surface of the cell. The principal bacterial species that are capable of causing meningitis (*Streptococcus pneumoniae, Haemophilus influenzae,* and *Neisseria meningitidis*) each secrete IgA proteases that cleave IgA and render it dysfunctional.[12,23,24] In vitro studies of human nasopharyngeal tissue in organ culture show that *N. meningitidis* and *H. influenzae* are capable of causing injury to ciliated epithelial cells, whereas nonpathogens are incapable of this damage. After the mucous barrier has been penetrated and ciliostasis occurs, the bacteria bind to nonciliated epithelial cells. The pattern of invasion across the epithelial cells appears to be distinct for different pathogens.[22] *N. meningitidis* enters nonciliated epithelial cells by endocytosis and traverses

**Table 8–1 PATHOGENETIC SEQUENCE OF
BACTERIAL NEUROTROPISM**

Neurotropic Stage	Host Defense	Strategy of Pathogen
1. Colonization or mucosal invasion	Secretory IgA	IgA protease secretion
	Ciliary activity	Ciliostasis
	Mucosal epithelium	Adhesive pili
2. Intravascular survival	Complement	Evasion of alternative pathway by polysaccharide capsule
3. Crossing of blood-brain barrier	Cerebral endothelium	Adhesive pili
4. Survival within CSF	Poor opsonic activity	Bacterial replication

Source: Quagliarello and Scheld. Reprinted, by permission of the New England Journal of Medicine (327:864–872, 1992).

the cell in membrane-bound vacuoles. On the other hand, *H. influenzae* traverses by an intercellular route after separating the apical tight junctions of columnar epithelial cells.[14,15] Current investigations are seeking to identify these specific binding epitopes on the bacterial surface as well as the cell surface receptors on epithelial cells.

The next stage of invasion requires survival in the intravascular space. Circulating complement is the initial host defense against bacteremia. The alternate complement pathway, which does not require specific antibody for activation, functions in the immunologically naive host as an early protective mechanism. The ability to evade this pathway differs for each organism.[14] Capsular sialic acid facilitates binding of complement regulatory protein for *N. meningitidis*.[5] *H. influenzae* type b evades the complement pathway because its polyribosyl phosphate capsule cannot interact with complement component C3.[14]

After bacteremia has been established in the intravascular space, the pathogen must then invade the central nervous system (CNS). The site and the mechanism of bacterial invasion of the meninges is poorly understood. One possibility arising from an infant rat model of *H. influenzae* suggests that the organism first invades the dural venous sinus system. Other studies, however, point to the possibility of invasion in the cribriform plate area after focal inflammation at that site. Finally, entry by way of the choroid plexus has been proposed as a possibility in other experimental studies.[10] The important principles that seem to have emerged after repeated experimental study are that (1) a sustained bacteremia is required before invasion of the meninges occurs; (2) bacterial adhesion to blood-brain barrier components may mediate CNS invasion; and (3) transport of the microorganisms within macrophages or other phagocytic cells entering the CNS by cell trafficking pathways may contribute to some forms of meningitis. Host humoral defense mechanisms are virtually absent in the brain, opsonic activity is undetectable or very low in infected CSF, and mechanisms to phagocytose bacterial pathogens within the fluid medium of the CSF are inefficient.[19,28] Because of these inefficiencies in major defense mechanisms, bacterial infection in the CSF progresses rapidly, and the large number of bacteria require that bactericidal agents be used for adequate therapy.

The presence of bacteria replicating within the CSF leads to subarachnoid space inflammation. This inflammation is largely responsible for the pathophysiologic consequences and the clinical syndrome of bacterial meningitis: increased permeability of the blood-brain barrier, cerebral edema, cerebral vasculitis, increased resistance to outflow of CSF, increased intracranial pressure, decreased cerebral blood flow with accompanying loss of autoregulation, cortical hypoxia, cerebral inflammation adjacent to the subarachnoid space, seizures, and so forth.[14–16] The response to bacterial replication and to inflammation in the CSF results in a

CSF neutrophilic pleocytosis. It is in this regard that the use of dexamethasone has been thought to be beneficial by reducing subarachnoid space inflammation. The CSF pleocytosis that follows the presence of live microorganisms results in further chemotactic attractants for leukocytes. The origin and mechanism by which neutrophils enter the CSF remains largely unknown (Fig. 8–1). It is known that neutrophils must first adhere to endothelial cells and that specific adhesion molecules, such as endothelial leukocyte adhesion molecule 1 (ELAM-1), are likely to be involved. Direct evidence in support of this has not been demonstrated in cerebral endothelium, however. This im-

portant interaction between leukocytes and the endothelial cell involves several families of adhesion molecules, including the immunoglobulin superfamily (ICAM-1 and ICAM-2),[1,20–22] the integrin family,[4,20] the CD-11/CD-18 subfamily, and the selectin family (ELAM-1).[2,3,13] Interestingly, neutrophil adhesion can be blocked by administration of monoclonal antibodies against the CD-11/CD-18 family of receptors, and this event can eliminate the CSF pleocytosis in experimental meningitis.[14] It is in this regard that the use of dexamethasone has been shown to be beneficial by enhancing monoclonal antibody effectiveness. The CSF pleocytosis that follows the presence of live microorgan-

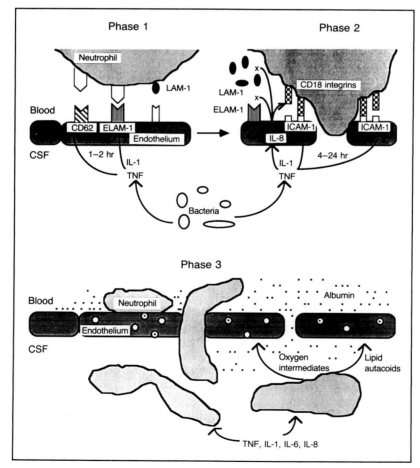

Figure 8–1. Schematic model of neutrophil exudation into CSF and breakdown of the blood-brain barrier (see text). (From Quagliarello and Scheld. Reprinted, by permission of the New England Journal of Medicine (327:864–872, 1992).

isms in the CSF results in further chemotactic attractants for leukocytes.

A number of cytokines are likely to be involved in this process (see Fig. 8–1). Bacteria in the CSF induce the local release of the inflammatory cytokines interleukin 1 (IL-1) and tumor necrosis factor (TNF). These cytokines induce expression of selectin molecules (ELAM-1 or CD62) on the membrane of endothelial cells.

In addition, locally secreted TNF can increase the affinity of another selectin molecule (LAM-1) on the neutrophil for its corresponding receptor on the endothelial-cell membrane. In phase 2 . . . , interleukin-8 (IL-8) is released by the endothelium, cleaves neutrophil LAM-1, inhibits the binding of ELAM-1, and increases the expression of β_2 (CD18) integrins on the neutrophils. Simultaneously, cytokines activate the endothelium to express ICAM-1, so that the selectin-mediated adherence event is replaced by integrin- and ICAM-mediated binding of the neutrophils to the endothelium and diapedesis. In phase 3, neutrophils within the CSF can be activated by local inflammatory cytokines to release vasoactive lipid autacoids (platelet-activating factor, leukotrienes, and prostaglandins) and toxic oxygen species to impair the blood-brain barrier. This process occurs through the slow vesicular uptake of macromolecules (albumin) by endothelium and by paracellular leakage through open intercellular junctions of the venules.[14]

The establishment of the inflammatory exudate in the subarachnoid space often leads to increased intracranial pressure, and this alone can cause life-threatening cerebral herniation. Brain edema occurs adjacent to the subarachnoid space, an effect that can be induced by live organisms or by cell wall fragments (of pneumococci) and by lipopolysaccharide[14,25] from Gram-negative organisms. The water content of the brain can also be increased by inflammatory cytokines.[17] The brain edema that occurs can be vasogenic, due to increased permeability of the blood-brain barrier; cytotoxic, caused by toxins released by bacteria or neu-

trophils; or interstitial, caused by CSF outflow resistance. Changes in cerebral blood flow accompany the meningitis. Experimental models show that blood flow increases at first and later decreases. This effect may result from the generation of oxygen intermediates in the microvasculature.[11] Loss of cerebrovascular autoregulation may occur and may result in fluctuation in cerebral blood flow as alterations occur in mean arterial blood pressure.[26] This loss of cerebrovascular autoregulation can lead to changes in substrate availability (oxygen and glucose).[15] It is likely that these events, together with increased intracranial pressure, contribute to a reduction in the level of consciousness, which commonly occurs with the progression of bacterial meningitis.

PATHOLOGY

The presence of bacteria or other organisms in the subarachnoid space leads to an inflammatory reaction in the pia and arachnoid; in pyogenic meningitis, pus accumulates in the space. Injury may occur to structures that lie within the subarachnoid space; inflammation within the ventricular system can lead to obstruction of the CSF flow; and inflammation of arteries, veins, and the adjacent cerebellar cortices can lead to local infarcts and inflammation within the cerebral tissues themselves. The outer arachnoid membrane is a remarkably effective barrier to extension of infection beyond the subarachnoid space, but subdural effusions may occur in response to the meningitis, particularly in infants.

On gross examination, the exudate has a grayish-yellow or yellowish-green appearance. It is most abundant at the base of the brain within the cisterns but also occurs over the convexities and within the rolandic and sylvian fissures. Exudate may extend along the spinal cord, may accompany the nerve sheaths, and may also be found within the ventricular system. On microscopic examination, large numbers of neutro-

Table 8–2 BACTERIAL CAUSES OF MENINGITIS, STRATIFIED BY AGE

Organism	Neonates (≤1 Month), %	Children (1 Month to 15 Years), %	Adults (>15 Years), %
H. influenzae	0–3	40–60	1–3
Strep. pneumoniae	0–5	10–20	30–50
N. meningitidis	0–1	25–40	10–35
Gram-negative bacilli	50–60	1–2	1–10
Streptococci	20–40*	2–4	5
Staphylococci	5	1–2	5–15
Listeria species	2–10	1–2	5

*Nearly all isolates are group B streptococci.

Source: Modified from Roos et al: Acute bacterial meningitis in children and adults. In WM Scheld et al (eds): Infections of the Central Nervous System. Raven Press, New York, 1991, pp. 335–409, with permission.

phils and bacteria are seen, and evidence of inflammation in the wall of small and medium-sized subarachnoid blood vessels may be present within 2 or 3 days. This combination of events can lead to hydrocephalus, cranial and spinal nerve deficits, focal neurologic deficits, seizure disorders, encephalopathy with coma, and subdural effusions.

EPIDEMIOLOGY

Bacterial meningitis is a common disease worldwide. Its approximate incidence is 4 to 10 cases per 100,000 persons per year in the United States, where more than 2000 deaths are reported annually. Approximately 25,000 cases occur in children younger than 5 years of age, but this frequency is declining rapidly in response to the introduction of H. influenzae type b polysaccharide-conjugate vaccines. The disease is even more common in developing countries. The relative frequency of isolation of the various bacterial species is shown in Table 8–2. The causative agents vary with the age of the patient. H. influenzae is still the principal cause of meningitis in children between the ages of 1 month and 15 years. It is a rare cause of meningitis in adults (1% to 3%). Strep. pneumoniae is the principal cause of meningitis in adults, although it occurs in 10% to 20% of meningitis patients between ages 1 month and 15 years. N. menin-

gitidis occurs both in children and in adults. Gram-negative bacilli are the major causes of meningitis in neonates, although streptococci and staphylococci are also important causes. Listeria is a rare cause of meningitis in any age group but is important because its early recognition is crucial for its proper treatment. In 1981, it was estimated that H. influenzae meningitis occurred in 1 in every 500 children during the first 4 years of life. The results of a recent study by Wenger and associates[27] are shown in Table 8–3. Mortality rates for all causes of meningitis except H. influenzae were approximately 20%; the mortality rate for H. influenzae meningitis was considerably less (3%). Although precise figures are not yet available, the impact of recent conjugate vaccines on the epidemiology of inac-

Table 8–3 BACTERIAL MENINGITIS IN FIVE STATES AND LOS ANGELES COUNTY, 1986

Organism	% of Total Cases	Case Fatality Rate, %
H. influenzae	45	3
Strep. pneumoniae	18	19
N. meningitidis	14	13
Group B streptococci	5	12
L. monocytogenes	3	22
Others	15	18

Source: Modified from Wenger et al: Bacterial meningitis in the United States, 1986—Report of a multistate surveillance study. J Infect Dis, 162:1316–1323, 1990. ©University of Chicago Press, with persmission.

**Table 8–4 CAUSES OF BACTERIAL MENINGITIS IN
FOUR GEOGRAPHIC AREAS**

Organism	PERCENTAGE OF TOTAL CASES			
	United States 1978–1981	United Kingdom 1980–1984	Dakar, Senegal 1970–1979	Salvador, Brazil 1973–1982
H. influenzae	48	29	20	23
Strep. pneumoniae	13	20	29	17
N. meningitidis	20	25	11	32
Group B streptococcus	3	7	4	2
L. monocytogenes	2	2	<0.5	
Other	8	16	9	8
Unknown	6		26	19

Source: Modified from Roos et al: Acute bacterial meningitis in children and adults. In WM Scheld et al (eds): Infections of the Central Nervous System. Raven Press, New York, 1991, pp. 335–409, with permission.

tive *H. influenzae* type b disease has been considerable. The causes of bacterial meningitis in four geographic areas is summarized in Table 8–4.

A number of factors predispose to the development of acute bacterial meningitis. Otitis media and mastoiditis occur in up to one quarter of patients with pneumococcal meningitis, and the lungs are the principal site of infection in another quarter of patients. In addition, a recent head injury, CSF rhinorrhea, chronic alcoholism, immunoglobulin deficiency, penetrating cranial wounds, and cerebral ventricular shunt may all contribute to the development of meningitis.

CLINICAL MANIFESTATIONS

The classic symptoms in adults are headaches, fever, stiff neck, and, with further progression, alterations in the level of consciousness, photophobia, seizures, vomiting, and back pain. Nausea and vomiting, profuse sweats, myalgia, and generalized malaise are common. The classic signs of Kernig and Brudzinski are present in about 50% of adults. Cranial nerve palsies, especially involving nerves III, IV, VI, and VII, occur in 10% to 20% of cases.[14,16] Visual field defects, dysphasia, and hemiparesis are less frequent. Seizures occur in up to 40% of cases. Papilledema is rare,

but later in the disease course patients may develop signs of increased intracranial pressure with coma, hypertension, and signs of impending temporal lobe herniation. Focal neurologic deficits, seizures, and encephalopathy probably arise from ischemia and infarction adjacent to the subarachnoid space. A subdural effusion may occur, particularly in children. The accompanying systemic manifestations may provide a clue to the cause of the meningitis. A rash is common with meningococcemia (50% of patients). The rash is erythematous and macular early in the disease course but later develops into a petechial phase, which after coalescence may appear as a gray, necrotic lesion. A petechial rash is not limited to *N. meningitidis* infection; similar findings have been reported with infection with the enteric cytopathic human orphan virus (Echovirus), *Staph. aureus*, *Acinetobacter* species, and *Rickettsia* species, and with sepsis due to encapsulated bacteria in asplenic hosts, vasculitides, and so forth.

The diagnosis of meningitis may be more difficult in children, particularly in very young infants, and in the elderly. In these patients, fever and vomiting may be more prominent than headache. In the elderly, signs of meningitis may be minimal, particularly in debilitated patients, who may show only a low-grade fever and altered mental status.

DIAGNOSIS AND LABORATORY FINDINGS

The most crucial diagnostic procedure for bacterial meningitis is lumbar puncture for examination of the CSF. If the neurologic examination reveals the possibility of focal signs and increased intracranial pressure, it may be necessary to defer the lumbar puncture until a CT scan or MRI study is performed. If suspicion of meningitis is high but immediate lumbar puncture is judged to be dangerous, it may be necessary to initiate antimicrobial therapy before the lumbar puncture can be performed. It must be emphasized, however, that the occurrence of herniation or complication of the neurologic picture from the lumbar puncture is relatively rare, and it is much more important to establish the diagnosis and initiate treatment than to procrastinate while awaiting imaging studies and subject the patient to a growing risk of increasing morbidity or mortality. When antimicrobial therapy must be initiated prior to examination of the CSF, empiric antimicrobial therapy must be continued to cover all the leading possibilities if specific cultural confirmation is lacking.

The CSF often contains between 1000 and 10,000 leukocytes/mL, although larger or smaller concentrations are also encountered. Neutrophilic leukocytes predominate, but increasing proportions of mononuclear cells are found in samples taken later in the disease course. As the exudate in the infection increases, CSF lymphocytosis may occur in up to one third of patients with lower CSF cell counts. The elevation in white cell count is accompanied, in almost all cases, by elevated protein concentration and a lowered CSF glucose (hypoglycorrhachia) level. The gross appearance of the fluid is often cloudy or turbid, particularly if the white cell count is markedly elevated. Xanthochromia may occur with meningitis but if marked suggests the possibility of subarachnoid hemorrhage. The CSF should be examined with a Gram stain, and cultures should be performed on all specimens, even if the CSF cell count is low. The CSF glucose concentration must be compared to simultaneous serum glucose concentrations. It is less than 40 mg/dL (less than 2.2 mmol/L) in about 60% of patients with bacterial meningitis, and the CSF-to-serum glucose ratio is less than 0.31 in approximately 70% of patients. A CSF glucose concentration of less than 1.9 mmol/L (34 mg/dL), a CSF-to-blood glucose ratio less than 0.23, a CSF protein concentration of greater than 2.2 g/L (220 mg/dL), and a total leukocyte count of more than 2×10^6/L or a neutrophil count of more than 1180×10^6/L are predictors of bacterial, as opposed to viral, meningitis with a certainty of 99% or better.[18]

Examination of the CSF by Gram stain can provide an accurate identification of the etiologic agent in up to 60% to 90% of cases. Contamination of the staining reagents or of collecting tubes can lead to false-positive results. Negative Gram stains are usually caused by prior antimicrobial therapy or by low CSF concentrations of the microorganisms. Culture of the CSF is positive in 70% to 85% of patients with bacterial meningitis, but positive cultures decrease with prior antimicrobial therapy. Blood cultures may also be positive and should always be sent together with the CSF for identification of the pathogen. Other tests can be performed on CSF to facilitate the diagnosis of bacterial meningitis if the Gram stain is negative. Countercurrent immunoelectrophoresis (CIE) may be helpful in the detection of specific microbial antigens and is reported to have a sensitivity of up to 60% to 95%. The test has been largely replaced by the coagglutination (COA) or latex agglutination (LA) techniques, which are more rapid and sensitive than CIE and require only small amounts of bacterial antigen for confirmation (a positive test).[15] Although a negative test will not rule out infections due to a particular meningeal pathogen, these rapid tests have facilitated early diagnosis. The limulus lysate test is highly sensitive for detection of lipopolysaccharide in the CSF, but does not yield specific etiologic information within the many Gram-negative organisms potentially present.

The vast majority of patients with bacterial meningitis do not require imaging studies with CT or MRI. Imaging may be important to detect complications such as hydrocephalus or a parameningeal site of infection and is important in patients with coma, seizure activity, or signs of increased intracranial pressure. The MRI is more sensitive in detection of complications of meningitis (subdural effusions, cerebritis, cortical infarction) but is more difficult to obtain in critically ill patients.

Because of complications that accompany systemic infection, most patients with meningitis should be treated in an intensive care unit. Shock, disseminated intravascular coagulation, syndrome of inappropriate secretion of antidiuretic hormone, and other complications may occur. It is important to assess for the possibility of a coexisting pneumonia (particularly with pneumococcal disease) and to continue to monitor renal function, coagulation function, and serum electrolytes during the course of therapy. Arthritis, pericarditis, or other distant manifestations may occur with infection by some organisms.

TREATMENT

Antimicrobial Therapy

After establishing through a lumbar puncture that the diagnosis of meningitis is likely, patients should receive empiric antimicrobial therapy based upon their age, underlying disease status, and other factors that might make the diagnosis of a specific bacterial agent most likely (see also Chapter 13).[15,17] Assuming normal renal function, the empiric regimens based upon age include the following: Neonates younger than 1 month of age, who are most likely to be infected with *Escherichia coli*, *Streptococcus agalactiae*,

and *Listeria monocytogenes*, should receive ampicillin (150 to 200 mg/kg per day intravenously in divided doses every 4 to 6 hours) plus a third-generation cephalosporin (usually cefotaxime 200 mg/kg per day intravenously in divided doses every 6 hours). An alternative choice may be ampicillin plus an aminoglycoside. Infants aged 4 to 12 weeks, who are more likely to be infected with *H. influenzae* or *Strep. pneumoniae*, in addition to the neonatal pathogens already mentioned, should receive ampicillin plus a third-generation cephalosporin. Children aged 3 months to 6 years, who are most likely to be infected with *H. influenzae*, may be treated only with a third-generation cephalosporin, although some authorities recommend ampicillin and chloramphenicol (100 mg/kg per day orally in divided doses every 6 hours) or chloramphenicol alone (cefuroxime should be avoided). In young adults, where the diagnosis is most likely to be *N. meningitidis* or *Strep. pneumoniae*, penicillin G or ampicillin are often used empirically (see caveat below). In patients older than age 50, where the incidence of Gram-negative aerobic bacilli and *L. monocytogenes* increases, the treatment should consist of ampicillin and a third-generation cephalosporin combination. In postneurosurgical patients, after head trauma and so forth, in whom there is a possibility of infection by staphylococci, diphtheroids, or Gram-negative bacilli including *P. aeruginosa*, treatment should consist of vancomycin (40 mg/kg per day intravenously in divided doses every 6 to 12 hours) plus ceftazidime (6 g/day intravenously in divided doses every 8 hours in the adult).

After identification of the infecting organism, treatment can be modified based on susceptibility results. Bacterial meningitides due to *Strep. pneumoniae* or *N. meningitidis* are usually adequately treated with penicillin G or ampicillin, but "relatively" penicillin-resistant pneumococci have increased in frequency in recent years and require that susceptibility testing of all pneumococcal isolates from sterile body fluids be undertaken. A third-generation cephalosporin should be used for these relatively resistant forms, and vancomycin may be required for highly resistant pneumococci.

Meningococcal strains that are relatively resistant to penicillin also have been reported, particularly in Spain, and a third-generation cephalosporin may be required for maximum benefit. Approximately one third of *H. influenzae* isolates in the United States produce beta-lactamase and are resistant to ampicillin. Chloramphenicol resistance is rare but has been reported in up to 50% of cases in some countries. Recently, the American Academy of Pediatrics endorsed third-generation cephalosporins as empiric therapy in children with bacterial meningitis. Ceftriaxone is superior to cefuroxime in this group. Third-generation cephalosporins have greatly improved the outcome of treatment for Gram-negative enteric bacillary meningitis, with cure rates of 78% to 94%. Patients with *Pseudomonas* meningitis may be treated with ceftazidime alone, although the addition of an aminoglycoside (systemic or directly into the CNS) may be required in selected cases.

The principles underlying these recommendations for treatment are based upon sound pathophysiologic studies as described by Quagliarello and Scheld.[14] These point out the importance of administering bactericidal, rather than bacteriostatic, therapy. However, because the infected CSF contains large numbers of organisms in a closed space, bactericidal treatment may cause massive bacteriolysis, with the release of high concentrations of inflammatory bacterial fragments.

Adjunctive Corticosteroid Therapy

The potential for bacterial cell-wall components to exacerbate inflammation and abnormalities in the cerebral microvasculature has fostered both experimental and clinical studies to test the efficacy of adjunctive agents that reduce inflammation.[14–16] Clinical trials in children indicate that adjunctive corticosteroid therapy reduces the complications of meningitis and improves the outcome. The efficacy of dexamethasone (0.15 mg/kg body weight, administered every 6 hours for 4 days) was the subject of the first study.[9] The first dose of dexamethasone was given 30 minutes to several hours after the first antibiotic dose. A significantly lower incidence of moderate to severe bilateral sensorineural hearing loss (3% versus 16%) was found 6 weeks after discharge from the hospital.[7] This benefit persisted; 4% of patients treated with dexamethasone and 12% of patients given placebo had neurologic sequelae (ataxia and hemiparesis) at 1 year.[8] A second clinical trial has been published more recently in which the first dose of dexamethasone was given 15 to 20 minutes before the first dose of antibiotic. Patients received dexamethasone 0.15 mg/kg every 6 hours for 4 days, plus cefotaxime. The patients who received corticosteroids had lower CSF pressures, lower CSF concentrations of cytokines (TNF-α and platelet-activating factor), and less inflammation 12 hours later than control patients. Survivors at 15-month follow-up had fewer neurologic and audiologic sequelae overall (14% as compared with 38% in the control group). These results have led to recommendations that children with *H. influenzae* meningitis receive glucocorticoids at the time of initiation of treatment. In another retrospective study,[6] 97 children with pneumococcal meningitis also had fewer neurologic sequelae when they were administered glucocorticoids. It is now common practice in pediatric infectious disease circles to recommend that glucocorticoids accompany antibiotic therapy.

The question of whether adults will benefit from adjunctive corticosteroid therapy was reviewed by Quagliarello and Scheld,[14] who state, "We suggest that the overwhelming experimental data and the documented clinical benefit to children support a similar approach in adults with bacterial meningitis, although decisions must be individualized and caution exercised in specific patients, for example those who are immunocompromised or who have granulocytopenia.''[14,p870] It is possible that other adjunctive anti-inflammatory agents will be used in the future. These are summarized by the above-named authors.

It is important in patients with meningitis to improve their likelihood of beneficial outcome by careful monitoring of increased intracranial pressure. Increased intracranial pressure may be treated with elevation of the head of the bed to 30°, hyperventilation to a $Paco_2$ of 27 to 30 mmHg, administration of hyperosmolar agents, and intravenous lidocaine to reduce transient rises in intracranial pressure during endotracheal suctioning. Seizures should be treated with benzodiazepines or phenytoin. The use of plasma exchange for meningococcemia is under investigation but remains experimental at this time.

PROGNOSIS

The overall fatality rates for meningeal pathogens for cases diagnosed in the United States in 1986 are summarized in Table 8–3. The mortality rate overall for *H. influenzae* is less than 5% but may exceed 20% to 25% in developing countries. As shown in Table 8–3, pneumococcal meningitis has a fatality rate of close to 20% and *N. meningitidis* 13%. The highest mortality rate is for meningitis due to *Listeria monocytogenes* (22%), *Staph. aureus*, or Gram-negative aerobic bacilli.

The major sequelae of meningitis are sensorineural injury with hearing loss and delayed language development, cerebral palsy due to infarction of brain, mental retardation, seizures, and behavioral difficulties.

SUMMARY

Bacterial meningitis is a common neurologic problem that occurs at all ages. Bacterial colonization of the nasopharyngeal mucosa is the most frequent pathogenetic mechanism. Entry into the cerebrospinal fluid requires traversal of the apical epithelium cell of the mucosal lining, intravascular survival, and transfer across the blood-brain barrier. Once the cerebrospinal fluid is entered, rapid replication occurs and the clinical manifestations develop rapidly. The principal bacterial species capable of causing meningitis are *Strep. pneumoniae*, *H. influenzae*, and *N. meningitidis*. Other bacterial pathogens to be considered are *Staph. aureus* and *P. aeruginosa* in patients with head trauma or neurosurgic intervention, and *L. monocytogenes*, particularly in immunocompromised patients. The diagnosis requires examination of the cerebrospinal fluid with appropriate attention to protein and glucose levels, Gram stain, and culture. Early treatment gives a favorable outcome in the majority of patients. Glucocorticoid adjunctive therapy is recommended in children and may also become the accepted treatment in adults, although controlled studies in the latter group have not been performed.

REFERENCES

1. Berendt AR, Simmons DL, Tansey J, Newbold CI, and Marsh K: Intercellular adhesion molecule-1 is an endothelial cell adhesion receptor for *Plasmodium falciparum*. Nature 341:57–59, 1989.
2. Bevilacqua MP, Stengelin S, Gimbrone MA Jr, and Seed B: Endothelial leukocyte adhesion molecule 1: An inducible receptor for neutrophils related to complement regulatory proteins and lectins. Science 243:1160–1165, 1989.
3. Geng J-G, Bevilacqua MP, Moore KL, et al: Rapid neutrophil adhesion to acti-

vated endothelium mediated by GMP-140. Nature 343:757–760, 1990.

4. Hynes RO: Integrins: A family of cell surface receptors. Cell 48:549–554, 1987.

5. Joiner KA: Complement evasion by bacteria and parasites. Annu Rev Microbiol 42:201–230, 1988.

6. Kennedy WA, Hoyt MJ, and McCracken GH Jr: The role of corticosteroid therapy in children with pneumococcal meningitis. Am J Dis Child 145:1374–1378, 1991.

7. Lebel MH, Freij BJ, Syrogiannopoulos GA, et al: Dexamethasone therapy for bacterial meningitis: Results of two double-blind, placebo-controlled trials. N Engl J Med 319:964–971, 1988.

8. McCracken GH Jr and Lebel MH: Dexamethasone therapy for bacterial meningitis in infants and children. Am J Dis Child 143:287–289, 1989.

9. Mustafa MM, Lebel MH, Ramilo O, et al: Correlation of interleukin-1β and cachectin concentrations in cerebrospinal fluid and outcome from bacterial meningitis. J Pediatr 115:208–213, 1989.

10. Parkkinen J, Korhonen T, Pere A, Hacker J, and Soinila S: Binding sites in the rat brain for *Escherichia coli* S fimbriae associated with neonatal meningitis. J Clin Invest 81:860–865, 1988.

11. Pfister HW, Koedel U, Haberl RL, et al: Microvascular changes during the early phase of experimental bacterial meningitis. J Cereb Blood Flow Metab 10:914–922, 1990.

12. Plaut AG: The IgA1 proteases of pathogenic bacteria. Annu Rev Microbiol 37:603–622, 1983.

13. Polley MJ, Phillips ML, Wayner E, et al: CD62 and endothelial cell-leukocyte adhesion molecule 1 (ELAM-1) recognize the same carbohydrate ligand, sialyl-Lewis x. Proc Natl Acad Sci U S A 88:6224–6228, 1991.

14. Quagliarello V and Scheld WM: Bacterial meningitis: Pathogenesis, pathophysiology, and progress. N Engl J Med 327:864–872, 1992.

15. Roos KL: Management of bacterial meningitis in children and adults. Semin Neurol 12:155–164, 1992.

16. Roos KL, Tunkel AR, and Scheld WM: Acute bacterial meningitis in children and adults. In WM Scheld, RJ Whitley, and DT Durack (eds): Infections of the Central Nervous System. Raven Press, New York, 1991, pp. 335–409.

17. Saukkonen K, Sande S, Cioffe C, et al: The role of cytokines in the generation of inflammation and tissue damage in experimental gram-positive meningitis. J Exp Med 171:439–448, 1990.

18. Scheld WM: Bacterial meningitis and brain abscess. In Isselbacher K, Braunwald E, Wilson J, Martin JB, Fauci A, Kasper D, (eds): Harrison's Principles of Internal Medicine, Ed 13. 1994 (in press).

19. Simberkoff MS, Moldover NH, and Rahal J Jr: Absence of detectable bactericidal and opsonic activities in normal and infected human cerebrospinal fluids: A regional host defense deficiency. J Lab Clin Med 95:362–372, 1980.

20. Springer TA: Adhesion receptors of the immune system. Nature 346:425–434, 1990.

21. Staunton DE, Marlin SD, Stratowa C, Dustin ML, and Springer TA: Primary structure of ICAM-1 demonstrates interaction between members of the immunoglobulin and integrin supergene families. Cell 52:925–933, 1988.

22. Staunton DE, Merluzzi VJ, Rothlein R, Barton R, Marlin SD, and Springer TA: A cell adhesion molecule, ICAM-1, is the major surface receptor for rhinoviruses. Cell 56:849–853, 1989.

23. Stephens DS and Farley MM: Pathogenic events during infection of the human nasopharynx with *Neisseria meningitidis* and *Haemophilus influenzae*. Rev Infect Dis 13:22–33, 1991.

24. Swartz MN: Bacterial meningitis: More involved than just the meninges. N Engl J Med 311:912–914, 1984.

25. Tauber MG: Brain edema, intracranial pressure and cerebral blood flow in bacterial meningitis. Pediatr Infect Dis J 8:915–917, 1989.

26. Tureen JH, Dworkin RJ, Kennedy SL, Sachdeva M, and Sande MA: Loss of cerebrovascular autoregulation in exper-

imental meningitis in rabbits. J Clin Invest 85:577–581, 1990.

27. Wenger JD, Hightower AW, Facklam RR, et al: Bacterial meningitis in the United States, 1986—Report of a multistate surveillance study. J Infect Dis 162:1316–1323, 1990.

28. Zwahlen A, Nydegger UE, Vaudaux P, Lambert P-H, and Waldvogel FA: Complement-mediated opsonic activity in normal and infected human cerebrospinal fluid: Early response during bacterial meningitis. J Infect Dis 145:635–646, 1982.

Chapter 9

CHRONIC MENINGITIS

Tarvez Tucker, M.D., **and**
Jerrold J. Ellner, M.D.

Chronic meningitis is defined as the persistence (for at least 4 weeks) of signs and symptoms of meningitis, sometimes with an encephalitis component, and an abnormal cerebrospinal fluid (CSF). A number of infectious and noninfectious diseases can cause chronic meningitis. The clinical presentation is virtually identical despite the diverse causes (Table 9–1). Patients present with the subacute to indolent onset of headache, fever, and stiff neck; associated signs of encephalitis may include confusion, disorientation, and lethargy. The CSF is almost invariably abnormal, with pleocytosis, usually mainly lymphocytic, and elevated protein; on occasion, the CSF glucose level is mildly to moderately depressed. Initial evaluation of the patient usually occurs before the 4 weeks required to satisfy the clinical definition has been achieved. As a consequence, major therapeutic decisions sometimes need to be made before the patient reaches this empirical point in the disease process.

The diagnosis of chronic meningitis warrants a thorough attempt to establish the underlying cause, with particular attention to treatable conditions.[7a,21,49,59] Recurrent meningitis usually can be distinguished from chronic meningitis by disease-free intervals in which CSF is normal, punctuated by acute clinical exacerbations with marked pleocytosis. Recurrent meningitis often is caused by a congenital or acquired dural defect or by a parameningeal infectious focus repeatedly discharging into the subarachnoid space. In the acquired immunodeficiency syndrome (AIDS) era, recognition that a patient is or may be from a group at high risk of infection with human immunodeficiency virus (HIV) results in a shift in the differential diagnosis of central nervous system (CNS) infection. This topic is considered in a separate section.

Before considering the approach to the individual patient, a few general principles should be stated.

1. Chronic meningitis often is not associated with findings on history or physical examination that assist in the differential diagnosis. Nonetheless, the clinician must focus on areas of the physical examination often given inadequate attention. The skin may show the characteristic rash of *erythema chronicum migrans* (ECM), virtually establishing the diagnosis of Lyme disease (see color insert, Fig. 10–1), or the palate may show lesions characteristic of disseminated histoplasmosis. The fundi may contain telltale signs of sar-

Table 9–1 COMMON CAUSES OF CHRONIC MENINGITIS IN THE OTHERWISE NORMAL HOST

Infectious	Noninfectious
Mycobacterium tuberculosis	Meningeal carcinomatosis
Cryptococcus neoformans	Sarcoidosis
Coccidioides immitis	Granulomatous angiitis
Histoplasma capsulatum	Systemic lupus erythematosus
Blastomyces dermatitidis	Behçet's syndrome
Sporothrix schenckii	Vogt-Koyanagi-Harada syndrome
Candida sp.	
Brucella sp.	
Treponema pallidum	
Borrelia burgdorferi	
Cysticercus cellulosae	

coidosis, tuberculosis, Behçet's syndrome, or Vogt-Koyanagi-Harada (VKH) syndrome, as is discussed below. Consultation with an ophthalmologist, and, where appropriate, a dermatologist, may be helpful.

2. Infectious meningitis should be at the top of the differential diagnosis because of its treatability. Nonetheless, infectious and noninfectious causes of chronic meningitis are not easily separable. The absence of exposure to certain infections virtually excludes them from consideration (e.g., cysticercosis, other parasitic agents). The exposure in certain instances may, however, be readily overlooked, such as the tick bite associated with Lyme disease.

3. Some forms of chronic meningitis may present without the extraneural manifestations that usually accompany a systemic disease. For example,

tuberculous infection may be limited clinically to the CNS. This is easily understood in the context of the natural history of tuberculosis, where the meningitis represents reactivation of a latent focus and is separated in time and space from the pulmonary portal of infection. Also confusing is CNS involvement that antedates characteristic systemic manifestations. Examples are hypothalamic dysfunction (e.g., diabetes insipidus) as a harbinger of sarcoidosis, and carcinomatous meningitis presenting before the primary tumor has been diagnosed.

4. The CSF abnormalities become particularly useful in organizing the approach to a patient in cases in which history and physical examination have not been helpful (Table 9–2).

APPROACH TO THE PATIENT

The history, physical examination, and laboratory data may focus the differential diagnosis around a few of the disease processes that can cause chronic meningitis, may indicate an extraneural site for biopsy, and may provide support for a therapeutic trial.

History

The travel and exposure history of the patient may suggest infection by an agent that is relatively restricted in its geographic distribution (Table 9–3). A few caveats are in order, however. The exposure and primary infection may have antedated development of chronic

Table 9–2 CSF ABNORMALITIES TYPICAL OF SPECIFIC CAUSES OF CHRONIC MENINGITIS

Lymphocytes, cells/μL	Glucose Level	Cause of Meningitis
<50; occasionally ≥50–100	Normal or low	Sarcoidosis, cerebrovascular syphilis
<50; occasionally ≥50–100	Normal	Vasculitis, Lyme disease, HIV
<50; occasionally ≥50–100	Low	Carcinoma
≥50–500	Normal or low	Fungal meningitis, syphilitic meningitis
≥50–500	Normal or low	Tuberculous meningitis
≥50–500	Normal	Chemical meningitis

Table 9–3 INFECTIOUS AGENTS ASSOCIATED WITH SPECIFIC EXPOSURES

Histoplasma capsulatum	Mississippi and Ohio river valleys
Blastomyces dermatitidis	Mississippi and Ohio river valleys, southeastern United States
Coccidioides immitis	Semiarid areas of southwestern United States
Borrelia burgdorferi	Northeastern United States; tick exposure peak in summer and early fall
Cysticercus cellulosae	Mexico, South America
Mycobacterium tuberculosis	Close contact with a patient with tuberculosis
Brucella sp.	Unpasteurized milk, dairy products
Angiostrongylus cantonensis	Far East—raw or undercooked mollusks, contaminated vegetables

meningitis by years or decades, for example, in histoplasmosis or tuberculosis. Also in diseases characterized by areas of high endemicity, such as Lyme disease, sporadic cases can occur in other areas as well. The history also reveals antecedent extraneural manifestations of a disease process currently involving the CNS, such as syphilis, systemic lupus erythematosus (SLE), Behçet's syndrome, and Lyme disease. In patients with a previously diagnosed adenocarcinoma, lymphoma, or melanoma, the current disease may represent spread of the tumor, an opportunistic infection, or a chemical reaction to intrathecal drug administration. A history of an opportunistic infection, Kaposi's sarcoma, or lymphoma also may indicate that a patient is infected with HIV.

Physical Examination

Findings on physical examination may suggest a specific diagnosis and/or identify a site for biopsy. The rash of ECM is pathognomonic of Lyme disease (see Fig. 10–1). Depigmentary choroidal tubercles are found in patients with tuberculosis and sarcoidosis; uveitis

also may be seen in Behçet's syndrome and VKH syndrome. Depigmentation of the skin and hair (vitiligo, poliosis) is suggestive of VKH syndrome. A skin rash consisting of macular- or papular-hyperpigmented lesions that also involves the palms and soles may be a manifestation of secondary syphilis. Sarcoidosis, tuberculosis, and disseminated mycoses may also present with skin lesions. Subcutaneous nodules, abscesses, draining sinuses, or ulcerative lesions are found in disseminated fungal infections and particularly suggest cryptococcosis or blastomycosis. Palatal lesions (nodular or ulcerative) and other lesions involving the oral mucosa are found in disseminated histoplasmosis.

An enlarged lymph node may provide a useful site for biopsy. The yield is greater if the involved node is large (> 1.5 to 2.0 cm), abnormal in consistency (firm or hard), noninguinal, and asymmetric. Hepatomegaly accompanied by an increase in the serum alkaline phosphatase level may suggest that liver biopsy will be useful.

An important issue on neurologic examination is whether features of encephalitis accompany the signs and symptoms of meningitis. Certain infectious diseases such as cysticercosis and toxoplasmosis commonly present with a clinical picture of meningoencephalitis. Alteration of consciousness is uncommon in fungal infections and rare in spirochetal infections such as Lyme disease. Diseases that affect the basilar meninges, causing cranial nerve palsies and hydrocephalus, include sarcoidosis and tuberculosis as well as some of the fungal meningitides. These conditions may present with signs and symptoms of hydrocephalus such as mental status change, ataxia, and nausea and vomiting.

Involvement of specific cranial nerves can be helpful diagnostically. Oculomotor palsies or eighth-nerve dysfunction suggests an inflammatory process, usually granulomatous, affecting the basilar meninges, such as tuberculosis, sarcoidosis, fungal infections, or syphilis. Some infectious processes show a predilection for involvement of specific cranial nerves; syphilis, for example, frequently affects cranial nerves II, VII, and VIII; sarcoidosis, cranial nerve VII. Nonlocalizing sixth-nerve palsies also may result from elevations of cerebral pressure due to causes other than local infection, such as parameningeal foci of infection or hydrocephalus.

Leptomeningeal carcinomatosis frequently presents with a constellation of neurologic signs and symptoms implicating multiple areas of involvement of the neuraxis: cranial nerves, nerve roots, and long tract signs. In this case, a clinical diagnosis may be suspected prior to obtaining a computed tomography (CT) scan or performing a lumbar puncture for confirmatory cytologies.

Laboratory Data

Certain laboratory tests and radiographic procedures should be performed in all patients with chronic meningitis. Complete blood cell count, serum chemistries, and presence of antinuclear antibody and antibody to HIV should be determined.

Cryptococcal polysaccharide antigen should be determined and serologic tests for syphilis and HIV performed in all patients (Table 9–4). The decision to perform other serologic tests should be based on the exposure history. Ancillary diagnostic tests, some of them still investigational, may be helpful in specific cases. For example, tuberculostearic acid in the CSF may be indicative of tuberculous meningitis;[14] a test is available from the Centers for Disease Control. Many infectious causes of chronic meningitis also are associated with selective compartmentalization of antigen-responsive lymphocytes and antibody-forming cells in the subarachnoid space. The ratio of lymphocyte reactivity to antigens and of antibody levels in CSF compared to blood or serum is of potential use diagnostically. Unfortunately, the data for individual patients may be difficult to interpret because of

Table 9–4 DIAGNOSTIC TESTS IN CHRONIC MENINGITIS

	Serum	*CSF*	*Comment*
Cryptococcosis	Antigen	Antigen	Together, 94% positive
		India ink	50% positive result, higher in acute presentations and in immunosuppressed patients
Syphilis	FTA-absorbed	VDRL	Negative serum FTA-ABS rules out syphilis
Histoplasmosis	Antibody	Antibody	Antibody in CSF; 50% specific
	Antigen*	Antigen*	High specificity; sensitivity is higher in HIV infection
Coccidioidomycosis	Antibody	Antibody	Serum complement fixation titer of at least 1:16 suggests dissemination
Brucellosis	Antibody	Antibody	Nonagglutinating antibody to *Brucella* sp. in CSF is most reliable
Blastomycosis	ELISA*	?	
Sporotrichosis	ELISA*	ELISA*	
Lyme disease	Acute stage: indirect IgM ELISA Convalescence: capture IgM ELISA	?	FTA-ABS should be performed in all patients because syphilis is associated with antibodies cross-reactive with *Borrelia*
			Atypical presentations require confirmatory Western blots; antibody is present in CSF in chronic stages

*Not routinely available. Requires special arrangements with investigators.

lack of sufficient validation of the assay.

Lumbar puncture should be repeated at weekly intervals or more often to assure adequate material for culture and cytologies and to follow the course of meningeal inflammation. India ink preparations of CSF are invaluable for the diagnosis of cryptococcal meningitis, particularly when the disease presents acutely, and also for immunosuppressed patients, in whom yeast may outnumber white blood cells. Optimal performance of this test requires mixing India ink with the sediment of 3 to 5 mL of CSF; if the mixture is correct, newsprint can be read through the slide. The entire slide should be scanned under low power by an experienced observer, and suspicious areas should be scanned under high dry and oil immersion. Cryptococci appear as refractile yeast with internal inclusions, sometimes budding, and most importantly surrounded by a large, round, regular capsule that is impermeable to ink particles (Fig. 9–1). *Cryptococcus neoformans* is the only pathogenic encapsulated yeast, so this "bedside test" is a means of establishing a definitive diagnosis and beginning therapy immediately. Multiple specimens of CSF for cytologic examination (at least three) are necessary to assess adequately the possibility of tumor. Most patients with chronic meningitis have a lymphocytic pleocytosis (see Table 9–2). A chronic neutrophilic pleocytosis is suggestive of some fungal infections; of infection with nocardia, actinomycetes, or brucella; of SLE; and of chemical meningitis. A chronic eosinophilic pleocytosis suggests Hodgkin's disease, tuberculosis, cysticercosis or infection by other parasites, or chemical meningitis. Staining of CSF lymphocytes with monoclonal antibodies can be used to determine whether the pleocytosis is monoclonal, as might arise from a lymphoma or leukemia.[28]

Staining of CSF for diagnosis of tuberculous meningitis has had a variable yield of acid-fast bacilli (AFB). The yield is optimized by centrifuging 10 to 20 mL of CSF and examining a thick smear of the resultant sediment. Wet preparations and stains of the sediment should also be examined for yeast.

Culture of CSF remains the mainstay of the diagnosis of chronic meningitis and should be repeated at regular intervals until a diagnosis is obtained. The yield of infectious agents may improve with the passage of time. CSF obtained by cisternal or ventricular taps will probably provide a higher yield than that obtained by lumbar puncture. All samples should be cultured for bacteria, mycobacteria, and fungi. Cultures of three samples of CSF are usually adequate for the detection of most bacteria and mycobacteria, although in the latter instance there may be a delay before cultures are positive. Anaerobic culture conditions and increased CO_2 tension are necessary to isolate actinomycetes and brucella, respectively. If initial cultures are negative, further specimens should be cultured for fungi. The yield of fungal cultures can be improved by inoculating Sabouraud's agar layered on the bottom of Erlenmeyer flasks with large volumes of CSF. This allows for long periods of culture and avoids desiccation. Fungal cultures should be examined for at least 4 to 6 weeks, since growth of some organisms is exceedingly slow, particularly with a low inoculum. The growth of even a single colony of an organism that is capable of

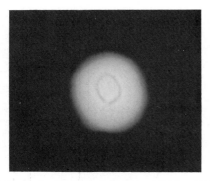

Figure 9–1. Encapsulated budding yeast on India ink preparation of CSF from a patient with cryptococcal meningitis.

causing chronic meningitis, such as sporothrix, cannot be ignored.[51]

Patients with chronic meningitis as a manifestation of tuberculosis, cryptococcosis, blastomycosis, and histoplasmosis frequently have occult systemic dissemination of the infection. Therefore, even in the absence of signs of systemic disease it is important to culture gastric washings (for mycobacteria) and blood, sputum, urine, and stool for mycobacteria and fungi. Biopsy specimens should be obtained from skin and mucosal lesions as well as from abnormal lymph nodes. Additionally, biopsy of the bone marrow and liver are useful if tuberculosis, histoplasmosis, or other granulomatous disease is suspected. Biopsy specimens should be divided for culture and histologic tests. If a craniotomy is performed for exploration of a mass lesion or to relieve symptomatic hydrocephalus, meningeal and brain biopsy specimens should be obtained together with a sample of ventricular fluid (see later).[37] Granulomas are a not-infrequent, nonspecific finding in biopsy specimens. Demonstration of AFB or yeast in a tissue is more helpful, because it provides a presumptive diagnosis and allows initiation of therapy pending culture results. The pathologic finding of granulomas with caseation is suggestive of tuberculosis, histoplasmosis, and coccidioidomycosis. Focal necrosis in granulomas may be seen in brucellosis, and a mixture of pyogenic and granulomatous inflammation in blastomycosis. Biopsy also may reveal unsuspected malignancy (Fig. 9–2), sarcoidosis, or vasculitis.

The presence of a positive skin test to intermediate-strength purified protein derivative (PPD) indicates that an individual is infected with *Mycobacterium tuberculosis*, thus increasing the likelihood that the chronic meningitis is tuberculous. A negative tuberculin skin test result is not useful, however, because up to 35% of patients with tuber-

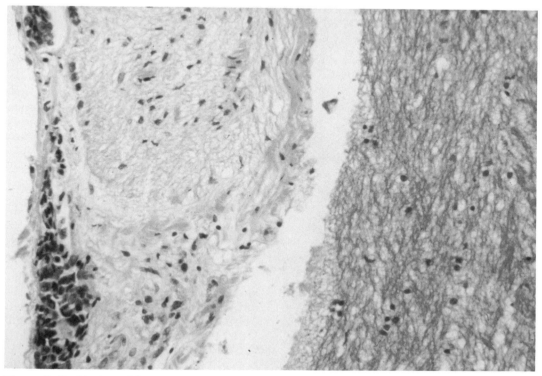

Figure 9–2. Meningeal biopsy in a patient with leptomeningeal carcinomatosis. The primary tumor was adenocarcinoma of the breast.

culous meningitis are nonreactive. If the initial skin test is nonreactive, tuberculin testing should be repeated after 2 weeks. Many anergic patients with tuberculosis will, for unknown reasons, have positive skin test results within the first 2 weeks of hospitalization, particularly if antituberculous therapy has been instituted.

CT scanning should be performed in all patients with chronic meningitis before the initial lumbar puncture, to exclude a mass lesion or hydrocephalus. Nonspecific findings may be present, such as increased contrast enhancement over the convexities and obscuration of the pontine and basilar cisterns by inflammatory cells (Fig. 9–3). The finding of contrast enhancement of granulomatous lesions (see Fig. 9–4) or larger parenchymal lesions may be helpful in diagnosis (see Fig. 9–5).[46a] CT scanning also may show calcified lesions, for example, in cysticercosis (see Fig. 9–6), cerebral infarction (due to

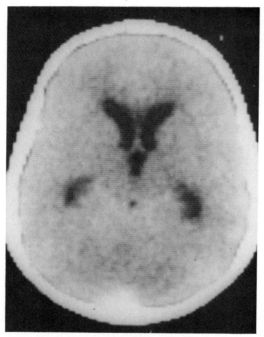

Figure 9–3. CT scan of a patient with chronic meningitis, showing partial obscuration of pontine cisterns by inflammatory cells.

vasculitis), or hydrocephalus. Hydrocephalus is potentially reversible with treatment of the chronic meningitis and does not constitute a sufficient indication for surgery. Cerebral angiography may demonstrate vasculitis, potentially obviating the need for a meningeal biopsy if the findings are typical of granulomatous angiitis.

Approach to Culture-Negative Cases of Chronic Meningitis

Serious or progressive functional impairment early in the course of chronic meningitis, before the results of cultures and serologic tests are available or after the initial test results have proven negative, prompts the choice between a neurosurgical biopsy procedure and empirical treatment. Certain general principles may assist in this decision.

If the history, physical examination, and laboratory data allow a presumptive clinical diagnosis, treatment of the entity, if treatment exists, should be instituted pending confirmatory tests. The clinician must weigh the certainty of the clinical diagnosis and the severity of the illness in deciding how to proceed. If the presentation is very suggestive of Lyme disease, for example, a therapeutic trial of ceftriaxone is appropriate unless the patient is so ill that a dire outcome is predictable should the diagnosis be wrong.

Management of the seriously impaired or deteriorating patient should be based, in part, on the CSF formula (see Table 9–2). If the pleocytosis is predominantly lymphocytic with 50 to 500 cells/μL and the CSF glucose level is depressed or normal, an infectious disease is extremely likely. If the diagnosis of tuberculosis is supported by a tuberculin skin test, empirical antituberculous treatment is appropriate pending the outcome of cultures. Should the tuberculin skin test result be negative, antituberculous drugs can be started and serologic tests conducted. Fungal meningitis is likely in this setting; histoplasma, blastomyces, and sporothrix often cause chronic meningitis in which lumbar CSF is culture-negative.[37,51] Untreated, fungal meningitis may progress rapidly to irreversible disease. Therefore, observing the patient for a response to antituberculous drugs is not an acceptable alternative unless a biopsy procedure is contraindicated because of bleeding diathesis, the patient's age, or underlying disease. Accordingly, arrangements should be made for an invasive procedure to be performed. It may be appropriate to begin with cerebral angiography if vasculitis seems a reasonable explanation for the patient's illness. The results of cryptococcal antigen and serologic tests for syphilis and HIV should be known before proceeding with meningeal biopsy. Serologic tests that are positive for syphilis or cryptococcal polysaccharide antigen should lead to a therapeutic trial. If these studies have negative results, a meningeal biopsy should be performed, possibly with aspiration of ventricular fluid for culture.

If the CSF pleocytosis is predominantly lymphocytic but is of a lower grade (<50 cells), infectious disease is unlikely, particularly diseases that can be diagnosed at meningeal biopsy. Some patients in this category will improve spontaneously without a specific diagnosis or therapy.[30] The impetus for meningeal biopsy is lessened by the lack of treatable causes likely to emerge from the invasive procedure and by the possibility of a self-limited idiopathic process. Certainly, biopsy should be delayed at least until the results of cultures and cytologic and serologic tests are available.

Empirical treatment with corticosteroids is contraindicated because of the deleterious effects on unsuspected and untreated tuberculous or fungal meningitis. Empirical treatment with antifungal therapy rarely is indicated in the absence of a defined infectious agent because of the toxicity of available agents and uncertainty about dose, duration, and route of administration.

SPECIFIC CAUSES OF CHRONIC MENINGITIS

The more common causes of chronic meningitis are now reviewed with particular attention to features important in establishing the diagnosis and guiding treatment. More detailed information concerning the treatment of fungal infections can be found in Chapter 13.

Infectious Causes

TUBERCULOUS MENINGITIS

Tuberculous meningitis often develops when an active or quiescent parameningeal tuberculous focus ruptures or leaks into the subarachnoid space.[48] Although the actual discharge of the so-called Rich focus is a chance event, the likelihood of tuberculous meningitis is influenced by the prevalence of tuberculous infection in the population. Where tuberculosis is common, meningeal involvement usually occurs in children aged 3 months to 5 years, as a consequence of miliary disease representing progressive primary tuberculosis.[44] Hilar adenopathy occurs in 50% to 90% of cases. In the United States, the declining prevalence of tuberculosis infection and the increasing age of patients with tuberculosis results in a greater proportion of cases in adults, usually representing delayed reactivation. In this setting, tuberculous meningitis may be isolated to the CNS, and chest x-rays frequently are normal.

The pathologic hallmarks of tuberculosis are exudative basilar meningitis and vasculitis involving vessels at the base of the brain, most prominently the middle or anterior cerebral arteries. Approximately one third of patients have strokes as a result of vasculitis. Hydrocephalus is a relatively common finding in tuberculous meningitis, although it may resolve with medical therapy alone.

Clinical Manifestations. The initial symptoms of tuberculous meningitis are nonspecific complaints that in about one half of patients are 2 weeks or less in duration. The most common symptoms are low-grade fever, lassitude, depression, confusion, and personality or behavioral changes.[1,34,35,38,63] These initial symptoms progress to headache and stiff neck. Involvement of cranial nerves I, III, IV, and VI is present in about one third of patients. Focal signs may result from the associated vasculitis and cerebral infarction.

Diagnosis. The CSF formula usually is typical of chronic meningitis. During the first few weeks after onset of symptoms, however, a neutrophilic pleocytosis may be present, later shifting to a mononuclear pleocytosis of 100 to 500 cells/μL.[32,42] Hypoglycorrhachia is found in 50% to 90% of patients; serial lumbar punctures usually show progressive depression of CSF glucose levels. Increased opening pressure and elevated CSF protein levels may be present; hyponatremia also may occur due to inappropriate secretion of antidiuretic hormone. CT scan findings consist of hydrocephalus, contrast enhancement of the basilar exudates sometimes obliterating the cisterns, ischemic infarction, and focal granulomas (Fig. 9–4).

The tuberculin skin test is particularly useful for diagnosis in geographic areas of low prevalence of *M. tuberculosis* infection. About one third of patients will, however, have a negative tu-

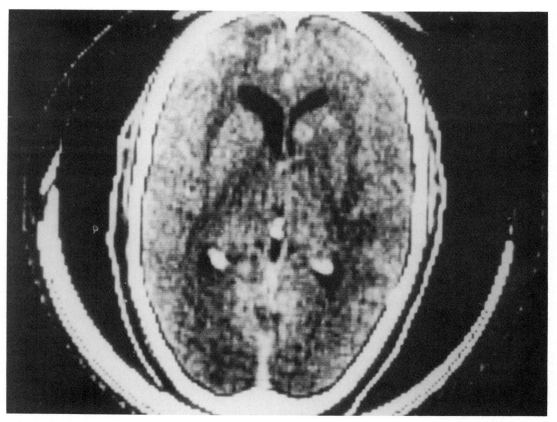

Figure 9–4. CT scan of patient with miliary tuberculosis, showing contrast-enhancing granulomatous lesions.

berculin skin test at the time of presentation with tuberculous meningitis. The demonstration of AFB in a stained sediment of CSF establishes the diagnosis. The yield has been extremely variable (10% to 87%), however, and is in large part technique-dependent (see page 192). The yield from culture of CSF ranges from 50% to 90%. Cultures of sputum and gastric aspirates are positive in 21% to 50% of cases, particularly (but not only) in the setting of an abnormal chest radiograph.

Treatment. Empirical therapy often is appropriate pending the results of cultures, which require 4 to 6 weeks. Combination therapy with isoniazid 5 to 10 mg/kg per day and rifampin 600 mg daily for 9 months should be effective unless drug resistance is present. If drug resistance is suspected because of previous treatment for tuberculosis or infection in Southeast Asia, for example, or if the patient is also infected with HIV, the addition of pyrazinamide 20 to 35 mg/kg daily and ethambutol 15 mg/kg daily is appropriate for the initial 2 months of treatment; the regimen then can be adjusted depending on the pattern of drug sensitivity. The efficacy of corticosteroids in the treatment of adults with tuberculous meningitis is uncertain. Possible indications are life-threatening illness with obtundation or coma, multiple cerebral infarctions, marked increases in intracranial pressure, and cranial neuropathies. If corticosteroids are to be used, moderate doses are appropriate for a limited period (approximately 4 weeks). As discussed above, if a patient presents with chronic meningitis and the CSF abnormalities are consistent with tuberculosis but the tuberculin skin test is negative, empirical antituberculous drugs should be started and a thorough attempt initiated concurrently to establish a definitive diagnosis.

The outcome of tuberculous meningitis depends on the extent of neurologic damage at the time of diagnosis. Mortality is 10% to 33%. Neurologic sequelae occur in 25% to 31% of adult cases and consist of hydrocephalus, learning disabilities, persistent cranial nerve damage, and focal signs such as hemiparesis.

CRYPTOCOCCAL MENINGITIS

Cryptococcal meningitis is the most common CNS infection in chronically immunosuppressed patients;[30] in those who do not have AIDS, approximately one half with cryptococcal meningitis have an underlying disease associated with immunosuppression. Exposure to *Crypt. neoformans,* a common environmental saprophyte, is widespread, but cryptococcal disease is infrequent. Hence, history of exposure is not helpful. Underlying diseases associated with depression of the cell-mediated immune response impose the greatest risk of cryptococcal disease. The classic associations with Hodgkin's disease, lymphosarcoma, and treatment with high doses of corticosteroids have been overshadowed by AIDS.[36,71] Patients with renal or other allografts or who are receiving treatment with high doses of corticosteroids also are at increased risk. Other individuals developing cryptococcal meningitis may have an underlying process associated with some degree of immunocompromise (sarcoidosis, diabetes mellitus, chronic hepatic or renal failure).

The portal of entry of cryptococcus is the lungs. Nodular pulmonary lesions may be present when the patient develops symptoms of CNS involvement. More commonly, the pulmonary infection is not demonstrable clinically and is presumably inactive. Invasive pulmonary cryptococcosis may occur in patients with immunosuppressive disease; occult dissemination to the CNS is likely in such patients. Patients with pulmonary cryptococcosis, therefore, require a lumbar puncture for determination of cryptococcal antigen, as well as other routine studies.

Clinical Manifestations. Cryptococcal meningitis usually presents as a subacute to chronic febrile syndrome with headache.[9,19,41,56,57] The onset of illness may be extremely indolent; in such cases, the major finding is dementia or subtle cognitive defects. Confusion, irritability, and other personality changes reflective of meningoencephalitis are found in about one half of patients with cryptococcal meningitis. Ocular abnormalities are present in 40% of patients and include papilledema due to direct invasion of the nerve, with or without loss of visual acuity, and cranial nerve palsies. Focal cryptococcomas may present as mass lesions with focal neurologic signs (Fig. 9–5).

Diagnosis. The CSF findings in patients with cryptococcal meningitis vary with the presence of an underlying disease and the nature of the CNS involvement. The cell count usually ranges from 40 to 400 per μL. In more than half of patients, the pleocytosis is mainly composed of mononuclear cells. The protein concentration is over 40 mg/dL and may be quite high. The glucose concentration is depressed in 55% of patients. In the immunocompromised host, signs of inflammation may be minimal. The density of organisms may exceed that of white blood cells.

The India ink preparation of CSF is positive for organisms in up to one half of patients with cryptococcal meningitis (see Fig. 9–1); it is more likely to be positive for organisms in patients presenting with acute infection or who are immunosuppressed. The India ink preparation should be performed routinely in all patients with meningitis and may reveal organisms even in the

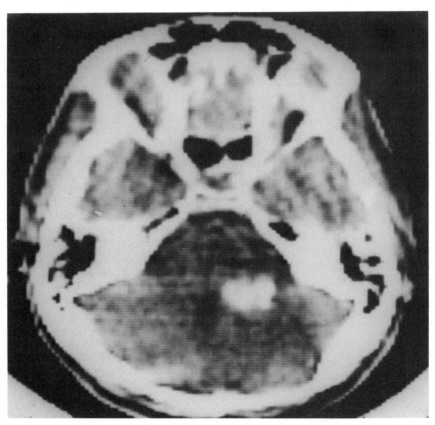

Figure 9–5. CT scan of a patient with cryptococcal meningitis, showing a contrast-enhancing cryptococcoma.

absence of a significant inflammatory response. Cryptococcal polysaccharide antigens must be determined in serum as well as CSF in all patients with chronic meningitis and should yield the diagnosis in about 94% of patients (see Table 9–4). The initial culture of CSF is positive for cryptococcus in three quarters of patients, but cultural yield may be delayed as long as 2 to 6 weeks. Additional cultures of CSF, as well as cultures of blood, sputum, urine, and stool are appropriate in all patients and may be positive for cryptococcus even in the absence of clinical signs of dissemination or local end-organ involvement.

Treatment. Currently, cryptococcal meningitis is treated with amphotericin B 0.3 mg/kg intravenously per day and flucytosine 150 mg/kg per day for 6 weeks. Renal function and flucytosine levels must be carefully monitored. Patients with AIDS will relapse without maintenance therapy. Fluconazole is an oral drug that may prove effective either in the initial therapy of cryptococcal meningitis or as maintenance therapy. Following termination of treatment, patients at risk for relapse, such as those with continuing high levels of polysaccharide antigen, should have repeated lumbar punctures for polysaccharide antigen determination and examination and culture of CSF.[9]

COCCIDIOIDAL MENINGITIS

Coccidioides immitis is a thermal dimorphic fungus that exists in nature as a mycelial form and in the tissues of infected animals and humans in a spherule (yeast)-like form. Endemic areas are at low altitudes, warm, and arid; in the United States, the areas of California, New Mexico, and Texas are endemic for *Coccidioides.*

Wind-borne arthrospores of *Cocci. immitis* infect through the respiratory route. Dissemination occurs in approximately 1 of 200 patients with symptomatic coccidioidomycosis, and one half of patients who disseminate develop meningitis. Dissemination to the meninges occurs early in the course of disease, often within the first 3 months. For unknown reasons, non-Caucasians, particularly Filipinos, are at higher risk of dissemination.[6]

Clinical Manifestations and Diagnosis. The presentation of coccidioidal meningitis varies from the acute to chronic stage.[6,10,16,70] The most common symptoms are fever, headache, and weight loss. About one half of patients develop disorientation, lethargy, confusion, or memory loss, and one third have a stiff neck. Papilledema, cranial nerve signs, and other focal findings also may occur. Extraneural lesions in the skin (one third of patients) or lung (two thirds of patients) are useful sites for establishing the diagnosis by culture and/or biopsy.

Usual CSF findings are lymphocytic pleocytosis, mean count 260 per μL (range 0 to 1200), with increased protein level and hypoglycorrhachia (in 76%). Rarely, the CSF may be normal. Culture of CSF is positive for organisms in up to 46% of patients. Blood and urine cultures also may yield the organism. Serologic tests are critical to the diagnosis. A serum complement fixation titer of greater than or equal to 1:16 is suggestive of disseminated coccidioidomycosis,[56] as is the presence of antibody of any titer in the CSF. Results of modified complement fixation tests of CSF are positive in up to 95% of patients. Most patients will have a negative coccidioidin skin test.

Treatment. Patients with coccidioidal meningitis must be treated with intravenous plus intraventricular amphotericin B.[70] The local amphotericin is given 3 times weekly for 3 months, through an indwelling reservoir, and then tapered. Therapy is discontinued only after the CSF has been normal for at least 1 year in patients receiving amphotericin B on a once-every-6-weeks regimen. The CSF must be followed at 6-week intervals for an additional 2 years to exclude relapse.

HISTOPLASMA MENINGITIS

Histoplasma capsulatum is a thermal dimorphic fungus found in its mycelial phase in the United States in the soil of the Ohio and Mississippi river valleys. Disturbances of soil containing the fungus result in the airborne spread of spores over wide areas. After inhalation, microconidia transform into yeast that disseminate hematogenously. The development of cell-mediated immunity usually leads to regression of infection, although delayed reactivation remains possible.

Clinical Manifestations and Diagnosis. Meningitis due to histoplasma is rare. When it occurs, meningitis may represent an isolated site of infection or it may be associated with progressive dissemination. In the latter case, associated findings include fever, anorexia, weight loss, and granulomatous lesions in multiple organs (hepatomegaly, splenomegaly, lymphadenopathy, mucosal or skin ulcers).[55] The presentation of chronic histoplasma meningitis usually consists of mental status abnormalities (reduced level of consciousness, confusion, personality changes, memory impairment) and headache.[26,27,60,64] Cranial nerve palsies and focal signs also occur commonly.

The CSF shows a lymphocytic pleocytosis (11 to 100 cells/μL) (rarely over 300 cells/μL) with increased protein and depressed glucose levels (in 79% of patients). Cultures of CSF are positive for histoplasma in up to 56% of patients. Large volumes of CSF may optimize the yield of culture.

Fungal cultures of blood, bone marrow, sputum, and urine also should be obtained, as well as biopsies of other tissues involved clinically. Although skin testing is contraindicated because it may falsely elevate serologic titers, detection of antibody in serum and CSF and of histoplasma in urine, CSF, and serum is useful and may support empirical use of amphotericin B pending the results of culture. A positive CSF culture or radioimmunoassay for antibodies to histoplasma in CSF is found in at least two thirds of patients; false-positive results occur, however, in one half of other chronic fungal meningitides, and serum antibodies may passively diffuse into the CSF.[65]

The radioimmunoassay for histoplasma antigen is highly specific. A polysaccharide antigen is found in the urine of 90% and in the blood of 50% of patients with disseminated histoplasmosis.[66] Antigen also has been found in the CSF of two of ten patients with histoplasma meningitis.[67] Sensitivity of antigen detection appears to be even higher in patients with AIDS.[67]

Treatment. Patients with histoplasma meningitis should be treated with amphotericin B for a total dose of 2.0 g. After treatment is completed, the CSF must be examined over a 2-year period for early recognition of relapse. Amphotericin B given intraventricularly is indicated in patients who fail to respond to intravenous drugs and in those who relapse more than once.

BLASTOMYCOTIC MENINGITIS

Blastomyces dermatitidis is a thermal dimorphic fungus that also causes disease around the Mississippi river basin and Great Lakes and in the southeastern United States. Its environmental niche seems to be the soil.[37] Blastomycosis disseminates from a pulmonary focus with associated involvement of the skin, bone, and prostate. CNS involvement may be isolated and usually occurs in the setting of dissemination.

Clinical Manifestations and Diagnosis. Blastomycotic meningitis usually presents as an acute and/or fulminant infection with headache, stiff neck, and focal signs.[8,37,68] The CSF usually shows a lymphocytic pleocytosis with cell counts that may exceed 1200 cells/μL. The CSF protein level is increased, and the glucose level may be depressed. Organisms may be seen on direct smear of the CSF; Because cultures are positive for *Blastomyces* in only about one fourth of patients, diagnosis usually requires culture from extraneural sites, particularly lung, skin, and biopsy material. Neither skin testing nor the generally available serologic assays are helpful because of their low sensitivity and specificity.

Treatment. Intravenous amphotericin B is the drug of choice for treatment of blastomycotic meningitis. Experience is insufficient to know the optimal dose of drug, but at least 2 g seems necessary.

SPOROTHRIX MENINGITIS

Sporothrix schenckii is a thermal dimorphic fungus isolated from a number of environmental sources. Infections usually have followed inoculation of the fungus from soil, plants, and timber, and, less frequently, from bites of animals, birds, and insects. Lymphocutaneous disease is most common and rarely disseminates. Pulmonary disease also is uncommon. The infection has been isolated to the CNS in most of the 15 patients reported with sporothrix meningitis.[23,51]

Headache is a uniform feature of the presentation; patients are generally afebrile. Gait disturbance and seizures have occurred. CSF pleocytosis is mainly lymphocytic (0 to 517 cells/μL), the protein level is increased, and the glucose level is depressed. The delay between onset of symptoms, first lumbar puncture, and diagnosis resulted in a mean 6.5-month delay in instituting treatment.[23,51] In a recent study, all patients showed CSF and serum antibodies to the causative agent by enzyme immunoassay and latex agglutination.[51]

The recommended treatment of sporothrix meningitis is amphotericin B intravenously for a total dose of at least 2.0 g. Some isolates are resistant to amphotericin B, and the meningitis may be refractory to therapy, with cultures persistently positive for sporothrix.

CANDIDA MENINGITIS

Candida meningitis is a manifestation of disseminated disease and is associated with intravenous drug use, indwelling venous catheters, abdominal surgery, and corticosteroid therapy.[3,17,58] Overall, 71% of patients with candida meningitis have active extraneural candida infections, and an additional 14% have had antecedent procedures that may have introduced yeast into the subarachnoid space (ventricular shunting, lumbar puncture).

The onset of symptoms may be abrupt or insidious. Fever is, however, an invariable part of the presentation. The major findings are headache and stiff neck; some patients have depressed mental status, confusion, and cranial neuropathies or other focal neurologic signs. CSF findings are quite variable; pleocytosis may range up to 2000 cells/μL, with a mean in one series of 600 cells. Lymphocytes predominate in approximately one half of patients. Protein levels are elevated in most patients, and glucose levels are depressed in 60%. Yeast is found on smears of CSF in 43% of the patients, and cultures of CSF usually are positive for candida. Extraneural culture may yield candida as well. The treatment of candida meningitis requires amphotericin B.[3,17]

BRUCELLA MENINGITIS

Brucellosis remains a common disease worldwide.[6,24,45] Most patients with CNS brucellosis report consumption of unpasteurized dairy products, contact with animals or animal products, or a previous episode of brucellosis; one third do not have a clear exposure history.

Clinical Manifestations. Approximately 3.5% of patients with brucellosis have predominant involvement of the CNS. Brucella meningitis may be associated with systemic symptoms (fever, arthralgia, myalgia, sweating, and malaise) or an entirely localized process.[7] In one third of patients with meningitis, CNS involvement is the first manifestation of brucellosis. The meningitis itself usually is subacute to chronic and may be transient or recurrent. Associated cranial neuropathies may occur with involvement of cranial nerves VI, VII, or most commonly VIII. Meningitis may be the predominant manifestation of CNS brucellosis, or there may be meningoencephalitis, myeloradiculitis, or neuritis. Most of the patients show motor abnormalities. Disordered mentation, sensory disturbances, spastic paraparesis, seizures, sciatica, or cervicobrachialgia also may be prominent. Occasionally vascular involvement associated with transient ischemic attacks or, rarely, subarachnoid hemorrhage occurs and has been attributed to vasculitis or spasm of intracerebral vessels.

Diagnosis. The CSF shows a mononuclear cell pleocytosis (20 to 500 cells/μL), with depressed glucose levels in two thirds of cases and increased protein levels. Brucella may be cultured from the CSF, particularly if the disease is localized, but rarely in this case is found concurrently in blood. The diagnosis hinges on demonstration of antibody to brucella in CSF. The most reliable serologic finding is the presence of nonagglutinating antibody to brucella in the CSF (and serum) by a modified Coombs' test.

Treatment. Optimal treatment of CNS brucellosis probably should consist of doxycycline plus rifampin and must be continued for prolonged periods (>4 months), ultimately gauging duration by changes in CSF. The response to antibiotics reflects in large measure the extent of irreversible neurologic disease before institution of therapy.

NEUROSYPHILIS (see Chapter 11)

Despite the general decline in the prevalence of syphilis in the antibiotic era, neurosyphilis remains an important diagnostic consideration in patients with signs of meningeal inflammation and neurologic deficits. The frequency of neurosyphilis, in fact, is likely to increase, reflective of the increase in the worldwide prevalence of primary and secondary forms of syphilis in the past decade and the increased

occurrence of syphilitic infections in HIV-positive individuals. Neurosyphilis may take a particularly aggressive clinical course in the HIV-infected patient. Even in immunocompetent hosts, however, the index of suspicion must remain high for syphilitic infection of the central nervous system, because atypical forms of the disease are common and because, in most cases, the disease is treatable.

Clinical Manifestations. Infection of the central nervous system occurs in about 10% of persons infected with *Treponema pallidum.* Although infection may be asymptomatic, more commonly it presents within 2 years of the initial primary stage, with clinical meningitis. Fever may be absent; headache, mental status changes, and signs of meningeal inflammation usually are present. Cranial nerve palsies, particularly of cranial nerves II, VII, and VIII, result from the basilar meningitis. Seizures may occur due to involvement of the meninges over the cerebral convexities. *Cerebrovascular syphilis* occurs after a longer latency of several years from primary infection, usually presenting with stroke syndromes, but preischemic prodromes also occur, with headache, lethargy, or behavioral changes developing from weeks to months before the acute ischemic event. Angiography is helpful as it may show "beading" and concentric narrowing of both large and medium-sized cerebral vessels.

General paresis refers to the dementia that occurs after an even longer latency (10 to 20 years) and may be indistinguishable from dementia of another cause. *Tabes dorsalis,* the fourth classic form of neurosyphilis, presents about 10 years after infection with a triad of "lightning" pains, urinary dysfunction, and ataxia. On examination, Argyll Robertson pupils frequently are present, as are areflexia and loss of posterior column function. General paresis or tabes dorsalis should be readily distinguishable from chronic meningitis.

All the clinical syndromes of neurosyphilis result from active meningeal inflammation. Abnormal CSF is the hallmark of this disease. In fact, the diagnosis of cerebrovascular syphilis or paretic neurosyphilis ("general paresis" or "dementia paralytica") cannot be made if the CSF is normal. Tabes dorsalis in the late stages, however, can present with normal CSF parameters. Unreactive CSF serologic tests for syphilis with normal CSF occurred in only 2 of 100 cases of tabes dorsalis reported by Merritt and coworkers in 1946.[43]

Diagnosis. The CSF in syphilitic meningitis usually shows lymphocytic pleocytosis with values of 500 cells/μL or greater; syphilitic vascular disease is associated with a less vigorous lymphocytic pleocytosis in the 50- to 200-cells/μL range. The protein level commonly is elevated in neurosyphilis, although it is usually less than 200 mg/dL. The fluorescent treponemal antibody absorption (FTA-ABS) test of serum is reactive in more than 95% of patients with late syphilis regardless of therapy. For practical purposes, therefore, a negative FTA-ABS on serum virtually excludes the diagnosis of neurosyphilis (see Table 9–4). The Venereal Disease Research Laboratory (VDRL) test on the CSF is more useful as a gauge of disease activity. Patients with negative CSF serologic test results probably most often represent meningitis due to causes other than syphilis.[54]

Treatment. The standard treatment regimens for neurosyphilis recently have been revised because of reports of recurrence or persistence of the infection following what was thought to be adequate antibiotic therapy for early primary syphilis. Treatment recommended for neurosyphilis now includes aqueous penicillin-G 600,000 units given intramuscularly every day for 15 days, or penicillin-G 2 to 4 million units given intravenously every 4 hours for 10 to 14 days. Treatment of the immunocompromised patient with neurosyphilis requires the more intensive intravenous regimen.

Assessment of the adequacy of treatment regimens for neurosyphilis involves repeat lumbar punctures at 6, 12, and 24 months. The CSF pleocytosis should show resolution to normal within a period of 6 months. Both the serum and CSF VDRL tests should return to nonreactive; occasionally a low-fixed VDRL titer is found in the serum. Relapse can occur, so any change in clinical status should prompt a repeat lumbar puncture.

LYME DISEASE (see Chapter 10)

Lyme disease, caused by a newly recognized spirochete, *Borrelia burgdorferi,* can cause meningoencephalitis in the early stage of the infection, and a clinical picture consistent with chronic meningitis during the later stages of the illness. CSF in patients with chronic neurologic involvement shows a lymphocytic pleocytosis consisting of a range of 6 to 700 cells/μL, with a median count of 166. A plasma cell reaction has been described in the CSF in early stages of neurologic involvement in Lyme disease. The total protein level is usually mildly elevated and antibody against *B. burgdorferi* is found in high titers in the more chronic neurologic stages of the disease.

CYSTICERCOSIS (see Chapter 12)

Cysticercosis is the most common parasitic infection of the CNS worldwide and is seen in the southwestern United States. Most patients present with seizures or increased intracranial pressure. Cysticercus racemosus produces multiple cysts near the basilar meninges that may result in chronic meningitis, sometimes with hydrocephalus. Fever and cranial neuropathy are, however, rare. The CSF is normal in one half of patients; the other half have a pleocytosis, sometimes with depressed glucose. The CT scan is helpful diagnostically since it may show 2 to 10 mm calcific lesions (Fig. 9–6; see Fig. 12–4) or cystic lesions that undergo enhancement with contrast. Results of serologic tests such as the indirect hemagglutination test performed by the Centers for Disease Control are positive in most patients with meningitis.

OTHER INFECTIONS OF THE CENTRAL NERVOUS SYSTEM

There is a group of organisms that most commonly causes brain abscesses or focal granulomas (see Table 9–5 and Chapter 7) the clinical syndrome may, however, resemble chronic meningitis with prominent focal findings (and focal lesions on neuroradiographic procedures), or, in rare instances, these organisms may cause an isolated meningitis. These organisms are considered in Table 9–5.

Sarcoidosis

Five percent of patients with sarcoidosis have neural involvement; in nearly half of them, the presenting manifestations of sarcoidosis are neurologic.[11a] Cranial nerve palsies are common, particularly a peripheral seventh-nerve palsy, due to the granulomatous inflammation of the meninges at the base of the brain. Eighth-nerve dysfunction takes the form of sensorineural hearing loss; the optic nerve also may be compressed by granulomas or affected by pressure due to hydrocephalus. Hypothalamic dysfunction occurs, producing neuroendocrine disease, most commonly affecting water balance. In fact, serum prolactin levels may be elevated in CNS sarcoidosis.

A chronic aseptic meningitis also can occur in sarcoidosis, both as the first neurologic manifestation and as a recurrent syndrome. Headache and meningeal signs are present, and the CSF shows a lymphocytic pleocytosis (in 70% of patients) in the range of 6 to 200 cells/μL; 70% have elevated protein levels, usually less than 200 mg/dL, and 20% have hypoglycorrhachia.[15,25]

Only the neuroendocrinologic features and the extent of cranial and peripheral neuropathies distinguish sarcoidosis from other forms of chronic meningitis. The diagnosis may be made by histologic examination of enlarged lymph nodes or tissue obtained by transbronchial biopsy or mediastinoscopy, and on some occasions by biopsy of salivary glands or conjunctiva. A finding of elevated serum angiotensin-converting enzyme levels sometimes is helpful. In some instances, however, sarcoidosis is limited to the CNS; in this case, it must be distinguished from infectious causes of chronic meningitis (which may occur with increased frequency in patients with sarcoidosis, particularly in the setting of treatment with high doses of corticosteroids). When mass lesions are present in the cerebrum, biopsy may yield definitive diagnosis. Pursuit of histologic confirmation of the diagnosis may require meningeal biopsy; exclusion of complicating infection is of paramount importance, since corticosteroids are used to treat CNS sarcoidosis.

Vasculitis and Rheumatologic Syndromes

CNS involvement may on occasion be the presenting feature of unrecognized systemic vasculitis. Rarely, neurologic syndromes may be the sole manifestation of vasculitis, as in granulomatous angiitis of the central nervous system.

GRANULOMATOUS ANGIITIS OF THE NERVOUS SYSTEM

Granulomatous angiitis is a disease of unknown cause characterized by granulomatous inflammation involving the small arteries and arterioles of the parenchymal and leptomeningeal vessels. Langhans'-type and foreign body giant cells may be found in association with intimal proliferation. Histologically the disease resembles giant cell arteritis, except that the media of the vessel may be spared.

The mean age of the patient at diagnosis is 46.[53] Clinically, patients present with headache and encephalopathy, followed by progression to a

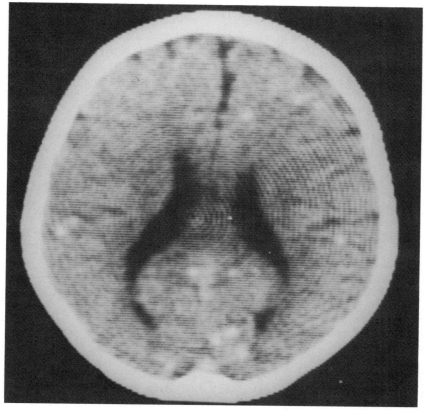

Figure 9–6. CT scan of a patient with cysticercosis showing multiple calcific densities.

**Table 9–5 ORGANISMS THAT USUALLY CAUSE
FOCAL LESIONS IN THE CENTRAL NERVOUS SYSTEM
BUT MAY PRESENT AS CHRONIC MENINGITIS**

Organism	Setting	Clinical Syndrome
Aspergillus sp.	Neutropenia, allograft recipient	CNS involvement is usually part of terminal dissemination
Zygomycetes sp.	Diabetic ketoacidosis	Rhinocerebral mucormycosis
Nocardia sp.	Impaired cellular immunity, high-dose corticosteroids	CNS involvement as part of dissemination
Cladosporium tritalchoides	Normal host	Meningitis; sometimes lesions in lung or ear
Phialophora sp.	Normal host	Chromoblastomycosis—CNS disease and skin lesions
Pseudallescheria boydii	Subtropical Central and South America	Young male laborers acquire disease through contact with soil. Intracranial pressure usually is increased
Actinomyces and *Arachnia* sp.	Normal host	Anaerobic mouth flora; produces mixed infection

strokelike syndrome with hemiparesis or other focal signs including cranial neuropathies.

The CSF frequently is abnormal, with elevated opening pressure, elevated total protein levels in approximately 80% and a lymphocytic pleocytosis (usually less than 100 cells/μL) in three quarters of patients. Glucose levels are depressed in only one third. The erythrocyte sedimentation rate is elevated in some patients. Similarly, other laboratory studies indicative of autoimmune disease are of no use diagnostically. Angiography may show evidence of the characteristic symmetrical or segmental narrowing, irregularity of vessels, or "beeding"; if not, leptomeningeal biopsy is necessary to establish the diagnosis. The prognosis is poor in most patients, with death occurring within weeks to months of diagnosis. The use of corticosteroids and immunosuppressive agents may improve the outcome.

VASCULITIS ASSOCIATED WITH HERPES ZOSTER OPHTHALMICUS

From 1 week to 2 years after ophthalmic zoster, patients may develop "crossed hemiplegia." At times, the facial nerve also is involved clinically. The CSF parameters and pathologic characteristics are similar to those seen in granulomatous angiitis of the central nervous system, with elevated numbers of lymphocytes and protein content. The prognosis usually is better, however, with significant resolution of neurologic deficits.

COGAN'S SYNDROME

Cogan's syndrome, vestibulo-auditory dysfunction and interstitial keratitis presenting in young adults, may on rare occasion present with a meningoencephalitis. A mild CSF pleocytosis may occur in a small percentage of patients. The diagnosis usually is established by associated eighth-nerve involvement as well as visual loss due to keratitis. Although rare, this syndrome is important to recognize because of its response in some cases to corticosteroids.[61]

SYSTEMIC VASCULITIDES AFFECTING THE CENTRAL NERVOUS SYSTEM

Polyarteritis Nodosa. The CNS may be involved in polyarteritis nodosa (PAN), although less commonly than the peripheral nervous system (PNS). (PAN is a cause of mononeuritis multiplex.) Initial symptoms include headache and fever with cognitive changes that have been described as "toxic delirium" with confusion and disorientation. Less commonly, CNS involvement begins abruptly with hemiparesis and seizures. Abdominal pain, myalgias, or arthralgias may be present upon initial diagnosis. Neurasthenic symptoms (weight loss, fatigue, anorexia, and generalized weakness) are present in some patients, as are sinusitis, mastoiditis, or otitis. The CSF may be normal or show a low-grade pleocytosis and elevated protein level, usually less than 100 mg/dL.[52] Interpretation of the CSF formula may be complicated by the occurrence of seizures, stroke, or subarachnoid hemorrhage, syndromes that also may produce inflammatory changes in the CSF.

Systemic Lupus Erythematosus. Disturbed mental function is a common neurologic manifestation of SLE. Encephalopathy occurs in 10% to 30% of patients, usually manifest as acute confusional states, affective disorders, and perceptual disturbances. At times, it is difficult to attribute mental status changes to SLE because metabolic dysfunction due to renal disease, ischemic events due to hypertension, and corticosteroid-related psychotic changes may produce cognitive changes. SLE also may present with seizures, migraine headache, stroke or transient ischemic attack (TIA) syndromes, transverse myelopathy, chorea, or peripheral neuropathies. The CSF is abnormal in approximately one fourth of patients with central nervous system dysfunction, usually showing a mild elevation of protein level and minimal pleocytosis. Rarely, the glucose level is depressed; hypoglycorrhachia is more common in transverse myelopathy associated with SLE.

Recent evidence suggests that magnetic resonance imaging (MRI) scans may be more sensitive than CT in detecting evidence of active CNS disease.[32] T_2-weighted images show focal high-intensity areas, often in the white matter, possibly representing vasculopathy and microinfarcts associated with SLE.

Sjögren's Syndrome. Sjögren's syndrome is a rheumatologic disorder with frequent central nervous system manifestations. Sjögren's syndrome is characterized by xerophthalmia (dry eyes), xerostomia (dry mouth), and drying of other mucous membranes and the skin. The sicca complex may also occur in association with other connective tissue disease such as rheumatoid arthritis, SLE, or progressive systemic sclerosis. Peripheral neuropathies occur in about 25% of patients. CNS dysfunction may be even more common, particularly if subtle cognitive change is assessed. Signs and symptoms of CNS disease include stroke or TIAs, seizures, movement disorders, encephalopathy, intermittent central nervous system dysfunction similar to multiple sclerosis, and recurrent aseptic meningitis.

In the subset of patients whose disease mimics demyelinating disease, the CSF profile in Sjögren's syndrome may look quite similar to multiple sclerosis, with an elevated immunoglobulin G (IgG) index, lymphocytic pleocytosis, and oligoclonal banding. Preliminary data, however, indicate the presence of anti-RO (SS-A) autoantibodies in the CSF of patients with Sjögren's syndrome and neurologic symptoms.[47] Oligoclonal bands are more frequently found in patients with Sjögren's syndrome and active CNS disease; they are infrequent in patients with Sjögren's

syndrome without neurologic symptoms or signs. The MRI scan is sensitive in demonstrating focal neurologic disease in Sjögren's syndrome. Even in patients with diffuse cognitive dysfunction, approximately 50% show abnormalities on MRI, most frequently small, hyperintense areas in subcortical white matter on T_2-weighted images.

Behçet's Syndrome. Behçet's syndrome is characterized by recurrent oral and genital ulceration with ocular lesions. In 5% to 10% of patients, it is also associated with neurologic complications, usually late in the illness. Seizures, encephalopathy, strokelike syndromes, cranial nerve paresis, and a meningitis-like picture may occur. Pleocytosis is present in most patients, although it is usually less than 60 cells/μL,[50] either with lymphocytic or neutrophilic predominance. Protein levels are usually mildly elevated. Glucose levels are normal.

The neurologic manifestations of Behçet's syndrome may follow an intermittent, exacerbating-remitting pattern similar to multiple sclerosis. It also may be difficult to distinguish the neurologic manifestations of Behçet's syndrome from those of stroke due to atherosclerotic vascular disease or syphilis, or from an infiltrative meningeal process. The presence of ocular lesions and oral and genital ulcerations usually clarifies the diagnosis.

Vogt-Koyanagi-Harada Syndrome. Inflammation affecting the uvea, retina, meninges, and skin occurs in the VKH syndrome. Findings on physical examination of vitiligo, poliosis (whitening of hair), and uveitis usually suggest the diagnosis. In one series, 61% of patients developed meningeal signs and symptoms.[44] Meningeal symptoms may either precede or postdate the onset of ocular inflammation. Because of the occurrence of meningoencephalitis in this syndrome, it has also been called the uveomeningoencephalitic syndrome.[46] Corticosteroid therapy appears to be effective in preserving vision and preventing systemic complications.

Migraine with CSF Pleocytosis. In a subset of patients with migraine and transient neurologic dysfunction with headache and focal symptoms, the CSF may be abnormal. A mononuclear pleocytosis occurs in a range from 40 to 233 cells/μL with an average of 121 cells/μL.[2] Protein level is increased, usually around 100 mg/dL, and the glucose level is normal. It is not clear whether the CSF abnormalities reflect an inflammatory process presenting as migraine or are due to the migraine itself.

Chemical Meningitis

The intrathecal injection and even the oral administration of several compounds may cause an inflammatory reaction in the leptomeninges, producing a chemical meningitis. Contrast agents for radiographic studies (the older, oil-based media such as Pantopaque were more likely to produce arachnoiditis than the newer, water-soluble agents such as metrizamide) and drugs such as chemotherapeutic agents, antibiotics, and local anesthetics may produce a chemical meningitis. Certain nonsteroidal anti-inflammatory drugs (ibuprofen is the prototype) may produce a similar syndrome. The CSF may reflect a partial or complete spinal block with low opening pressure, elevated protein level, and a lymphocytic pleocytosis; glucose level usually is normal. At times, fever and signs of meningeal irritation are prominent. The CSF abnormalities generally resolve in 1 to 2 weeks.

Chronic Meningitis Associated with Malignancies

PRIMARY BRAIN TUMORS

Current neuroradiographic procedures are such that brain tumor usually can be distinguished from chronic meningitis. Malignant gliomas that are necrotic, however, particularly those that invade ventricular walls, may be associated with very high CSF cell counts. Of the primary brain tumors, oligodendrogliomas also may be responsible for subarachnoid bleeding. Rarely, leptomeningeal infiltration by a glioma may produce a syndrome indistinguishable from meningeal carcinomatosis.

MENINGEAL CARCINOMATOSIS

Diffuse leptomeningeal spread of solid tumors without parenchymal lesions can produce the clinical syndrome of chronic meningitis. Patients with breast or lung tumors or melanoma are most susceptible to meningeal spread of metastases (see Fig. 9–2). Among the solid tumors, adenocarcinomas most commonly seed the leptomeninges. In a series of 90 patients from Memorial Sloan-Kettering Cancer Center, 73% suffered from adenocarcinoma.[62]

The diagnosis of malignancy as the cause of chronic meningitis is suggested clinically when neurologic deficits appear at multiple levels of the neuraxis: the cerebrum, cranial nerves, and spinal roots. Headache and encephalopathy as well as seizures also may be present. Cranial nerve deficits are common, particularly those involving extraocular muscles causing diplopia; eighth-nerve dysfunction with hearing loss, dizziness, or vertigo; and seventh and second nerve involvement, causing facial numbness and diminished visual acuity. Radicular symptoms also are common, with back pain radiating down one or both legs, leg weakness, and sphincteric dysfunction. Paresthesias may be present. A cauda equina syndrome also may be the presenting neurologic abnormality.

In the series from Memorial Sloan-Kettering Cancer Center, the CSF obtained from initial lumbar puncture was abnormal in all but three patients.[62] The cell count, predominantly lymphocytes, was elevated in 51 of 90 patients, and the protein level was increased to approximately 50 mg/dL in 73 patients. The finding of low-grade pleocytosis (usually <50 cells/μL) and markedly depressed glucose level is very suggestive of meningeal carcinomatosis. Definitive diagnosis is confirmed by the finding of malignant cells within the CSF. Results of cytologic tests of the CSF obtained from initial lumbar puncture were positive in 49 of 90 patients (54%), but on subsequent spinal taps cytologic test results eventually became positive in 82%. Larger volumes of CSF increase the chance of finding the yield of malignant cells. Because the recovery of malignant cells unequivocally establishes the diagnosis of leptomeningeal carcinomatosis, repeated lumbar punctures, at times six or more, may be appropriate if the clinical suspicion is high.

Supporting radiographic studies include myelography, CT scanning, and MRI.[46a] Myelograms may show characteristic thickening and nodularity of the nerve roots, resulting from tumor seeding of the meninges in these areas. MRI also is sensitive to these nodules and may suggest actual tumor involvement of thickened nerve roots. CT scans of the head may show hydrocephalus, possibly reflecting occlusion of CSF absorptive pathways in the subarachnoid space, or contrast enhancement of the basilar cisterns (see Fig. 9–4).

Treatment for leptomeningeal metastases, when attempted, may complicate the picture, as intraventricular drugs may produce a chemical meningoencephalitis or meningitis. After the administration of intraventricular methotrexate via an Ommaya reservoir, for example, an acute meningoencephalopathy may occur with headache, fever, cognitive changes, and meningeal signs. The CSF shows an increased pleocytosis (greater than that associated with the tumor) with elevated protein level, suggesting methotrexate toxicity. Chemotherapy may result in improvement or stabilization of neurologic symptoms in some patients, however, on occasion prolonging survival.

CHRONIC BENIGN LYMPHOCYTIC MENINGITIS

This term mainly is useful as a reminder that some individuals presenting with headache and low-grade lymphocytic pleocytosis will resolve their symptoms and CSF abnormalities within 7 to 25 weeks.[30] Patients with focal signs or symptoms and high CSF protein and low glucose levels are more likely to have a progressive process.

CHRONIC MENINGITIS IN THE IMMUNOCOMPROMISED PATIENT

The differential diagnosis of chronic meningitis shifts dramatically in the presence of overt immunocompromise.[31] Not only is the relative frequency of infectious agents altered, but progression of the underlying disease and complications of its therapy must be considered as potential causes of the neurologic syndromes. The number of immunocompromised patients clearly is increasing because of the AIDS epidemic, the increasing number of organ transplantation recipients, and the increasing number of immunosuppressive therapies used to treat patients with cancer and autoimmune disease. CNS infections in the chronically immunosuppressed individual also may differ in presentation, course, and response to treatment. In one recent series, 30 of 49 immunosuppressed patients died as a result of their CNS infection, in contrast to the otherwise favorable prognosis of the underlying disease in 41 of these 49 immunocompromised patients.[31]

Several principles can be cited concerning the diagnosis and management of chronic meningitis in the immunocompromised patient.

1. With sufficient immunosuppression, as in transplant recipients and

patients with AIDS, *infections with more than one organism may occur* simultaneously. For example, contrast-enhancing lesions on cerebral CT scan in an HIV-positive individual may be due to infection with toxoplasma, cryptococci, and candida. In one series,[40] 30% of patients with more than one abscess on cerebral CT scan were infected with organisms other than or in addition to toxoplasma. The same patient also may have sequential infections with different infectious agents.

2. The *depressed immune and inflammatory response* may dampen the CSF profile in cryptococcal meningitis in the immunosuppressed patient, in which case it is characterized by a less dramatic pleocytosis and correspondingly normal chemistries. As another example, the toxoplasma abscess in the immunocompromised patient may show less of a surrounding inflammatory response on histopathologic examination. The dearth of inflammatory changes also affects the clinical manifestations of chronic meningitis. Symptoms and signs of meningeal irritation may be minimal or absent. The clinician's vigilance must be high in immunosuppressed patients because early diagnosis and treatment of chronic meningitis is required to mitigate the otherwise poor prognosis.

3. The immunocompromised patient manifests *susceptibility to infection with opportunistic organisms that normally do not cause disease.* The precise nature of the underlying disease impacts on the nature of the susceptibility. For example, patients with AIDS differ from other individuals with depressed cellular immunity in that they have a relatively greater occurrence of infection with *M. avium* and a decreased development of *Listeria* and *Nocardia* infections.

Acquired Immunodeficiency Syndrome

AIDS requires special consideration because it accounts for an increasing proportion of patients presenting with the clinical syndrome of chronic meningitis. The impact of AIDS on the diagnosis and management of chronic meningitis is so great that serologic tests for HIV now should be included among the routine laboratory tests recommended for all patients with chronic meningitis.

Acute meningitis or meningoencephalitis may occur following infection with HIV, at about the time of seroconversion. This aseptic meningitis has been considered "atypical" because of the frequent occurrence of long tract signs and cranial nerve deficits. Although the syndrome usually is self-limited, on rare occasions meningitis can persist or recur. Patients periodically manifest headache or fever with mild CSF pleocytosis over a period of months from the initial symptoms. The recovery of HIV in neurologically asymptomatic HIV-seropositive patients suggests that the CNS is invaded by the retrovirus.[29,52]

The main infectious complications of AIDS that present as a subacute-to-chronic meningitis are toxoplasmosis, cryptococcosis, and syphilis, as discussed below. Additionally, *M. tuberculosis*,[70] *Candida albicans*, *Histoplasma capsulatum*, *Coccidioides immitis*, *Aspergillus fumigatus*, and cytomegalovirus cause meningeal inflammation.

TOXOPLASMA GONDII

The most commonly encountered neurologic opportunistic infection, affecting 28% of AIDS patients,[39] is caused by *Toxoplasma gondii*. Because most adults in the United States have antibodies to this protozoan, and because toxoplasmosis is rare in children with HIV infection, it is assumed that cerebral toxoplasmosis in the HIV-infected population represents reactivation of latent infection.

Clinical Manifestations. Cerebral toxoplasmosis generally presents with headache accompanied by focal signs and symptoms including hemiparesis, aphasia, hemisensory loss, or seizures.[11] Less commonly, meningoencephalitis may be characterized by mental status changes, lethargy, and cognitive decline indistinguishable from that of AIDS dementia complex or other causes of chronic meningitis. CT scan is quite helpful in diagnosis, showing contrast-enhancing lesions with a predilection for the basal ganglia, the gray-white junction of the cerebral hemispheres, and the cerebellum. Ring enhancement of these lesions is characteristic but is not invariable. MRI is more sensitive than CT; multiple lesions may be seen on MRI scans when CT scans show only a solitary abscess. As noted, however, sometimes multiple lesions may be due to multiple pathogens.

In toxoplasma meningoencephalitis, CSF protein level usually is mildly elevated and there is a mononuclear pleocytosis of mild degree. Although negative IgG titers make the diagnosis of toxoplasmosis unlikely, blood CSF serologic tests are not reliable. For example, specific IgG may be undetectable in the CSF in patients with biopsy- or autopsy-proven CNS toxoplasmosis.

Treatment. Most physicians caring for AIDS patients in whom toxoplasmosis is a diagnostic consideration will begin an empirical course of therapy with pyrimethamine and sulfadiazine. Support for this approach is based upon the high prevalence of this infection in AIDS patients with CNS symptoms and appropriate radiographic lesions.[13] Initial response to therapy can be expected in up to 90% of patients treated with two-drug therapy.[42] It may be necessary to substitute clindamycin for sulfadiazine, however, because of toxicity. Lifelong maintenance therapy with pyrimethamine is recommended after 6 to 8 weeks of full-dose therapy. If the patient does not improve clinically or radiographically after 1 to 2 weeks of empirical therapy, consideration should be given at that time to brain biopsy to establish the diagnosis definitively.

CRYPTOCOCCUS NEOFORMANS

Cryptococcus neoformans is the third most common infectious agent that causes neurologic disease in patients with AIDS, following HIV itself and *Toxoplasma gondii.* Although fever, headache, and lethargy are common presenting symptoms, meningeal signs occur only in a minority, and stiff neck, papilledema, and photophobia usually are absent. As noted, the CSF is less likely to be abnormal in AIDS patients with cryptococcal meningitis than in other hosts. In the majority of patients in several series,[20,36] the pleocytosis was less than 5 cells/μL. Although modest protein level elevations occur, the CSF glucose level usually is greater than 40 mg/dL. In some patients, all CSF parameters are normal. The presence of underlying HIV infection does not, however, alter the yield of CSF in terms of cryptococcal antigen and cultures. Cryptococcal antigen titer in the CSF, in fact, was greater than 1:8 in all 16 patients in the Kovacs and coworkers' series,[36] and in 20 of 22 patients in the Zuger and coworkers' series.[71] Serum cryptococcal antigen frequently is markedly elevated, with a median titer of 1:400 in Dismukes' 21 patients,[20] and may exceed that of the CSF.[12]

High relapse rates and therapeutic failures complicate the management of cryptococcal meningitis in patients with AIDS. Long-term maintenance therapy usually is necessary. The initial response to amphotericin B is favorable in only 58% of cases,[18] and sustained clinical improvement occurs in only 20%. CSF cryptococcal antigen titers greater than 1:8 after therapy are associated with a higher relapse rate and worse prognosis.[20] Recent experience with fluconazole indicates that it is an effective agent for the maintenance phase of treatment.[58]

TREPONEMA PALLIDUM

Treponema pallidum infection takes a clinically aggressive course in HIV-seropositive persons.[33] The meningitic and meningovascular forms of early neurosyphilis are seen with increased frequency in the HIV-positive population.

Several reports have documented the development of neurosyphilis in patients treated for early syphilis with benzathine penicillin.[5,22] Most physicians now recommend higher doses of antibiotics for longer periods to treat syphilis in HIV-infected subjects. Repeat CSF examinations with serologic tests are required to assess whether or not treatment has been adequate. Differentiating true relapse from reinfection in this sexually active population may be difficult.[4]

LYMPHOMA

Non-Hodgkin's systemic lymphoma is the most important noninfectious consideration in the HIV-infected population, because it can spread to the leptomeninges to cause a lymphomatous meningitis. Patients present with symptoms and signs referable to many levels of the neuraxis. Multiple cranial neuropathies, spinal root radicular syndromes, and pyramidal tract signs often signal the diagnosis. This neurologic picture is quite characteristic of leptomeningeal spread of malignancy and may in fact warrant a thorough search for signs of lymphoma elsewhere. The CSF may show a modest lymphocytic pleocytosis with slightly elevated protein and lowered glucose levels. Initial CSF cytologic test results may be negative; the yield is improved, however, by obtaining larger quantities of fluid at repeat lumbar punctures and perhaps by obtaining cisternal fluid.

SUMMARY

Chronic meningitis is the persistence for more than 4 weeks of meningitis that produces headache, fever, stiff neck, CSF abnormalities, and sometimes signs of encephalitis. Therapeutic efforts often must begin before the precise cause has been identified, because a number of different diseases can cause virtually identical clinical presentations and some are readily treatable. Diagnosis is aided by the patient's history, the physical examination, radiographic procedures, and laboratory tests that may include biopsy or examination of the blood and CSF. The different patterns of CSF abnormalities can be especially helpful in suggesting a diagnosis.

The causes of chronic meningitis include a variety of infectious agents, sarcoidosis, vasculitides, an inflammatory reaction to contrast agents or drugs, and malignancy. The immunocompromised patient is especially at risk and often differs from the immunocompetent patient in presentation, course, and response to treatment. These patients may be infected with more than one organism or with organisms that ordinarily do not cause disease and may display a depressed response to infection that may hinder the early diagnosis required to mitigate their poor prognosis.

REFERENCES

1. Barrett-Connor EB: Tuberculous meningitis in adults. South Med J 60:1061–1067, 1967.
2. Bartleson JD, Swanson JW, and Whisnant JP: A migrainous syndrome with cerebrospinal fluid pleocytosis. Neurology 31:1257–1262, 1981.
3. Bayer AS, Edwards JE Jr, Seidel JS, et al: Candida meningitis. Medicine 55:477–486, 1976.
4. Bayne LL, Schmidley JW, and Goodin DS: Acute syphilitic meningitis: Its occurrence after clinical and serologic cure of secondary syphilis with penicillin G. Arch Neurol 43:137–138, 1986.
5. Berry CD, Hooton TM, Collier AC, and Lukehart SA: Neurologic relapse after benzathine penicillin therapy for secondary syphilis in a patient with HIV infection. N Engl J Med 316:1587–1589, 1987.

6. Bouza E, Dreyer JS, Hewitt WL, and Meyer RD: Coccidioidal meningitis. An analysis of 31 cases and review of the literature. Medicine 60:139–172, 1981.

7. Bouza E, Garcia de la Torre M, Parras F, et al: Brucellar meningitis. Rev Infect Dis 9:810–822, 1987.

7a. Bruyn RPM and Bruyn GW: Chronic meningitis. In McKendall RR (ed): Handbook of Clinical Neurology, Vol 12, Viral Disease. Elsevier, Amsterdam, 1989, pp 643–650.

8. Buechner HA and Clawson CM: Blastomycosis of central nervous system. II. A report of nine cases from the Veterans Administration Cooperative Study. Am Rev Respir Dis 95:820–826, 1967.

9. Butler WT, Alling DW, Spickard A, et al: Diagnostic and prognostic value of clinical and laboratory findings in cryptococcal meningitis. A follow-up study of forty patients. N Engl J Med 270:59–67, 1964.

10. Candill RG, Smith CE, and Reinarz JA: Coccidioidal meningitis. A diagnostic challenge. Am J Med 49:360–365, 1970.

11. Carranzana EJ, Rossitch EJ, and Samuels MA: Cerebral toxoplasmosis in the acquired immunodeficiency syndrome. Clin Neurol Neurosurg 91:291–301, 1989.

11a. Chapelon C, Ziza J-M, Piette, JC, et al: Neurosarcoidosis: Signs, course and treatment in 35 confirmed cases. Medicine 69:261–276, 1990.

12. Chuck SL and Sande MA: Infections with cryptococcus neoformans in the acquired immunodeficiency syndrome. N Engl J Med 321:794–799, 1989.

13. Cohn JA, McMeekiny A, Cohen W, et al: Evaluation of the policy of empiric treatment of suspected toxoplasma encephalitis in patients with the acquired immunodeficiency syndrome. Am J Med 86:521–527, 1989.

14. Daniel TM: New approaches to the rapid diagnosis of tuberculous meningitis. J Infect Dis 155:599–602, 1987.

15. Delaney P: Neurological manifestations in sarcoidosis. Ann Intern Med 87:336–345, 1977.

16. Deresinski SC and Stevens DA: Coccidioidomycosis in compromised hosts. Medicine 54:377–395, 1974.

17. DeVita VT, Utz JP, Williams T, et al: Candida meningitis. Arch Intern Med 117:527–535, 1966.

18. DeVita VT Jr, Broder S, Fauci AS, et al: Developmental therapeutics and the acquired immunodeficiency syndrome. Ann Intern Med 106:568–581, 1987.

19. Diamond RD and Bennett JE: Prognostic factors in cryptococcal meningitis. A study of 111 cases. Ann Intern Med 80:176–181, 1974.

20. Dismukes WE: Cryptococcal meningitis in patients with AIDS. J Infect Dis 157:624–628, 1988.

21. Ellner JJ and Bennett JE: Chronic meningitis. Medicine 55:341–369, 1976.

22. Emskotter Th, Jenzevski H, Pulz M, and Spehn J: Neurosyphilis in HIV infection—persistence after high-dose penicillin therapy. J Neuroimmunol 20:153–155, 1988.

23. Ewing GE, Bosl GJ, and Peterson PK: *Sporothrix schenckii* meningitis in a farmer with Hodgkin's disease. Am J Med 68:455–457, 1980.

24. Fincham RW, Sahs AL, and Joynt RJ: Protean manifestations of nervous system brucellosis. JAMA 184:269–275, 1963.

25. Gaines JD, Eckman PM, and Remington JS: Low CSF glucose level in sarcoidosis involving the central nervous system. Arch Intern Med 125:333–336, 1970.

26. Gelfand JA and Bennett JE: Active *Histoplasma* meningitis of 22 years duration. JAMA 233:1294–1295, 1975.

27. Gilden DH, Miller EM, and Johnson WG: Central nervous system histoplasmosis after rhinoplasty. Neurology 24:874–877, 1974.

28. Goodson JD and Strauss GM: Diagnosis of lymphomatous leptomeningitis by cerebrospinal fluid lymphocyte cell surface markers. Am J Med 66:1057–1059, 1979.

29. Ho DD, Rota TR, Schooley RT, et al: Isolation of HTLV-III from cerebrospinal fluid and neural tissues of patients with neurologic syndromes related to the acquired immunodeficiency syndrome. N Engl J Med 313:1493–1497, 1985.

30. Hopkins AP and Harvey PKP: Chronic benign lymphocytic meningitis. J Neurol Sci 18:443–453, 1973.

31. Hooper DC, Pruitt AA, and Rubin RH: Central nervous system infection in the chronically immunosuppressed. Medicine 61:166–188, 1982.

32. Jacobs L, Kinkel PR, Costello PB, et al: Central nervous system lupus erythematosus: The value of magnetic resonance imaging. J Rheumatol 15:601–606, 1988.

33. Johns DR, Tierney M, and Felsenstein D: Alteration in the natural history of neurosyphilis by concurrent infection with the human immunodeficiency virus. N Engl J Med 316:1569–1572, 1987.

34. Johnson J and Ellner JJ: Tuberculous meningitis. In: Evans RW, Baskin DS, and Yatsu FM (eds): Prognosis in Neurological Disease. Oxford University Press, 1992.

35. Kennedy DH and Fallon FJ: Tuberculous meningitis. JAMA 241:264–268, 1979.

36. Kovacs JA, Kovacs AA, Polis M, et al: Cryptococcosis in the acquired immunodeficiency syndrome. Ann Intern Med 103:533–538, 1985.

37. Kravitz GR, Davies SF, Eckman MR, and Sarosi GA: Chronic blastomycotic meningitis. Am J Med 71:501–505, 1981.

38. Lepper MH and Spies HW: The present status of the treatment of tuberculosis of the central nervous system. Ann N Y Acad Sci 106:106–123, 1963.

39. Levy RM, Bredesen DE, and Rosenblum ML: Neurological manifestations of the acquired immunodeficiency syndrome (AIDS): Experience at UCSF and review of the literature. J Neurosurg 62:475–495, 1985.

40. Levy RM, Bredesen DE, and Rosenblum ML: Multiple coexistent intracranial pathologies in the acquired immunodeficiency syndrome. In: Proceedings of the International Conference on Acquired Immunodeficiency Syndrome (AIDS), Paris, France, June 23–25, 1986, p 56. Abstract.

41. Littman ML and Walter JE: Cryptococcosis: Current status. Am J Med 45:922–923, 1968.

42. McArthur JC: Neurologic manifestations of AIDS. Medicine 66:407–437, 1987.

43. Merritt HH, Adams RD, and Solomon HC: Neurosyphilis. Oxford University Press, New York, 1946.

44. Molavi A and LeFrock JL: Tuberculous meningitis. Med Clin North Am 69:315–331, 1985.

45. Pascual J, Combarios O, Polo JM, and Verciano J: Localized CNS brucellosis: Report of 7 cases. Acta Neurol Scand 78:282–289, 1988.

46. Pattison EM: Uveomeningoencephalitic syndrome (Vogt-Koyanagi-Harada). Arch Neurol 12:197, 1965.

46a. Phillips ME, Ryals TJ, Kambhu SA, et al: Neoplastic versus inflammatory meningeal enhancement with Gd-DTPA. J Comput Assist Tomogr 14:536–541, 1990.

47. Provost TT, Vasily D, and Alexander E: Sjögren's syndrome. Neurol Clin 5:405–426, 1987.

48. Rich AR and McCordock HA: The pathogenesis of tuberculous meningitis. Bull Johns Hopkins Hosp 52:5, 1933.

49. Salaki JS, Louria DB, and Chmel H: Fungal and yeast infections of the central nervous system: A clinical review. Medicine 63:108–113, 1984.

50. Schotland DL, Wolf SM, White HH, and Dubin HV: Neurologic aspects of Behçet's disease. Case report and review of the literature. Am J Med 34:544–553, 1963.

51. Scott EN, Kauman L, Brown AC, et al: Serologic studies in the diagnosis and management of meningitis due to *Sporothrix schenckii*. N Engl J Med 317:935–945, 1987.

52. Scully RE, Mark EJ, and McNeely BU: Case 43-1986. Case Records of the Massachusetts General Hospital 315:1143–1154, 1986.

53. Sigal LH: The neurologic presentation of vasculitis and rheumatologic syndromes. A review. Medicine 66:157–180, 1987.

54. Simon RP: Neurosyphilis. Arch Neurol 42:606–613, 1985.

55. Smith CE, Saito MT, and Simons SA: Pattern of 39,500 serologic tests in coccidioidomycosis. JAMA 160:546–552, 1956.

56. Spickard A, Butler WT, Andriole V, et al: The improved prognosis of cryptococcal meningitis with amphotericin B therapy. Ann Intern Med 58:66–83, 1963.

57. Stocksill MT and Kauffman CA: Comparison of cryptococcal and tuberculous meningitis. Arch Neurol 40:81–85, 1983.

58. Sugar AM and Saunders C: Oral fluconazole as suppressive therapy of disseminated cryptococcosis in patients with acquired immunodeficiency syndrome. Am J Med 85:481–489, 1988.

59. Swartz M: Chronic meningitis—many causes to consider. N Engl J Med 317:957–959, 1987.

60. Tynes BS, Crutcher JC, and Utz JP: Progressive disseminated histoplasmosis. Ann Intern Med 76:557, 1972.

61. Vollertsen RS, McDonald TJ, Younge BR, et al: Cogan's syndrome: 18 cases and a review of the literature. Mayo Clin Proc 61:344–361, 1986.

62. Wasserstrom WR, Glass JP, and Posner JB: Diagnosis and treatment of leptomeningeal metastases from solid tumors: Experience with 90 patients. Cancer 49:759–772, 1982.

63. Weiss W and Flippin HF: The changing incidence and prognosis of tuberculous meningitis. Am J Med Sci 50:46–59, 1965.

64. Wheat LJ, Batteiger BE, and Sathapatayavongs B: *Histoplasma capsulatum* infections of the central nervous system. A clinical review. Medicine 69:244–260, 1990.

65. Wheat J, French M, Batteiger B, et al: Cerebrospinal fluid *Histoplasma* antibodies in central nervous system histoplasmosis. Arch Intern Med 145:1237–1240, 1985.

66. Wheat LJ, Kohler RB, and Tewari RP: Diagnosis of disseminated histoplasmosis by detection of *Histoplasma capsulatum* antigen in serum and urine specimens. N Engl J Med 314:83–88, 1986.

67. Wheat LJ, Kohler RB, Tewari RP, et al: Significance of *Histoplasma* antigen in the cerebrospinal fluid of patients with meningitis. Arch Intern Med 149:302–304, 1989.

68. Wilhelmj CM: The primary meningeal form of systemic blastomycosis. Am J Med Sci 169:712–721, 1925.

69. Winn WA: The treatment of coccidioidal meningitis. The use of amphotericin B in a group of 25 patients. Calif Med 101:78–89, 1964.

70. Woolsey RM, Chambers TH, Chung HD, and McGarry JD: Mycobacterial meningomyelitis associated with human immunodeficiency virus infection. Arch Neurol 45:691–693, 1988.

71. Zuger A, Louie E, Holzman RS, et al: Cryptococcal disease in patients with the acquired immunodeficiency syndrome. Diagnostic features and outcome of treatment. Ann Intern Med 104:234–240, 1986.

Chapter 10

NEUROLOGIC MANIFESTATIONS OF LYME DISEASE

John J. Halperin, M.D.

DIAGNOSIS
NERVOUS SYSTEM INVOLVEMENT
TREATMENT

Even though *Borrelia burgdorferi*, the organism responsible for Lyme borreliosis, was first identified less than a decade ago, many of the neurologic disorders it causes have been well known for many years. Reports of tick bite–associated lymphocytic meningitis, often with Bell's palsy or focal neuropathic pain or weakness, appeared early in this century. Initial descriptions[72] did not clearly differentiate between this disorder and tick bite paralysis. In 1922, however, Garin and Bujadoux[23] clearly established the existence of a distinct syndrome when they described a patient who developed a large red rash at the site of a tick bite, followed 3 weeks later by severe sciatica in the same limb. The patient proceeded to develop severe neuropathic pain in both legs and the trunk, and focal arm weakness and atrophy. On examination, he had marked wasting and weakness of the deltoid but otherwise good strength, normal reflexes, and no objective sensory alterations. His cerebrospinal fluid (CSF) had 75 white cells per mm^3 and a protein level of 130 mg/dL. A Wassermann test was slightly positive. The authors concluded that the causative agent was a tick-borne spirochete (but not syphilis), which had attacked the central nervous system (CNS), primarily the anterior horns of the spinal cord and the meninges. In 1941, Bannwarth[7] described a similar neurologic syndrome (without realizing that it was associated with tick bites or dermatologic manifestations) in association with "rheumatism." The rash that Garin and Bujadoux noted (actually described initially by Afzelius[3]) has come to be known as erythema chronicum migrans (ECM) (Fig. 10–1; see color insert); more recently it has become apparent that both the rash and the neurologic manifestations improve following antibiotics.

This disease, under somewhat different guise, first gained prominence in North America in 1975, when an epidemic of childhood arthritis was recognized in Lyme, Connecticut. Extensive epidemiologic studies by Steere and colleagues[66] led to the discovery that this also seemed to develop after tick bites and that many patients also recalled having had a peculiar, large circular rash. In 1982, the causative organism, *Borrelia burgdorferi*, was identified,[10] and it soon became apparent that the European syndrome of Garin-Bujadoux-Bannwarth and the American disease known as Lyme disease were caused by closely related, if not identical, organisms.[4,8,65] In both instances it was found that the causative bacterium, a spirochete related to the treponeme, was transmitted by bites of a small, hard-shelled *Ixodes* tick. In the

216

late 1970s, reports started to appear describing nervous system abnormalities in North American patients with Lyme disease;[56] a few years later, European investigators began to reemphasize the occurrence of joint involvement in their patients with *B. burgdorferi* infection.[9,40] During the past decade it has become increasingly clear that the European and North American forms of this infection share more similarities than differences.

It has also become apparent that this disorder is far more widespread than initially thought, and it is now the most commonly reported vector-borne infection in the United States.[73] Cases have been reported from an ever-increasing number of states (46 at the time of this writing), as well as from Canada, Europe, Russia, China, Japan, Australia, and South America. In the United States, the disease is most prevalent in the Northeast (particularly southeast Massachusetts, Connecticut, Rhode Island, New Jersey, and Long Island and Westchester in New York), the North Central states (Wisconsin, Minnesota), and in northern California, as well as Oregon. The disease is transmitted almost exclusively by bites of *Ixodes* ticks: *I. dammini* in the northern United States (referred to colloquially as the deer tick in the Northeast and as the bear tick in the North Central states); the closely related, if not identical, *I. scapularis* in the South; and *I. pacificus* on the West Coast. In much of the rest of the world, *I. ricinus* is the primary carrier. The Lone Star tick also may be capable of transmitting this infection; other species of blood-ingesting insects have been reported to carry *B. burgdorferi* but probably are not capable of transmitting infection. (Of note, *Ixodes* ticks are not able to transmit Rocky Mountain Spotted Fever, the other common tick-borne disease in the United States; the Lone Star tick can.)

Ixodes ticks generally go through a 2-year life cycle, starting as larvae, maturing to nymphs, and then to adults. At each stage they have a single blood meal. If they become infected at one stage, they may transmit spirochetes at the next feeding. Generally, they feed on small vertebrates at the most immature stages (*I. dammini* being particularly fond of white-footed field mice) and on larger animals (deer, bears, raccoons, humans) at later stages, though they can bite humans at any stage of development. Although it is not invariably true, spirochete transmission generally only occurs after the tick has been feeding for several hours (usually at least 6 to 8 hours). Even when infected ticks feed longer than this, infection of the host is by no means certain. For this reason, prophylactic antibiotic treatment after tick bites is not generally recommended; the usual recommendation is to wait for some sign of infection to develop.[15]

In the first few years following the characterization of Lyme arthritis, the concept was introduced that, by analogy to syphilis, Lyme disease could be thought of as occurring in three stages. Primary, stage I Lyme disease consisted of the rash and flulike illness; stage II, secondary disease, occurred somewhat later, when the organisms disseminated, with involvement of the heart (cardiac conduction abnormalities) and nervous system (lymphocytic meningitis, painful radiculitis, Bell's palsy); stage III, tertiary disease, consisted of late-developing arthritis. This schema provided a useful framework for the development of our understanding of this disease, and the terms are still widely used. Because many patients fail to follow this pattern, however, developing swollen joints within days of the bite, or encephalitis months later, for example, these terms may now have outlived their utility. It seems more useful to divide the disease simply into early localized infection, early disseminated infection, and late disseminated infection (Table 10–1). It is true that there is a tendency for more severe neurologic manifestations to occur early (painful radiculitis, cranial neuritis, meningitis, encephalitis) and more indolent forms (milder neuropathy, milder encephalitis) to occur later, but this simply may

Table 10–1 LYME BORRELIOSIS PHASES

ACUTE, LOCALIZED
Unifocal ECM
Flulike illness

ACUTE, DISSEMINATED
Multifocal ECM
Cardiac conduction abnormalities
Arthralgias
Arthritis
Lymphocytic meningitis
Headache without meningitis
Bell's palsy
Radiculitis
Encephalitis

CHRONIC
Arthritis
Arthralgias
Encephalitis
Chronic neuropathy
Encephalopathy

reflect the fact that patients with severe, dramatic illness seek medical attention quickly, while those with milder, more insidious involvement only present when symptoms persist and progress over an extended period of time. Although some patients with rheumatologic involvement may develop a form of arthritis, presumably immune-mediated, that persists after apparently adequate antimicrobial treatment,[64] most observations to date suggest that the pathophysiology of nervous system involvement is less heterogeneous.[25]

With the identification of the causative organism and the development of serologic testing to demonstrate exposure to it, numerous reports began to appear describing a multitude of additional neurologic and extraneurologic disorders in association with Lyme disease. For example, it is now clear that hepatitis (usually asymptomatic) may occur with some frequency;[24] one case of possible *B. burgdorferi* pneumonia has been reported.[41] Anecdotal reports have attributed essentially every imaginable neuropsychiatric disorder to *B. burgdorferi* infection.[51,52] Despite all these reports, our understanding of the pathogenesis of this disease remains very rudimentary. Fortunately for patients, this illness is rarely if ever fatal. However, the absence of any pathologic material has made it very difficult to advance our understanding of its pathophysiology and to learn what manifestations really are caused by *B. burgdorferi* infection. Some of the reported associations do appear to be causal; others may represent somewhat overlapping clinical presentations of disorders that are superficially similar; and others clearly represent the chance occurrence of two unrelated disorders in the same patient. This review analyzes the basis for the different reported associations and to provide a rational basis for analysis of future work in this area.

DIAGNOSIS

Prior to the development of serologic tests, the diagnosis of Lyme disease could be made definitively only in the setting of an appropriate history. At least one third of patients never develop the pathognomonic skin rash, however, and many do not develop frank arthritis, Bell's palsy, or painful radiculitis. The ticks responsible for spreading the infection are so small that the majority of patients do not recall having been bitten. In the absence of these "classic" clinical manifestations, diagnosis was difficult. Unfortunately, even with the identification of *B. burgdorferi* and the development of serodiagnostic tests, the definitive diagnosis of Lyme disease still remains difficult in many cases.

Routine culture of the organism is not yet practical; the bacterium is difficult to culture from patients, both because there appear to be few organisms present and because the spirochete is technically difficult to grow. Serologic tests have been developed, but these have not yet been standardized. Laboratories vary widely in the technology used. Some use immunofluorescence assays (IFAs); although this is a widely used technique, it is difficult to standardize and requires meticulous attention to technical detail to produce reliable, reproducible results (particularly if large numbers of samples are being processed). Many laboratories use enzyme-linked immunosorbent assays (ELISAs), which are easier to standardize and eliminate subjective operator error. A small number of research labs are using capture ELISAs,[39,62] but this technology is not yet either standardized or widely available.

Probably even more important than the variability in technique employed is the wide range of antigen preparations used. Most are "homegrown" and vary considerably in the relative proportions of different antigenic determinants included. Several groups have begun using preparations consisting of well-characterized specific fractions of the organism. Using a purified flagellin fraction, Hansen and associates[38] have reduced broad background cross-reactivity, improving the signal-to-noise ratio, thereby improving sensitivity. The trade-off has been that the selected antigen is common to many other spirochetes; therefore, although in general there is less cross-reactivity with antibodies against other types of bacteria, specificity is diminished in the presence of other spirochetal infections (e.g., syphilis, periodontal disease caused by *Treponema dentola,* and other borrelial infections such as relapsing fever). Similarly, using a selected combination of partially purified fractions of the organism[47] has been shown to improve specificity in some instances, but this incurs a loss of sensitivity, because not all patients produce antibody to the same selected antigens. As if this were not producing enough confusion, laboratories even vary in their definitions of positive and negative test results. Some use a statistical analysis of simultaneously processed normal controls; others use an empirically derived "cutoff" valve below which all results are considered negative, which does not vary from one run to the next. Finally, the infection is often a very chronic one, so antibody titers may not change rapidly; this

makes it difficult to base a diagnosis on a rising or falling titer, a criterion used in many other, more acute diseases. For the same reason it is often difficult to use serologic data to determine if a patient has been adequately treated, because the titer often drops only very slowly.

Even when serologic tests are performed under optimal conditions, there are at least two circumstances in which negative results may be misleading. Very early in the disease, before or while the rash is apparent, patients usually will be seronegative, because it typically takes 2 to 6 weeks for a measurable antibody response to develop after infection. Patients with ECM are usually seronegative, but this should not be misinterpreted as evidence that they are not infected. Rather the presence of ECM should be considered pathognomonic of Lyme disease, and the patient should be treated immediately. In the presence of other, less unique clinical disorders that might be associated with Lyme disease early in its course (e.g., Bell's palsy), if a serologic test is negative, it should be repeated after 6 weeks, to detect possible seroconversion.[27]

The other circumstance in which antibody may not be detectable, despite the presence of persistent infection, is in patients who have been partially treated (perhaps inadvertently) early in the course of infection.[17] Early partial treatment appears to attenuate the antibody response, although infection may remain. In these patients it has been possible to measure the specific T lymphocyte response to *B. burgdorferi* in vitro. This extremely cumbersome assay has been used experimentally to provide evidence of *B. burgdorferi* exposure in antibody-negative patients.[17,45] Because many of these patients have shown objective improvement following antimicrobial therapy, the assumption has been that they have had active persistent infection. Unfortunately, this test is so labor-intensive that it seems unlikely it will ever be widely used.

False-positive results also occur. Other spirochetes (*T. pallidum, T. dentola,* other *Borrelia* sp.) share enough antigens with *B. burgdorferi* that cross-reactive antibodies are quite common. Occasional patients with antinuclear antibodies, rheumatoid factors, or hypergammaglobulinemia may also have nonspecific false-positive results. Immunoblotting can be helpful in differentiating these false-positive results from true-positive results. Probably the biggest problem, though, is positives that are not false but are irrelevant. Several studies have demonstrated seroprevalence rates of 10% to 15% in hyperendemic areas.[36,68] A recent study[44] suggests that in one hyperendemic area, half the population may be seropositive. When these seropositive patients develop other unrelated illnesses, the presence of anti–*B. burgdorferi* antibodies can give rise to a great deal of confusion.

This technical difficulty in providing clear-cut answers, coupled with the great interlaboratory variability in technique and conclusions, as well as the often confusing and somewhat nonspecific nature of the symptoms described by many patients with Lyme disease, has fostered the notion that it is virtually impossible either to make a firm diagnosis of Lyme disease or ever to exclude it. This has produced a great deal of confusion and anxiety on the part of patients and physicians, many of whom are left with the impression that there are no valid diagnostic tools for this disorder and no objective measures of disease response to therapy. In fact, if a reasonably reliable laboratory is available, and it is known that the patient has not previously received antibiotics, the serologic results can be quite useful.

In the not-too-distant future it is likely that newer technologies, such as those based on deoxyribonucleic acid (DNA) polymerase chain reaction (PCR) will be used to diagnose this disorder.[33a,40a,57] Until such additional organism-based diagnostic tools are brought to bear, however, the laboratory diagnosis of this infection will remain difficult. Until then, it would seem most appropriate to adopt two different sets of criteria to establish the diagnosis of neuroborreliosis: (1) extremely stringent criteria to be used for research purposes to link new clinical syndromes to this infection, and (2) less restrictive criteria to be used for clinical diagnosis and as a guide for therapy. For clinical diagnosis, the typical rash, ECM, is so unusual that it can be considered pathognomonic regardless of any laboratory findings. Serologic testing should be used with caution. It is essential that the sample be processed in a laboratory that has demonstrated proficiency in the technology it uses (ELISA, IFA, or capture ELISA). Positive results occurring in endemic areas must be viewed as indicative of exposure; whether active infection is occurring must be judged clinically. In all instances, causes of false-positive results must be considered and excluded, including syphilis, lupus, hypergammaglobulinemic states, and other borrelial infections. If necessary, Western blots can be used to differentiate false-positive results from true-positive results. Rare patients, with histories of antibiotic use, may be infected despite negative serologic test results; in such individuals, assessment of T-cell–specific immune responsiveness may be informative. If CNS infection is suspected, the demonstration of intrathecal antibody production can be extremely helpful (see later discussion). This measure appears to have so few false-positive results that, in the absence of a history of prior antimicrobial treatment, a positive result should be considered proof of CNS infection. In the absence of such a clear-cut result, laboratory findings must be combined with clinical observations. If a patient's symptoms and findings are consistent with the disorders already described in Lyme borreliosis, and serologic testing is indicative of exposure, treatment appears justified.

NERVOUS SYSTEM INVOLVEMENT

The earliest reports of this illness suggested that the nervous system was its most important target. In the European literature, the disease was felt to be predominantly neurologic,[23] and even though Bannwarth described "rheumatism" in his patients,[7] this has only been reemphasized quite recently. The initial identification of the disorder in North America was triggered by recognition of its rheumatologic consequences, and for that reason this aspect has been heavily emphasized. With each passing year, however, it has become increasingly apparent that neurologic abnormalities are a major element of this illness in North America as well. Although it is probable that there are differences between the clinical presentations of this illness on the two sides of the Atlantic, the similarities are becoming increasingly striking.

The initial neurologic emphasis in North American Lyme disease was on a dramatic triad[56] of manifestations—lymphocytic meningitis, Bell's palsy, and painful radiculitis. As experience grew and serologic testing made diagnosis appear simpler, the number of reported neurologic manifestations grew explosively, such that by the mid 1980s the feeling was widespread that this disease could mimic virtually any neurologic disorder. Many of these anecdotal reports are methodologically flawed, however; in endemic areas (the regions from which these reports arose), large numbers of patients have positive serologic test results but no symptoms. In such a setting, only a rigorous epidemiologic study will resolve whether other syndromes are causally related to *B. burgdorferi* infection or are only chance coincidental occurrences. Only in the past several years, as objective quantitative tools have been used to study these patients in a systematic fashion, has it begun to be possible to discern the unifying threads of these different disorders and deter-mine what this infection can and cannot cause.

Peripheral Nervous System Manifestations

Since the earliest European reports, the most common site of neurologic involvement has appeared to be the peripheral nervous system (PNS). Garin and Bujadoux,[23] and subsequently Bannwarth,[7] described acute, usually painful but primarily motor neuropathies, often with profound weakness but minimal sensory abnormalities on examination. Most of the patients had a striking CSF pleocytosis at the same time, and this, coupled with the marked pain, led to the concept that this was primarily a polyradiculitis. More recent reports have described a tremendous variety of PNS disorders (Table 10–2) in patients with *B. burgdorferi* infection—so much so that it has become customary to refer to the "protean manifestations" of this disease. However, a close examination of published data and of patients with these protean manifestations suggests the presence of unifying themes.

The best-studied entity has been Bannwarth's syndrome, or acute painful polyradiculitis. These symptoms most often involve the lower extremities but can affect either an upper extremity or the trunk. Although Euro-

Table 10–2 PERIPHERAL NERVOUS SYSTEM LYME BORRELIOSIS

MULTIFOCAL AXONAL NEUROPATHY
Painful radiculitis
Guillain-Barré-like (acute motor > sensory neuropathy; CSF pleocytosis)
Brachial neuritis
Mononeuritis multiplex
Chronic, mild sensorimotor neuropathy
Bell's palsy
Motor neuropathy (?)

ENTRAPMENT NEUROPATHIES
Carpal tunnel syndrome

MYOSITIS

pean reports have suggested that the pain often develops in the limb that was bitten by the tick, this has not been observed consistently in North American series. Neurophysiologic studies have generally demonstrated widespread abnormalities, including evidence of nerve root involvement.[25,45] Sural nerve biopsies have demonstrated moderate to severe axon loss with prominent perivascular inflammatory infiltrates, particularly in the epineurium.[11,30,75] Notably, no reports have demonstrated blood vessel wall destruction to suggest a true vasculitis. Also of note, no compelling pathologic or neurophysiologic findings typical of primary demyelination have been published. Beyond simply describing the pathologic alterations due to this disorder, these studies also provide an important inference about the site of PNS damage. Because sensory axons arise from dorsal root ganglia, which are located peripheral to the subarachnoid space, sensory nerve biopsies (and sensory nerve conduction studies) are usually normal in patients with disorders of the nerve roots. The fact that sural sensory nerve biopsies demonstrate severe abnormalities strongly supports the notion that Bannwarth's syndrome actually is a disseminated neuropathy that does not attack nerve roots exclusively.

Whereas some patients present with acute, rapidly progressive, painful paralysis, far more will develop a more gradually progressive, less debilitating neuropathy with mild sensorimotor signs and symptoms.[30] These patients, who typically have had untreated *B. burgdorferi* infection for several years, have more insidious but persistent, mild sensorimotor symptoms, often describing a variety of fluctuating positive and negative sensory symptoms. Neurophysiologic studies in these patients also provide evidence of a widespread but patchy multifocal axonal neuropathy, and sural nerve biopsies have demonstrated changes qualitatively similar to—though quantitatively less severe than—those seen in Bannwarth's syn-

drome.[30] As in biopsies from patients with Bannwarth's syndrome, efforts to find spirochetes, or deposition of antibody, immune complexes, or complement, have consistently given negative results, leaving the pathogenesis of these disorders unknown. Importantly, patients at both ends of this spectrum improve following antibiotic treatment.

One infrequent association that has been reported in patients with evidence of *B. burgdorferi* infection has been a disorder clinically resembling the Guillain-Barré syndrome[14,69] [acute inflammatory demyelinating polyneuropathy (AIDP)]. Because AIDP occurs uncommonly following bacterial infections, such an association would be somewhat surprising. In most of these reports, however, a careful analysis suggests that the similarities between these patients' syndromes and AIDP is rather superficial. In virtually all instances, patients have had a prominent CSF lymphocytic pleocytosis, much more typical of Bannwarth's syndrome than of AIDP. Moreover, neurophysiologic studies have generally demonstrated neither slowing of conduction into the demyelinating range nor evidence of conduction block. Clinically, this syndrome has resembled AIDP, in the sense that it is a rapidly progressive, primarily motor neuropathy, but the laboratory findings suggest that this is much more similar to the well-known *B. burgdorferi*–associated polyradiculoneuritis than to AIDP. Whether the small number of remaining cases of typical AIDP reported in patients with Lyme borreliosis really are causally related to this infection, or whether they represent chance coincidental occurrences, remains to be determined.

Another PNS manifestation that has been emphasized is the occurrence of "brachial neuritis" (which occurred in Garin and Bujadoux's first case). Detailed neurophysiologic studies in a small number of such patients have demonstrated disseminated neurophysiologic abnormalities at sites unrelated to their presenting symptoms.[25] For example, patients with brachial neuritis in one arm may have abnormalities in the opposite, asymptomatic one. Similarly, many patients with painful radiculoneuritis will have evidence of disseminated neurophysiologic abnormalities at sites far removed from their painful symptoms.

Cranial nerve involvement also occurs quite frequently in patients with Lyme borreliosis. Although the cranial neuropathies are considered separately, it is worth emphasizing that in many patients with Bell's palsy (just as in patients with Lyme disease–related painful radiculitis, brachial neuritis, mild sensorimotor neuropathies, and fulminant AIDP-like neuropathies) neurophysiologic testing demonstrates disseminated lesions of multiple sensory and motor fibers throughout the body.[25] In fact, it is quite striking that patients with all these different clinical presentations have neurophysiologic abnormalities that are qualitatively quite similar, suggesting that all are merely differing manifestations of a shared pathophysiologic process.

In addition to these primary neuropathic syndromes, entrapment neuropathies (particularly carpal tunnel syndrome) also appear to occur frequently in patients with Lyme disease.[33] This should not be surprising given the frequency of entrapment neuropathies in patients with other polyneuropathies, and the fact that Lyme disease can often cause arthritis, which may involve the wrist.

Finally, a few case reports have been published describing a polymyositis-like illness in patients with Lyme disease.[5,59,80] These cases are rare and anecdotal, but at least one patient appeared to respond to antibiotics. Because Lyme infection is associated with a prominent inflammatory reaction in many other tissues (heart, nerve, liver), an inflammatory myositis would not be unexpected. In view of the very small number of reports that have appeared to date, it would seem wise to reserve judgment for now as to whether a causal relation exists.

Cranial Nerve Manifestations

In a disseminated disease such as Lyme borreliosis, the cranial nerves could theoretically be damaged at any of three different sites. The origins could be involved by an inflammatory lesion within the neuraxis, the roots could be involved by a meningitis as they cross the subarachnoid space, or the peripheral processes themselves could be damaged, presumably by the same process that affects other peripheral nerves. Although all three mechanisms are possible, the literature suggests that most cranial nerve involvement occurs in the context of a meningitis. Certainly, this would be the easiest mechanism to envision, because meningitis is common in Lyme borreliosis and cranial nerves are often involved in other meningitides. It is perhaps surprising, however, that so few reports of cranial neuropathies (other than Bell's palsy) have appeared; for many of these lesions, the data still only can be considered anecdotal and unproven. Over the next few years these possible associations may be clarified.

Cranial nerve I (olfactory): Loss of the sense of smell has yet to be reported in the literature. Although several patients have reported that their perception of smell and/or taste was distorted or absent (in the absence of hepatitis), diminished olfaction has not been demonstrable on examination.

Cranial nerve II (optic): Several case reports of optic neuritis in patients with *B. burgdorferi* infection have appeared.[20,58,63,81] In none has there been compelling evidence that there was CNS infection with *B. burgdorferi* nor has the response to antimicrobials been clearly different from the spontaneous improvement usually seen following idiopathic optic neuritis. Whether optic neuritis could be caused in these patients by a noninfectious mechanism, or whether these reports constitute coincidental occurrences, remains to be determined.

Cranial nerves III (oculomotor), IV (trochlear), and VI (abducens): Many published series of patients with Lyme borreliosis[19,61] include patients with meningitis and extraocular muscle paresis. This combination of findings seems to occur with sufficient frequency to be a valid association. Rare instances of Argyll-Robertson pupils have also been reported.

Cranial nerve V (trigeminal): Many patients with Lyme disease describe a variety of abnormal facial sensations, e.g., paresthesias, numbness, stiffness. A few instances of atypical facial pain have also been described. Involvement of this nerve also seems to be so frequent that this association seems valid.[19,56,82]

Cranial nerve VII (facial): Bell's palsy probably occurs in up to 10% of patients with Lyme borreliosis.[13,53] This infection is one of the few disorders (along with sarcoidosis, other basilar meningitides, and the Guillain-Barré syndrome) that is associated with bilateral facial nerve paresis. In addition to facial paresis, many patients describe twitching (fasciculations versus myokymia) of facial muscles. These patients may have a CSF pleocytosis, depending on the site of involvement. Many patients with peripherally located lesions have neurophysiologic evidence of a disseminated neuropathy.[25] Interestingly, although patients with Bell's palsy often are found to have subclinical lesions of other peripheral nerves on neurophysiologic testing, the converse does not seem to hold: Patients with *B. burgdorferi*–associated peripheral neuropathies rarely if ever have subclinical lesions of the seventh cranial nerve.[26]

Cranial nerve VIII (vestibulocochlear): Several published series of patients with nervous system Lyme disease have described patients with dizziness that improved following antibiotics (although it is difficult to judge whether this was any different from the usual spontaneous improvement in this symptom). A few patients with hearing dysfunction have also been described.[34,35,56,70]

Cranial nerves IX (glossopharyngeal), X (vagus), XI (accessory), and XII (hypoglossal): It is very difficult to find reports of abnormal function of the lowest cranial nerves in these patients.[56,70] Although a few seropositive patients with vocal cord paralysis have been described,[60] a causal relationship to *B. burgdorferi* infection has been difficult to prove. Similarly, several seropositive patients have developed a clinical picture resembling bulbar amyotrophic lateral sclerosis (ALS); as in other patients with disorders resembling different forms of motor neuron disease (see later discussion), a cause-and-effect relationship has been difficult to establish.

Central Nervous System Manifestations (Table 10–3)

Since the first case reported by Garin and Bujadoux, it has been apparent that many patients with this infectious disease develop a clinical syndrome in-

Table 10–3 CENTRAL NERVOUS SYSTEM LYME BORRELIOSIS

LYMPHOCYTIC MENINGITIS
With secondary cranial neuropathies

FOCAL ENCEPHALOMYELITIS
Severe, with focal findings
Mild, with encephalopathy

REMOTE EFFECTS
Mild encephalopathy
Fatigue

distinguishable from aseptic meningitis. This is in all ways typical of other lymphocytic meningitides: patients present with headache, photophobia, stiff neck, and fever. CSF usually has a lymphocytic pleocytosis, elevated protein level, normal glucose level, and negative cultures. (Occasional patients have the identical clinical picture, but normal CSF.) In rare instances it has been possible to culture *B. burgdorferi* from the CSF, using special medium, but this is usually not possible. Several authors have emphasized the appearance of somewhat unusual-appearing plasmacytoid cells in the CSF;[78] these are not always found, however. Meningitis may occur in isolation or in association with painful radiculoneuritis, Bell's palsy, or other neurologic processes. Like these other manifestations, the lymphocytic meningitis may resolve spontaneously, without antibiotic treatment. However, as in several other infections in which there is an early, self-limited meningitis (e.g., syphilis, HIV-1), it is not unreasonable to assume that even when the host's inflammatory response subsides, infectious organisms may remain behind in the CNS, where they could cause future problems. The long-term effects of such CNS seeding remain to be determined. Because Lyme disease is so often difficult to diagnose with certainty, however, and because so many other neurologic diseases are without a known pathogenesis and "gold standard" diagnostic tests, there has been considerable interest in determining whether *B. burgdorferi* infection might be responsible for a variety of idiopathic CNS disorders.

Assessment of intrathecal production of anti–*B. burgdorferi* antibody has provided a highly sensitive and specific method of diagnosing CNS invasion. As in many other infections (e.g., HIV, herpes, toxoplasmosis), the presence of organisms within the CNS triggers the local production of specific antibody. In each of these disorders, the proportion of total immunoglobulin in the CSF that is specific for the causative organism can be measured; after making a similar determination of the proportion of serum immunoglobulin that is specific for the infectious agent, an index that is a measure of the relative concentrations of specific antibody in the two compartments, normalized for total immunoglobulin concentration (CSF:serum), can be calculated. If there is selective intrathecal synthesis of specific antibody, the proportion of specific antibody will be greater in the CSF, and this index will be greater than 1. Several studies have now validated this approach in Lyme borreliosis.[31,45,71,79] In some patients, this local production of specific antibody results in the appearance of oligoclonal bands in the CSF; it has been demonstrated both that these bands are specific to *B. burgdorferi*[37,49] and that clones of *B. burgdorferi*–recognizing B cells are concentrated in the CSF.[6]

One consequence of this compartmentalization of infection and immune response behind the blood-brain barrier is that it is possible to treat a systemic infection partially, eradicate bacteria outside the CNS, have the peripheral blood antibody response subside, but still have an ongoing infection and antibody response within the neuraxis. In this setting, the patient may have a negative peripheral blood serologic test result but a positive CSF test result. In the Swedish experience,[71] this was initially thought to occur in as many as 20% to 25% of patients with CNS *B. burgdorferi* infection; recent European data more closely approximate North American experience (perhaps 5% to 7%; unpublished observations), although this is a very difficult number to ascertain reliably.

Using this antibody index as a guide, it is clear that there are rare patients with CNS *B. burgdorferi* infection who develop a severe, unifocal or multifocal encephalomyelitis.[1,21,31] These patients present with significant abnormalities on neurologic examination (ranging from hemiparesis or spastic gait to coma), have focal areas of what appears to be inflammation on magnetic reso-

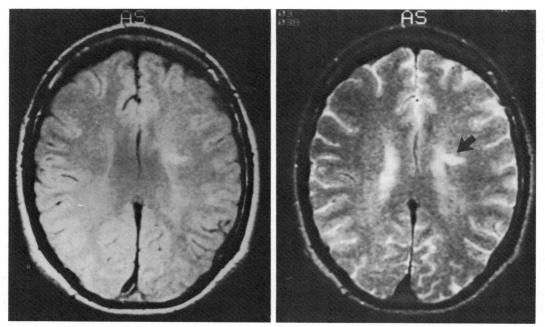

Figure 10–2. MRI, horizontal section, proton-weighted image on the left, T_2-weighted image on the right. Patient is a 29-year-old man who, 2 weeks after exposure in a Lyme-endemic area, developed a febrile illness with difficulty voiding, lower extremity weakness and paresthesias, and a CSF pleocytosis. Arrow indicates area of presumed leukoencephalitis.

nance imaging (MRI)[32] (Fig. 10–2), and have inflammatory CSF findings. Some may recover nearly completely following appropriate, aggressive antibiotic therapy; others will be left with significant neurologic residua. Many of these patients, who may present with a somewhat gradually progressive focal neurologic disease (evolving over weeks to a few months), have been mistakenly diagnosed as having either demyelinating disease or brain tumors. In general, appropriate studies of the CSF readily differentiate this infectious process from other disorders; differentiation from a mass lesion may occasionally be more difficult if the lesion's location makes a lumbar puncture seem ill-advised. Although some patients with particularly chronic CNS infection with this organism have had CSF oligoclonal bands,[1,2,37] none has had elevated concentrations of myelin basic protein.[31] It is important to note that this illness is not readily confused with relapsing-re-

mitting multiple sclerosis (MS). In the absence of intercurrent antibiotics, these patients follow a progressive course without spontaneous remissions. They also seem quite different from patients with MS in that only rarely are there unexplained abnormalities on evoked-potential testing.[31] One potential source of confusion, though, is that the CSF Lyme antibody index may remain elevated after treatment. The chronically elevated antibody concentration in the CSF may decrease very slowly like that in peripheral blood. It often will drift down in parallel to the concentration in the blood, resulting in a persistently elevated CSF:serum antibody ratio. Although it is still somewhat controversial, most workers in the field believe that persistent elevation of this ratio after treatment does not, in and of itself, mean that active CNS infection remains. However, one is frequently confronted with a situation in which a patient has been partially treated, has persistent CNS signs or symptoms, and is found to have proportionately more specific antibody in the CSF than in serum. Without knowing the pretreatment measures of CSF antibody, it may be impossible to decide if the patient has been adequately treated or not. Faced with this possibility, CSF is being examined in an ever-increasing proportion of patients with possible CNS Lyme disease, prior to initial antibiotic treatment.

In addition to concerns about possible confusion between Lyme neuroborreliosis and demyelinating disease, there has been a great deal of attention paid to the possibility of a dementing illness being caused by this infection.[12] It is clear that many Lyme disease patients develop a low-grade encephalopathy,[29,32,42] which is probably no different from the encephalopathy seen in many other infectious illnesses. In contrast, occasional patients probably do develop a more severe encephalopathy, secondary to a mild version of the multifocal encephalitis described above. Regardless of the mechanism in an individual patient, however, there is usually a measurable improvement after antimicrobial treatment, although, as with other signs and symptoms of this disease, improvement may require several months to evolve following successful therapy. Other more severe and irreversible forms of dementia seem unlikely, if for no other reason than that this disease has been recognized in its neurotropic forms in Europe for decades, without any significant evidence that such a problem occurs. (In fact, in Europe B. burgdorferi infection is generally felt to be a benign, self-limited disease, which only very rarely produces long-term complications, other than occasional, late dermatologic problems, even if untreated.) Theoretically it might be argued that this disorder, like other meningitides, might be a risk factor for the subsequent development of normal-pressure hydrocephalus; a few suggestive cases have been

seen (unpublished observation), but the evidence has never been wholly convincing that Lyme disease was responsible for the patients' difficulties.

Recently there has been considerable controversy regarding the possibility that B. burgdorferi may produce a disorder that could mimic ALS.[22,28,48,77] Two patients have been described[22,28] with what was diagnosed as primary lateral sclerosis but was probably actually Lyme neuroborreliosis. Several patients with a lower motor neuropathy in association with B. burgdorferi infection[28] have appeared to improve following antibiotic therapy. Whether in the long run this will turn out to be a real entity will require considerable additional study.

Isolated reports have raised a number of other interesting possibilities. Several seropositive patients with stroke[50] or CNS vasculitis (but probably without evidence of intrathecal production of specific antibody) have been reported.[74,76] If it turns out that this infectious disease actually does cause such a vasculitis (which is not inconceivable in view of the pathologic changes seen elsewhere in the body), and if it can be demonstrated that any of the other CNS manifestations are due to a similar pathophysiologic process, this would provide a means of unifying many of the PNS and CNS manifestations of this rather protean disease.

Finally, several anecdotal reports have suggested an association between B. burgdorferi infection and psychiatric disease. Most systematic data suggest that psychiatric illness—in particular, depression—is neither more common nor more severe in patients with Lyme disease than it is in those with other chronic medical disease.[43] Moreover, of the small number of cases of severe psychiatric disease occurring in Lyme-seropositive patients that have been completely evaluated, none has had evidence of intrathecal synthesis of specific antibody, suggesting that these syndromes were not caused by CNS infection.[31]

TREATMENT

In thinking about patients with Lyme borreliosis, it is most convenient to divide them conceptually into two groups—those with early, localized disease (e.g., a unifocal ECM, perhaps with a flulike febrile illness), and those with disseminated infection (either multifocal ECM or evidence of multiple-organ-system involvement) (Table 10–4). In its earliest, localized form, treatment is almost always successful with oral antibiotics. Usually a 3-week course of either doxycycline (100 mg 2 or 3 times a day) or amoxicillin (500 to 1000 mg 3 times a day, with or without probenecid 500 mg 3 times a day) will suffice. Patients with more disseminated infection, particularly those with CNS infection, may be considerably more difficult to treat. Of note, a significant fraction of patients with ECM present with a multifocal rash; this does represent a disseminated infection, and some prelimi-

Table 10–4 TREATMENT

ACUTE, LOCALIZED
Amoxicillin 500–1000 mg 3 times per day for 3 weeks
or
Doxycycline 100 mg twice a day for 3 weeks
(*not* in children < 8 years old, pregnant or lactating women)

ACUTE, DISSEMINATED
Amoxicillin 500–1000 mg 3 times a day with probenecid 500 mg 3 times a day for 3 weeks
or
Doxycycline 100 mg 2 or 3 times a day for 3 weeks
(*not* in children < 8 years old, pregnant or lactating women)
or
Ceftriaxone 2 g IV once a day for 2 weeks
or
Cefotaxime 2 g IV 3 times a day for 2 weeks

CHRONIC, DISSEMINATED
Ceftriaxone 2 g IV once a day for 2–4 (? 4 +) weeks
or
Cefotaxime 2 g IV 3 times a day for 2–4 (? 4+) weeks
or
Penicillin 4 million units IV every 4 hours for 2–4 (? 4 +) weeks

IV = intravenous.

nary evidence (Asbrink, personal communication) suggests that a significant proportion of these patients will have a CSF pleocytosis! Despite this observation, high-dose oral antibiotics appear to be effective in most such patients. Other patients may present with cardiac conduction abnormalities or with swollen joints. In these instances, high-dose oral antibiotics may be effective in mild cases, but in the face of third-degree heart block or markedly swollen joints, parenteral antibiotics are usually used. Similarly, in patients with PNS involvement, a long course (3 to 6 weeks) of oral antibiotics may be useful in mild cases, but for more severe, fulminant neuropathies (Bannwarth's syndrome, Bell's palsy with a CSF pleocytosis) parenteral antibiotics are probably more effective. As should be clear from this discussion, many of these treatment issues remain to be resolved; the systematic studies have not yet been completed.

The optimal form of parenteral therapy has yet to be determined, particularly when CNS infection is probable. The organism responsible for this disease, *B. burgdorferi,* has several unusual properties.[46] It divides very slowly both in vivo and in vitro; effective killing requires exposure to adequate levels of antibiotics for an extended period of time. In vitro, brief exposure to very high levels of effective antibiotics usually accomplishes nothing; in contrast, sustained exposure to a constant, but much lower concentration of the same antibiotic for 48 to 96 hours may be extremely effective. For this reason, pharmacokinetic properties become very important. The ideal agent would be one with an easily attainable minimal inhibitory concentration (MIC), adequate blood-brain barrier penetration, and a relatively long half-life, with sustained CSF levels. The earliest studies on patients with CNS infection used meningeal doses of intravenous penicillin.[67] This was effective in many patients but by no means in all. Since that time, isolated reports have appeared describing the efficacy of chloramphenicol[18] and of cefotaxime[54,55] in penicillin-resistant cases. In theory, most third-generation cephalosporins should be effective. Ceftriaxone, 2 g given once a day, is currently the most widely used regimen.[16] This agent was initially chosen because of its long half-life and because the CSF levels generally attained (even in the absence of inflamed meninges) greatly exceed the in vitro MIC;[46] clinical studies have suggested that this agent is highly effective. Its once-a-day dosing regimen also makes it very convenient to use on an outpatient basis. The optimal duration of therapy remains to be established. Most centers have started with a 2-week course; it is clear that this is inadequate for some patients, who will need longer courses. One of the difficulties in treating patients with this disease is that even when the infection is eradicated, symptoms may persist and only gradually subside over several months. In the absence of any accurate, objective indicators of disease activity, it is impossible to know with certainty when treatment has been adequate.

SUMMARY

Lyme borreliosis is a multisystem infectious disease caused by the tick-borne spirochete *B. burgdorferi*. In addition to neurologic problems, it can cause cardiac conduction abnormalities, arthritis, and occasionally hepatitis. If the nervous system is involved, the clinical manifestations are highly varied. PNS involvement can be manifest as a diffuse peripheral neuropathy (either acute, disseminated, and predominantly motor; or quite indolent, patchy, and mixed sensorimotor in character), as a cranial neuropathy (usually cranial nerve VII), or as a clinically focal and painful radiculitis. Demyelinating neuropathies occur rarely. In patients with any of these disorders, neurophysiologic studies demonstrate disseminated abnormalities, at sites remote from the presenting symptoms. Biopsied sensory nerves generally dem-

onstrate an axonal neuropathy, with prominent perivascular inflammatory infiltrates, although without evidence of a true vasculitis. The most common CNS manifestation is a lymphocytic meningitis. Occasional patients develop a unifocal or multifocal encephalitis that may present in its most severe form with severe CNS dysfunction, or in a mild, indolent form as an encephalopathy. Many other patients with *B. burgdorferi* infection develop a mild encephalopathy, but this probably is nonspecific and does not represent CNS infection in most instances. A few case reports of CNS vasculitis have been published; such a process might underlie changes that have been thought to represent an encephalitis in some of these patients and might provide a unifying hypothesis, providing evidence of similar pathogenic mechanisms in both the PNS and CNS.

Although the definitive diagnosis of *B. burgdorferi* infection may be difficult, it is generally possible to identify CNS infection by determining whether there is evidence of intrathecal synthesis of specific antibody. Using this technique, it has been possible to demonstrate that there is virtually no overlap between Lyme neuroborreliosis and relapsing-remitting MS. Although several cases of Lyme encephalitis have been misdiagnosed as progressive MS, determination of CSF anti–*B. burgdorferi* antibody readily separates most patients with this infectious encephalitis from those with demyelinating disease. There is little if any compelling evidence to suggest that Lyme disease causes an irreversible dementia; there is some suggestive evidence that it may cause a motor neuropathy. Treatment of this infectious disease requires a rational approach to antibiotic selection, and an appreciation that the neuraxis is often involved early on. Interestingly, even patients with severe CNS infections can do quite well, with near-complete recovery, if treated aggressively.

Many questions remain to be answered. The organism responsible for this infection is highly unusual: infection can persist for months or years, despite the presence of a vigorous antibody- and cell-mediated immune response. How it does so remains a mystery. Why it is that some patients develop severe CNS disease and others remain asymptomatic is unknown. The optimal antimicrobial agents and the correct duration of treatment are yet to be determined. Even such simple questions as how to improve diagnostic accuracy require a great deal of additional study. Finally, our understanding of the pathogenesis of this disorder remains extremely rudimentary. In the next few years, as more powerful diagnostic tools are applied in the systematic study of large numbers of affected individuals, many of these dilemmas should be resolved.

REFERENCES

1. Ackermann R, Gollmer E, and Rehse KB: Progressive *Borrelia* encephalomyelitis. Chronic manifestation of erythema chronicum migrans disease of the nervous system. Dtsch Med Wochenschr 110(26):1039–1042, 1985.
2. Ackermann R, Rehse KB, Gollmer E, and Schmidt R: Chronic neurologic manifestations of erythema migrans borreliosis. Ann N Y Acad Sci 539:16–23, 1988.
3. Afzelius A: Verhandlugen der Dermatorischen Gesellshaft zu Stockholm. Arch Derm Syphiligr 101:404, 1910.
4. Asbrink E, Hederstedt B, and Hovmark A: The spirochetal etiology of acrodermatitis chronica atrophicans Herxheimer. Acta Derm Venereol 64:506–512, 1984.
5. Atlas E, Novak SN, Duray PH, and Steere AC: Lyme myositis: Muscle invasion by *Borrelia burgdorferi*. Ann Intern Med 109(3):245–246, 1988.
6. Baig S, Olsson T, and Link H: Predominance of *Borrelia burgdorferi* specific B cells in cerebrospinal fluid in neuroborreliosis. Lancet 2(8654):71–74, 1989.
7. Bannwarth A: Chronische lymphocy-tare Meningitis, entzundliche Polyneuritis und "Rheumatismus." Arch Psychiatr Nervenkr 113:284–376, 1941.
8. Benach JL, Bosler EM, Hanrahan JP, et al: Spirochetes isolated from the blood of two patients with Lyme disease. N Engl J Med 308:740–742, 1983.
9. Bianchi G, Rovetta G, Monteforte P, et al: Articular involvement in European patients with Lyme disease. A report of 32 Italian patients. Br J Rheumatol 29(3):178–180, 1990.
10. Burgdorfer W, Barbour AG, Hayes SF, et al: Lyme disease: A tick borne spirochetosis? Science 216:1317–1319, 1982.
11. Camponovo F and Meier C: Neuropathy of vasculitic origin in a case of Garin-Bujadoux-Bannwarth syndrome with positive *Borrelia* antibody response. J Neurol 233:69–72, 1986.
12. Carlsson M and Malmvall B-E: *Borrelia* infection as a cause of presenile dementia. Lancet 2:798, 1987.
13. Clark JR, Carlson RD, Sasaki CT, Pachner AR, and Steere AC: Facial paralysis in Lyme disease. Laryngoscope 95:1341–1345, 1985.
14. Clavelou P, Beytout J, Vernay D, et al: Neurologic manifestations of Lyme disease in the northern part of the Auvergne. Neurology 39(Suppl 1):350, 1989.
15. Costello CM, Steere AC, Pinkerton RE, and Feder HMJ: A prospective study of tick bites in an endemic area for Lyme disease. Conn Med 53(6):338–340, 1989.
16. Dattwyler RJ, Halperin JJ, Volkman DJ, and Luft BJ: Treatment of late Lyme disease. Lancet 1:1191–1193, 1988.
17. Dattwyler RJ, Volkman DJ, Luft BJ, Halperin JJ, Thomas J, and Golightly MG: Seronegative Lyme disease. Dissociation of specific T- and B-lymphocyte responses to *Borrelia burgdorferi*. N Engl J Med 319(22):1441–1446, 1988.
18. Diringer MN, Halperin JJ, and Dattwyler RJ: Lyme meningoencephalitis—report of a severe, penicillin-

resistant case. Arthritis Rheum 30:705–708, 1987.

19. Dupuis M, Mertens C, Gonsette RE, Nuytten W, Bouffioux J, and Dobbelaere F: Meningoradiculite par spirochete (Borrelia burgdorferi) apres piqure d'arthropodes. Rev Neurol (Paris) 141:780–785, 1985.

20. Farris BK and Webb RM: Lyme disease and optic neuritis. J Clin Neuro Ophthalmol 8:73–78, 1988.

21. Feder HMJ, Zalneraitis EL, and Reik LJ: Lyme disease: Acute focal meningoencephalitis in a child. Pediatrics 82(6):931–934, 1988.

22. Fredrikson S and Link H: CNS-borreliosis selectively affecting central motor neurons. Acta Neurol Scand 78(3):181–184, 1988.

23. Garin and Bujadoux: Paralysie par les tiques. J Med Lyon 71:765–767, 1922.

24. Goellner MH, Agger WA, Burgess JH, and Duray PH: Hepatitis due to recurrent Lyme disease. Ann Intern Med 108(5):707–708, 1988.

25. Halperin J, Luft BJ, Volkman DJ, and Dattwyler RJ: Lyme neuroborreliosis. Peripheral nervous system manifestations. Brain 1990:1207–1222, 1990.

26. Halperin JJ and Dattwyler RJ: Peripheral nervous system manifestations of Lyme disease. Neurology 39(Suppl 1):234, 1989.

27. Halperin JJ, Golightly M, and Long Island Neuroborreliosis Collaborative Study Group. Lyme borreliosis in Bell's palsy. Neurology 40(Suppl 1):342, 1990.

28. Halperin JJ, Kaplan GP, Brazinsky S, et al: Immunologic reactivity against Borrelia burgdorferi in patients with motor neuron disease. Arch Neurol 47:586–594, 1990.

29. Halperin JJ, Krupp LB, Golightly MG, and Volkman DJ: Lyme borreliosis-associated encephalopathy. Neurology 40:1340–1343, 1990.

30. Halperin JJ, Little BW, Coyle PK, and Dattwyler RJ: Lyme disease—a treatable cause of peripheral neuropathy. Neurology 37:1700–1706, 1987.

31. Halperin JJ, Luft BJ, Anand AK, et al:

Lyme neuroborreliosis: Central nervous system manifestations. Neurology 39(6):753–759, 1989.

32. Halperin JJ, Pass HL, Anand AK, Luft BJ, Volkman DJ, and Dattwyler RJ: Nervous system abnormalities in Lyme disease. Ann N Y Acad Sci 539:24–34, 1988.

33. Halperin JJ, Volkman DJ, Luft BJ, and Dattwyler RJ: Carpal tunnel syndrome in Lyme borreliosis. Muscle Nerve 12(5):397–400, 1989.

33a. Halperin JJ, Volkman DJ, and Wu P: Central nervous system abnormalities in Lyme neuroborreliosis. Neurology 41:1571–1582, 1991.

34. Hanner P, Rosenhall U, Edstrom S, and Kaijser B: Hearing impairment in patients with antibody production against Borrelia burgdorferi antigen. Lancet 1(8628):13–15, 1989.

35. Hanny PE and Hauselmann HJ: Die Lyme-Krankheit aus der Sicht des Neurologen. Schweiz Med Wochenschr 117:901–915, 1987.

36. Hanrahan JP, Benach JL, Coleman JL, et al: Incidence and cumulative frequency of endemic Lyme disease in a community. J Infect Dis 150:489–496, 1984.

37. Hansen K, Cruz M, and Link H: Oligoclonal Borrelia burgdorferi-specific IgG antibodies in cerebrospinal fluid in Lyme neuroborreliosis. J Infect Dis 161:1194–1202, 1990.

38. Hansen K, Hindersson P, and Pedersen NS: Measurement of antibodies to the Borrelia burgdorferi flagellum improves serodiagnosis in Lyme disease. J Clin Microbiol 26(2):338–346, 1988.

39. Hansen K, Pii K, and Lebech A-M. Improved immunoglobulin M serodiagnosis in Lyme borreliosis by using μ capture enzyme-linked immunosorbent assay with biotinylated Borrelia burgdorferi flagella. J Clin Micribiol 1991; 29:166–173

40. Huaux JP, Bigaignon G, Stadtsbaeder S, Zangerle PF, and Nagant DC: Pattern of Lyme arthritis in Europe: Report of 14 cases. Ann Rheum Dis 47(2):164–165, 1988.

40a. Keller TJ, Halperin JJ, and Whitman

M. PCR detection of *Borrelia burgdorferi* DNA in cerebrospinal fluid of Lyme neuroborreliosis patients. Neurology 1992; 42:32.

41. Kirsch M, Ruben FL, Steere AC, Duray PH, Norden CW, and Winkelstein A: Fatal adult respiratory distress syndrome in a patient with Lyme disease. JAMA 259(18):2737–2739, 1988.

42. Krupp LB, Masur D, Scwartz J, et al. Cognitive functioning in late Lyme borreliosis. Arch Neurol 1991; 48:1125–1129.

43. Krupp LB, LaRocca NG, Luft BJ, and Halperin JJ: Comparison of neurologic and psychologic findings in patients with Lyme disease and chronic fatigue syndrome. Neurology 39(Suppl 1):144, 1989.

44. Lastavica CC, Wilson ML, Berardi VP, Spielman A, and Deblinger RD: Rapid emergence of a focal epidemic of Lyme disease in coastal Massachusetts. N Engl J Med 320(3):133–137, 1989.

45. Logigian EL, Kaplan RF, and Steere AC: Chronic neurologic manifestations of Lyme disease. N Engl J Med 323(21):1438–1444, 1990.

46. Luft BJ, Volkman DJ, Halperin JJ, and Dattwyler RJ: New chemotherapeutic approaches in the treatment of Lyme borreliosis. Ann N Y Acad Sci 539:352–361, 1988.

47. Magnarelli LA and Anderson JF: Enzyme-linked immunosorbent assays for the detection of class-specific immunoglobulins to *Borrelia burgdorferi*. Am J Epidemiol 127(4):818–825, 1988.

48. Mandell H, Steere A, Reinhardt B, Yoshinari N, and Munsat T: Lack of antibodies to *Borrelia burgdorferi* in patients with amyotrophic lateral sclerosis. N Engl J Med 320:255–256, 1989.

49. Martin R, Martens U, Sticht GV, Dorries R, and Kruger H: Persistent intrathecal secretion of oligoclonal, *Borrelia burgdorferi*-specific IgG in chronic meningoradiculomyelitis. J Neurol 235(4):229–233, 1988.

50. May EF and Jabbari B: Stroke in neuroborreliosis. Stroke 21:1232–1235, 1990.

51. Pachner AR: Neurologic manifestations of Lyme disease, the new "great imitator." Rev Infect Dis 6:S1482–1486, 1989.

52. Pachner AR, Duray P, and Steere AC: Central nervous system manifestations of Lyme disease. Arch Neurol 46(7):790–795, 1989.

53. Pachner AR and Steere AC: The triad of neurologic manifestations of Lyme disease. Neurology 35:47–53, 1985.

54. Pal GS, Baker JT, and Wright DJM: Penicillin resistant borrelia encephalitis responding to cefotaxime. Lancet 1:50–51, 1988.

55. Pfister HW, Preac MV, Wilske B, and Einhaupl KM: Cefotaxime vs penicillin G for acute neurologic manifestations in Lyme borreliosis. A prospective randomized study. Arch Neurol 46(11):1190–1194, 1989.

56. Reik L, Steere AC, Bartenhagen NH, Shope RE, and Malawista SE: Neurologic abnormalities of Lyme disease. Medicine (Baltimore) 58(4):281–294, 1979.

57. Rosa PA and Schwan TG: A specific and sensitive assay for the Lyme disease spirochete *Borrelia burgdorferi* using the polymerase chain reaction. J Infect Dis 160(6):1018–1029, 1989.

58. Schechter S: Lyme disease associated with optic neuropathy. Am J Med 81:143–145, 1986.

59. Schmutzhard E, Willeit J, and Gerstenbrand F: Meningopolyneuritis Bannwarth with focal nodular myositis. Klin Wochenschr 64:1204–1208, 1986.

60. Schroeter V, Belz GG, and Blenk H: Paralysis of recurrent laryngeal nerve in Lyme disease. Lancet 2(8622):1245, 1988. Letter.

61. Sindic CJM, Depre A, Bigaignon G, et al: Lymphocytic meningoradiculitis and encephalomyelitis due to *Borrelia burgdorferi*. J Neurol Neurosurg Psychiatry 50:1565–1571, 1987.

62. Steere AC, Berardi VP, Weeks KE, Logigian EL, and Ackermann R: Evaluation of the intrathecal antibody response to *Borrelia burgdorferi* as a diagnostic test for Lyme neuroborreliosis. J Infect Dis 161(6):1203–1209, 1990.

63. Steere AC, Duray PH, Danny JH, et al.

Unilateral blindness caused by infection with Lyme disease spirochete, *Borrelia burgdorferi*. Ann Intern Med 103:382–384, 1985.

64. Steere AC, Dwyer E, and Winchester R: Association of chronic Lyme arthritis with HLA-DR4 and HLA-DR2 alleles. N Engl J Med 323(4):219–223, 1990.

65. Steere AC, Grodzicki RL, Kornblatt AN, et al: The spirochetal etiology of Lyme disease. N Engl J Med 308:733–740, 1983.

66. Steere AC, Malawista SE, Hardin JA, et al. Erythema chronicum migrans and Lyme arthritis. Ann Intern Med 86:685–698, 1977.

67. Steere AC, Pachner AR, and Malawista SE: Neurologic abnormalities of Lyme disease: Successful treatment with high-dose intravenous penicillin. Ann Intern Med 99:767–772, 1983.

68. Steere AC, Taylor E, Wilson ML, et al: Longitudinal assessment of the clinical and epidemiologic features of Lyme disease in a defined population. J Infect Dis 154:295–300, 1986.

69. Sterman AB, Nelson S, and Barclay P: Demyelinating neuropathy accompanying Lyme disease. Neurology 32:1302–1305, 1982.

70. Stiernstedt G, Gustafsson R, Karlsson M, Svenungsson B, and Skoldenberg B: Clinical manifestations and diagnosis of neuroborreliosis. Ann N Y Acad Sci 539:46–55, 1988.

71. Stiernstedt GT, Granstrom M, Hederstedt B, and Skoldenberg B: Diagnosis of spirochetal meningitis by enzyme linked immunosorbent assay and indirect immunofluorescence assay in serum and cerebrospinal fluid. J Clin Microbiol 21:819–825, 1985.

72. Strickland C: Note on a case of "tick paralysis" in Australia. Parasitology 7:379, 1915.

73. Tsai TF, Bailey RE, and Moore PS: National surveillance of Lyme disease, 1987–1988. Conn Med 53(6):324–326, 1989.

74. Uldry PA, Regli F, and Bogousslavsky J: Cerebral angiopathy and recurrent strokes following *Borrelia burgdorferi* infection. J Neurol Neurosurg Psychiatry 50:1703–1704, 1987.

75. Vallat JM, Hugon J, Lubeau M, et al: Tick bite meningoradiculoneuritis. Neurology 37:749–753, 1987.

76. Veenedaal-Hilbers JA, Perquin WVM, Hoogland PH, and Doornbos L: Basal meningovasculitis and occlusion of the basilar artery in two cases of *Borrelia burgdorferi* infection. Neurology 38:1317–1319, 1988.

77. Waisbren B, Cashman N, Schell R, and Johnson R: *Borrelia borgdorferi* antibodies and amyotrophic lateral sclerosis. Lancet 2:332–333, 1987.

78. Walshe TM and Szyfelbein W: Case records of the Massachusetts General Hospital. N Engl J Med 319:1654–1662, 1988.

79. Wilske B, Scierz G, Preac-Mursic V, et al: Intrathecal production of specific antibodies against *Borrelia burgdorferi* in patients with lymphocytic meningoradiculitis. J Infect Dis 153:304–314, 1986.

80. Wokke JHJ, de Koning J, Stanek G, and Jennekens FGI: Chronic muscle weakness caused by *Borrelia burgdorferi* meningoradiculitis. Ann Neurol 22:389–392, 1987.

81. Wu G, Lincoff H, Ellsworth RM, and Haik BG: Optic disc edema and Lyme disease. Ann Ophthalmol 18:252–255, 1986.

82. Yagnik PM and Dhaduk V: Polyneuritis cranialis in Lyme disease. J Neurol Neurosurg Psychiatry 49(8):963–964, 1986. Letter.

EDITORS' COMMENTARY:

Issues Surrounding Management of Suspected Lyme Disease

The rapid emergence of Lyme disease, now the most common vector-borne human disease (epizooenosis) in the United States and Europe, has given rise to considerable public and medical concerns regarding prevention, diagnosis, and treatment. Halperin's excellent summary of central nervous system infection by *Borrelia burgdorferi* indicates the protean nature of the clinical symptoms and signs. Several controversial issues concern the clinician, who must determine when and how to treat suspected cases.

Epidemiology: The source of infection is the deer tick (*Ixodes dammini* in the northeastern United States, *I. pacificus* in the western United States, and *I. ricinus* in Europe), which belongs to a species of "black-legged" ticks that are found worldwide. In addition to Lyme disease (borreliosis), the ticks transmit babesiosis *(Babesia microti)* in the United States and tick-borne encephalitis in Asia and Europe. The ticks exist in larval, nymph, and adult forms; the mouse is the common reservoir, except on the western coast of the United States where the wood rat has been shown to be the reservoir for *I. pacificus*. Infected ticks (nymphs) appear early in the spring and summer (May to mid-July). They are tiny, about the size of a poppy seed. The adult tick is larger, about the size of an apple seed, but is smaller than the common dog tick (which is never infected with *Borrelia burgdorferi*). It is estimated that in high-risk areas of Maine, Massachusetts, and New York, up to one third of the nymph population and one half of the adult tick population are infected.

Prevention. The risk of exposure can, of course, be greatly reduced by avoiding outdoor activities in heavily infested areas (not entirely practical for everyone), or by wearing protective clothing, applying insect repellents, or recognizing and promptly removing ticks discovered by examination of the body, head, and limbs. The best data from animal experiments suggest that infection with *B. burgdorferi* is highly unlikely if ticks are removed before 48 hours.[10]

The possibility of developing an effective vaccine is being explored, but actual attempts at development are not likely to be successful soon.[1] The issues surrounding who should receive a vaccine, if available, and how often it would be required to establish immunity must await these advances. In the meantime, the practical concerns for the patient and physician focus on methods to establish the diagnosis, when and whether prophylactic treatment should be given in cases of possible or suspected infection, and the approaches to management of the later chronic forms of illness, which commonly involve the CNS.

The discovery of a tick fixed to the skin of a patient who lives in an area of high risk raises the question of whether prophylactic treatment should be given. As summarized by Kassirer,[3] the factors to be considered include the probability that the tick is infected, the length of time the tick has been attached, and the chance that the disease will occur without a telltale rash. Many clinicians familiar with Lyme disease in susceptible areas prescribe doxycycline or amoxicillin after any tick bite because the treatment is safe and effective. In contrast, many expert investigators believe that this approach represents "overkill" and advise that because the risk is small, treatment be given only after signs of infection (e.g., rash, flulike symptoms) appear or after a more serious manifestation of the disease appears (e.g., Bell's palsy, joint involvement). An effort to define these issues and to provide a cost-benefit analysis by "decision analysis" was reported by Magid and colleagues,[7] who concluded that a calculated risk of 1% to 3.5% warrants prophylactic treatment with doxycycline, whereas a risk of less than 1% warrants no treatment. Shapiro and colleagues[12] examined the risk of infection and the efficacy of prophylactic antimicrobal treatment after documented bite by the deer tick. In a double-blind, placebo-controlled study of 387 subjects, they concluded that even in an area of high risk (Connecticut), the risk of infection after a documented deer-tick bite is so low that "prophylactic treatment is not routinely indicated."[12]

Diagnosis. Another concern is the reliability of methods for establishing a diagnosis in patients who present with symptoms consistent with Lyme disease and who live in or recently visited an area of high risk. Fewer than two thirds of patients develop the erythema migrans, the typical rash (see Fig. 10–1 on color insert). The question then arises as to how reliable the diagnostic laboratory tests are. These tests are based primarily on antibody measurement by enzyme-linked immunosorbent assay (ELISA) or immunoblot.[2] Fewer than 1% of patients have positive results of standard laboratory tests 1 week after infection, fewer than 50% show any rise in antibody 1 to 3 weeks after exposure, and only 90% show detectable increases after 4 weeks. False-positive results are common in patients with syphilis, acute mononucleosis, DLE, rheumatoid arthritis, or septicemia, and in human immunodeficiency virus (HIV)–positive, AIDS-affected patients. Furthermore, the prevalence of asymptomatic carriers whose serologic test results are positive, or of previously infected individuals further reduces the usefulness of the test. Newer methods of antigen determination by polymerase chain reaction (PCR) promise more accurate diagnosis but are plagued by false-positive results arising from DNA contamination. These issues have been addressed in several recent communications.[4,5,8,11]

We recommend application of the principles described by Magid and associates,[7] and we emphasize that the risk of acquiring the disease is less than commonly believed by both patients and physicians who live in high-risk areas. Nevertheless, prophylactic treatment in patients with a greater than 1% likelihood of infection is more cost-effective than repeated visits to the physician, multiple diagnostic tests, and in many cases, the other tests that the physician is tempted to order and that are unnecessary in asymptomatic individuals.

References

1. Fikrig E, et al: A recombinant vaccine for Lyme disease. In Schutzer S (ed): Lyme Disease: Molecular and Immunologic Approaches, Cold Spring Harbor Press, New York, 1992.

2. Golightly MG and Ciciana AL: ELISA and immunoblots in the diagnosis of Lyme borreliosis: Sensitivities and sources of false-positive results. In Schutzer S (ed): Lyme Disease: Molecular and Immunologic Approaches. Cold Spring Harbor Press, New York, 1992.

3. Kassirer JP: Is a tick's bark worse than its bite—formulating an answer with decision analysis. N Engl J Med 327:562–563, 1992.

4. Keller TL, Halperin JJ, and Whitman M: PCR detection of *Borrelia burgdorferi* DNA in cerebrospinal fluid of Lyme neuroborreliosis patients. Neurology 42:32–42, 1992.

5. Kruger WH and Pulz M: Detection of *Borrelia burgdorferi* in cerebrospinal fluid by the polymerase chain reaction. J Med Microbiol 35:98–102, 1991.

6. Luft BJ, Bosler EM, and Dattwyler RJ: Diagnosis of Lyme borreliosis. In Schutzer S (ed): Lyme Disease: Molecular and Immunologic Approaches. Cold Spring Harbor Press, New York, 1992.

7. Magid D, Schwartz B, Craft J, and Schwartz JS: Prevention of Lyme disease after tick bites—a cost-effective analysis. N Engl J Med 327:534–541, 1992.

8. Pachner AR: CNS Lyme disease [letter]. Neurology 42: 1849, 1992.

9. Persing DH, Barthold SW, and Malawista SE: Molecular detection of *Borrelia burgdorferi*. In Schutzer S (ed): Lyme Disease: Molecular and Immunologic Approaches. Cold Spring Harbor Press, New York, 1992.

10. Piesman J, Maupin GO, Campos EG, and Happ CM: Duration of adult female *Ixodes dammini* attachment and transmission of *Borrelia burgdorferi*, with description of a needle aspiration isolation method. J Infect Dis 163:895–897, 1991.

11. Schutzer S (ed): Lyme Disease: Molecular and Immunologic Approaches. Cold Spring Harbor Press, New York, 1992.

12. Shapiro ED, Gerber MA, Holabird NB, et al: A controlled trial of antimicrobial prophylaxis for Lyme disease after deer-tick bites. N Engl J Med 327:1769–1773, 1992.

Chapter 11

NEUROSYPHILIS

Roger Simon, M.D., and
Lydia Bayne, M.D.

THE CLINICAL SPECTRUM OF
 NEUROSYPHILIS
LABORATORY DIAGNOSIS AND
 CEREBROSPINAL FLUID
 ANALYSIS
TREATMENT
HIV INFECTION AND
 NEUROSYPHILIS

A decade ago, nervous-system syphilis was a rarity on hospital wards; since 1980 its incidence has increased dramatically[4,16] following the resurgence of primary and secondary syphilis (Fig. 11–1), now estimated at 14.7 cases per 100,000 people.[8,34] This rise in primary and secondary syphilis was first seen in the promiscuous homosexual male population[6] but more recently has spread to the heterosexual community through contact with the prostitute pool.[10] The natural history of untreated syphilis is well known from syphilitic population cohorts specifically followed without therapy and from the broad experience of the prepenicillin era. Approximately 7% of untreated patients with primary or secondary syphilis will develop some form of symptomatic neurosyphilis.[24]

Neurosyphilis may take many clinical forms (Table 11–1, Fig. 11–2), but each of the neurologic manifestations of syphilis is the result of chronic, insidious inflammation in the subarachnoid space, occurring as a reaction to treponemal invasion of the central nervous system (CNS). It is unknown whether this invasion, which presumably occurs at the time of the bacteremia, is universal; the inflammatory response in the cerebrospinal fluid (CSF) is seen in 34% of asymptomatic syphilitic patients.[48] The peak of CSF abnormalities comes at 13 to 18 months after the primary infection, but in 10% of cases is coincident with secondary manifestations.[44] Thus, the risk of neurosyphilis is determined early in the course of the disease. Adams and colleagues[1,44,46] noted that the overall risk of neurosyphilis (both symptomatic and asymptomatic) following primary infection is 30% but is reduced to 1% if the CSF examination is normal 5 years after primary infection.

Some investigators have challenged these basic premises of CNS invasion, with CNS inflammation dictating the presence of, and the activity of, nervous-system syphilis. "Modern" criteria and "atypical" presentations have been suggested,[29] but such atypical features have not been found in other recent large clinical series,[53] and tests of CSF from patients with "modern" criteria have failed to demonstrate the presence of spirochetes using the sensitive testicular inoculation technique.[36]

THE CLINICAL SPECTRUM OF NEUROSYPHILIS

The clinical syndromes of neurosyphilis are conventionally divided into four

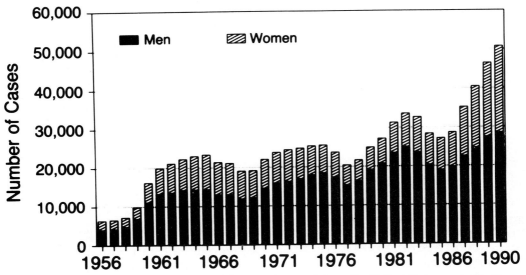

Figure 11–1. Number of cases of primary and secondary syphilis in the United States, according to sex, 1956 to 1990. Data were obtained from the Public Health Service (Division of STD-HIV Prevention. Sexually transmitted disease surveillance, 1990. Centers for Disease Control, Atlanta, 1991). (From Hook EW III and Marra CM: Acquired syphilis in adults. N Engl J Med 326:1061, 1992, with permission.)

entities: acute syphilitic meningitis, cerebrovascular syphilis, syphilitic dementia (general paresis), and tabes dorsalis. These syndromes are not singularly distinct entities but often form an overlapping spectrum. Syphilitic meningitis, for instance, comprises some portion of vascular syphilis, dementia, and tabes dorsalis, because each is the result of the prolonged inflammatory

Table 11–1 CLINICAL
MANIFESTATIONS OF
NEUROSYPHILIS

Manifestations	Percent
Asymptomatic	31
Tabetic	30
Paretic	12
Vascular	10
Meningeal	6
Taboparetic	3
Optic neuritis	3
Spinal cord syndromes	3
Eighth-nerve syndrome	1
Miscellaneous	1

Source: Based on 676 cases from Merritt, Adams, and Solomon.[44]

process in the subarachnoid space. Syphilitic meningitis may be associated with rare forms of nervous-system involvement such as syphilitic polyradiculopathy[38] or gumma.[37] Some features of dementia may be seen in vascular syphilis (e.g., Argyll-Robertson pupils), and clinical features of tabes dorsalis and dementia commonly overlap and are referred to by the term *taboparesis.* Nonetheless, in pure form, each of these syndromes has a different time course, different presentation, and different pathology.

To a substantial degree the clinical subtypes of neurosyphilis follow a predictable time course (see Fig. 11–2) after primary infection. It should be noted, however, that because of the frequently occult nature of the painless primary lesion, the time of initial infection may not be known; neurosyphilis must often be diagnosed on serologic grounds rather than by history.

Acute syphilitic meningitis occurs earliest following primary infection, often at the time of the secondary rash. The meningeal inflammation extend-

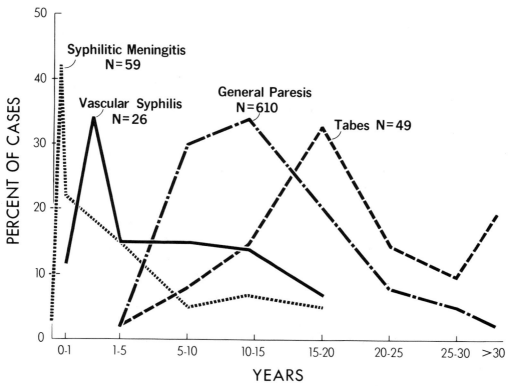

Figure 11–2. Interval between primary syphilitic infection and symptomatic neurosyphilis. (From Simon: Neurosyphilis. Arch Neurol 42:607, with permission. Copyright 1985 American Medical Association.)

ing to involve cerebral blood vessels results in cerebrovascular neurosyphilis, which is usually seen within the first 5 years following primary infection. The so-called parenchymal forms of neurosyphilis, dementia and tabes, occur after a more protracted interval. Because of this time frame, the syndromes of neurosyphilis most commonly encountered in recent years are syphilitic meningitis and cerebral vascular syphilis, these being the earliest forms of CNS syphilis and therefore most likely to be seen in a new epidemic.

Acute Syphilitic Meningitis

Symptomatic meningeal syphilis is usually seen during the first months to 2 years following the primary infection: 10% of cases occur concurrent with the secondary rash. Patients are afebrile with positive meningeal signs, headache, and often some degree of confusion; the course is subacute, and the spinal fluid is reactive with a lymphocytic pleocytosis.

The inflammatory process producing this syndrome may be preferentially concentrated either at the base or vertex of the brain. Vertex involvement results in impairment of CSF drainage through the sagittal sinus, with resultant acute communicating hydrocephalus (Fig. 11–3). With involvement of the base of the brain, cranial nerve abnormalities are prominent. The most frequently involved cranial nerves are those at the cerebellar-pontine angle (VI, VII, and VIII) and the optic and oculomotor nerves (Table 11–2). Asymmetry is the rule; this is especially helpful in regard to optic nerve abnor-

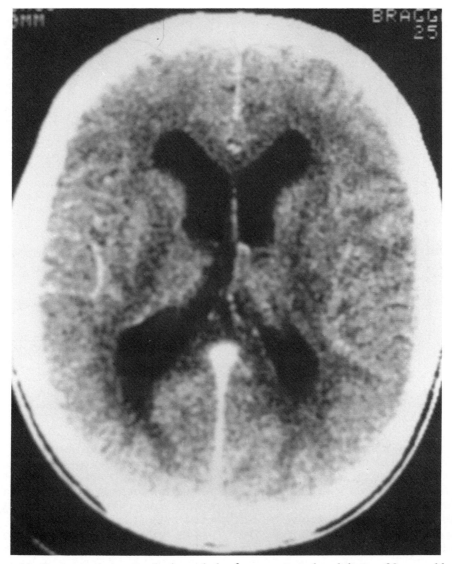

Figure 11–3. Acute obstructive hydrocephalus from meningeal syphilis in a 32-year-old man.

malities, where ophthalmoscopic examination will reveal papillitis that is generally unilateral.

The diagnosis of acute syphilitic meningitis is based on clinical suspicion in the setting of a meningeal syndrome with cranial nerve abnormalities, and a lymphocytic inflammatory CSF with a positive serologic test result. A negative CSF Venereal Disease Research Laboratory (VDRL) test result might theoretically occur in the setting of far-advanced immune suppression, as a prozone phenomenon, or as a manifestation of the CSF inflammatory response in early syphilis preceding seropositivity.[18,19] An accurate diagnosis is particularly important, as the relatively mild symptoms may resolve without treatment but leave the patient at risk for progression to the fixed deficits associated with the later forms of neurosyphilis. The specific incidence of residual abnormality and disease pro-

Table 11–2 CRANIAL NERVE INVOLVEMENT IN ACUTE SYPHILITIC MENINGITIS*

Cranial Nerves	Percent of Abnormalities
I	1
II	15
III	12
IV	2
V	6
VI	12
VII	23
VIII	23
IX–X	3
XI	0.2
XII	2

*340 cranial nerve abnormalities from 195 patients with acute syphilitic meningitis.
Source: Modified from Merritt, Adams, and Solomon: Neurosyphilis. Oxford University Press, 1946, p 39, with permission.

gression unfortunately is unclear, as the only large series from the prepenicillin era, that of Merritt and Moore in 1935,[46] is contaminated with patients with viral meningitis (a syndrome unrecognized at that time) who incidentally had reactive blood serologic tests.

Cerebrovascular Syphilis

The syndrome of meningovascular syphilis occurs when the inflammatory process in the subarachnoid space causes compromise of cerebral arteries traversing the subarachnoid space. Accordingly, a syndrome of middle-sized–vessel vasculitis is seen (Fig. 11–4), which produces ischemia in the distribution of the involved vessels. According to Merritt and associates,[44] the middle cerebral artery is most commonly affected, but any cerebral or spinal vascular bed may be involved in isolation or in combination.[28,33,40] The inflammatory process in the CSF, although resulting in vascular occlusion, produces a clinical syndrome that is distinct from thromboembolic stroke in both presentation and time course. Patients frequently have prodromal symptoms of headache, personality change, or emotional lability, which are the results of diffuse meningeal or meningovascular

inflammation. When the vascular occlusion occurs, it frequently evolves and progresses over hours or days, producing a temporal profile distinct from the apoplectic onset of stroke.

The clinical diagnosis is assisted by the universal occurrence of an inflammatory CSF with a positive serologic test result. Patients with normal CSF, reported in the prepenicillin era, undoubtedly represented patients with atherosclerotic carotid and vertebral artery disease not recognized as clinical entities at that time.[20]

Neuroradiologic abnormalities in meningovascular syphilis often show early and prominent involvement in the deep penetrating arteries supplying the central white matter. This computed tomography (CT) or magnetic resonance imaging (MRI) finding (Fig 11–5) is especially suggestive of vasculitis affecting medium-sized vessels, as the lenticulostriate arteries originate from intracerebral vessels of such caliber. Angiography demonstrates concentric constriction of medium-caliber vessels. The differential diagnosis of such angiographic findings includes subarachnoid hemorrhage, tuberculous meningitis, and drug-induced vasculitis,[55,65] as well as other systemic or isolated CNS necrotizing vasculitides.

Syphilitic Dementia (General Paresis)

Syphilitic dementia, also known as general paresis or dementia paralytica, is the parenchymal meningoencephalitic form of CNS syphilis. The symptoms generally begin 10 to 20 years after the primary infection, with a range from 3 to 30 years.[68] There is a striking male predominance (men affected 4 to 7 times more often than women), which has classically been explained by the decreased infectivity of *Treponema pallidum* during pregnancy. In the days before penicillin, this form of the disease was rampant; it then virtually disappeared but is now beginning to re-emerge.

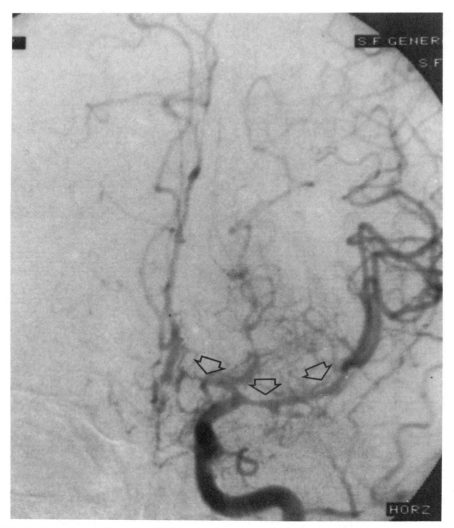

Figure 11–4. Anteroposterior view of left carotid angiogram showing constriction *(arrows)* of anterior and medial segments of the middle carotid artery in a 26-year-old man with meningovascular syphilis. (From Lowenstein et al,[40] p 337, with permission.)

The symptoms of syphilitic dementia are notoriously nonspecific, being those of any organic brain syndrome (Table 11–3). Disease progression is associated with intellectual decline. The classic features of psychosis and grandiose delusional states were well known in the old literature,[44] but these colorful syndromes were less common than the simple dementing type. Tremors of the hands, producing disordered handwriting, and of the tongue and lips, producing dysarthria, were stated by older authors as highly characteristic of advancing syphilitic dementia.[44] Modern experience with the disease is insufficient to provide confirmation.

The most useful features in differentiating syphilitic paresis from other causes of dementia are the relatively early age of onset (most commonly between the ages of 30 and 50)[68] and the fact that, in the great majority of cases, the untreated disease was fatal within months to a few years. An inflammatory CSF is always found, and the blood and CSF serologic test results are always positive. Accordingly, in any subacute dementing illness, a serum fluorescent treponemal antibody absorbed (FTA-ABS) evaluation, with examination of the spinal fluid if the FTA is reactive, is essential.

Tabes Dorsalis

The onset of tabes dorsalis is delayed following primary infection, with intervals of 10 to 20 years most often cited. The range of disease onset is broad, however, encompassing a 5- to 50-year spread after primary syphilis. There is some suggestion in the older literature that younger patients and patients treated for primary or secondary syphilis (prepenicillin) may have had a shorter incubation period.[44] As with general paresis, a marked male predominance is noted in the classic literature, with ratios of 7 to 1 often cited.[44,68]

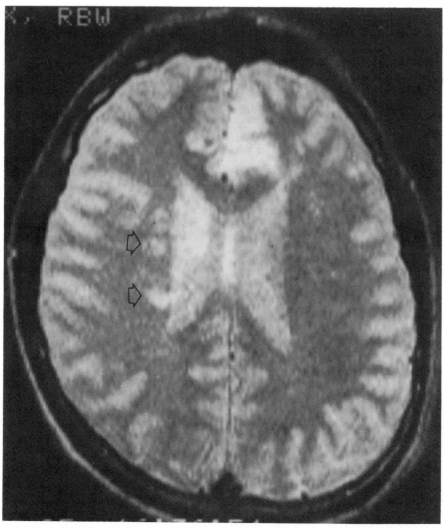

Figure 11–5. MRI of brain of patient from Figure 11–4. Note small areas of high signal in right deep white matter *(arrows)*, characteristic of meningovascular syphilis. (Right front polar high signal abnormality can be seen as well.) (From Lowenstein et al,[40] p 335, with permission.)

Table 11–3 SIGNS AND SYMPTOMS OF SYPHILITIC DEMENTIA (GENERAL PARESIS)

SYMPTOMS
Irritability
Fatigability
Personality changes
Impaired judgment and insight
Depression or elation
Confusion and delusions

SIGNS
Expressionless face
Facial, lingual, and labial movement tremors
Dysarthria
Disordered handwriting (due to intention tremor)
Hyperactive reflexes
Rare focal signs

Source: Data from Merritt.[43]

The symptoms are shown in Table 11–4. The classic triad of symptoms is tabetic lightning pain, sensory ataxia, and dysuria, combined with the triad of signs: pupillary abnormalities, areflexia, and Romberg's sign. The earliest findings are those of tabetic lightning pains, pupillary abnormalities, and loss of lower-extremity reflexes. Accordingly, these signs should be sought when the issue of parenchymal syphilis is raised.

Lightning pains eventually occur in 75% to 90% of all patients, even those with mild disease. These are most commonly felt in the lower extremities but may affect any region of the body. Each pain is brief and lancinating, perhaps best described by Wilson[68] by the phrase "the twanging of a single fiddle string." The pains can vary from region to region, persist from minutes to hours, and vanish for months, only to recur. As the disease progresses, susceptibility to deep pain declines. This results in the classic absence of pain when the Achilles tendon is squeezed (Abadie's sign) or the absence of pain in the upper extremity when pressure is applied over the ulnar nerve (Biernacki's sign). Both hypesthesia and hyperesthesia also may occur in a pseudo-radicular distribution that may involve the extremities, chest, or malar region of the face. These regions have been referred to as the zone of Hitzig.[68]

The predominant sensory loss, however, is in the large nerve fibers carrying joint position and vibratory information into the posterior column, resulting in sensory ataxia and a positive Romberg's sign (see Table 11–4). Either vibratory or position sense may be affected out of proportion to the other in any given patient, so both sensory modalities are important to test on examination. The primary pathologic site for this sensory neuropathy, whether in the proximal dorsal root segments within the root entry zone or in the dorsal root ganglion nuclei, remains an unsettled issue. Nevertheless, only during the phase of active syphilitic inflammation, when the CSF is reactive, can the disease process be halted.

Table 11–4 SYMPTOMS AND SIGNS OF TABETIC NEUROSYPHILIS*

	Percent
SYMPTOMS	
Lancinating pains	75
Ataxia	42
Bladder disturbance	33
Paresthesias	24
Gastric or visceral crises	18
Visual loss	16
Rectal incontinence	14
Deafness	7
Impotence	4
SIGNS	
Abnormal pupils	94
Argyll-Robertson	48
Other	64
Reflex abnormalities	
Absent ankle jerks	94
Absent knee jerks	81
Absent biceps and triceps reflexes	11
Romberg's sign	55
Impaired sensation	
Vibratory	52
Position	45
Touch and pain	13
Optic atrophy	20
Ocular palsy	10
Charcot's joints	7

*Analysis of 150 cases.
Source: Merritt, Adams, and Solomon: Neurosyphilis. Oxford University Press, 1946, p 2, with permission.

Abnormal pupils are highly characteristic, but classic Argyll-Robertson (AR) pupils occur in only half of patients (see Table 11–4). These classic AR pupils demonstrate a dissociation between constriction to light and accommodation (so-called light-near dissociation). The pupils are characteristically small, irregular, and bilateral.[39] A host of other pupillary abnormalities that occur in tabes dorsalis may be unilateral or marked by mydriasis or an absent pupillary light reflex.[22] A lesion involving the midbrain tectum was proposed by Merritt[45] to be the pathologic basis for classic AR pupils. The differential diagnosis of light-near dissociation is small, the most common mimicry being found in diabetic autonomic neuropathy (so-called pseudotabes) as well as with pineal region tumors or any lesion involving the midbrain tectum.[13,39]

As the disease progresses, bladder disturbances and sensory ataxia become prominent. Optic atrophy, oculomotor nerve palsies, gastric crises, distal ulceration, and Charcot's joints are seen. The sensory ataxia is characteristically worse in the lower extremities than the upper. The ensuing gait abnormality is wide-based and unsteady and differentiated from cerebellar ataxia by the marked exacerbation of instability with cessation of visual clues (Romberg's sign). Involvement of the upper extremity produces a pseudoathetotic movement of the fingers of the outstretched hand.

Involvement of the low sacral nerve roots produces bladder hypotonia with overflow incontinence. Rectal incontinence is uncommon, but distention of the colon due to insensitivity is frequent in established cases. Genital sensory impairment results in impotence and a loss of the cremasteric and bulbocavernosus reflexes.

Sensory impairment also results in the trophic lesions of Charcot's hips, knees, and ankles, as well as distal extremity ulcerative perforations. Many of the symptoms and signs resulting from sensory alteration are not corrected or may even progress, following eradication of active disease with penicillin therapy. Such progressive symptoms may include lightning pains, gastric crises, urinary incontinence, Charcot's joints, and, rarely, optic atrophy.

LABORATORY DIAGNOSIS AND CEREBROSPINAL FLUID ANALYSIS

The clinical syndromes of neurosyphilis occur as a result of CNS invasion by the spirochetes and the consequent inflammatory process in the CSF. Accordingly, CSF abnormalities are the hallmark of each stage of neurosyphilis. Representative examples of modern cases from the authors' experiences and recent literature are given in Table 11–5, and summaries from the classic literature in Table 11–6. Lymphocytic pleocytosis with the maximum cell counts (many hundreds to over a thousand cells per mL) is characteristically found in the most acute form, syphilitic meningitis. Decreasing numbers of cells were reported[44] in syphilitic vascular disease, paresis, and tabes dorsalis (see parts b to d of Table 11–6). The glucose content may be mildly reduced in syphilitic meningitis but is otherwise normal. The protein concentration is rarely over 200 mg/dL in syphilitic meningitis, syphilitic vascular disease, and paresis. Protein concentrations of less than 100 mg/dL are the rule in tabes dorsalis. The gamma globulin portion of the protein content is commonly elevated and oligoclonal bands may be present.[44,59] The correlate of gamma globulin elevation in the classic literature is that of abnormal colloidal gold curves. In late, "burnt out" tabes dorsalis, the CSF may be normal, although positive serologic test results are usually retained. The diagnosis of active neurosyphilis, then, is based on a compatible clinical syndrome of meningeal, vascular, dementing, or tabetic

Table 11–5 RECENT EXAMPLES OF CSF FINDINGS IN VARIOUS NEUROSYPHILITIC SYNDROMES

Syndrome	OP	WBC Count (per mL)	Glucose Level (mg per dL)	Protein Level (mg per dL)	Gamma Globulin, IgG Index*	VDRL Blood	VDRL CSF
Meningitis	170	154 (94%L)	29	95		1:64	1:4
Cerebrovascular	192	58 (87%L)	41	119	0.93	1:512	1:16
Paresis		220	49	305	1.99	1:128	1:8
Tabes							
Active		62		140		1:15[†]	1:28[†]
Inactive		2	76	43		1:16[‡]	1:2[‡]

Key: IgG = immunoglobulin G; OP = opening pressure; %L = % of total WBC that are lymphocytic; WBC = white blood cell.
  *Normal IgG index = 0.23–0.64.
  [†]Data from Giles.[23]
  [‡]Data from Yoder.[64]

symptoms in the setting of an inflammatory CSF. Reactive treponemal blood serologic test results (positive FTA-ABS or *Treponema pallidum* hemagglutination assay [TPHA]) are universal. Negativity of these blood serologic test results excludes the diagnosis.

A positive CSF VDRL test result is essentially universal, although multiple samples occasionally may be required. Persistent negative results rarely have been reported in neuro-ophthalmologic presentations.[12] The issue of negative CSF serologic test results and the occurrence of active neurosyphilis is difficult to address from the older literature, in which the relatively insensitive Wassermann test was used and the series were contaminated by the inclusion of nonsyphilitic syndromes of cerebral vascular disease and viral meningitis. Where clinical diagnoses were clear in the older literature (e.g., paresis and tabes dorsalis), however, the large number of reported cases suggest that seronegativity (even with the

Table 11–6 CSF FINDINGS IN NEUROSYPHILIS BY TYPE, SUMMARIZED FROM THE CLASSIC LITERATURE

	Value	Percent
A. SYPHILITIC MENINGITIS*		
Opening pressure, mm H_2O	<200	34
	210–400	51
	>400	15
Cells/mL	<10	1
	11–100	24
	101–500	35
	501–2000	40
Glucose level, mg/dL	<20	3
	20–29	7
	30–39	33
	40–49	1
	50–80	43
	>81	3
Protein level, mg/dL	<45	12
	40–100	40
	101–200	38
	201–381	10

(continued)

Table 11–6—*Continued*

	Value	Percent
Serologic tests (Wassermann)		
CSF	+	86
	−	14
Blood	+	65
	−	35
B. SYPHILITIC VASCULAR DISEASE†		
Opening pressure, mm H_2O	<200	85
	210–240	15
Cells/mL	<10	37
	11–100	60
	>100	3
Protein level, mg/dL	15–45	34
	46–100	41
	101–200	22
	201–260	3
Wassermann	+	81
	−	19
C. GENERAL PARESIS‡		
Opening pressure, mm H_2O	<200	>90
	200–300	<10
Cells/mL	0–10	10
	11–100	80
	>100	10
Protein level, mg/dL	29–44	25
	45–100	50
	101–498	25
Serologic tests (Wassermann)		
CSF	+	100
	−	0
	+	>95
Blood	−	<5
D. TABES§		
Opening pressure, mm H_2O	Normal	90
	200–300	10
Cells/mL	0–5	53
	5–50	31
	50–100	16
	100–165	9
Protein level, mg/dL	14–45	47
	45–100	50
	100–25C	3
Serologic tests		
CSF	+	72
	−	28
Blood	+	88
	−	12

*Based on 80 cases (n = 30 for glucose) reported by Merritt and Moore.[46] Patients with negative serologic test results probably have viral meningitis and not syphilis (see text).

†From data of Merritt, Adams, and Solomon.[44] Glucose level is not reported. Patients with negative Wassermann test probably have nonsyphilitic cerebrovascular disease (see text).

‡Based on 100 cases of untreated paresis from Merritt, Adams, and Solomon.[44] Glucose levels were "normal or moderately reduced."

§From data of Merritt, Adams, and Solomon.[44] Glucose levels were "normal as a rule."

Wassermann reaction) must be exceedingly rare. In 100 paretic patients of Merritt, serologic tests of the CSF had positive results in every case;[44] a universal CSF positivity in paresis was also reported in 77 cases by Wilson.[68]

The role of the more sensitive treponemal test (FTA) of the CSF[15] remains uncertain, as the unabsorbed FTA test produces an unacceptably false-positive response in 4.5% of normal patients and the addition of sorbent (FTA-ABS) markedly decreases the sensitivity to 75%.[42] Accordingly, Jaffe and colleagues[31] concluded that "without other supporting clinical or laboratory data, the diagnostic value of a reactive CSF FTA is unknown."

In neurologically normal, non–HIV-infected patients with positive blood serologic test results, when is a lumbar puncture indicated? A positive nontreponemal serologic test (VDRL) result with a negative treponemal serologic test (FTA-ABS) result excludes the diagnosis of neurosyphilis and constitutes a false-positive VDRL test result. In such cases, a VDRL titer of less than 1:8 is found and the reactivity is often absent on repeated testings. Transient biologic false-positive reactions are associated with pregnancy, recent inoculations, or viral infections. A substantial proportion of idiopathic cases occur as well.[5] Chronic false-positive reactions are found in patients with a group of autoimmune diseases in which a positive antinuclear antibody (ANA) rheumatoid factor or lupus erythematosus (LE) preparation are also found.[5] In some patients, the FTA-ABS result may be falsely positive as well.[11,25] Such studies are often normal with repetition or occur in patients with abnormal plasma globulin levels, as associated with rheumatoid arthritis, autoimmune hemolytic anemia, alcoholic cirrhosis, and pregnancy.[35,60] In the absence of such associated diseases and of neurologic abnormalities on examination, the results of routine lumbar puncture in patients with a positive blood FTA-ABS will usually be normal or nonspecific.[63]

In non–immune-suppressed patients with a known history of syphilis, or in patients with a true-positive blood FTA-ABS test result who remain asymptomatic, a consensus has never been reached as to whether lumbar puncture is indicated. Further, because of the wide range of time over which maximum CSF abnormalities might be seen (months to 5 years following infection), the optimum timing for lumbar puncture is unclear. On a population basis, the low probability of finding abnormalities is overwhelmed by the great number of patients eligible for such a screen. Therefore, as a general rule, we do not recommend a lumbar puncture for an asymptomatic patient.

TREATMENT

Clinical neurosyphilis of all varieties is due to the inflammatory process in the CSF. This inflammatory process is the indicator of disease activity and therefore the ultimate monitor of effective therapy. Although a number of aspects of antibiotic treatment for neurosyphilis are incompletely established, normalization of the CSF is the requirement of any treatment regimen. Further, this normalization of the CSF documents eradication of active disease. Relapses have not been seen with normalization persistent for 2 years.[14]

Penicillin remains the drug of choice. Numerous regimens have been recommended as "adequate treatment," although the clinical outcome is not different using widely varying penicillin doses.[53,67] The supportive data are uncertain, but it is generallly accepted that the treponemicidal CSF levels of penicillin are 0.03 IU/mL (0.018 μg/mL). Intramuscular benzathine penicillin produces levels well below this accepted limit, with 12 of 13 patients reported by Moore as having no detectable CSF concentrations when this intramuscular regimen was used.[48] CSF penicillin concentrations reported from other regimens are found in Table 11–7. A recent study reported peak and

Table 11–7 CSF PENICILLIN CONCENTRATIONS IN VARIOUS TREATMENT REGIMENS FOR NEUROSYPHILIS

Pencillin Dose*	CSF Concentration $\mu g/mL$
Aqueous penicillin G 5 MU/day	0.3
Aqueous penicillin G 10 MU/day	2.4
Benzathine penicillin G 7.2 MU/day	0
Penicillin G procaine 12 MU, intramuscularly	0
Aqueous penicillin G 400,000 U intravenously, every 4 hours	0
Aqueous penicillin G 24 MU/day	0.018
Aqueous penicillin G 2 MU/day (with 2 g probenecid)	0.018

*MU = mouse unit.
Sources: Data from Mohr et al[47]; Polnikorn et al[54]; and Dunlop et al.[17a,17b]

nadir levels of CSF penicillin concentrations well above 0.03 IU/mL with 12 million units of intravenous penicillin given daily in four divided doses.[57] The use of probenecid as an adjunct to slow reabsorption of penicillin through the choroid plexus has also been recommended. Although probenecid increases the concentration of penicillin in CSF, it may (ironically) decrease the parenchymal concentration by competing for uptake at membrane transport sites.[21]

Accordingly, data indicate that neurosyphilis should not be treated with intramuscular therapy but can be adequately treated with 12 million units or greater of intravenous penicillin daily. Although they have not been vigorously studied, alternate treatment regimens for penicillin-allergic patients have been recommended or reported (Table 11–8). Investigational therapies for neurosyphilis currently being studied include ceftriaxone.

Although the dosage of penicillin for neurosyphilis appears relatively clear, the optimal duration of treatment is uncertain. It has been standard practice to treat with intravenous penicillin for 2

to 3 weeks while documenting a fall in CSF cell count and protein content.[30] Complete normalization of CSF is uncommon during this period of time, but without additional therapy (or additional hospitalization) the CSF usually continues to clear over the next weeks to months (Table 11–9). A normal cell count and falling protein content at 6 months is requisite for cure. Repeated CSF examinations should then be performed over the next 2 years to document continued reduction in protein content and a normal cell count. The VDRL titer in the CSF usually falls but

Table 11–8 TREATMENT REGIMENS FOR NEUROSYPHILIS

ESTABLISHED
Aqueous crystalline penicillin G, 12 to 24 million units IV daily (divided doses every 4 hours) for 10–14 days

APPROVED
Aqueous procaine penicillin G, 2.4 million units IM daily, plus probenecid 500 mg PO 4 times daily for 10–14 days

UNDER STUDY
Ceftriaxone 1 g IV every 12 hours

ALTERNATE DRUG REGIMENS FOR PENICILLIN-ALLERGIC PATIENTS
Desensitize to penicillin (preferred alternative)
Tetracycline hydrochloride 500 mg PO 4 times a day for 30 days*
Doxycycline 200 mg PO twice a day for 21 days†
Erythromycin 500 mg PO 4 times a day for 30 days
Chloramphenicol 1 g IV 4 times a day for 14 days
Ceftriaxone 1 g every 12 hours (under study)

RECOMMENDED TREATMENT REGIMENS FOR SYPHILIS IN HIV-COINFECTED PATIENTS
No change in therapy for early syphilis (CSF examination may be a useful guide to adequate treatment)
Benzathine penicillin should not be used
Examine CSF before and following treatment as a treatment guide
Aqueous crystalline penicillin G IV, 12–24 million units daily (2–4 million units every 4 hours)
Aqueous or procaine penicillin G, 2.4 million units IM daily plus probenecid 500 mg PO 4 times daily

IV = intravenous, IM = intramuscular, PO = per os (by mouth).
*Data from Romanowski, Starreveld, and Jarema.[56]
†Data from Whiteside, Flynn, and Fitzgerald.[66]

Table 11–9 CSF RESPONSE TO PENICILLIN TREATMENT*

	Admission	Day 7	Day 21	6 Months
Opening pressure, mL CSF	120			Normal
Cells/mL	207 (94% L)	100 (100% L)	24 (100% L)	0
Glucose level, mg/dL	51	66	54	66
Protein level, mg/dL	50 (14.4% gamma globulin)	38	48	34
Serologic tests (VDRL)				
CSF	1:2	1:1		
Blood	1:64	1:64	1:64	1:64

*Meningovascular syphilis treated with aqueous penicillin G, 24 million units daily for 21 days.
Source: Data from Holmes, Brant, Zawadski, and Simon.[28]

may not become unreactive. Any deviation from this scenario, especially an elevated cell count, demands retreatment.[14] Intravenous penicillin, 2 to 4 million units every 4 hours for 10 to 14 days, is to date the only known effective treatment. Table 11–8 lists options for those patients with a known, potentially life-threatening hypersensitivity reaction to penicillin. Ceftriaxone 1 g/day for 2 weeks is now being advocated, but its efficacy in controlled population studies is not yet proven. A follow-up lumbar puncture at 3 months and 6 months is mandatory if a regimen other than penicillin was used.

HIV INFECTION AND NEUROSYPHILIS

Some association between neurosyphilis and HIV infection is clear, as both diseases can be a consequence of promiscuous sexual behavior. It is likely that syphilis can predispose to the acquisition of the AIDS virus. Genito-ulcerative lesions such as syphilitic chancres are a substantial risk factor for the acquisition of HIV infection because the skin break provides an avenue of entry for the virus.[61] In theory, also, the concentration of T cells at the site of the skin lesion magnifies the possibility that the virus will find its intended host cell. In addition, the transient suppression of cellular immunity associated with a new syphilitic infec-

tion may make concomitant HIV infection more likely.[49] It is not yet clear whether the reverse is the case, that is, whether HIV infection predisposes to the acquisition of syphilis.

Recent case reports and reviews have suggested that, in patients coinfected with HIV, the neurosyphilis progresses in an unusually rapid, atypical, and aggressive manner.[3,27,32,38,50,58,69] Even in the pre-AIDS era, however, it was well recognized that it was not unusual for meningitic symptoms to appear as early as at the time of the secondary rash, that there was wide variability in the rate of progression, and that the clinical presentation was protean.[44] Further, none of the symptoms in recently reported cases were unusually severe in the context of the known spectrum of the disease. To date, the single postmortem study examining this issue did not find the incidence, time course, or neuropathologic evidence of neurosyphilis to be associated with HIV seropositivity.[7] Given the remarkable variability in the natural history of syphilis both before and after penicillin, only the accumulation of considerable numbers of modern cases will allow significant comparison between the pre-AIDS and post-AIDS disease.

It has been suggested that standard penicillin regimens for primary or secondary syphilis are less effective in HIV-coinfected patients.[32,50] Such reported cases often were those treated with benzathine penicillin, which is known to produce subtherapeutic concentrations in the CSF. Recently, isolation of treponemes from the CSF of three HIV-positive patients following penicillin treatment was suggested as a confirmation of penicillin insensitivity in HIV-infected patients.[41] Recovery of treponemes following clinically successful penicillin therapy for neurosyphilis, with documented resolution of CSF abnormalities, was also reported in the pre-AIDS era, however,[62] and the significance of these treponemes remains uncertain.[17] Further, penicillin has been successful in treating syphilis in patients immune-suppressed by chemotherapy.[34]

The issue of "penicillin failure" in HIV-coinfected patients also is complicated by the CSF pleocytosis that frequently accompanies AIDS. A recent study of 114 asymptomatic early HIV-positive patients found that 57 had abnormal CSF (either pleocytosis or elevated protein level or both) without evidence of other CNS infection.[2] An increase in oligoclonal bands or in CSF gamma globulin production may occur as well. Accordingly, patients with a persistent CSF pleocytosis resistant to multiple doses of penicillin may have CSF inflammation secondary to HIV itself (now suspected to invade the CNS routinely very early in the infection) rather than persistent, active neurosyphilis.

Seronegative neurosyphilis in HIV-coinfected patients has also been recently suggested.[27] Late serologic conversions in secondary syphilis[27] and the fact that the cellular response of the CSF may precede serologic positivity in early syphilis[19] may explain these cases; in other cases of initially negative serologic test results, the prozone phenomenon has been invoked. Alternatively, some experimental evidence exists that impaired cellular immunity (e.g., secondary to cytotoxic drugs) permits a shortening of the incubation time and the more rapid dissemination of secondary lesions in experimental models of syphilis.[52] Syphilis also produces a transient decrease of T lymphocytes in lymph nodes in both the primary and secondary stages, with a resultant increase in the number of circulating T-suppressor cells. Conceivably, this combination could affect CSF expression of syphilis in HIV-coinfected patients, but such an association has not been demonstrated. In regard to the issue of seronegativity, antibody production by the plasma cells requires the collaboration of the appropriate T4 helper cells to bring about differentiation and activation of the precursor B cell. Fourteen of 110 previously FTA-ABS–positive HIV-infected patients have recently been documented to lose FTA reactivity coincident with a fall in their T4/T8 blood ratios, but not before.[26] A decrease in antibody production in HIV-infected patients following routine vaccination has also been reported.[51] Accordingly, a decline in the immune capacity of patients with HIV does occur late, but its association with the occurrence of nervous-system syphilis in such patients remains speculative.[11a]

Specific Treatment Regimens for HIV-Coinfected Patients

Treatment regimens for syphilis in HIV-coinfected patients have been recently recommended by the Centers for Disease Control (CDC) (see Table 11–8).[9] The principle remains the same as treatment for nervous system syphilis in any patient: intravenous penicillin should be used in spirocheticidal doses and the CSF monitored as an index of therapy. Additionally, the current CDC recommendation is that all HIV-coinfected patients with latent syphilis (syphilis of greater than 1 year's duration) have their CSF examined, whether or not they have neurologic symptoms.

SUMMARY

The incidence of neurosyphilis has been rising since the beginning of the AIDS pandemic. The disease can appear in several clinical forms, but each is the result of chronic inflammation of the CNS. The clinical spectrum includes acute syphilitic meningitis, cerebrovascular syphilis, syphilitic dementia (general paresis), and tabes dorsalis. Overlapping syndromes are common. CSF abnormalities remain the hallmark of laboratory diagnosis. Lymphocytic pleocytosis (cell counts of 100 to 1000 per mL) is found in acute syphilitic meningitis and may be accompanied by lowered CSF glucose concentrations. Fewer cells are found in syphilitic cerebrovascular disease and in the general paresis. Protein level elevation in the CSF is common in all forms. Serologic tests for the treponemal antibody in the blood are universally positive in neurosyphilis; CSF serologic test results are almost always positive, although repeated testing is sometimes required. Routine CSF examination in *asymptomatic* HIV-negative patients with positive blood serologic test results is not recommended.

Penicillin remains the drug of choice for treatment of neurosyphilis. A daily dosage regimen of intravenous penicillin (12 million units) administered in divided doses (every 4 hours) achieves treponemicidal CSF levels. Treatment is continued for 2 to 3 weeks. Intramuscular penicillin treatment should not be given because of failure to achieve adequate CSF levels. Ceftriaxone or amoxicillin is usually given to penicillin-sensitive patients. Repeated CSF examinations are made over the subsequent 2 years. Retreatment is required if cell count and protein level do not return to and remain normal.

Concurrent syphilitic infection may predispose to HIV infection, and patients coinfected with HIV and *Treponema pallidum* may show a more rapid and virulent form of neurosyphilis. Treatment protocols are the same in coinfected patients, although monitoring of CSF changes is complicated by HIV-associated abnormalities that may not return to normal with successful eradication of neurosyphilis. HIV and treponemal coinfected patients who are neurologically asymptomatic should have CSF examination if the duration of syphilis exceeds 1 year; if the CSF is abnormal, such patients should be treated for neurosyphilis.

REFERENCES

1. Adams RA and Victor M: *Principles of Neurology,* Ed 4. McGraw-Hill, New York, 1989.
2. Appleman ME, Marshall DW, Brey RL, et al: Cerebrospinal fluid abnormalities in patients without AIDS who are seropositive for the human immunodeficiency virus. J Infect Dis 158:193–199, 1988.
3. Berry CD, Hooton TM, Collier AC, and Lukehart SA: Neurologic relapse after benzathine penicillin therapy for secondary syphilis in a patient with HIV infection. N Engl J Med 316:1587–1589, 1987.
4. Burke JM and Schaberg DR: Neurosyphilis in the antibiotic era. Neurology 35:1368–1371, 1985.
5. Catterall RD: Systemic disease and the biological false positive reaction. *Br J Vener Dis* 48:1–10, 1972.
6. Centers for Disease Control: Syphilis trends in the United States. MMWR (9/11/81) 30:441–444, 1981.
7. Centers for Disease Control: Tertiary syphilis deaths—South Florida. MMWR (7/31/87) 36:488–491, 1987.
8. Centers for Disease Control: Continuing increase in infectious syphilis—United States. MMWR (1/29/88) 37:35–38, 1988.
9. Centers for Disease Control: Diagnosis of syphilis in HIV-infected patients. MMWR (10/7/88) 37:601–608, 1988.
10. Centers for Disease Control: Relationship of syphilis to drug use and prostitution—Connecticut and Philadelphia, Pennsylvania. MMWR (12/16/88) 37:755–758, 1988.
11. Cohen P, Stout G, and Ende N: Serologic reactivity in consecutive patients admitted to a general hospital. Arch Intern Med 124:364–367, 1969.

11a. Courevitch MN, Selwyn PA, Davenny K, et al: Effects of HIV infection on the serologic manifestations and response to treatment of syphilis in intravenous drug users. Ann Intern Med 118:350–355, 1993.

12. Currie JN, Coppeto JR, and Lessell S: Chronic syphilitic meningitis resulting in superior orbital fissure syndrome and posterior fossa gumma. J Clin Neuro Ophthalmol 8:145–155, 1988.

13. Dacso CC and Bortz DL: Significance of the Argyll Robertson pupil in clinical medicine. Am J Med 86:199–202, 1989.

14. Dattner B, Thomas EW, and De Melio L: Criteria for the management of neurosyphilis. Am J Med 10:463–467, 1951.

15. Davis LE and Schmitt JW: Clinical significance of cerebrospinal fluid tests for neurosyphilis. Ann Neurol 25:50–55, 1989.

16. Dorfman DH and Glaser JH: Congenital syphilis presenting in infants after the newborn period. N Engl J Med 323:1299–1302, 1990.

17. Dunlop EMC: Persistence of treponemes after treatment. Br Med J 2:577–580, 1972.

17a. Dunlop EMC, Al-Egaily SS, Houang, E: Production of treponemicidal concentration of penicillin in cerebrospinal fluid. Br Med J 283:646, 1981.

17b. Dunlop EMC, Al-Egaily SS, Houang E: Penicillin levels in blood and CSF achieved by treatment of syphilis. JAMA 241:2538–2540, 1979.

18. Feraru ER, Aronow HA, and Lipton RB: Neurosyphilis in AIDS patients: Initial CSF VDRL may be negative. Neurology 40:541–543, 1990.

19. Fildes P, Parnell RJG, and Maitland HB: The occurrence of unsuspected involvement of the central nervous system in unselected cases of syphilis. Brain 41:255–301, 1918.

20. Fishman RA: *Cerebrospinal Fluid in Diseases of the Nervous System.* WB Saunders, Philadelphia, 1980, pp 225–285.

21. Fishman RA: Blood-brain and CSF barriers to penicillin and related organic acids. Arch Neurol 15:113–124, 1966.

22. Fletcher WA and Sharpe JA: Tonic pupils in neurosyphilis. Neurology 36:188–192, 1986.

23. Giles AJH: Tabes dorsalis progressing to general paresis after 20 years despite routine penicillin therapy. Br J Vener Dis 56:368–371, 1980.

24. Gjestland T: The Oslo study of untreated syphilis. Acta Derm Venereol 35(Suppl 34):1–368, 1955.

25. Goldman JN and Lantz MA: FTA-ABS and VDRL slide test reactivity in a population of nuns. JAMA 217:53–55, 1971.

26. Haas J, Bolan G, Clement M, Larsen S, and Moss A: Sensitivity of treponemal tests for detecting prior treated syphilis during HIV infection. J Infect Dis 162:862–866, 1990.

27. Hicks CB, Benson PM, Lupton GP, and Tramont EC: Seronegative secondary syphilis in patients infected with the human immunodeficiency virus (HIV) with Kaposi sarcoma. Ann Intern Med 107:492–495, 1987.

28. Holmes MD, Brant-Zawadski MM, and Simon RP: Clinical manifestations of meningovascular syphilis. Neurology 34:553–556, 1984.

29. Hooshmand H, Escobar MR, and Kopf SW: Neurosyphilis: A study of 241 patients. JAMA 219:726–730, 1972.

30. Idsøe O, Guthe T, and Wilcox RR: Penicillin in the treatment of syphilis: The experience of three decades. Bull World Health Organ 47:1–68, 1972.

31. Jaffe HW, Larsen SA, Peters M, et al: Tests for treponemal antibody in CSF. Arch Intern Med 138:252–255, 1978.

32. Johns DR, Tierney M, and Feisenstein D: Alteration in the natural history of neurosyphilis by concurrent infection with the human immunodeficiency virus. N Engl J Med 316:1569–1572, 1987.

33. Johns DR, Tierney M, and Parker SW: Pure motor hemiplegia due to meningovascular neurosyphilis. Arch Neurol 44:1062–1065, 1987.

34. Johnson PC, Norris SJ, Miller GPG, et al: Early syphilitic hepatitis after

renal transplantation. J Infect Dis 158:236–237, 1988.

35. Jones RR, Pusey C, Shifferli J, et al: Essential mixed cryoglobulinemia with false-positive serologic test for syphilis. Br J Vener Dis 59:33–36, 1983.

36. Jordan KG: Modern neurosyphilis—A critical analysis. West J Med 149:47–57, 1988.

37. Kaplan JG, Sterman AB, Horoupian D, Leeds NE, Zimmerman RD, and Gade R: Luetic meningitis with gumma: Clinical, radiographic, and neuropathologic features. Neurology 31:464–467, 1981.

38. Lanska MJ, Lanska DJ, and Schmidley JW: Syphilitic polyradiculopathy in an HIV-positive man. Neurology 38:1297–1301, 1988.

39. Lowenfeld IE: The Argyll Robertson pupil 1869–1969, a critical survey of the literature. Surv Opththalmol 14:199–299, 1969.

40. Lowenstein DH, Mills C, and Simon RP: Acute syphilitic transverse myelitis: An unusual presentation of meningovascular syphilis. Genitourin Med 63:333–338, 1987.

41. Lukehart SA, Hook EW, Baker-Zander SA, Collier AC, Critchlow CW, and Handsfield HH: Invasion of the central nervous system by Treponema pallidum: Implications for diagnosis and treatment. Ann Intern Med 109:855–862, 1988.

42. Mahoney JDH: Evaluation of CSF FTA-ABS test in latent and tertiary treated syphilis. Acta Derm Venereol 52:71–74, 1972.

43. Merritt HH: A Textbook of Neurology, Ed 2, Lea & Febiger, Philadelphia, 1959, pp 129–153.

44. Merritt HH, Adams RD, and Solomon HC: Neurosyphilis, Ed 2, Oxford University Press, New York, 1946.

45. Merritt HH and Moore M: The Argyll Robertson pupil. Arch Neurol Psychiatry 30:357–373, 1933.

46. Merritt HH and Moore M: Acute syphilitic meningitis. Medicine 14:119–183, 1935.

47. Mohr JA, Griffiths W, Jackson R, et al: Neurosyphilis and penicillin levels in cerebrospinal fluid. JAMA 236:2208–2209, 1976.

48. Moore JE: The Modern Treatment of Syphilis, Ed 2, CC Thomas, Springfield, 1943.

49. Musher DM and Schell RF: The immunology of syphilis. Hosp Pract December: 45–50, 1975.

50. Musher DM, Hamill RJ, and Baughn RE: Effect of human immunodeficiency virus (HIV) infection on the course of syphilis and on the response to treatment. Ann Intern Med 113:872–881, 1990.

51. Nelson KE, Clements ML, Miotti P, et al: The influence of human immunodeficiency virus (HIV) infection on antibody responses to influenza vaccines. Ann Intern Med 109:383–388, 1988.

52. Pacha J, Metzger M, Smogor W, Michalska E, Podwinska J, and Ruczkowska J: Effect of immunosuppressive agents on the course of experimental syphilis in rabbits. Arch Immunol Ther Exp 27:45–51, 1979.

53. Perdrup A, Jørgensen BB, and Pedersen NS: The profile of neurosyphilis in Denmark. A clinical and serological study of all patients in Denmark with neurosyphilis disclosed in the years 1971–1979 incl. by Wasserman reaction (CWRM) in the cerebrospinal fluid. Acta Derma Venereol 96(Suppl):3–14, 1981.

54. Polnikorn N, Witoonpanich R, Varachit M, et al: Penicillin concentrations in cerebrospinal fluid after different treatment regimens for syphilis. Br J Vener Dis 56:363–367, 1980.

55. Rabinov KR: Angiographic findings in a case of syphilis. Radiology 80:622–624, 1963.

56. Romanowski B, Starreveld E, and Jarema AJ: Treatment of neurosyphilis with chloramphenicol. Br J Vener Dis 59:225–227, 1983.

57. Schoth PEM and Wolters EC: Penicillin concentrations in serum and CSF during high-dose intravenous treatment for neurosyphilis. Neurology 37:1214–1216, 1987.

58. Shulkin D, Tripoli L, and Abell E: Lues

maligna in a patient with human immunodeficiency virus infection. Am J Med 85:425–427, 1988.

59. Simon RP: Neurosyphilis. Arch Neurol 42:606–613, 1985.

60. Sparling PF: Diagnosis and treatment of syphilis. N Engl J Med 284:642–653, 1971.

61. Stamm WE, Handsfield H, Rompalo AM, Ashley RL, Roberts PL, and Corey L: The association between genital ulcer disease and acquisition of HIV infection in homosexual men. JAMA 260:1429–1433, 1988.

62. Tramont EC: Persistence of *Treponema pallidum* following penicillin G therapy. JAMA 236:2206–2207, 1976.

63. Traviesa DC, Prystowsky SD, Nelson BJ, et al: Cerebrospinal fluid findings in asymptomatic patients with reactive serum fluorescent treponemal antibody absorption tests. Ann Neurol 4:524–530, 1978.

64. Yoder FW: Penicillin treatment of neurosyphilis: Are recommended dosages sufficient? JAMA 232:270–271, 1975.

65. Vata K, Scheibel R, Keiffer S, et al: Neurosyphilis and diffuse cerebral angiopathy. A case report. Neurology 24:472–476, 1974.

66. Whiteside YC, Flynn NM, and Fitzgerald FT: Penetration of oral doxycycline into the cerebrospinal fluid of patients with latent or neurosyphilis. Antimicrob Agents Chemother 28:347–348, 1985.

EDITORS' COMMENTARY:

Syphilis in HIV Infection

The number of cases of both primary and secondary syphilis reported to the Public Health Service has increased dramatically over the last 5 years.[3] Coincident with this trend has been a striking incidence of cases of neurosyphilis in human immunodeficiency virus (HIV)–positive individuals. Detailed reviews of the neurology of HIV infection and of neurosyphilis are found in Chapters 3 and 11. This commentary is directed at specific aspects of the diagnosis, clinical presentation, and management of neurosyphilis in HIV-positive individuals.

Diagnosis

Serologic tests have long been the mainstay in the specific diagnosis of syphilis. There are two basic diagnostic issues: (1) Which test results can be used to exclude or minimize the possibility that neurosyphilis is present? (2) Which test results establish the diagnosis of neurosyphilis? Although there has been concern that the HIV-induced immunodeficiency might make serologic testing unreliable, this has generally not proved to be the case.[7,11,13] Similarly, the basic cerebrospinal fluid (CSF) profile in HIV-positive patients with neurosyphilis resembles that found in HIV-negative individuals.[9]

A negative serum Venereal Disease Research Laboratory (VDRL) test does not reliably exclude neurosyphilis in either HIV-positive or HIV-negative individuals. However, the fluorescent treponemal antibody absorption (FTA-ABS) test is sensitive and specific for syphilis, and a negative result of the serum FTA-ABS test essentially excludes the diagnosis of active neurosyphilis.

Patients with syphilis require further evaluation to determine whether they have neurosyphilis. The VDRL test on the CSF is highly specific, and a reactive result of the test on CSF not grossly contaminated with blood establishes the diagnosis of neurosyphilis.[1] The CSF VDRL test is not particularly sensitive, however, and a negative test result does not exclude the presence of active neurosyphilis.[1,4] By contrast, the FTA-ABS test on CSF is highly sensitive, and a negative result essentially excludes the diagnosis of neurosyphilis.[1] Unfortunately, because of the test's high sensitivity, a positive result does not always indicate the presence of neurosyphilis. We consider patients to have presumptive neurosyphilis if they have (1) a reactive CSF VDRL, (2) a reactive CSF FTA-ABS and an elevation of CSF protein or pleocytosis, or (3) a reactive serum FTA-ABS test result and elevated CSF protein or a pleocytosis. HIV-positive patients with syphilis who refuse to undergo a CSF examination should be treated as if they have neurosyphilis (see later).

Clinical Manifestations

The most commonly encountered symptomatic neurosyphilitic syndromes in HIV-positive patients are acute syphilitic meningitis (seen in approximately 50% to 60% of HIV-positive patients with neurosyphilis) and meningovascular syphilis (seen in approximately 25% to 30%).[14] To date, reports of syphilitic gumma, tabes dorsalis, and general paresis in HIV-positive individuals are exceedingly rare. Since these complications are among the last manifestations of neurosyphilis to occur, their rarity may simply reflect the failure of HIV-positive individuals to survive for the requisite period of time. Alternatively, it may reflect the fact that the AIDS epidemic is not yet old enough for HIV-positive individuals with syphilis to have developed these complications. The incidence of asymptomatic neurosyphilis (a positive result of the VDRL test of CSF and/or abnormalities in protein or cell count) has been as high as 50% in some recently reported series of patients.[2]

Increasing experience has suggested that the temporal course of syphilis may be accelerated in HIV-positive individuals, with the result that the various forms of neurosyphilis occur earlier during the course of infection than in immunocompetent (HIV-negative) individuals.[5] The basic presentations of both meningovascular syphilis and acute syphilitic meningitis are generally similar to those found in HIV-negative individuals (see Chapter 11). One exception to this rule is the increased frequency with which syphilitic cranial nerve dysfunction, particularly of the optic nerve, occurs in HIV-positive individuals. Ocular syphilis may present as uveitis, chorioretinitis, optic perineuritis and optic neuritis.[12] Nearly 80% of HIV-positive patients with evidence of ocular syphilis develop co-existing syphilitic meningitis.[12] Conversely, approximately 40% to 50% of HIV-positive patients with neurosyphilis develop evidence of syphilitic eye disease.[7] In addition, we have been impressed with the frequency with which meningovascular syphilis initially presents as an acute stroke, often involving small vessels supplying the brainstem,[6,8,15] in HIV-positive individuals.

Treatment

Most physicians who regularly treat HIV-positive patients with syphilis have adopted an aggressive stance to therapy. In treating HIV-positive patients with syphilis, we routinely use recommended treatment regimens for neurosyphilis (e.g., 12 to 24 million units of intravenous penicillin G sodium per day is administered as 2 to 4 million units every 4 hours for a 10- to 14-day course). In an alternative therapeutic regimen, probably equally efficacious, 2 g of ceftriaxone is administered intravenously every 12 hours for a 10- to 14-day course. We also treat patients with diphenhydramine hydrochloride (Benadryl) (50 mg daily) and prednisone (60 mg daily) for 3 days as prophylaxis against a Jarisch-Herxheimer reaction. Ideally, patients should show a fourfold decline in serum VDRL titer within 6 months and an eightfold decline within 12 months of completing therapy.[3] It appears, however, that HIV-positive patients may show slower serologic declines than their HIV-negative counterparts.[10,16] CSF pleocytosis should disappear within 6 months, although protein elevations and reactivity with VDRL testing of CSF may persist for a longer period.[10] We monitor serum VDRL test results at monthly intervals for the first 3 months following therapy, and then every 3 months thereafter. CSF should be checked after 6 months and again at 6-month intervals until it normalizes.[10] A particularly disturbing feature of the treatment of neurosyphilis in HIV-positive patients is the failure and relapse rate, which approaches 20% to 30% regardless of the regimen employed.[2] This may reflect the fact that adequate treatment of neurosyphilis requires not only appropriate antibiotic therapy but also a functional immune system.

References

1. Davis LE and Schmitt JW: Clinical significance of cerebrospinal fluid tests for neurosyphilis. Ann Neurol 25:50–55, 1989.
2. Dowell ME, Ross PG, Musher DM, et al: Response of latent syphilis or neurosyphilis to ceftriaxone therapy in persons infected with human immunodeficiency virus. Am J Med 93:481–488, 1992.
3. Hook EW and Marra CM: Acquired syphilis in adults. N Engl J Med 326:1060–1069, 1992.
4. Jaffe HW and Kabins SA: Examination of cerebrospinal fluid in patients with syphilis. Rev Infect Dis 4(Suppl 2):S842–S847, 1982.
5. Johns DR, Tierney M, and Felsenstein D: Alteration in the natural history of neurosyphilis by concurrent infection with the human immunodeficiency virus. N Engl J Med 315:1569–1572, 1987.
6. Johns DR, Tierney M, and Parker SW: Pure motor hemiplegia due to meningovascular neurosyphilis. Arch Neurol 44:1062–1065, 1987.
7. Katz DA and Berger JR: Neurosyphilis in acquired immunodeficiency syndrome. Arch Neurol 46:895–898, 1989.
8. Labauge R, Pages M, Tourniaire D, et al: Infarctus pontique, syphilis nerveuse et infection par le VIH. Rev Neurol (Paris) 147:406–408, 1991.
9. Lukehart SA, Hook EW, Baker-Zander SA, et al: Invasion of the central nervous system by *Treponema pallidum*: Implications for diagnosis and therapy. Ann Intern Med 109:855–862, 1988.
10. Marra CM: Syphilis and human immunodeficiency virus infection. Semin Neurol 12:43–50, 1992.
11. Matlow AG and Rachlis AR: Syphilis serology in human immunodeficiency virus infected patients with symptomatic neurosyphilis: Case report and review. Rev Infect Dis 12:703–707, 1990.
12. McLeish WM, Pulido JS, Holland S, et al: The ocular manifestations of syphilis in the human immunodeficiency virus type 1–infected host. Ophthalmology 97:196–203, 1990.
13. Musher DM: Syphilis, neurosyphilis, penicillin, and AIDS. J Infect Dis 163:1201–1206, 1991.
14. Musher DM, Hamill RJ, and Baughn RE: Effect of human immunodeficiency virus (HIV) infection on the course of syphilis and on the response to treatment. Ann Intern Med 113:872–881, 1990.
15. Rosenberg NL and Hughes RL: Angiography in pure motor hemiparesis due to meningovascular syphilis (letter). Arch Neurol 46:10–11, 1989.
16. Telzak EE, Greenberg MSZ, Harrison J, et al: Syphilis treatment response in HIV-infected individuals. AIDS 5:591–595, 1991.

Chapter 12

PARASITIC AND RICKETTSIAL INFECTIONS OF THE NERVOUS SYSTEM

James F. Bale, Jr., M.D.

PROTOZOA
CESTODES
NEMATODES
TREMATODES (FLUKES)
ROCKY MOUNTAIN SPOTTED FEVER
CAT-SCRATCH DISEASE

This chapter summarizes the neurologic complications of several different infestations or infections, including parasitic disorders, Rocky Mountain spotted fever, and cat-scratch disease. Although many of the parasitic diseases discussed in this chapter constitute medical curiosities in the United States or western Europe, certain disorders, such as malaria, schistosomiasis, and trypanosomiasis, constitute serious public health issues for millions of persons throughout many areas of Asia, Africa, and Latin America. More than 40 species of protozoa and over 100 different helminths can potentially infect humans,[143] and many directly invade the nervous system and produce neurologic dysfunction.

Because physicians in developed nations such as the United States infrequently encounter parasite-induced neurologic disorders, the treating physician must carefully pursue historical clues regarding the patient's age, travel history, dietary habits, or national ori-

gin. To accomplish this effectively, physicians must possess a basic knowledge regarding the worldwide epidemiology of infectious diseases.[86a]

The acquired immune deficiency syndrome (AIDS) has influenced substantially the epidemiology or clinical presentation of several disorders discussed in this and other chapters. Patients with AIDS have a well-established propensity to develop cerebral toxoplasmosis, a complication that may respond favorably to medical therapy. Patients with AIDS are also at risk for disseminated cat-scratch disease, although neurologic complications are uncommon.

The diagnostic evaluation, treatment, and prevention of parasitic disorders continues to be an arena of considerable change,[3,136,221] reflecting development of novel diagnostic procedures such as the polymerase chain reaction (PCR),[134a] new antimicrobial agents, and changing patterns of drug resistance. Consequently, the treating physician should consult local or regional public health officials when unusual parasitic disorders are encountered. In addition, the Centers for Disease Control (CDC) in Atlanta, Georgia (phone numbers are contained in the appropriate sections of the chapter) is a valuable resource for consultation.

PROTOZOA

Toxoplasma gondii

BIOLOGY AND EPIDEMIOLOGY

Toxoplasma gondii, an obligate intracellular parasite, infects birds and most mammals worldwide, but wild and domestic cats serve as the principal host.[60,102] Ingested orally, *T. gondii* replicates in the feline gastrointestinal tract, producing trophozoites, and is subsequently excreted in feces as oocysts. After acute infection, cats can shed millions of oocysts daily for 1 to 3 weeks. The oocysts later transform extracorporeally into infectious sporulated forms, a process that depends on favorable ambient conditions. Oocysts can remain dormant in soil for as long as 1 year.

Other mammals, including humans, usually acquire *T. gondii* via the oral route. Domestic meat-producing animals, such as sheep, pigs, and cattle, ingest infectious organisms, and after a proliferative phase, tissue cysts of *T. gondii* can be identified at many sites, such as in brain and skeletal muscle.[102] Carnivores, including humans, become infected by consuming cyst-containing meat from infected animals. Direct ingestion of infectious oocysts from cat feces or contaminated soils also contributes to transmission and presumably accounts for *T. gondii* infection among vegetarians. *T. gondii* can also be acquired congenitally,[37,45,46] and rarely via blood transfusion, organ transplantation,[122] or laboratory contamination.

Seroepidemiologic studies indicate that humans throughout the world have evidence of prior *T. gondii* infection. Infection rates vary considerably, according to factors such as age, geographic location, and dietary practices. Using the toxoplasma dye test, Feldman observed seroprevalence rates ranging from 4% among Navajo Indians to 68% among inhabitants of Tahiti.[58-60] The overall incidence of *T. gondii* infection in the United States is 0.25% to 1.2% annually among persons between the ages of 15 and 35 years.[189] Among women of childbearing age, rates between 1.1 and 1.3 infections per 1000 pregnant women have been observed in Norway,[194] and an incidence of nearly 10 per 1000 pregnant women has been reported in France.[40,45,46] The United States rate of approximately 1 congenitally infected infant per 1000 live births suggests that over 3000 infants with congenital toxoplasmosis are born annually in this country alone.[189]

CLINICAL DISORDERS

Congenital Infection. When acute toxoplasma infection occurs in a pregnant woman, the parasite can disseminate hematogenously to the placenta and fetus. Timing of maternal infection plays a critical role in transmission of the parasite and in fetal outcome. Epidemiologic studies indicate that transmission rates range from 30% to 45% for the entire gestation, with the rate of transmission highest during the third trimester.[40,45,46] First-trimester infections may lead to spontaneous abortion, whereas infections during the second through sixth months often produce fetal death or severe disease. By contrast, infections during the third trimester are usually subclinical.[45]

As one would predict based on the above observations regarding transmission and fetal outcome, most congenital toxoplasma infections do not cause symptoms in the infected newborn.[45,160] A small proportion of infected neonates, approximately 10%, have overt symptoms at birth with hepatosplenomegaly, jaundice, and rash, features that mimic those of congenital viral infection or erythroblastosis fetalis. Most of these infants also have central nervous system (CNS) involvement, consisting of hydrocephalus or microcephaly, chorioretinitis, or cerebral calcifications.[37,100,160] An additional group of congenitally infected infants, approximately 15%, have isolated chorioretinitis.[51,82]

In a prospective study, Desmonts and

Couvreur identified primary *T. gondii* infection in 183 pregnant women, a rate of 6.3 per 100 pregnancies.[45] Of 59 infants with definite congenital toxoplasmosis (an overall transmission rate of approximately 35%), 9 (15%) had adverse outcomes (death or severe disease), 11 (19%) had mild disease, and 39 (66%) had subclinical infections. Severe disease was observed in congenitally infected infants only when maternal infections occurred during the first two trimesters, but these authors emphasized that long-term observation was necessary to confirm that infants lacked sequelae attributable to toxoplasmosis.

The same authors also reviewed their experience with 300 patients with serologically confirmed, symptomatic congenital toxoplasmosis and observed ocular involvement in 76% of the children and neurologic disorders in 52%.[37] Approximately one third had intracranial calcifications, and 26% had hydrocephalus or microcephaly. Ocular disorders, principally chorioretinitis, can be evident at birth or develop subsequently in infants who were asymptomatic as neonates.[51,190,215] Chorioretinitis, bilateral in most infants, usually consists of a large, posterior lesion with vitreal spillover.[51,82] Additional ophthalmologic features associated with congenital toxoplasmosis include blindness, strabismus, amblyopia, and, rarely, microphthalmia.[82,190]

Congenital toxoplasmosis can be strongly suspected when an infant exhibits the clinical triad of chorioretinitis, hydrocephalus, and intracranial calcifications. The differential diagnosis consists primarily of other congenital infections grouped as the TORCH syndrome, an acronym referring to the causative organisms *T. gondii, O*ther, *R*ubella, *C*ytomegalovirus (CMV), and *Herpes simplex* viruses.[16a,138a] Common features of this syndrome include chorioretinitis, splenomegaly, jaundice, hepatomegaly, microcephaly, or petechial rash.

Congenital CMV infection and congenital toxoplasmosis share several clinical features, including chorioretinitis and intracranial calcifications. However, hydrocephalus occurs more commonly after congenital *T. gondii* infection, whereas microcephaly and sensorineural hearing loss suggest CMV infection.[16] Aicardi's syndrome,[213] a noninfectious disorder associated with lacunar retinal lesions, microcephaly, and psychomotor retardation, can be distinguished from toxoplasmosis by the presence of costovertebral anomalies and agenesis of the corpus callosum.

Infants with disseminated congenital toxoplasmosis can have thrombocytopenia, elevated serum bilirubin levels, anemia, or elevated serum transaminases. The cerebrospinal fluid (CSF) or neuroradiographic findings vary and depend on the nature of the cerebral involvement. Common CSF abnormalities include xanthochromia, an elevated protein content, and a pleocytosis consisting of lymphocytes or neutrophils.[100] Computed tomography (CT), more sensitive than plain skull radiography, often reveals hydrocephalus (obstructive or ex vacuo), parenchymal lesions, or intracranial calcifications that involve the periventricular regions, basal ganglia, or parenchyma diffusely.[47] These abnormalities correspond, at least in part, to the timing of maternal toxoplasma infection.

The primary neuropathologic lesion associated with congenital toxoplasmosis consists of a granulomatous meningoencephalitis.[5] On gross examination the brain has multifocal areas of cerebral softening, thickened pia-arachnoid, and dystrophic calcifications. Hydrocephalus results from aqueductal stenosis or ex vacuo from tissue destruction. Rarely, the destructive process is sufficiently severe to produce hydranencephaly. Microscopic examination of neural tissues reveals necrosis, mononuclear inflammation, calcification, and occasionally encysted or free parasites (Fig. 12–1).

The microbiologic diagnosis of congenital toxoplasmosis can be established using serologic studies or by

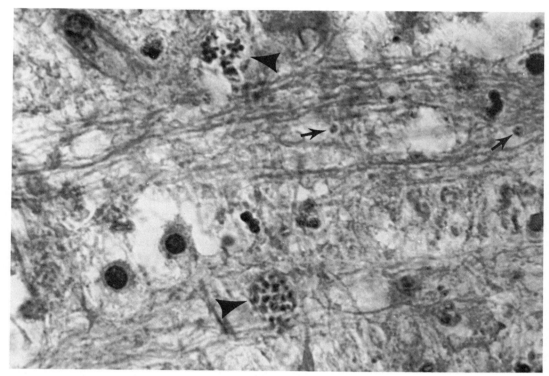

Figure 12–1. *Toxoplasma gondii* within cysts *(arrowheads)* or free *(arrows)* within the cerebral parenchyma of a congenitally infected infant (hematoxylin and eosin; original magnification ×400).

identifying organisms in tissues or body fluids such as CSF.[124] Of the various serologic assays, the Sabin-Feldman dye test, which measures immunoglobulin G (IgG), has gradually been supplanted by other methods, including enzyme-linked immunosorbent assay (ELISA), indirect hemagglutination, latex agglutination, immunofluorescence, or complement fixation, that allow quantitative or qualitative assay of either IgG or immunoglobulin M (IgM).[124,139,216] Congenital infection is supported by detection of specific antitoxoplasma IgM or persistence of toxoplasma IgG in the infant's sera as compared with paired maternal sera. Antitoxoplasma IgM becomes detectable within 2 weeks of infection and typically persists for approximately 6 months.[139] The antitoxoplasma IgG level peaks approximately 4 to 8 weeks after infection and persists indefinitely.

Acquired Infection. In immunocompetent children and adults, acquired toxoplasmosis rarely causes recognizable illness.[102,159] Some infected persons experience a self-limited disorder characterized by lymphadenopathy, fever, maculopapular rash, malaise, myalgias, hepatosplenomegaly, and, occasionally, pneumonia or myocarditis.[59,102] Eosinophils or atypical lymphocytes may be seen in the peripheral smear, the latter an additional similarity between acquired toxoplasmosis and mononucleosis syndromes induced by the Epstein-Barr virus or CMV.[16,87,195]

Rarely, acquired *T. gondii* infection causes acute, potentially fatal CNS disorders in otherwise healthy children and adults. Among the 45 cases of CNS toxoplasmosis reviewed by Townsend and colleagues,[201] approximately half had no identified predisposing medical condition. These patients ranged in age from 4½ to 82 years, and the spectrum of CNS involvement varied from diffuse encephalopathy or encephalitis to single or multiple mass lesions. CSF findings consisted of normal or mildly increased protein content, normal glucose concentration, and a lymphocytic pleocytosis ranging from 0 to 500 cells/mm³. Electroencephalograms (EEGs), when obtained, usually revealed diffuse or focal abnormalities.

T. gondii can be a particularly virulent pathogen in children or adults with impaired cell-mediated immunity.[167,201] Individuals at risk for serious toxoplasmosis include patients with malignancies, individuals undergoing immunosuppressive therapy for organ transplantation or connective tissue disorders, and, most recently, persons with AIDS.[64,110,130,141,178] In such patients, toxoplasmosis reflects newly acquired infection or recrudescence of latent T. gondii infestation. T. gondii infects at least 5% to 15% of patients with AIDS[131,141,153] and produces diffuse meningoencephalitis,[64,110,141] focal or multifocal mass lesions,[55,141] or, rarely, myelitis.[130]

CNS toxoplasmosis in AIDS patients begins subacutely with headache, lethargy, seizures, focal neurologic abnormalities, and signs of increased intracranial pressure.[77,141,153] In a multicenter review of 68 histologically confirmed cases of toxoplasma encephalitis in AIDS patients, 44% of the patients had headache, 37% were disoriented, 35% had seizures, and 58% had focal neurologic signs, consisting of hemiparesis, ataxia, or impaired speech or vision.[77] Abnormalities were identified on CT in 58 patients (92% of those studied by CT). Many patients had intercurrent infections with other opportunistic agents, including CMV, Mycobacterium tuberculosis, Pneumocystis carinii, M. avium-intracellulare, Cryptococcus neoformans, herpes simplex virus, or varicella-zoster virus.

In AIDS patients with neurologic signs or symptoms, the diagnostic and microbiologic evaluation is necessarily extensive.[54,141,178] Because many secondary complications, including CNS toxoplasmosis, produce macroscopic CNS lesions, neuroimaging studies, particularly CT (Fig. 12–2), have an important role.[55,64] Additional useful diagnostic studies include examination of the CSF and, possibly, brain biopsy. Toxoplasma infection is supported serologically by a positive antitoxoplasma IgM, a dye test exceeding 1:1024, or a fourfold or greater rise in antitoxoplasma IgG levels and can be confirmed by demonstrating organisms histologically in tissues or CSF. Potasman and co-workers detected intrathecal production of antibodies against T. gondii in patients with toxoplasma encephalitis and AIDS,[153] suggesting that analysis of paired CSF and serum samples has diagnostic utility. The PCR has been used to detect toxoplasma nucleic acids,[81a,168a] indicating a potential role for PCR in the diagnosis of CNS toxoplasmosis.

THERAPY

Several different therapeutic strategies have been developed to address the problem of congenital toxoplasmosis.[16a] In France, an endemic area where prenatal screening for toxoplasma infection is mandatory, the diagnosis of congenital infection has been achieved prenatally by detecting parasites or antitoxoplasma IgM in fetal blood samples.[40,46] Among 278 pregnant women at risk for fetal infection, Desmonts and co-workers identified nine congenitally infected fetuses.[46] These pregnancies were terminated, and toxoplasma encephalitis was confirmed histologically and parasitologically in the eight cases available for study. The false-negative rate for prenatal screening was less than 0.5% (1 case of congenital toxoplasmosis among 209 cases with negative results). A subsequent report from the same center suggested that maternal antiparasitic therapy using spiramycin and/or pyrimethamine plus sul-

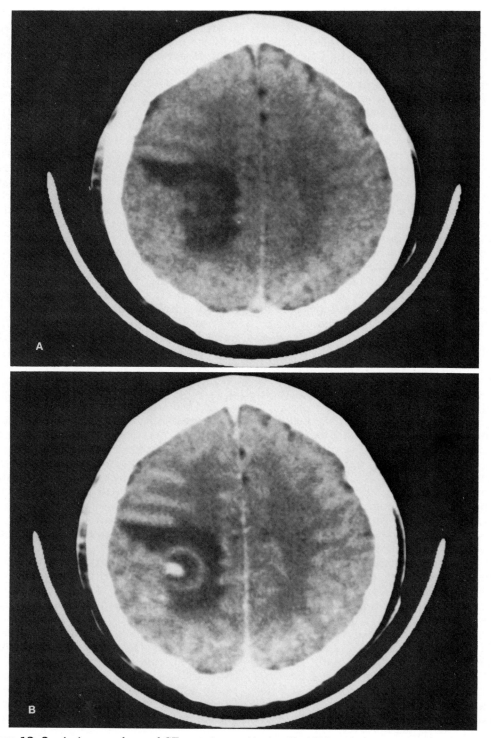

Figure 12–2. *A*, An unenhanced CT scan in a patient with AIDS and presumed CNS toxoplasmosis shows a large, hypodense lesion of the right parietal white matter. *B*, The corresponding contrast CT scan demonstrates ring enhancement, a common finding in CNS toxoplasmosis.   *Continued*

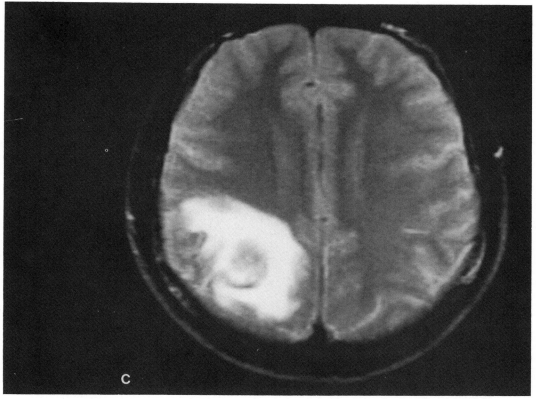

Figure 12–2 *continued.* *C*, T_2-weighted MRI performed on the same day confirms focal white matter edema. The clinical and neuroimaging abnormalities improved considerably during anti-toxoplasma drug therapy.

fadoxine or sulfadiazine reduced the fetal infection rate and improved the outcome of live-born infants.[40]

In the United States and other countries where prenatal screening for toxoplasma infection has not been performed routinely, treatment of congenitally infected infants remains problematic.[100,125] Although no randomized studies regarding the effectiveness of postnatal antimicrobial therapy of congenitally acquired infections have been reported, therapy with pyrimethamine, 1 mg/kg per day, and sulfadiazine, 100 mg/kg per day, has been advocated[3,100] (Table 12–1). Folinic acid must be given concurrently to diminish the marrow suppressive effects of pyrimethamine and sulfadiazine. One U.S. study suggested that postnatal treatment improves outcome.[196a]

The majority of infants with congenital toxoplasmosis and neurologic symptoms at birth have substantial long-term disabilities.[37,47,99,100] Among children diagnosed with congenital toxoplasmosis during the first year of life, Couvreur and Desmonts reported that only 14% had intelligence quotients of 90 or higher.[37] Progressive hydrocephalus, often requiring shunt placement, and seizures, partial or generalized, are additional common sequelae. In one survey of 31 infants with congenital toxoplasmosis, nearly 40% had seizures, beginning at a median age of 16 months.[47]

When acquired CNS toxoplasmosis in older children or adults is proven or strongly suspected by clinical or radiographic findings, therapy should consist of pyrimethamine, given as a loading dose of 100 to 200 mg daily for the first 1 or 2 days followed by 25 to 100

Table 12–1 DRUG THERAPY OF PARASITIC DISORDERS

Disorder	Drug	Regimen
Toxoplasmosis*	Pyrimethamine†	Adult: 100 to 200 mg as a loading dose, followed by 25 to 100 mg daily Child: 1 mg/kg per day (max. 25 mg/day)
	plus Sulfadiazine	Adult: 2 to 6 g/day Child: 100 mg/kg per day
Amebiasis	Metronidazole	Adult: 750 mg 3 times daily for 10 days Child: 35 to 50 mg/kg per day divided in 3 doses for 10 days
	followed by Iodoquinol	Adult: 650 mg 3 times daily for 20 days Child: 30 to 40 mg/kg per day divided in 3 doses for 20 days
Amebic meningitis (*Naegleria*)	Amphotericin B	Adult or Child: 1 mg/kg per day‡
Trypanosomiasis—African		
Hematogenous stage	Suramin	Adult: 100 mg IV test dose; if tolerated, 1 g IV on days 1, 3, 7, 14, and 21 Child: 20 mg/kg per day IV using similar test dose and schedule
Neurologic stage	Melarsoprol	Adult: 2 to 3.6 mg/kg per day IV given on 3 consecutive days, followed in 1 week by 3.6 mg/kg per day for 3 more days. Repeat in 10 to 21 days. Child: 18 to 25 mg/kg total divided in 9 or 10 doses over 1 month (see text)
Trypanosomiasis—American	Nifurtimox	Adult: 8 to 10 mg/kg per day divided (four times daily) for 120 days Child: Varies with age (see text)
Cysticercosis	Praziquantel	Adult or child: 50 mg/kg per day divided in 3 doses for 14 days
Visceral larva migrans§	Diethylcarbamazine	Adult or child: 6 mg/kg per day divided 3 times daily for 7 to 10 days
	or Thiabendazole	Adult or child: 50 mg/kg per day divided twice daily for 5 days (max. 3 g/day)
Trichinosis§	Mebendazole	Adult or child: 200 to 400 mg 3 times daily for 3 days, then 400 to 500 mg 3 times daily for 10 days
Strongyloides	Thiabendazole	Adult or child: 50 mg/kg per day divided twice daily for 2 days (max. 3 g/day)
Schistosomiasis	Praziquantel	Adult or child: 40 to 60 mg/kg per day divided 2 to 3 times daily for 1 day
Paragonimiasis	Praziquantel	Adult or child: 75 mg/kg per day divided 3 times daily for 2 days

*Duration of therapy variable (see text).
†Folinic acid, 5 to 50 mg, should be given concurrently.
‡Duration of therapy uncertain. Consider both intravenous (IV) and intrathecal therapy.
§Corticosteroids should be considered for severe cases.
Sources: Adapted from Abramowicz[3] and from the Report of the Committee on Infectious Diseases, Ed. 22: Peter G, Hall CB, Lepow ML, McCracken GH, Phillips CF (eds). The American Academy of Pediatrics, 1991, pp 589–605.

mg daily thereafter, and sulfadiazine, approximately 2 to 6 g daily.[3,100,110] Folinic acid should be given concurrently at a dose of 5 to 50 mg/day. The exact duration of therapy depends on the clinical and CT response; patients typically require 4 or more weeks of therapy. Patients with AIDS require lifelong maintenance therapy consisting of pyrimethamine 25 to 50 mg/day and sulfadiazine 2 to 3 g/day.[77,141]

The majority of patients treated with pyrimethamine and sulfadiazine exhibit some drug-related toxicity, usually consisting of thrombocytopenia, leukopenia, or skin rash. Modifications of the drug regimen may be necessary. Clindamycin, in doses ranging from 1.2 to 2.4 g/day, has been used effectively in patients who have sulfonamide hypersensitivity or relapse during conventional therapy with pyrimethamine and sulfadiazine.[165]

The outcome of acquired CNS toxoplasmosis depends greatly on the underlying condition. Although CNS toxoplasmosis can be fatal even in normal hosts, most immunocompetent patients survive when treated with pyrimethamine and sulfadiazine. By contrast, overall outcome in immunocompromised patients is considerably less favorable. In patients with AIDS and toxoplasma encephalitis reviewed by Haverkos,[77] 92% died, although not all deaths were directly attributable to toxoplasmosis. Patients who were alert when therapy was initiated fared better than those with altered consciousness. A subsequent study reported more encouraging results, noting improvement during acute therapy in 31 of 35 (89%) patients with AIDS and CNS toxoplasmosis and complete resolution in 14 of 24 patients (58%) after 2 or more months of antitoxoplasma therapy.[110]

Amebae

BIOLOGY AND EPIDEMIOLOGY

Various species of amebae, single-cell organisms, infect humans worldwide,
and at least three, *Entamoeba histolytica*, *Naegleria fowleri*, and *Acanthamoeba* species, can invade the CNS.[18,32,36,39,63] *E. histolytica*, which causes amebic dysentery, hepatic abscess, and, very rarely, CNS abscess, produces considerable morbidity and mortality in developing nations with poor sanitation.[72] Walsh estimated that at least 40,000 deaths occur annually from amebiasis, ranking it third behind malaria and schistosomiasis in numbers of parasite-induced deaths.[207]

Epidemiologic surveys indicate that the prevalence of *E. histolytica* infection, as measured by stool sampling, exceeds 30% in many regions of the world.[72] In Mexico, an endemic area with a high rate of invasive disease, *E. histolytica* causes approximately 15% of the diarrheal illnesses requiring hospitalization.[48] Infection spreads from person to person by the fecal-oral route, via contaminated water, or as a sexually transmitted disease. In developed nations such as the United States, *E. histolytica* has infected travelers to endemic regions, military personnel, residents of chronic care facilities, and homosexual men.[9]

Naegleria and *Acanthamoeba*, freeliving amebae, can be detected in soils or water and contribute to the microbiologic flora of the human respiratory tract.[207a] In one study, various amebae, including *Naegleria*, were detected in the nasal passages of 4.2% of 1250 persons living in Zaria, Nigeria.[2] *Naegleria* frequently inhabit warm, stagnant fresh water, particularly waters populated by coliform bacteria, throughout the southern United States,[211] and human infections have been reported in the United States[31d] as well as in Australia, Africa, and Europe. *Naegleria* enter the CNS directly by invading the nasal mucosa and penetrating the cribriform plate. *Acanthamoeba* species, common soil contaminants, presumably infect humans via contact with the skin, lungs, or gastrointestinal tract and reach the CNS hematogenously.

CLINICAL DISORDERS

Entamoeba histolytica. Most *E. histolytica* infections do not produce symptoms, a feature related to strain virulence.[9,72,103] Approximately 10% of infected persons experience gastrointestinal illnesses, ranging from mild, watery to severe, bloody diarrhea. Severe cases can be associated with fever, tenesmus, abdominal pain, or signs of gastrointestinal tract obstruction. Invasive disease of other organs, such as the liver, can develop several days later or be a late complication months or years after dysentery.[72] However, as many as 50% of patients with invasive disease lack an apparent history of gastrointestinal amebiasis.

Although amebic dysentery occurs commonly throughout many regions of the world, CNS amebiasis remains an exceptionally rare complication.[4,18,85,146] Adams and Macleod reported only one probable case of amebic brain abscess among over 2000 South African patients with invasive amebiasis.[4] Two cases of CNS disease were reported in US residents who had signs of hepatic or intestinal amebiasis but had no history of travel outside the eastern United States.[18] CNS amebic cerebritis or abscess usually affects patients who have also had liver abscesses and results from hematogenous dissemination of amebae. Signs indicating CNS involvement include headache, altered sensorium, fever, convulsions, and focal neurologic deficits.

Naegleria and Acanthamoeba. Symptomatic infections due to *Naegleria fowleri* or *Acanthamoeba* species typically involve the CNS. *Naegleria* produce primary amebic meningoencephalitis,[13,32,41,63] a fulminant illness that usually occurs in previously healthy children or young adults during the summer months. The disorder begins abruptly, heralded by headache, stiff neck, vomiting, and fever. Coma ensues rapidly, and occasional patients convulse. A history of aquatic activities, swimming, diving, or waterskiing, during the preceding week is usually elicited, although cases without an aquatic exposure have been reported,[185] particularly in arid regions where *Naegleria* may be a dust-borne pathogen.[2] Despite supportive and antimicrobial therapy, the disease progresses to death in virtually all cases.

Acanthamoeba species produce a subacute CNS disorder and frequently affect patients with underlying medical conditions.[36,39,71,86,120] Martinez reviewed 15 such cases and identified predisposing factors that included broad-spectrum antibiotic or immunosuppressive therapy, radiation therapy, alcoholism, or pregnancy.[120] Typical clinical features consist of altered mental status, convulsions, headache, fever, and focal neurologic deficits, such as aphasia or hemiparesis. The disease usually progresses more slowly than primary amebic encephalitis and produces a granulomatous encephalitis that simulates the clinical course of a CNS neoplasm.[144] Rapidly fatal cases have also been reported.[71]

LABORATORY FINDINGS AND DIAGNOSIS

Patients with amebic CNS infections may have peripheral leukocytosis, eosinophilia, or elevations of serum transaminases. The CSF abnormalities in primary amebic encephalitis due to *Naegleria* usually mimic those of bacterial disease, consisting of a neutrophilic pleocytosis, increased protein content, and diminished glucose content.[41] By contrast, the CSF of *Acanthamoeba* infection appears "viral" in character, with a lymphocytic pleocytosis, modest elevations of protein content, and normal or low glucose content.[123] CT or magnetic resonance imaging (MRI) can reveal cerebritis, cerebral edema, brain abscess (single or multiple), or enhancing mass lesions.[149]

The parasitologic diagnosis of amebic infections can be established by detecting serologic responses or identifying organisms in tissues or body fluids. Cysts or trophozoites of *E. histolytica* can be detected in feces, and indirect hemagglutination titers exceeding 1:256 suggest invasive disease. Virulent and avirulent strains of *E. histolytica* can be distinguished by their isoenzyme patterns (zymodemes).[9,72] The diagnosis of *Acanthamoeba* infection is usually made histologically by examining biopsy or autopsy specimens. In primary amebic encephalitis, *Naegleria* can be identified on wet-mount or stained preparations of CSF.[31d] Serologic tests of *Acanthamoeba* or *Naegleria* or examination of CSF samples for *Naegleria* can be performed by the CDC, Atlanta, GA.

The neuropathologic features of primary amebic meningoencephalitis consist of cerebral edema, purulent meningeal exudate, and hemorrhagic necrosis of the olfactory nerves, inferior frontal and temporal lobes, brainstem, cerebellum, and occasionally the cervical spinal cord.[41] *Naegleria* trophozoites can be identified by light microscopy in the meningeal exudate using hematoxylin and eosin stains. In *Acanthamoeba* infections, the characteristic lesion consists of a necrotizing granulomatous encephalitis, and meningeal involvement tends to be less extensive.[120] Light microscopic examination of cerebral tissues usually reveals trophozoites and cysts, particularly in perivascular regions.

TREATMENT

Treatment of amebic CNS infections generally remains less than satisfactory (see Table 12–1).[3,41,120] Metronidazole, an antimicrobial agent that penetrates brain readily, has been used with some success in patients with liver or brain abscesses caused by *E. histolytica*.[154] Patients with suspected or proven *Naegleria* meningoencephalitis should be treated aggressively with amphotericin B.[31d] One US survivor received this drug plus miconazole intravenously and intrathecally and rifampin orally.[162,171a] Sulfadiazine or ketoconazole may be of benefit in *Acanthamoeba* infections.[123,144] Cure of *Acanthamoeba* CNS infections has

been described using surgical and antiparasitic therapy, but *Acanthamoeba* infections, like those of *Naegleria,* are frequently fatal.

Malaria

BIOLOGY AND EPIDEMIOLOGY

Despite more than 3 decades of global eradication programs, malaria still causes considerable morbidity and mortality among inhabitants of endemic regions and remains a constant threat to travelers to these areas.[221] As recently as 1983, it was estimated that malaria affected as many as 300 million humans in the world per year and contributed to the deaths of more than 1 million persons annually in tropical Africa alone.[223] The endemic region for malaria currently encompasses most of Africa, Asia, and Latin America. In the United States, indigenous malaria was eradicated in the 1940s, but the disease continues to be imported into the United States and other nonendemic countries by immigrants, military personnel, and visitors to endemic regions.[31,112,223]

Four species of obligate intracellular protozoa in the genus *Plasmodium (P. malariae, P. ovale, P. falciparum,* and *P. vivax)* infect humans and produce malaria. The protozoa vary somewhat in their geographic distribution, and *P. falciparum,* the principal cause of cerebral malaria,[49,221] is particularly prevalent in Africa. Humans acquire malaria via several mechanisms: (1) from the bite of an infected female anopheline mosquito,[223] (2) after blood transfusion from an infected donor, (3) congenitally,[157] or (4) by sharing infected needles. After inoculation, the *Plasmodium* sporozoites travel hematogenously to the liver where they infect and multiply in hepatic parenchymal cells. Within approximately 2 weeks numerous merozoites egress from the liver into the circulation where they infect erythrocytes. In severe *P. falciparum* infections, 5% or more of the circulating erythrocytes contain parasites.[221]

CLINICAL DISORDERS

The incubation period for malaria ranges from approximately 6 to 16 days.[161] During the prodromal phase, patients may have vague constitutional complaints that include headache, malaise, abdominal pain, or myalgias. Fever, rigor, and chills, the cardinal signs of malaria, ensue and are usually accompanied by diaphoresis, intense headache, backache, cough, tachycardia, nausea, or vomiting.[221] Chills and fever, 40°C or higher, typically occur in paroxysms at varying intervals, and patients may seem relatively well in between. Physical signs at this stage can include hepatosplenomegaly, rash, or jaundice.

Cerebral malaria, the most common complication of severe malaria due to P. falciparum, usually begins abruptly with generalized convulsions and an altered level of consciousness.[7,49,161,221] The neurologic examination typically discloses diffuse and symmetric signs of hyperreflexia with flexor or extensor posturing in severely ill patients. Occasional patients have focal signs consisting of hemiparesis, monoparesis, or cranial nerve palsies.[7] Retinal hemorrhages have been reported in approximately 15% of cases, but papilledema or other signs of increased intracranial pressure are unusual.[221] Most neurologic symptoms persist for 24 to 72 hours and proceed either to death or to complete recovery. Severe malaria due to P. falciparum can be complicated by extreme hyperthermia, renal failure, pulmonary edema, hypovolemia, disseminated intravascular coagulopathy, or intercurrent infections.[221]

Several mechanisms have been proposed to explain the pathophysiology of severe malaria. Sequestration of infected erythrocytes presumably alters tissue perfusion or oxygenation and would account for most cerebral features, since sequestration is greatest within cerebral vasculature (Fig. 12–3). Overall cerebral blood flow is not altered, but elevations of CSF lactate levels in patients with severe coma suggest disturbances of CNS metabolic pathways.[221]

DIFFERENTIAL DIAGNOSIS

The differential diagnosis of cerebral malaria includes metabolic encephalopathies secondary to uremia, drugs or toxins, and meningitis or encephalitis due to viruses or bacteria.[221] Malaria can mimic typhoid fever, trypanosomiasis, or noninfectious disorders such as traumatic encephalopathy or brain tumor. Infants who acquire malaria congenitally or via blood transfusion may develop a sepsislike illness, with fever, lethargy, and decreased appetite, which mimics viral or bacterial diseases.[157] Disorders other than cerebral malaria should be considered when the patient exhibits prominent focal findings.[221]

LABORATORY FINDINGS

The laboratory findings of malaria vary according to the severity of the illness. Patients with severe malaria have anemia (hematocrit less than 20%), elevations of serum transaminase levels, mild hyponatremia (serum sodium concentrations ranging between 125 and 135 mEq/L), hypoglycemia, or thrombocytopenia.[221] The CSF is nearly always normal, although modest elevations of CSF protein content or mild pleocytosis can be compatible with cerebral malaria. CT of the head is usually normal.[221]

The parasitologic diagnosis can be established rapidly, specifically, and quantitatively by identifying parasites in thick smears of peripheral blood.[23,136] An experienced microscopist can detect as few as 1 infected cell per 10^6 erythrocytes, but parasites can be absent early in the course of infection. Thus, serial blood samples should be examined in patients with suspected malaria. The diagnosis of malaria can also be established serologically using indirect immunofluorescence or ELISAs,[23] but these tests are frequently negative in the early stages of infection. More re-

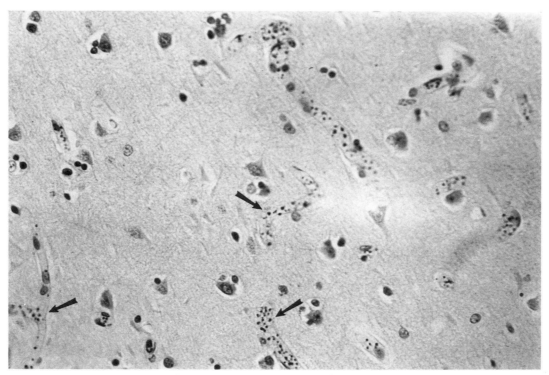

Figure 12–3. Cerebral tissues from a patient with *Plasmodium falciparum* malaria contain numerous parasites within cerebral vessels *(arrows)* (hematoxylin and eosin; original magnification ×160).

cently, nucleic acid hydridization methods have been applied to the diagnosis of malaria and have sensitivity that approaches that of microscopic examination of thick blood smears.[23,220]

PREVENTION AND TREATMENT

Strategies for the control of malaria must address several issues, including prevention of disease through chemoprophylaxis or physical measures, treatment of symptomatic malaria, and the emergence of antimicrobial resistance.[3,31,136,161,223] Clinicians should be aware that recommendations regarding malaria change periodically. Updated information regarding preventive or therapeutic strategies can be obtained from the Malaria Branch of the CDC [Malaria Hotline (404) 639-1610, 24-hour service].

As of March 1990, travelers to endemic regions where chloroquine-resis-

tant *P. falciparum* has not been reported should take chloroquine orally [adults: chloroquine phosphate salt 500 mg once per week; children: chloroquine phosphate salt 8.3 mg/kg once per week (to a maximum dose of 300 mg per week)] beginning 1 to 2 weeks before travel and continuing for 4 weeks after departure from the endemic region.[31,161] Although chloroquine may produce headache, gastrointestinal disturbance, blurred vision, pruritus, or dizziness, serious reactions are uncommon.[31]

Travelers to regions with chloroquine resistance, such as sub-Saharan Africa, South America, India, or southeast Asia, should take mefloquine.[31,31b,149a] Adults should take 250 mg once per week beginning 1 week before and for 4 weeks after travel in endemic areas. Childhood dosages are based on weight: 15 to 19 kg: ¼ tablet/week; 20 to 30 kg: ½ tablet/week; 31 to 45 kg: ¾ tablet/

week; > 45 kg: adult doses. Mefloquine is not recommended for pregnant women, children weighing less than 15 kg, persons with epilepsy or psychiatric disorders, persons taking beta-blockers or drugs that alter cardiac conduction, or persons requiring skilled fine motor coordination.[31] Alternatives to mefloquine include doxycycline or chloroquine [pyrimethamine–sulfadoxine (Fansidar) should be carried by persons who elect to use chloroquine in regions with chloroquine-resistant *P. falciparum*[31]]. Travelers should also use insect repellents [N,N-diethylmetatoluamide (DEET)], mosquito netting, and protective clothing.

Treatment for symptomatic *P. falciparum* malaria must be tailored to the severity of the disease and the likelihood of chloroquine resistance (Table 12–2).[65,149a,161,223] Therapy should begin with quinine or chloroquine orally unless the patient is unarousable or cannot swallow tablets. In severe malaria, patients can be treated with quinidine gluconate, 10 mg/kg as an intravenous loading dose (maximum 600 mg) over

1–2 hours, followed by a constant intravenous infusion of 0.02 mg/kg/min.[31c,132a] Therapy is continued intravenously for approximately 72 hours, followed by oral therapy as tolerated. Patients must be observed for other complications of malaria, including hypoglycemia, hypovolemia, hyponatremia, convulsions, or coagulopathy. Although quinidine gluconate is well-tolerated, patients require electrocardiographic monitoring during intravenous administration. Cinchonism, a syndrome characterized by tinnitus, nausea, and blurred vision can occur.

Trypanosomiasis

AFRICAN

Biology and Epidemiology. African trypanosomiasis, or sleeping sickness, a disease endemic within Africa between the latitudes of 15° north and 20° south, results from infection with the protozoan hemoflagellates *Trypanosoma brucei rhodesiense* or *T.*

Table 12–2 DRUG TREATMENT OF FALCIPARUM MALARIA

	Chloroquine-Sensitive	*Chloroquine Resistant*
If arousable	Chloroquine phosphate orally Adult: 600-mg base, then 300-mg base 6 hours later, then 300-mg base once per day for 2 days Child: 10-mg base/kg (max. 600-mg base), then 5-mg base/kg 6 hours later, then 5-mg/base/kg once per day for 2 days	Quinine sulfate orally Adult: 650 mg 3 times daily for 3 days Child: 25 mg/kg divided 3 times daily for 3 days *plus* Pyrimethamine-sulfadoxine (Fansidar) orally Adult: single dose of 3 tablets Child: <1 year– $\frac{1}{4}$ tablet 1 to 3 years– $\frac{1}{2}$ tablet 4 to 8 years– 1 tablet 9 to 14 years– 2 tablets as a single dose
If unarousable or cannot take oral medication	Quinidine gluconate IV Adult: 10 mg/kg loading dose IV (max. 600 mg) over 1 hour, then 0.02 mg/kg/min constant infusion until oral therapy with chloroquine is tolerated Child: Same as adult dose	Quinidine gluconate IV. (Same regimen as for chloroquine-sensitive strains, except that quinine sulfate in combination with pyrimethamine/sulfadoxine or mefloquine is used for oral therapy)[149a]

*Available in the United States from the Centers for Disease Control, Atlanta, Ga. Quinine sulfate can also be used for parenteral therapy of severe *P. falciparum* malaria.[161]

Sources: Adapted from Abramowicz,[3] Panisko and Keystone,[149a] Report of the Committee on Infectious Disease,[161] and World Health Organization.[221]

brucei gambiense.[43,118] Transmitted to humans by the bites of infected tsetse flies (genus *Glossina*), these pathogens produce several thousand cases of trypanosomiasis per year among inhabitants of endemic areas and constitute an important risk to travelers to these regions.[186] In the United States, one or two cases of African trypanosomiasis are reported annually among persons who have visited Africa or immigrated to the United States from endemic regions.[29,118,152,187]

T. brucei rhodesiense and *T. brucei gambiense* display important differences in their epidemiologic features and clinical consequences.[118,152,186] *T. brucei gambiense* usually infects humans in west-central Africa and is maintained by a human–tsetse fly–human transmission cycle. By contrast, *T. brucei rhodesiense* infection occurs more commonly in east-central Africa and involves wild animals, including bushbuck and hartebeest, as reservoirs.[217] Humans become infected with the metacyclic forms of trypanosoma contained within the saliva of the biting male or female tsetse fly. Organisms subsequently multiply in the skin and disseminate hematogenously or lymphatically. In rare instances, African trypanosomiasis has been acquired congenitally via maternal-fetal transmission.[118]

The incubation period of human African trypanosomiasis varies according to the form of disease and the origin of the infected host. Among native Africans, the rhodesian form has an incubation period ranging from 14 to 21 days, whereas symptoms of gambian trypanosomiasis may not appear for several weeks or even years.[6,118] Among Europeans and Americans, both forms cause acute disease with an incubation period ranging between 5 and 15 days.[50,152,186]

Clinical Manifestations. The clinical manifestations of African trypanosomiasis tend to parallel the human life cycle of the trypanosoma.[118,214] The initial signs, the trypanosoma chancre and skin lesions (pain, swelling, erythema, and nodule formation), reflect entry of organisms into the skin and local multiplication. The chancre develops in approximately 70% of infected Europeans but is infrequently reported in native Africans.[50,118] Skin nodules persist for approximately 2 weeks and usually resolve completely.

During the subsequent hematogenous and lymphatic dissemination of trypanosoma, patients experience high fever, headache, and lymphadenopathy, particularly of the posterior cervical chain during gambian trypanosomiasis (Winterbottom's sign). In acute rhodesian trypanosomiasis, neurologic symptoms, resulting from trypanosomal invasion of the CNS, appear within 2 to 6 weeks and consist of insomnia, severe headache, loss of concentration, personality changes, and altered sensation.[118] Patients also lose weight and exhibit tachycardia, a sign of myocarditis.

In chronic gambian trypanosomiasis, neurologic complications may not appear for months or years after initial infection.[6] Such patients experience the insidious onset of personality change, hallucinations, headache, and progressive somnolence and apathy, symptoms that indicate trypanosomal meningoencephalitis.[6,74] Patients with gambian trypanosomiasis may also exhibit ataxia and extrapyramidal signs of tremor, choreiform movements, shuffling gait, or rigidity.[118,152]

The initial clinical manifestations of trypanosomiasis in non-Africans tend to differ from those in native Africans. The American patients reported by Spencer and colleagues commonly experienced transient morbilliform rash, splenomegaly, localized edema, irritability, and insomnia.[187] Neurologic signs consisted of increased or decreased deep tendon reflexes, nystagmus, and frontal release phenomena. Only 20% of 119 Europeans with trypanosomiasis had mood or personality changes.[50]

Laboratory Features. The laboratory features of African trypanosomiasis can include a microcytic anemia, peripheral leukocytosis, an elevated sedimentation rate, and markedly elevated serum levels of IgM.[118] The CSF examination can be normal or show an elevated protein content or a lymphocytic pleocytosis.[6] Examination of fresh CSF or Giemsa-stained CSF sediment will frequently reveal trypomastigotes. In addition, organisms can be identified reliably in thick smears of peripheral blood or in aspirates from enlarged lymph nodes. Serologic studies using ELISA methods may also be useful. CT studies, performed on a limited number of patients, have disclosed mild hydrocephalus, diffuse lesions of white matter, or focal involvement of the basal ganglia.[129]

The neuropathologic lesions in fatal gambian trypanosomiasis consist of meningoencephalitis, cerebral edema, hypoxic injury, cerebral atrophy, or hemorrhagic leukoencephalopathy.[6] The meningoencephalitis varies in severity and can involve the cerebral white matter, basal nuclei, cerebellar white matter, or brainstem. Some of these pathologic features, notably cerebral edema, hypoxic injury, or leukoencephalopathy, may be attributable to arsenical encephalopathy[74] and melarsoprol-induced convulsions.[6]

Treatment. Suramin remains the drug of choice for the hematogenous stage of either form of African trypanosomiasis.[118,212] Because idiosyncratic responses (shock) can occur with suramin, patients should receive a test dose of 100 mg intravenously. Adults can then receive 1 g intravenously on days 1, 3, 7, 14, and 21, and children should be treated with 20 mg/kg intravenously using a similar schedule. Potential toxicities consist of rash, pruritus, and renal damage, and the patient's urine should be examined the day after each dose of the drug. The presence of marked proteinuria, hematuria, or casts contraindicates further therapy with suramin. Pentamidine has also been used in patients with early, symptomatic African trypanosomiasis.[152,212]

Patients with neurologic symptoms or signs should be treated with melarsoprol,[3,118,212] an organic arsenical compound (melarsen oxide and dimercaprol in propylene glycol) available from the CDC drug service [(404) 639-3670 or (404) 639-2888 (evenings, weekends, or holidays)]. The recommended adult dosage is 2 to 3.6 mg/kg per day given intravenously on 3 consecutive days, followed 1 week later by 3.6 mg/kg per day for an additional 3 days. This regimen should then be repeated 10 to 21 days later. Children should receive a total of 18 to 25 mg/kg divided into 9 or 10 doses given over a 1-month period, beginning with 0.36 mg/kg per day and increasing gradually every 1 to 5 days to a maximum dose of 3.6 mg/kg per day. Potential toxicities of arsenical compounds include dermatitis and encephalopathy.[6,74] In one review of 16 fatal cases of African trypanosomiasis due to *T. brucei gambiense*, arsenical encephalopathy, manifested by convulsions and coma, contributed to the deaths of 10 patients.[6] Eflornithine, a less toxic antitrypanosomal agent, has also been used successfully to treat African trypanosomiasis with CNS involvement.[152,197]

Patients treated with the above regimens usually recover completely, although relapses can occur and require retreatment. When untreated, both forms of trypanosomiasis progress to death from complications of heart failure, malnutrition, and secondary infections. At present, chemoprophylaxis of African trypanosomiasis with drugs such as pentamidine is not routinely recommended. Although difficult to quantitate precisely, the risk of trypanosomiasis among visitors to endemic regions of Africa appears to be low.[118,187]

AMERICAN

Biology and Epidemiology. American trypanosomiasis or Chagas' disease, caused by infection with *T. cruzi*, constitutes an important source of morbidity or mortality throughout Latin America.[96,114] Humans acquire *T. cruzi* from the contaminated feces of the hematophagous reduviid bugs. While biting, the insects defecate, and the parasites enter humans through the mucosa, conjunctiva, or broken skin. The trypanosoma multiply locally in the reticuloendothelial system and ultimately disseminate hematogenously. In addition, infection can be acquired congenitally or via blood transfusion, the latter being a significant problem in endemic areas and a potential complication in nonendemic areas, such as the United States, with large numbers of South American immigrants.[97]

Clinical Manifestations. The vast majority of T. cruzi infections occur asymptomatically.[22,96] When clinical disease does develop, children are more often affected by acute Chagas' disease than are adults. The earliest but not invariable sign, a red nodule or chagoma, can develop on the face or extremity at the site of T. cruzi inoculation. When the inoculation site is conjunctival, patients can have Romaña's sign,[96] edema of the eyelids with conjunctivitis and enlargement of the adjacent lymph nodes. Subsequently, constitutional symptoms begin and include fever, malaise, anorexia, headache, vomiting, and diarrhea. Examination at this time may reveal hepatosplenomegaly, generalized edema or lymphadenopathy, or signs of meningeal irritation.

Potentially severe complications of Chagas' disease include gastrointestinal or cardiac involvement.[96] Patients with chronic disease can develop megaesophagus and megacolon, which lead to dysphagia, reflux with the potential for aspiration, and severe constipation or impaction. Acute Chagas' disease is frequently associated with cardiac arrhythmias, such as tachycardia, premature ventricular contractions, or atrial fibrillation, which are manifestations of myocarditis. During the chronic stages, Chagas' disease can produce intractable congestive heart failure.[96,97]

Congenital Chagas' disease causes a disseminated disorder associated with hepatosplenomegaly, anemia, jaundice, edema, petechiae, and neurologic involvement.[20,84] Symptoms or signs may be present at birth, thus mimicking congenital TORCH infections,[16a] or develop a few months postnatally. The prognosis for symptomatic infants, as reviewed by Bittencourt,[20] was generally poor, and 37 of 67 (55%) of the infants were dead by 24 months of age. However, most survivors had no apparent long-term sequelae, other than parasitemia.

Neurologic complications can occur directly from meningoencephalitis[81,176,188] or indirectly as a consequence of cardiomyopathy.[97] Meningoencephalitis, most common in young patients with acute Chagas' disease, produces convulsions or altered levels of consciousness. Rarely, CNS granulomas develop and induce focal neurologic signs.[109a] The peripheral nervous system can also be affected during chronic Chagas' disease.[176] Congenitally infected infants exhibit tremors or convulsions, and neuropathologic examinations of fatal congenital cases reveal perivascular granulomatous lesions consisting of microglial proliferation and mononuclear infiltration.[20] Patients with chronic chagastic cardiomyopathy can have mural thrombi that may cause cerebral emboli, ischemia or infarction, and focal neurologic deficits.[96]

Diagnosis. The diagnosis of Chagas' disease can be established by demonstrating parasitemia, using Giemsa staining, wet-mount preparations, culture, or xenodiagnosis. Rarely, T. cruzi have been identified in the CSF of children[81] or congenitally infected infants.[20,84] Serologic studies, using complement fixation, immunofluorescence, or ELISA methods, also have diagnostic utility,[96] and immunocytochemistry can be used to detect T. cruzi antigens in pathologic specimens.[107] PCR can also be used to detect T. cruzi deoxyribonucleic acid (DNA).[134a]

Treatment. Treatment of acute symptomatic Chagas' disease currently consists of oral nifurtimox (adults: 8 to 10 mg/kg per day in four divided doses for 120 days; children 1 to 10 years: 15 to 20 mg/kg per day in four divided doses for 90 days; children 11 to 16 years: 12.5 to 15 mg/kg per day in four divided doses for 90 days).[21,22,73] Because parasites can persist in blood or be secreted in human milk, patients with proven or suspected Chagas' disease should not donate blood and, if female, should not breast-feed their infants.

CESTODES

Cysticercosis

BIOLOGY AND EPIDEMIOLOGY

Cysticercosis, the most common parasitic disease affecting the CNS,[15,151,170,174,181,191] results from infestation with larvae of the pork tapeworm *Taenia solium*. Although the disorder is endemic throughout much of Africa, Asia, eastern Europe,[191] and Central and South America,[181] numerous patients migrating to nonendemic regions, such as the United States, have been reported.[127,170,174] Humans, both definitive and intermediate hosts for *T. solium*, acquire the tapeworm by ingesting undercooked pork containing encysted larvae. The larvae mature in the human gastrointestinal tract, and the resulting adult tapeworms produce vast quantities of eggs that subsequently appear in the feces. When humans ingest the ova, either by consuming contaminated food or via fecal-oral autoinfection, the eggs hatch, and embryos penetrate the intestinal mucosa and disseminate hematogenously to eye, skeletal muscle, or brain. There, the larvae mature, become cysticerci, ranging in size from 3 mm to 2 cm or more.

CLINICAL MANIFESTATIONS

Patients with symptomatic CNS cysticercosis have varied neurologic signs and symptoms, features that reflect several factors, including the number and location of the cysts, their size, and the intensity of the evoked inflammatory response.[15,108,151,170,174] Cysts can invade cerebral parenchyma and induce seizures,[127,170,174] obstruct the flow of CSF and produce hydrocephalus,[182] involve the meninges and produce meningitis, occlude vascular structures and cause stroke,[126] or, rarely, involve the spinal cord and cause paraparesis.[8] Seizures, the most frequent neurologic complication, and hydrocephalus, the next most common problem, develop in approximately 50% and 30%, respectively, of patients with cerebral cysticercosis.

Sotelo and colleagues reviewed over 700 patients with neurocysticercosis seen during a 5-year period in Mexico City and noted a peak incidence in individuals 25 to 35 years of age.[181] Patients ranged in age from 5 to 76 years, with a mean age of 31 years, and men and women were affected equally. Approximately 50% of the patients had seizures, 43% had headache, 28% had papilledema, 27% had vomiting, 21% had pyramidal tract signs, and nearly 16% had intellectual deterioration. Additional features present in 1% to 10% of patients included ataxia, visual loss, optic atrophy, psychosis, diplopia, vertigo, tremor, and cranial nerve palsies.

In studies from the United States, McCormick and colleagues reported cysticercosis in 127 patients seen in Los Angeles between 1970 and 1980.[127] Although nearly all the patients were immigrants, six had no history of travel outside the United States, and thirteen of the affected immigrants had resided in the United States for 10 or more years prior to the onset of neurologic symptoms. Clinical manifestations, similar to those described by Sotelo and colleagues, consisted of seizures, hydrocephalus, meningitis, and stroke, either singly or in combination.

Scharf subsequently accumulated an additional 238 cases from the same hospital in Los Angeles and noted that only three patients were native-born Americans.[170] Common countries of origin were Mexico, El Salvador, and Guatemala. A seizure disorder was the most frequent primary diagnosis, present in 56% of the patients, and 21% had acute increases in intracranial pressure, due to obstructive hydrocephalus. Altered mental status was an additional common complaint. In another report of 52 children and adolescents,[134] ages 21 months to 20 years, with cerebral cysticercosis, 51 (98%) had seizures, and one child presented with headache and visual complaints. Seizure types included simple partial (29%), complex partial (20%), and generalized or mixed disorders (51%).

DIAGNOSIS

The diagnosis of cerebral cysticercosis can be suspected clinically in any patient from an endemic region who presents with acute or chronic neurologic complaints. Routine laboratory studies are usually unremarkable.[127,174,181] Modest peripheral leukocytosis or occasionally, eosinophilia can be seen, but the latter may reflect coinfection with other parasites.[134] The electroencephalogram (EEG) may reveal focal or generalized slowing, spike or sharp wave discharges, or be normal.

The CSF findings vary considerably and depend, in part, on whether cysticerci are present in the cerebral parenchyma or in the ventricular or subarachnoid spaces.[127,174,181] The CSF can be normal or show elevated protein content, hypoglycorrachia, or pleocytosis. Approximately half of the patients reported by Sotelo and colleagues had elevated CSF protein and/or more than 6 leukocytes/mm^3.[181] The pleocytosis is predominantly mononuclear, but neutrophils or eosinophils can be present. The protein content has been as high as 1.6 g/dL in an occasional patient.

Neuroimaging studies, particularly CT, have an extremely important role in the evaluation and management of patients with suspected or proven cerebral cysticercosis.[24,33,113,196] Most patients with CNS symptoms due to cysticercosis have CT or MRI lesions that, like the CSF features, depend on the activity of the disease and the location of cysticerci. Cystic lesions, an active lesion identified by CT in approximately half of the children reported by Mitchell and Crawford,[134] can be single or multiple, may enhance with contrast, and are frequently associated with varying degrees of edema. Using T_1-weighted MRI, pedunculated larvae can be identified within the cystic lesions.[113,158,196] The most common inactive or late lesion, present in approximately two thirds of adult patients, consists of small, punctate calcifications in the cerebral parenchyma (Fig.12–4). When cysticerci invade the spinal subarachnoid space or cord,[8] lesions can be detected by myelography, CT, or MRI.[28]

The diagnosis of cerebral cysticercosis can be supported by detecting serologic responses or established by identifying cysticerci on direct microscopic examination of biopsy tissues. Serologic studies have variable sensitivity and specificity, and the probability of detecting antibodies depends largely on the stage of the disorder.[33,127,174] In active disease cysticercus-specific IgG or IgM antibodies can frequently be detected in serum or CSF using complement fixation, hemagglutination inhibition, or ELISA.[166] McCormick and colleagues, for example, identified diagnostic hemagglutination titers in the CSF or serum of approximately 60% of patients with cerebral cysticercosis.[127] Titers were more frequently elevated in patients with meningitis (84% had positive results) than in patients without signs of CSF inflammation (only 42% had positive results). Chang and colleagues reported diagnostic serum or CSF ELISA results in 93% of patients with CT abnormalities attributed to cerebral cysticercosis.[33]

The characteristic histologic appearance of cerebral cysticercosis consists of the larva (Fig. 12–5) and a surrounding capsule with varying degrees of inflammation. When alive, the cysticerci induce only modest inflammation or gliosis, whereas larval death stimulates mononuclear cell inflammatory responses, gliosis, and the production of a well-defined fibrous capsule. In the late stages, larva and capsule calcify, and gliosis or neuronal atrophy can be observed in the adjacent cerebral parenchyma.[113] When cysticerci involve the cisterna magna, arachnoid spaces, or basal cisterns, clusters of organisms, the racemose form of cerebral cysticercosis, induce intense local inflammation and fibrosis.[113,182]

TREATMENT

Therapeutic strategies for neurocysticercosis (see Table 12–1) must be tailored to the location or activity of the cysticerci and the nature of the neurologic disorder. Anticysticercus drugs, such as praziquantel or albendazole,[180] should be considered for active disease, as evidenced by arachnoiditis or the presence of parenchymal cysts.[109,140,181] Praziquantel, currently considered an investigational drug by the US Food and Drug Administration, can be given 50 mg/kg per day in three divided doses for 14 days.[3,179] Efficacy of praziquantel has been suggested by a shortened duration of symptoms and resolution of CT lesions,[179,180,184] but improvement or resolution of CT abnormalities or clinical symptoms can occur spontaneously.[132,134]

Praziquantel therapy is frequently associated with headache, exacerbation of seizures, or signs of increased intracranial pressure, particularly during the first few days of therapy.[179] These changes have been attributed to death

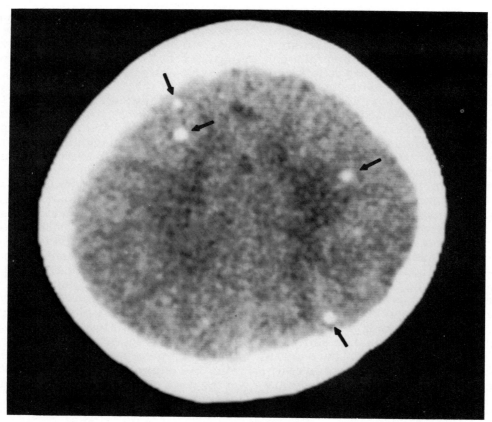

Figure 12–4. Punctate calcifications (arrows) consistent with cerebral cysticercosis identified by CT in a Mexican adolescent with a seizure disorder.

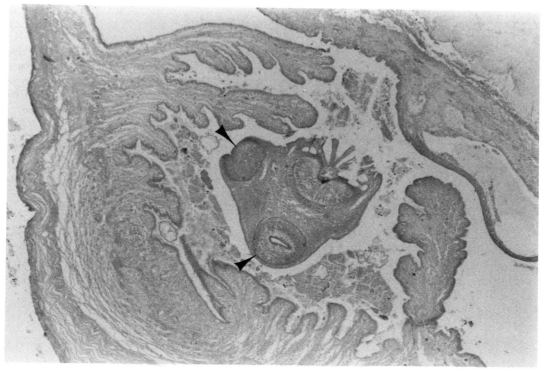

Figure 12–5. Cerebral cysticercus (*arrowheads* indicate suckers) identified in a 50-year-old woman from Texas who had made several trips to Mexico (hematoxylin and eosin; original magnification ×48). (Courtesy of Dr. R. Schelper, Department of Pathology, The University of Iowa, College of Medicine, Iowa City.)

of the cysticerci and can be alleviated by corticosteroid therapy. Plasma levels of praziquantel can decrease substantially, however, during concurrent dexamethasone administration.[203]

Surgical therapy is generally reserved for patients with fourth-ventricular cysts, spinal lesions, or large mass lesions that obstruct CSF flow or simulate neoplasms.[109,127,140,182,192] Patients with progressive hydrocephalus may respond favorably to ventriculoperitoneal shunt placement, but the long-term prognosis for such patients appears highly variable.[127,182] Inactive disease, as indicated by parenchymal calcifications, requires only symptomatic therapy such as anticonvulsants for seizures. Freezing of pork has been reported to kill cysticerci,[183] suggesting that prevention may be possible.

Other Cestode Infestations

BIOLOGY AND EPIDEMIOLOGY

Migrating larvae of several other cestodes, including *Echinococcus granulosus*, *Taenia multiceps*, and *Diphyllobothrium* or *Spirometra* species, can potentially invade the brain and induce neurologic complications.* The distribution of these disorders in the world corresponds to the geographic distribution of the intermediate animal hosts. Infestations with *Echinococcus* and *T. multiceps* usually occur in sheepherding regions of Africa, South America, the former Soviet Union, and

---

*References 57, 78a, 133, 133a, 149b, 150.

Mediterranean or eastern European countries.[143] By contrast, most cases of sparganosis, infection with *Diphyllobothrium* or *Spirometra* larvae, have been reported in Asian nations.[57,133a] However, sporadic cases of cestode infestation occur worldwide.

The pathogenesis of these parasitic infections strongly resembles that of cysticercosis. Adult tapeworms reside in the intestinal tracts of various animal hosts, including sheep, cats, and dogs, and produce ova that are excreted liberally in feces. Humans become infected by ingesting the ova or larvae of the cestodes. In sparganosis, the parasitic life cycle involves a second intermediate host: fish, frog, or snake. Sparganosis can be acquired by consumption of water contaminated by larvae-infected *Cyclops* species or,

rarely, by application of poultices of intermediate hosts to open human wounds.[57]

The embryos or larvae penetrate the intestinal walls and migrate to various tissues, particularly the liver (Fig. 12–6), lung, and skeletal muscle. Fortunately, dissemination to brain constitutes a rare event. Hydatid cysts involve the CNS in only 1% to 2% of *Echinococcus granulosus* infections.[62,150] As of 1990, only 12 cases of cerebral sparganosis and 55 cases of intracranial coenurosis, *T. multiceps* infection, had been reported in the medical literature.[11,57,133,133a,149b] Patients with cerebral hyatid cysts are usually younger than 30 years of age, whereas cerebral sparganosis and coenurosis tend to occur in the third through sixth decades of life.

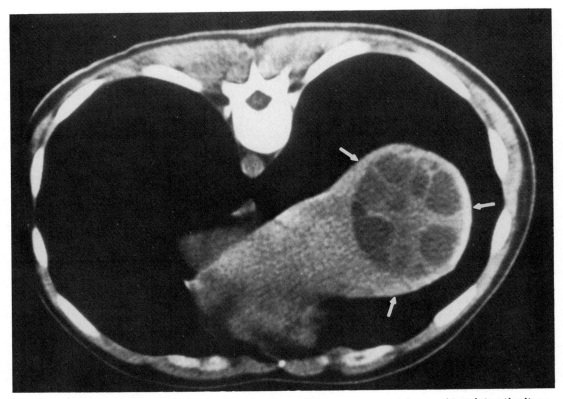

Figure 12–6. A low thoracic CT scan reveals a large *Echinococcus* cyst *(arrows)* involving the liver. (Courtesy of Dr. R. D. Andersen, Department of Pediatrics, The University of Iowa, College of Medicine, Iowa City.)

CLINICAL MANIFESTATIONS

The larvae of these various parasites usually produce single, mass lesions within brain parenchyma that cause headache, convulsions, personality changes, memory loss, or focal neurologic deficits. In cerebral hydatid cysts, symptoms or signs of increased intracranial pressure, headache, vomiting, or papilledema predominate, and approximately 50% of patients have seizures.[150] *T. multiceps* can also involve the posterior fossa, leading to signs of increased intracranial pressure or obstructive hydrocephalus.[149b] Rarely, the brainstem or spinal cord can be affected.[57] The neurologic features of each of these infestations tend to develop insidiously over several months and thus mimic a CNS neoplasm.

DIAGNOSIS

Except for modest increases in the numbers of circulating eosinophils, systemic laboratory studies tend to be normal. The CSF can show an increased protein content or a mild lymphocytic pleocytosis, but lumbar punctures should be avoided in patients with suspected CNS mass lesions. Imaging studies, such as CT or MRI, have an extremely important diagnostic role in cerebral cestode infestations. In cerebral hydatid disease, the CT usually reveals a single, large hypodense mass lesion that involves the temporoparietal region and exerts considerable mass effect on the adjacent cerebral parenchyma.[62,149] Cerebral sparganosis and coenurosis tend to produce solitary hypodense lesions that show ring or nodular enhancement.[11,57,133,149b] The parasitologic diagnosis of cerebral cestode infestations usually requires examination of biopsy or autopsy tissues.

TREATMENT

Treatment consists largely of surgical removal of the cerebral lesion. For hydatid cysts, mebendazole, an experimental echinoccocal drug in the United States, has been recommended when cysts rupture[1] or cannot be surgically removed. Although fatalities have been reported, most patients recover completely after surgical therapy.[57,149b,150]

NEMATODES

Visceral Larva Migrans

BIOLOGY AND EPIDEMIOLOGY

Toxocara canis, the principal cause of visceral larva migrans, infects domestic dogs and other canines, including wolves and foxes, throughout the temperate and tropical climatic zones of the world.[66,68,169] Seroepidemiologic studies indicate that 7% to 50% or more of domestic dogs in endemic regions have evidence of *T. canis* infection.[169] Dogs frequently acquire *T. canis* larvae transplacentally or postnatally via breast milk, such that 80% or more of young puppies become infected by 3 months of age.[66] Larvae migrate to the bronchioles and trachea of infected puppies, are swallowed, and mature within the small intestines into adult worms. The female adult worms subsequently produce vast quantities of ova, as many as 200,000 per day. These thick-shelled ova are shed in feces and develop extracorporally during the next 3 to 4 weeks into forms that become infective for other canines or humans. Ova can survive in moist soils for many months, but are usually killed by desiccation or temperatures below $-15°C$.[68]

Humans become infected by ingesting eggs present in contaminated soils or on fomites.[66] In endemic areas 10% to 30% of soil samples contain *T. canis* larvae.[66,68,169] The percentage of humans in endemic regions who possess antibodies to *T. canis,* evidence of prior infection, varies considerably, from approximately 3% among random blood donors in the United Kingdom[66] to as high as 80% among children in St. Lucia.[199] In the United States visceral larva migrans has been reported more commonly in southeastern and south central states.[169]

CLINICAL MANIFESTATIONS

The life cycle of T. canis infection in humans parallels that of adult dogs, except that mature worms are not produced.[66,68] Ova hatch in the small intestine, and larvae penetrate the intestinal lumina and migrate to the liver, lung, and systemic circulation. Most infected humans, particularly those with a small parasite load, do not experience symptoms that can be attributed directly to T. canis.[66] Symptomatic infections usually occur in young children, an epidemiologic characteristic linked to age-related pica. Infected children may exhibit cough, fever, malaise, weight loss, pallor, lymphadenopathy, hepatosplenomegaly, or skin rash, features that reflect larval-induced tissue injury and the associated inflammatory responses. Among adult and pediatric patients with high toxocara antibody titers, abdominal pain, lethargy, nausea, and anorexia are also common complaints.

Ocular infiltration by T. canis larvae represents the most frequent, serious complication of visceral larva migrans.[225] Patients affected by ocular larva migrans tend to be older than those with visceral involvement and usually lack systemic signs or symptoms of T. canis infection.[169] Ocular involvement induces several different ophthalmologic conditions, including posterior granuloma, chronic endophthalmitis, retinal detachment, uveitis, vitreous abscess, pars planitis, optic neuritis, or keratitis.[68] Posterior granuloma, the most common ocular manifestation, produces vision loss or strabismus and resembles retinoblastoma, a similarity that has frequently led to enucleation of the infected eye.

Neurologic complications, rare but potentially serious manifestations of visceral larva migrans include headache, convulsions, or behavioral changes.[68,169,170b,198] A single case report also suggested an association between T. canis infection and acute infantile hemiplegia.[12] These complications presumably reflect direct invasion of the CNS, a pathogenetic mechanism supported by detection of T. canis larvae in CNS tissues.[80,143a,170b] At least two studies have also noted a higher seropositivity rate for T. canis among patients with chronic epilepsy of uncertain cause.[38,218] Although this finding suggests a potential etiologic role for T. canis infection, a similar study attributed these differences in toxocaral seropositivity to confounding variables such as a higher rate of pica among epileptic children.[67]

DIAGNOSIS

Patients with systemic visceral larva migrans typically have persistent eosinophilia, ranging from 25% to 90% of the circulating leukocytes, and a panhyperimmunoglobulinemia of IgG, IgM, and especially immunoglobulin E (IgE).[52] By contrast, patients with isolated ocular involvement frequently lack such findings. When patients develop CNS complications, the CSF may show a modest pleocytosis with eosinophilia. The parasitologic diagnosis of T. canis infection can be established by detecting antibodies in serum using ELISA methods.[44] Stool cultures for ova or parasites are characteristically negative, however. In rare instances, infections with T. cati or with Baylisacaris procyonis, the cat and raccoon ascarids, mimic those of T. canis infection.[63a]

TREATMENT

Although antihelminthic agents, including diethylcarbamazine (6 mg/kg per day in three divided doses for 7 to 10 days) and thiabendazole, have been used clinically or experimentally (see Table 12–1), no drug has been uniformly effective in visceral larva migrans.[3] Patients with severe pulmonary disease or cardiac symptoms may respond to corticosteroids, and such therapy should be considered for patients with acute ocular involvement. Most patients with visceral larva migrans have a benign, albeit protracted course. Eosinophilia and complaints of nausea or abdominal pain can persist for many months, but fatalities, although reported, are exceptionally uncommon.

Eosinophilic Meningitis

BIOLOGY AND EPIDEMIOLOGY

Angiostrongylus cantonensis, the lung worm of rats, is the principal cause of eosinophilic meningitis in humans, an association first reported in Taiwan in 1945.[17,98a] Subsequently, numerous cases have been observed in many regions of the world, such as India, Southeast Asia, Cuba, Egypt, and the Pacific Islands, including Australia and Hawaii.[35,98a,155] Rats serve as the definitive host for the parasite, but the life cycle also includes intermediate hosts, snails and slugs, and transport hosts, fish, shrimp, and crabs. Humans acquire infection with *A. cantonensis* or related species by ingesting raw or undercooked intermediate or transport hosts.[98a]

CLINICAL MANIFESTATIONS

After an average incubation period of approximately 16 days (range of 2 to 13 days), humans develop symptoms and signs consisting of headache, vomiting, stiff neck, paresthesias, and fever.[106] The fever tends to be low grade and inconsistent, although temperatures of 40°C or higher have been observed in children.[35] Occasional patients experience convulsions or cranial nerve palsies usually involving the sixth or seventh cranial nerves. Neurologic dysfunction results from direct invasion and death of *A. cantonensis* within the CNS.[98a]

DIAGNOSIS

The cardinal laboratory feature of *A. cantonensis* infection is an eosino-

philic CSF pleocytosis. In patients described by Kuberski and Wallace,[106] CSF leukocyte counts ranged from 29 to 3410 per cubic millimeter, with eosinophils comprising 10% to 92% (mean of 38%) of the cells. The CSF protein content can be modestly elevated, averaging 100 mg/dL, and the glucose content tends to be in the low-normal range. Most patients also have a circulating eosinophilia exceeding 3% of the peripheral white blood cell count. CT may be normal or reveal ventricular enlargement or focal edema.[84a,98a] A gadolinium-enhanced MRI study of a single patient with *A. cantonensis* infection showed meningeal and parenchymal enhancement.[84a]

A. cantonensis infection can be strongly suspected in individuals who inhabit or visit endemic areas and develop an eosinophilic meningitis. Larvae can occasionally be detected in CSF,[105] and serologic studies of serum or CSF may reveal evidence of infection.[151a] Because the disorder remains rare outside the Western Pacific, other disorders must be considered more likely in patients from nonendemic regions who exhibit an eosinophilic CSF pleocytosis.[98a,104] Disorders that are potentially associated with CSF eosinophilia include foreign body, CNS malignancy,[94] *Coccidioides immitis* meningitis, cysticercosis, and infections with several other parasites, including *Paragonimus westermani*,[175] *Gnathostoma spinigerum*,[154a,156] or *Schistosoma* species.[104]

In certain regions, such as Thailand, eosinophilic meningitis is frequently due to *G. spinigerum* infection, a disorder appropriately labeled eosinophilic myeloencephalitis by Punyagupta and colleagues.[154a] When compared with *A. cantonensis*, infection with *G. spinigerum* is more likely to be associated with radicular pain, signs of cord or cerebral dysfunction, and bloody or xanthochromic CSF. This disorder appears to carry a substantially higher mortality rate (approximately 12%) than does infection with *A. cantonensis*.[154a]

TREATMENT

Because most patients have a self-limited disorder and recover completely, therapy consists of supportive care. In many patients, the lumbar puncture is both diagnostic and therapeutic. Therapy with agents such as penicillin, tetracycline, thiabendazole, or prednisone has not altered the clinical course of eosinophilic meningitis due to A. cantonensis.[98a] Occasional fatalities have been described, due in some instances to intercurrent pneumonia.

Trichinosis

BIOLOGY AND EPIDEMIOLOGY

Trichinosis, infestation with the larvae of Trichinella species, remains an important public health concern throughout the world.[90,135,143] At least three species of Trichinella cause human infections, T. spiralis in temperate climates, T. nelsoni in Africa, and T. nativa in the Arctic. Maintained in the wild by various carnivores, including bears, foxes, wolves, hyenas, leopards, or lions, Trichinella infect humans and pigs as incidental hosts.[143] Most human trichinosis, due to T. spiralis, is acquired by consuming undercooked, larvae-infested pork, but sporadic outbreaks of human disease have also followed consumption of meat from bear,[135] walrus,[143] horse,[10] or wild pig. In the United States approximately 0.1% of domestic pigs and 0.1% to 6% of black bears contain T. spiralis larval cysts.[135]

After ingestion, larvae emerge during digestion of cysts in the stomach and mature into adult worms during the subsequent 1 to 2 days. Ova from female adult worms appear within approximately 5 days and develop into new larvae that penetrate the intestinal mucosa and invade the systemic circulation. Larvae then disseminate hematogenously to various tissues, including the lungs, heart, skeletal muscle, and occasionally the CNS.

CLINICAL MANIFESTATIONS

Human trichinosis ranges from an asymptomatic infestation with Trichinella larvae to a severe, occasionally fatal disorder, a clinical spectrum that corresponds largely to the parasitic load.[90,135] Most patients with low-level Trichinella infection have no recognizable illness. In symptomatic patients, the earliest features, nausea, diarrhea, or occasionally vomiting, reflect the gastrointestinal phase of infection. Within 2 to 3 weeks, symptomatic patients typically have fever, myalgias, malaise, weakness, and periorbital edema, which can be accompanied by chemosis or conjunctival hemorrhages. Subungual splinter hemorrhages may also be seen. Myalgias and weakness, due to larval-induced myositis, typically involve muscles that subserve eye movement, mastication, deglutination, and neck movement. In severe cases, weakness can be diffuse and debilitating, reflecting a parasite load that can exceed 50 larvae per gram of muscle.

Neurologic complications, affecting approximately 10% of patients with symptomatic trichinosis,[101,135,137] usually appear during the second and third weeks of the illness and indicate direct larval involvement of the brain (encephalitis) or CSF spaces (meningitis). Signs initially tend to be diffuse and include personality change, headache, meningismus, or lethargy.[70,101] Later, focal signs, consisting of motor or cranial nerve paralysis, predominate and correlate with larval encystment. Additional potential neurologic complications reported in association with symptomatic trichinosis include cerebellar dysfunction, convulsions, or peripheral neuropathies.[70] This broad spectrum of neurologic complications emphasizes that trichinosis should be considered in patients with acute neurologic disorders of uncertain cause.

DIAGNOSIS

The combination of myalgias, periorbital edema, and fever should suggest strongly the possibility of trichinosis.[90] Other than eosinophilia and variable elevations of creatine phosphokinase, systemic laboratory studies in patients with trichinosis tend to be unremarkable. In patients with neurologic involvement, the CSF is usually normal but can contain an elevated protein content, lowered glucose level, or a modest lymphocytic pleocytosis. Larvae can be identified within CSF in approximately one fourth of patients with *Trichinella*-induced neurologic dysfunction.[137] The EEG may show diffuse or focal slowing.

The parasitologic diagnosis of trichinosis can be established by microscopic examination of muscle biopsy specimens or by serologic means. Examination of compressed samples of striated muscle is a rapid and effective means of detecting trichinosis, or larvae can be identified by routine histologic tests (Fig. 12–7). Serum antibodies to *T. spiralis* usually appear during the third or fourth week of the illness and can be detected using the bentonite agglutination test.[135]

TREATMENT

Treatment consists principally of supportive care, although a brief course of corticosteroids (e.g., 1 to 2 mg/kg for 1 day) has been recommended for patients with cardiac, pulmonary, or neurologic complications. Thiabendazole has also been used, in dosages of 50 mg/kg per day for approximately 5 days, not to exceed 3 g/day[3] (see Table 12–1). Proper cooking of potentially infected meat, particularly pork, remains the most effective means to prevent human trichinosis. Most patients recover from trichinosis uneventfully, but convalescence may take several weeks or more.[101,135] Some fatalities still occur, usually in patients who have cardiac or severe neurologic involvement.[135]

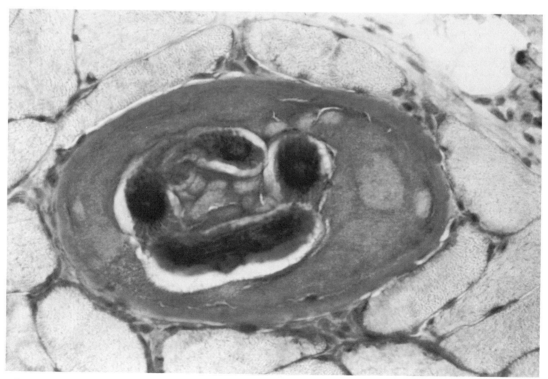

Figure 12–7. *Trichinella spiralis* larva identified in the striated muscle of an adult with trichinosis (periodic acid–Schiff; original magnification ×400). (Courtesy of Dr. R. Shelper, Department of Pathology, The University of Iowa, College of Medicine, Iowa City.)

Strongyloides Stercoralis

BIOLOGY AND EPIDEMIOLOGY

Strongyloides stercoralis, a nematode endemic in tropical and subtropical regions, has in rare instances invaded the CNS, producing meningitis, infarction, or brain abscess.[121,142,148] Infections have been described worldwide, and studies of US inhabitants indicate that 0.4% to 4% excrete *S. stercoralis* in their stools.[64a] Larvae infect humans by penetrating the skin and subsequently migrate to the intestines, lung, or, rarely, CNS.[121,148] Immunocompromised patients are at risk for severe, disseminated infections.[171]

CLINICAL MANIFESTATIONS, DIAGNOSIS, AND TREATMENT

Although infections are frequently asymptomatic, systemic features of *Strongyloides* infection can include abdominal pain, vomiting, diarrhea, or malabsorption syndromes.[64a,142] Neurologic complications, which may be the presenting features, consist of headache, hemiparesis, impaired consciousness, focal seizures, or meningeal signs.[121,142] Parasitic infection may be suggested by peripheral blood eosinophilia. Stool examinations can reveal *Strongyloides* larvae, but repeated sampling is frequently necessary to confirm infection.[64a] The string test or duodenal aspirate can also be used to identify larvae. In one instance, CT revealed multiple ring enhancing lesions compatible with cerebral abscesses,[121] findings that were later confirmed at autopsy. Therapy currently consists of thiabendazole, 50 mg/kg per day (maximum of 3 g/day) for 2 days[3,163] (see Table 12–1).

TREMATODES (FLUKES)

Schistosomiasis

BIOLOGY AND EPIDEMIOLOGY

Humans can be infected with several different *Schistosoma* species, but *S. mansonia, S. japonicum,* and *S. haematobium* cause the majority of cases of human schistosomiasis. Endemic in 74 countries of Africa, South America, the Caribbean, and Asia,[31a] schistosomiasis has been estimated by Mahmoud to affect more than 200 million people worldwide.[117] Although rare in Europe or North America, several outbreaks of schistosomiasis have occurred among US and European citizens traveling to endemic regions.[31a]

The three principal *Schistosoma* species utilize humans as their primary host and chronically inhabit the vascular system in the mesenteric veins (*S. mansoni* and *S. japonicum*) or vesical plexus *(S. haematobium).* Adult worms produce hundreds of eggs daily, which appear in urine or feces or remain within the liver, intestines, or urinary tract of the infected host. The life cycle of *Schistosoma* species continues when eggs enter fresh water, hatch into miracidia, and infect their intermediate hosts, various species of snails.[117] This stage amplifies the numbers of parasites dramatically, and within 6 weeks vast quantities of *Schistosoma* cercariae emerge. Humans become infected by cutaneous contact with cercariae-infested waters.[31a] Cercariae invade the skin and migrate to the lungs, liver, and eventually to blood vessels.

CLINICAL MANIFESTATIONS

The systemic signs of human schistosomiasis correspond to the stages of parasitic infection but can be absent with light infestations.[117] During cutaneous penetration, cecariae produce a pruritic, papular skin rash (swimmer's itch), and maturation and migration of the worms during the subsequent 1 to 3 months lead to fever, headache, malaise, cough, diarrhea, abdominal pain, and anorexia (Katayama syndrome).[31a] Heavy infestations induce considerable inflammation and fibrosis, causing portal hypertension, ascites, hepatosplenomegaly, and esophageal varices. *S. haematobium* primarily affects the bladder and produces hematuria, dysuria, urgency, and bladder pain.

Neurologic complications have been

most frequent following infections with S. japonicum* but can also occur with schistosomiasis due to S. haematobium or S. mansoni. Based on cases reported by several authors,[34,89,200] approximately 3.5% of patients with S. japonicum infections experience neurologic complications. In 1948 Kane and Most reviewed 51 cases of CNS schistomiasis identified between 1889 and the end of World War II.[89] Of these, 27 involved US army personnel stationed during World War II on Leyte in the Philippines, an endemic region for S. japonicum.

CNS schistosomiasis usually begins 6 to 25 weeks after presumed exposure to the parasite.[89,138] Virtually all patients have fever and most have prodromal symptoms of cough, gastrointestinal complaints, or urticaria. Neurologic symptoms usually begin abruptly and include, in order of decreasing frequency, altered sensorium, extremity weakness, visual disturbances, incontinence, sensory disturbances, altered speech, ataxia, vertigo, and neck stiffness.[14,89,200] Focal or generalized seizures can also occur. Patients typically have hyperreflexia, motor paralysis (hemiplegia, monoplegia, or quadriplegia), and frequently exhibit papilledema or palsies of cranial nerves III, IV, VI, VII, X, or XII. Transverse myelitis can also be seen.[29a] These neurologic complications result from direct involvement of the CNS by Schistosoma eggs and the resulting inflammatory responses.

DIAGNOSIS

Laboratory studies in schistosomiasis usually reveal leukocytosis, ranging from 7000 to 33,000 white blood cells per mm^3, and eosinophilia, constituting from 7% to 80% of the total leukocyte count.[89,138,200] The sedimentation rate may also be elevated. The CSF is abnormal in approximately one third of patients with CNS schistosomiasis, showing an elevated protein content or a

mild pleocytosis of lymphocytes or, occasionally, eosinophils.[89,200] The EEG may reveal focal slowing or epileptiform activity, and CT in one patient showed multiple hypodense cerebral lesions with adjacent enhancing nodules.[95]

The parasitologic diagnosis of schistosomiasis can be established by detecting eggs in feces or urine or, occasionally, in biopsy specimens of rectal mucosa. However, the majority of patients reviewed by Kane and Most had negative stool specimens at the onset of their neurologic symptoms.[89] Histologic examination of CNS tissues can disclose eggs and granulomatous reactions (Fig. 12–8), and serologic responses to Schistosoma can be detected by immunofluorescence or ELISA methods.[116] Although detection of antibody may not correlate with disease activity, serologic studies can be useful in patients with suspected schistosomiasis who are not yet excreting ova.

TREATMENT

Praziquantel, 40 to 60 mg/kg given in a single day, can be used to effectively treat all species of Schistosoma.[3] Alternatives include oxamniquine for S. mansoni and metrifonate for S. haematobium. In one patient, resolution of CNS lesions was observed during a 10-week course of dexamethasone,[95] suggesting an adjunctive role for corticosteroids. Prior to the availability of praziquantel, the outcome for patients with CNS schistosomiasis was quite variable. Although only 1 death occurred among the 27 World War II military personnel with cerebral schistosomiasis japonica reviewed by Kane and Most, 88% of the survivors had residual neurologic deficits when examined several months after the onset of the disorder.[89]

Paragonimiasis

BIOLOGY AND EPIDEMIOLOGY

Paragonimiasis, a disorder endemic in various areas of Asia, Africa, and Latin America, results from infection

---

*References 14, 34, 89, 117, 138, 164, 200.

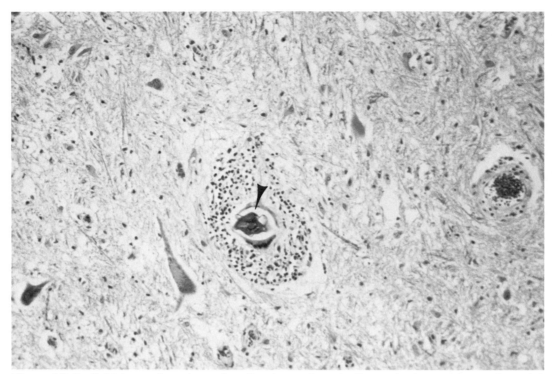

Figure 12–8. Schistosomal egg *(arrowhead)* and granuloma in the cerebral parenchyma of an adult with CNS schistosomiasis (hematoxylin and eosin; original magnification ×100). (Courtesy of Dr. R. Schelper, Department of Pathology, The University of Iowa, College of Medicine, Iowa City.)

with the lung fluke *Paragonimus westermani.* Humans acquire paragonimiasis by consuming raw or undercooked fresh-water crabs or crayfish infected with *Paragonimus* larvae. The ingested larvae migrate from the small intestine to the lungs via the peritoneal cavity and diaphragm. There the larvae mature into adult worms that produce eggs that may appear in sputum or feces. Several different carnivores, including wolves, cats, foxes, leopards, and tigers, act as reservoirs for the fluke. Most cases of cerebral disease have been reported among inhabitants of endemic areas,[93,177] but systemic paragonimiasis has been observed in the United States among southeast Asian refugees.

CLINICAL MANIFESTATIONS

Most infections do not produce recognizable illnesses, but when symptoms do appear, they usually reflect pulmonary or abdominal involvement. Patients commonly experience fever, productive cough, hemoptysis, and pleuritic chest pain, and abdominal pain or jaundice may also be present. Chest radiographs during this phase of the illness can reveal pleural effusions, nodular densities, or lung abscess, features that often mimic pulmonary tuberculosis.[145]

Potential neurologic complications of paragonimiasis consist of convulsions, either focal or generalized, or focal neurologic deficits.[79,93,145,175] These complications can begin in childhood or adulthood and result from direct invasion of the CNS by immature or mature worms. The parasite enters the cranium along perivascular tissues and resides in cerebral parenchyma. When alive, the worms produce eggs, may migrate within the brain or spinal cord, and induce gliosis and granulomatous inflammatory reactions. Eventually, the worms die and calcify.

DIAGNOSIS

Patients with paragonimiasis usually have peripheral eosinophilia, and eggs can frequently be identified in sputum or feces. Antibodies to *P. westermani* and other species can be detected using ELISA.[203a] In cerebral paragonimiasis, CT reveals hypodense and calcific lesions of parietal, occipital, or temporal lobes.[177,202,224] The calcific lesions tend to be multiple and have a multilobulated, cavitated appearance that is considered pathognomonic for the disorder. Biopsy of these lesions can yield eggs or more mature forms.

TREATMENT

Praziquantel, the current drug of choice for symptomatic paragonimiasis, can be given at a dose of 25 mg/kg 3 times daily for 2 days. Surgical therapy may also be necessary for hydrocephalus or lesions that are large or mimic neoplasms.[202] Although most patients gradually recover, long-term sequelae can include hemiparesis, mental retardation, hydrocephalus, or chronic convulsive tendencies.

ROCKY MOUNTAIN SPOTTED FEVER

Biology and Epidemiology

Rocky Mountain spotted fever (RMSF), a disorder caused by the obligate intracellular microorganism *Rickettsia rickettsii*, remains the most common rickettsial disorder in the United States. Between 1920 and 1960 the CDC received reports of approximately 100 to 200 cases annually.[75] After 1960, however, the incidence of RMSF increased significantly, ranging from 500 to more than 1000 cases annually in the United States, an overall incidence of 0.2 to 0.5 cases per 100,000 population.[30,61,76] Although this disorder was initially described in Idaho and Montana,[74a,215a] most affected persons live in suburban or rural areas of the eastern United States, particularly from Maryland south to Georgia and west to Kansas and Oklahoma.[30] Rarely, persons living in Canada, Central America, or urban areas of the United States such as New York City[168] have contracted RMSF. In 1988, RMSF was reported in 38 states, with North Carolina and Oklahoma having the highest incidence.[30a,97a]

RMSF is transmitted to humans via contact with the wood tick, *Dermacentor andersoni;* the dog tick, *Dermacentor variabilis;* and the Lone-Star tick, *Amblyomma americanum,* which serve as the natural reservoir for the rickettsia.[128] Over 80% of human RMSF cases begin in April through July, when ticks are most active.[30a] However, 20% or more of affected persons lack a clear history of tick exposure. Aerosol transmission of *R. rickettsii* has occurred in laboratory workers,[147] suggesting that this route could theoretically contribute to RMSF transmission. The median age of persons with RMSF was 15 years for cases reported between 1977 and 1980,[78] and nearly 60% of affected patients were younger than 21 years of age.

Clinical Manifestations

The incubation period from tick exposure to onset of disease ranges from 1 to 14 days, with an average of approximately 7 days.[78] RMSF usually begins abruptly with fever to 40°C or higher, headache, malaise, vomiting, myalgias, and arthralgias, although as many as one third of patients with proven RMSF will have a more gradual onset,[173] and initial symptoms can mimic neurologic,[83] respiratory, or acute gastrointestinal disorders.[42,206]

Rash, the most characteristic clinical feature of RMSF, often appears on the second through the fourth day of the illness but may not be evident until day 15.[78,92] The exanthem, first erythematous macules and then papules or petechiae, begins on the wrists and ankles and spreads distally to the palms and soles and centripetally to the extremities and trunk. Among cases reviewed by the CDC in 1987, 76.5% had rash, and 50% of patients had rash involving the palms and soles,[30] but the rash can be faint, evanescent, or never develop in 10% or more of serologically proven cases.

Approximately half of the patients with RMSF have severe myalgias, and conjunctivitis, splenomegaly, hepatomegaly, and jaundice can also be present. Severe or untreated cases can be associated with shock, arrhythmias, impaired renal function, disseminated intravascular coagulation, and death. In a CDC review of 262 cases, hepatomegaly, jaundice, blood urea nitrogen concentration exceeding 25 mg/dL, or atypical initial symptoms (e.g., absence of rash) were more frequent among patients who died.[78]

The usual neurologic features of RMSF consist of headache, meningismus, altered sensorium, and convulsions.[19,30,78,83,91] Headache, present in 60% to 75% of cases, is diffuse and intractable, although young children may not directly identify headache as the source of their discomfort. Encephalitis occasionally predominates, producing hallucinations, convulsions, focal neurologic deficits, and progressive coma, features that may reflect cerebral edema.[91] Other neurologic abnormalities reported in RMSF include ataxia, aphasia, sensorineural hearing loss, peripheral neuropathy, and papilledema.[19,78] The neuropathologic findings of fatal cases consist of cerebral edema, perivascular and meningeal lymphocytic infiltration, glial nodule formation, and an extensive necrotizing vasculitis, the fundamental pathologic lesion of RMSF.[19]

Diagnosis

The acute onset of fever and rash during the summer months should indicate a high probability of RMSF, especially when accompanied by thrombocytopenia and hyponatremia. Disorders that may be considered in the differential diagnosis of RMSF include other infectious illness, such as meningococcemia, measles, enteroviral infections, or infectious mononucleosis.[88,195,222] Summer season and a rash that involves the palms and soles argue in favor of RMSF. Ehrlichiosis, another tick-borne disorder, shares several epidemiologic and clinical features with RMSF, but patients with this disorder infrequently have rash involving the palms and soles.[127a]

Laboratory abnormalities in persons with RMSF include thrombocytopenia, hyponatremia, anemia, azotemia, elevated serum transaminase levels, or an elevated creatine kinase.[78] The CSF can show a lymphocytic or polymorphonuclear pleocytosis or be normal despite the presence of meningeal signs.[19,83,91] In severe cases, evidence of myocardial damage can be detected by electrocardiography.[78]

The diagnosis of RMSF can be confirmed by serologic assays, immunofluorescence studies of tissue specimens, or isolation of R. rickettsii.[204] The Weil-Felix reaction, a traditional serologic test, relies on cross-reactivity to Proteus OX-19 and OX-2 antigens but has generally been supplanted by more accurate and specific assays. The CDC criteria for the serologic diagnosis of RMSF include (1) a fourfold rise in antibody titer by complement fixation, indirect fluorescence antibody, latex agglutination, microagglutination, or indirect hemagglutination methods, or (2) a single high titer of antibody of 1:64 or higher by immunofluorescence or 1:16 or higher by complement fixation.[30a,61,78] Immunofluorescence studies of skin biopsy material are highly specific[205,219] but have relatively low sensitivity. PCR has promise as a sensitive and rapid means to detect rickettsial infection.[26a]

Treatment

Because delay in appropriate antibiotic administration is strongly linked to adverse outcome in RMSF, therapy should be initiated as soon as the disorder is suspected. Therapy for RMSF consists of (1) tetracycline 20 to 50 mg/kg per day for children older than 8 years of age or 500 mg 4 times daily for nonpregnant adults or (2) chloramphenicol 50 to 100 mg/kg per day.[53,88] The antibiotic can be given orally or intravenously, depending on the severity of the illness, and continued for 2 to 3 days after resolution of fever (a total of 7 to 10 days).[88] Mortality rates remain between 3% and 7% in the United States,[30,61,78] with highest fatality rates among elderly patients. Although most patients recover completely, children with RMSF may have sequelae consisting of behavioral disturbances and learning disabilities.[69]

CAT-SCRATCH DISEASE

Biology and Epidemiology

Cat-scratch disease (CSD) is a relatively benign disorder usually associated with subacute or chronic regional lymphadenopathy in childhood.[208] Previously of unknown cause, CSD has now been attributed to infection with a small gram-negative bacterium, identified initially by Warthin-Starry stains of lymph node biopsies from patients with CSD.[56,209,210] Now classified as *Afipia felis*, this bacterium has been cultured from the lymph nodes of patients with CSD.[22a] Additional evidence supporting this bacterium as a cause of CSD includes (1) detection of elevated antibody titers against the bacterium in patients with CSD, and (2) production of skin lesions and reisolation of the bacterium from an armadillo inoculated with bacteria from a known CSD patient.[56,210] CSD has also been linked to a rickettsial-like organism *Rochalimaea henselae*.[145a] This organism was originally isolated from the blood of persons with bacillary angiomatosis, a disorder that shares features with disseminated CSD in immunocompromised hosts.[118a,158a] Patients with CSD commonly have elevated antibody titers to this organism.[145a]

Although most reports describe patients from the United States, the disorder apparently occurs worldwide. Two large clinical series, including over 1000 patients and encompassing 30 or more years of experience with CSD, indicate that the disorder has several epidemiologic or clinical characteristics.[26,119] These include (1) a young age of affected patients (approximately 85% are less than 18 years of age), (2) a history of exposure to cats, often young kittens, (3) an onset in the fall or winter in the majority of patients, (4) an inoculation site, usually indicated by a papule, pustule, or mucous membrane lesion, and (5) regional lymphadenopathy, typically involving axillary, inguinal, or cervical lymph nodes.

Clinical Manifestations

The incubation period between cat encounter and onset of a skin lesion at the inoculation site is approximately 3 to 5 days, and within 1 to 2 weeks regional lymphadenopathy develops. Associated symptoms in typical cases include malaise, anorexia, and low-grade fever that rarely exceeds 39°C. The oculoglandular syndrome of Parinaud, the most common atypical manifestation of CSD, consists of a granuloma of the palpebral or rarely global conjunctiva and involvement of the preauricular lymph nodes.[25,27,119] Other unusual complications of CSD include erythema nodosum, bony involvement, atypical pneumonia, and thrombocytopenic purpura.[119]

Occasionally, CSD produces a more severe illness associated with myalgias, arthralgias, weight loss, splenomegaly, and pleurisy.[119] Disseminated CSD has been described in patients with AIDS.[98,118a,170a] Clinical features of CSD in such patients included fever, weight loss, splenomegaly, arthritis, synovitis, adenopathy, and skin eruptions.[118a]

Neurologic complications have been reported in approximately 2% to 3% of immunocompetent patients with CSD.[26,111,115,119,193] Encephalopathy, the most common neurologic feature, usually begins 1 to 6 weeks after the onset of CSD and is associated with headache, convulsions, and an altered level of consciousness.[111,115] Status epilepticus can be the initial sign of CSD, and focal neurologic abnormalities have occasionally been identified. Rarely, patients with CSD have signs compatible with spinal cord involvement, consisting of paraparesis, quadriparesis, or the Brown-Sequard syndrome.[111] Of four such patients reviewed by Lewis and Tucker,[111] three also had cerebral involvement, with stupor or coma. CNS signs typically resolve spontaneously within 2 to 6 days. To date, neurologic complications have not been reported in patients with AIDS and CSD.

The pathogenesis of CNS complications of CSD has not been determined and could reflect direct invasion of the CNS or secondary effects. In a 7-year-old girl with aphasia and a right hemiparesis, arteriography revealed abnormalities of the internal carotid and middle cerebral arteries,[172] suggesting that a primary vasculitis could account for certain CNS features of CSD.

Diagnosis

Nearly any disorder that produces lymphadenopathy and mild systemic symptoms must be considered in the differential diagnosis of CSD. Disorders that might mimic CSD include infections with viruses or atypical mycobacteria and neoplastic conditions such as lymphoma or histiocytosis X. Certain viruses, notably the Epstein-Barr virus or CMV, may produce lymphadenopathy and neurologic complications similar to those of CSD, but can be differentiated from CSD by serologic or virologic studies.

The systemic laboratory findings in CSD consist of nonspecific elevations of the white blood cell count or erythrocyte sedimentation rate. The CSF is usually normal, although mild elevations of the white blood cell count (typically <100 cells/mm^3) or protein content (typically <100 mg/dL) are compatible with CSD.[111] EEGs obtained during the encephalopathic phase of CSD reveal diffuse slowing, but focal abnormalities have been reported. In children with CSD encephalopathy and hemiparesis, CT has occasionally disclosed lesions compatible with cerebral infarction.[111,172]

The diagnosis of CSD relies on (1) a history of contact with a cat, (2) a positive skin test for CSD, (3) negative laboratory tests for other disorders associated with lymphadenopathy, or (4) characteristic histopathologic features in skin or lymph node biopsies. Margileth and colleagues suggest that the diagnosis can be made reliably when three of these four criteria are satisfied.[119] Characteristic histopathologic features of lymph nodes consist of central necrosis, epithelioid granuloma formation, and lymphocytic infiltration. Tissues should be examined for bacilli using Warthin-Starry and Brown-Hopps staining.[56,118a] Serologic studies of *Rochalimaea* species may also be useful.[145a] Additional information regarding serologic studies for CSD or detection of *Rochalimaea henselae* can be obtained from the CDC [(404) 639-1075].

Treatment

The majority of immunocompetent patients with CSD have a benign, self-limited illness, and therapy does not seem to alter the course of CSD.[119] By contrast, antibiotics should be considered strongly in immunocompromised patients or patients with disseminated CSD. The disorder appears to respond to several antibiotics, including erythromycin, doxycycline, isoniazid, rifampin, or ethambutol.[98,118a]

SUMMARY

Although uncommon in the United States and western Europe, invasion of the CNS by various parasites should be considered prominently in the differential diagnosis of patients who have visited or lived in endemic regions of Asia, Africa, or Latin America. Some of these conditions also may be congenital or may be spread by diet or other means, such as the tick bite of Rocky Mountain spotted fever. Immunocompromised patients have a propensity to develop certain of these disorders, especially cerebral toxoplasmosis.

Because effective treatment often depends on a prompt and accurate diagnosis, physicians should be thorough in examining the history of patients with symptoms that suggest these infections. Public health officials or the CDC may offer advice on rapidly changing diagnostic procedures, antimicrobial agents, and drug resistance.

REFERENCES

1. Abdulla K, Tapoo AK, and Agha HSA: Ruptured cerebral hydatid cyst: A case report. J Trop Med Hyg 91:302–305, 1988.
2. Abraham SN and Lawande RV: Incidence of free-living amoebae in the nasal passages of local population in Zaria, Nigeria. J Trop Med Hyg 85:217–222, 1982.
3. Abramowicz M (ed): The medical letter on drugs and therapeutics. The Medical Letter 30:15–22, 1988.
4. Adams EB and MacLeod IN: Invasive amebiasis. Medicine (Baltimore) 56:325–334, 1977.
5. Adams JH: Toxoplasmosis. In Blackwood W, Corsellis JAN (eds): Greenfields Neuropathology. Year Book Medical Publishers, Chicago, 1976, pp 269–270.
6. Adams JH, Haller L, Boa FY, Doua F, Dago A, and Konian K: Human African trypanosomiasis *(T. b. gambiense):* A study of 16 fatal cases of sleeping sickness with some observations on acute reactive arsenical encephalopathy. Neuropathol Appl Neurobiol 12:81–94, 1986.
7. Ahmad SH, Moonis R, Kidwai T, Khan TA, Khan HM, and Shahab T: Cerebral malaria in children. Indian J Pediatr 53:409–413, 1986.
8. Akiguchi I, Fujiwara T, Matsuyama H, Muranaka H, and Kameyama M: Intramedullary spinal cysticercosis. Neurology 29:1531–1534, 1979.
9. Allason-Jones E, Mindel A, Sargeaunt P, and Williams P: *Entamoeba histolytica* as a commensal intestinal parasite in homosexual men. N Engl J Med 315:353–356, 1986.
10. Ancelle T, Dupouy-Camet J, Bougnoux M, et al: Two outbreaks of trichinosis caused by horsemeat in France in 1985. Am J Epidemiol 127:1302–1311, 1988.
11. Anders K, Foley K, Stern WE, and Brown WJ: Intracranial sparganosis: An uncommon infection. J Neurosurg 60:1282–1286, 1984.
12. Anderson DC, Greenwood R, Fishman M, and Kagan IG: Acute infantile hemiplegia with cerebrospinal fluid eosinophilic pleocytosis: An unusual case of visceral larva migrans. J Pediatr 86:247–249, 1975.
13. Anderson K and Jamieson A: Primary amebic meningoencephalitis. Lancet 1:902–903, 1972.
14. Ariizumi M: Cerebral schistosomiasis japonica: Report of one operated case and fifty clinical cases. Am J Trop Med Hyg 12:40–45, 1963.
15. Arseni C and Samitca DC: Cysticercosis of the brain. Br Med J 1:494–497, 1957.
16. Bale JF Jr: Human cytomegalovirus infection and disorders of the nervous system. Arch Neurol 41:310–320, 1984.
16a. Bale JF Jr and Murph JR: Congenital infections and the nervous system. Pediatr Clin North Am 39:669–690, 1992.
17. Beaver PC and Rosen L: Memorandum on the first report of angiostrongylus in man, by Nomura and Lin, 1945. Am J Trop Med Hyg 13:589–590, 1964.
18. Becker GL, Knep S, Lance KP, and Kaufman L: Amebic abscess of the brain. Neurosurgery 6:192–194, 1980.

19. Bell WE and Lascari AD: Rocky Mountain spotted fever. Neurology 20:841–847, 1970.

20. Bittencourt AL: Congenital Chagas disease. Am J Dis Child 130:97–103, 1976.

21. Brener Z: Present status of chemotherapy and chemoprophylaxis of human trypanosomiasis in the western hemisphere. Pharmacol Ther 7:71–90, 1979.

22. Brener Z: Recent developments in the field of Chagas' disease. Bull World Health Organ 60:463–473, 1982.

22a. Brenner DJ, Hollis DG, Moss CW, English CK, et al: Proposal of *Afipia* gen. nov., with *Afipia felis* sp. nov. (formerly cat-scratch disease bacillus), *Afipia clevelandensis* sp. nov. (formerly Cleveland Clinic Foundation Strain), *Afipia broomeae* sp. nov., and three unnamed genospecies. J Clin Microbiol 29:2450–2460.

23. Bruce-Chwatt LJ: From Laveran's discovery to DNA probes: New trends in diagnosis of malaria. Lancet 1:1509–1511, 1987.

24. Byrd SE, Locke GE, Biggers S, and Percy AK: The computed tomographic appearance of cerebral cysticercosis in adults and children. Neuroradiology 144:819–823, 1982.

25. Carithers HA: Oculoglandular disease of Parinaud: A manifestation of cat-scratch disease. Am J Dis Child 132:1195–1200, 1978.

26. Carithers HA: Cat-scratch disease. Am J Dis Child 139:1124–1133, 1985.

26a. Carl M, Tibbs CW, Dobson ME, Paparello S, and Dasch GA: Diagnosis of acute typhus infection using the polymerase chain reaction. J Infect Dis 161:791–793, 1990.

27. Cassady JV and Culbertson CS: Cat-scratch disease and Parinaud's oculoglandular syndrome. Arch Ophthalmol 50:68–74, 1953.

28. Castillo M, Quencer RM, and Post MJD: MR of intramedullary spinal cysticercosis. AJNR 9:393–395, 1988.

29. Centers for Disease Control: An outbreak of African trypanosomiasis—California. MMWR 18:385–386, 1969.

29a. Centers for Disease Control: Acute schistosomiasis with transverse myelitis in American students returning from Kenya. MMWR 33:445–447, 1984.

30. Centers for Disease Control: Rocky Mountain spotted fever—United States, 1987. MMWR 37:388–390, 1988.

30a. Centers for Disease Control: Rocky Mountain spotted fever—United States, 1988. MMWR 38:513–515, 1989.

31. Centers for Disease Control: Recommendations for the prevention of malaria among travelers. MMWR 39:1–10, 1990.

31a. Centers for Disease Control: Acute schistosomiasis in U.S. travelers returning from Africa. MMWR 39:141–148, 1990.

31b. Centers for Disease Control: Change in dosing regimen for malaria prophylaxis with mefloquine. MMWR 40:72–73, 1991.

31c. Centers for Disease Control, Treatment of severe *Plasmodium falciparum* malaria with quinidine: Discontinuation of parenteral quinine from CDC drug service. MMWR 40:240, 1991.

31d. Centers for Disease Control: Primary amebic meningo-encephalitis—North Carolina, 1991. MMWR 41:437–490, 1991.

32. Cerva L and Novak K: Amoebic meningoencephalitis: Sixteen fatalities. Science 160:92, 1968.

33. Chang KH, Kim WS, Cho SY, Han MC, and Kim C: Comparative evaluation of brain CT and ELISA in the diagnosis of neurocysticercosis. AJNR 9:125–130, 1988.

34. Chang YC, Chu CC, and Fan W: Cerebral schistosomiasis. Chin Med J 75:892–907, 1957.

35. Char DFB and Rosen L: Eosinophilic meningitis among children in Hawaii. J Pediatr 70:28–35, 1967.

36. Cleland PG, Lawande RV, Onyeme-

lukwe G, and Whittle HC: Chronic amebic meningoencephalitis. Arch Neurol 39:56–57, 1982.

37. Couvreur J and Desmonts G: Congenital and maternal toxoplasmosis. Med Child Neurol 4:519–530, 1962.

38. Critchley EMR, Vakil SD, Hutchinson DN, and Taylor P: Toxoplasma, toxocara, and epilepsy. Epilepsia 23:315–321, 1982.

39. Culbertson CG, Ensminger PW, and Overton WM: *Hartmanella (Acanthamoeba):* Experimental chronic, granulomatous brain infections produced by new isolates of low virulence. Am J Clin Pathol 46:305–314, 1966.

40. Daffos F, Forestier F, Capella-Pavlovsky M, et al: Prenatal management of 746 pregnancies at risk for congenital toxoplasmosis. N Engl J Med 318:271–275, 1988.

41. Darby CP, Conradi SE, Holbrook TW, and Chatellier C: Primary amebic meningoencephalitis. Am J Dis Child 133:1025–1027, 1979.

42. Davis AE Jr and Bradford AD: Abdominal pain resembling acute appendicitis in Rocky Mountain spotted fever. JAMA 247:2811–2812, 1982.

43. De Raadt P: African sleeping sickness today. Trans R Soc Trop Med Hyg 70:114–116, 1976.

44. De Savigny DH, Voller A, and Woodruff AW: Toxocariasis: Serologic diagnosis by enzyme immunoassay. J Clin Pathol 32:284–288, 1979.

45. Desmonts G and Couvreur J: Congenital toxoplasmosis. N Engl J Med 290:1110–1116, 1974.

46. Desmonts G, Forestier F, Thulliez PH, Daffos F, Capella-Pavlovsky M, and Chartier M: Prenatal diagnosis of congenital toxoplasmosis. Lancet 1:500–504, 1985.

47. Diebler C, Dusser A, and Dulac O: Congenital toxoplasmosis. Neuroradiology 27:125–130, 1985.

48. Donta ST, Wallace RB, Whipp SC, and Olarte J: Enterotoxigenic *Escherichia coli* and diarrheal disease in Mexican children. J Infect Dis 135:482–485, 1977.

49. Droff RB, Deller J, Kastl A, and Blocker WW: Cerebral malaria. JAMA 202:679–682, 1967.

50. Duggan AJ and Hutchinson MP: Sleeping sickness in Europeans: A review of 109 cases. J Trop Med Hyg 69:124–131, 1966.

51. Dunn SA, Schwartz D, Brinkley J, and Wright KW: Congenital toxoplasmosis presenting as isolated acute chorioretinitis in the neonate. J Pediatr Ophthalmol Strabismus 25:30–32, 1988.

52. Dunne K and Gill D: Toxocariasis: Diagnosis and dilemmas. Br J Clin Pract 41:681–683, 1987.

53. DuPont HL, Hornick RB, Weiss CF, Snyder MJ, and Woodward TE: Evaluation of chloramphenicol acid succinate therapy of induced typhoid fever and Rocky Mountain spotted fever. N Engl J Med 282:53–57, 1970.

54. Elder GA and Sever JL: Neurologic disorders associated with AIDS retroviral infection. Rev Infect Dis 10:286–302, 1988.

55. Elkin CM, Leon E, Grenell SL, and Leeds NE: Intracranial lesions in the acquired immunodeficiency syndrome. JAMA 253:393–396, 1985.

56. English CK, Wear DJ, Margileth AM, Lissner CR, and Walsh GP: Cat-scratch disease. JAMA 259:1347–1352, 1988.

57. Fan K and Pezeshkpout GH: Cerebral sparganosis. Neurology 36:1249–1251, 1986.

58. Feldman HA: Nationwide serum survey of United States military recruits, 1962. Am J Epidemiol 81:385–391, 1965.

59. Feldman HA: Toxoplasmosis. N Engl J Med 279:1370–1375, 1431–1437, 1968.

60. Feldman HA and Miller LT: Serological study of toxoplasmosis prevalence. Am J Hyg 64:320–335, 1956.

61. Fishbein DB, Kaplan JE, Bernard KW, and Winkler WG: Surveillance of Rocky Mountain spotted fever in the United States, 1981–1983. J Infect Dis 150:609–611, 1984.

62. Fleta J, Sarria A, Villagrasa J, et al:

Computed tomography in the diagnosis of brain hydatidosis in children. Acta Paediatr Scand 76:835–836, 1987.

63. Fowler M and Carter RF: Acute pyogenic meningitis probably due to *Acanthamoeba* sp.: A preliminary report. Br Med J 2:740–742, 1965.

63a. Fox AS, Kaszacos KR, Gould NS, Heydemann PT, Thomas C, and Boyer KM: Fatal eosinophilic meningoencephalitis and visceral larva migrans caused by the raccoon ascarid *Baylisascaris procyonis*. N Engl J Med 312:1619–1623, 1985.

64. Gaston A, Gherardi R, N'Guyen JP, et al: Cerebral toxoplasmosis in acquired immunodeficiency syndrome. Neuroradiology 27:83–86, 1985.

64a. Genta RM: Global prevalence of strongyloidiasis: Critical review with epidemiologic insights into the prevention of disseminated disease. Rev Infect Dis 11:755–767, 1989.

65. Gilles HM: The treatment and prophylaxis of malaria. Ann Trop Med Parasitol 81:607–617, 1987.

66. Gillespie SH: Human toxocariasis. J Appl Bacteriol 63:473–479, 1987.

67. Glickman LT, Cypess RH, Crumrine PK, and Gitlin DA: *Toxocara* infection and epilepsy in children. J Pediatr 94:75–78, 1979.

68. Glickman LT and Schantz PM: Epidemiology and pathogenesis of toxocariasis. Epidemiol Rev 3:230–250, 1981.

69. Gorman RJ, Saxon S, and Snead OC III: Neurologic sequelae of Rocky Mountain spotted fever. Pediatrics 67:354–357, 1981.

70. Gray DF, Morse BS, and Phillips WF: Trichinosis with neurologic and cardiac involvement. Ann Intern Med 57:230–243, 1962.

71. Grunnet ML, Cannon GH, and Kushner JP: Fulminant amebic meningoencephalitis due to *Acanthamoeba*. Neurology (NY) 31:174–177, 1981.

72. Guerrant RL: The global problem of amebiasis: Current status, research needs, and opportunities for progress. Rev Infect Dis 8:218–227, 1986.

73. Gutteridge WE: Chemotherapy of Chagas' disease. Tran R Soc Trop Med Hyg 70:123–124, 1976.

74. Haller L, Adams H, Merouze F, and Dago A: Clinical and pathological aspects of human African trypanosomiasis *(T. b. gambiense)* with particular reference to reactive arsenical encephalopathy. Am J Trop Med Hyg 35:94–99, 1986.

74a. Hammarsten JF: The contributions of Idaho physicians to knowledge of Rocky Mountain spotted fever. Trans Am Clin Climatol Assoc 94:27–43, 1982.

75. Hattwick MAW: Rocky Mountain spotted fever in the United States, 1920–1970. J Infect Dis 124:112–114, 1971.

76. Hattwick MAW, O'Brien RJ, and Hanson BF: Rocky Mountain spotted fever: Epidemiology of an increasing problem. Ann Intern Med 84:732–739, 1976.

77. Haverkos HW: Assessment of therapy for toxoplasma encephalitis. Am J Med 82:907–914, 1987.

78. Helmick CG, Bernard KW, and D'Angelo LJ: Rocky Mountain spotted fever: Clinical, laboratory, and epidemiological features of 262 cases. J Infect Dis 150:480–488, 1984.

78a. Hermos JA, Healy GR, Schultz MG, and Barlow J: Fatal human cerebral coenurosis. JAMA 213:1461–1464, 1970.

79. Higashi K, Aoki H, Takebayashi K, Morioka H, and Sakata Y: Cerebral paragonimiasis. J Neurosurg 34:515–528, 1971.

80. Hill IR, Denham DA, and Scholtz CL: *Toxocara canis* larvae in the brain of a British child. Trans R Soc Trop Med Hyg 79:351–354, 1985.

81. Hoff R, Teixeira RS, Carvalho JS, and Mott KE: *Trypanosoma cruzi* in the cerebrospinal fluid during the acute stage of Chagas' disease. N Engl J Med 278:604–606, 1978.

81a. Holliman RE, Johnson JD, and Savva D: Diagnosis of cerebral toxoplasmosis in association with AIDS using the polymerase chain reaction. Scand J Infect Dis 22(2):243–244, 1990.

82. Hogan M: Ocular toxoplasmosis. Trans Am Acad Ophthalmol Otolaryngol 62:7–37, 1958.

83. Horney LF and Walker DH: Meningoencephalitis as a major manifestation of Rocky Mountain spotted fever. South Med J 81:915–918, 1988.

84. Howard JE: La Enfermedad de Chagas Congenita. Santiago, Universidad de Chile, 1962.

84a. Hsu WY, Chen JY, Chien CT, Chi CS, and Han NT: Eosinophilic meningitis caused by *Angiostrongylus cantonensis*. Pediatr Infect Dis J 9:443–445, 1990.

85. Hughes FB, Faehnle SF, and Simon JL: Multiple cerebral abscesses complicating hepatopulmonary amebiasis. J Pediatr 86:95–96, 1975.

86. Jager BV and Stamm WP: Brain abscesses caused by free-living amoeba probably of the genus *Hartmannella* in a patient with Hodgkin's disease. Lancet 2:1343–1345, 1972.

86a. Jones TC: Protozoal diseases. In Mandell GL, Douglas RG, and Bennet JE (eds): Principles and Practices of Infectious Diseases. John Wiley & Sons, New York, 1979, pp 2085–2087.

87. Jordan MC, Rousseau WE, Stewart JA, Noble GR, and Chin TDY: Spontaneous cytomegalovirus mononucleosis. Ann Intern Med 79:153–160, 1973.

88. Kamper CA, Chessman KH, and Phelps SJ: Rocky Mountain spotted fever. Clin Pharm 7:109–116, 1988.

89. Kane CA and Most H: Schistosomiasis of the central nervous system. Arch Neurol Psychiatry 59:141–183, 1948.

90. Kasper DL, Kass EH (Weller PF, discussant): Infectious disease rounds: Headache, fever, and periorbital edema. Rev Infect Dis 9:804–809, 1987.

91. Katz DA, Dworzack DL, Horowitz ED, and Bogard PJ: Encephalitis associated with Rocky Mountain spotted fever. Arch Pathol Lab Med 109:771–773, 1985.

92. Kelsey DS: Rocky Mountain spotted fever. Pediatr Clin North Am 26:367–376, 1979.

93. Kin SK: Cerebral paragonimiasis. Arch Neurol 1:30–37, 1959.

94. King DK, Loh KK, Ayala AG, and Gamble JF: Eosinophilic meningitis and lymphomatous meningitis. Ann Intern Med 82:228, 1975.

95. Kirchhoff LV and Nash TE: A case of schistosomiasis japonica: Resolution of CAT-scan detected cerebral abnormalities without specific therapy. Am J Trop Med Hyg 33:1155–1158, 1984.

96. Kirchhoff LV and Neva FA: *Trypanosoma* species (Chagas' disease). In Mandell GL, Douglas RG Jr, and Bennett JE (eds): Principles and Practice of Infectious Diseases, Ed 2. John Wiley & Sons, New York, 1985, pp 1531–1537.

97. Kirchoff LV and Neva FA: Chagas' disease in Latin American immigrants. JAMA 254:3058–3060, 1985.

97a. Kirk JL, Fine DP, Sexton DJ, and Muchmore HG: Rocky Mountain spotted fever. A clinical review based on 48 confirmed cases, 1943–1986. Medicine 69:35–45, 1990.

98. Koehler JE, LeBoit PE, Egbert BM, and Berger TG: Cutaneous vascular lesions and disseminated cat-scratch disease in patients with the acquired immunodeficiency syndrome (AIDS) and AIDS-related complex. Ann Intern Med 109:449–455, 1988.

98a. Koo J, Pien F, and Kliks MM: *Angiostrongylus* (parastrongylus) eosinophilic meningitis. Rev Infect Dis 10:1155–1162, 1988.

99. Koppe J, Loewer-Sieger D, and De Roever-Bonnet H: Results of 20-year follow-up of congenital toxoplasmosis. Lancet 1:254–256, 1986.

100. Koskiniemi M, Lappalainen M, and Hedman K: Toxoplasmosis needs

evaluation. Am J Dis Child, 143:724–728, 1989.

101. Kramer MD and Aita JF: Trichinosis with central nervous system involvement. Neurology 22:485–491, 1972.

102. Krick JA, and Remington JS: Toxoplasmosis in the adult—an overview. N Engl J Med 298:550–553, 1978.

103. Krogstad DJ, Spencer HC, and Healy GR: Amebiasis. N Engl J Med 262–265, 1978.

104. Kuberski T: Eosinophils in the cerebrospinal fluid. Ann Intern Med 91:70–75, 1979.

105. Kuberski T, Bart RD, Briley JM, and Rosen L: Recovery of *Angiostrongylus cantonensis* from cerebrospinal fluid of a child with eosinophilic meningitis. J Clin Microbiol 9:629–631, 1979.

106. Kuberski T and Wallace GD: Clinical manifestations of eosiniophilic meningitis due to *Angiostrongylus cantonensis.* Neurology 29:1566–1570, 1979.

107. Landman G, Correa-Alves A, Mendes NF and Mendes E: Identification of *Trypanosoma cruzi* in human tissues using an immunoperoxidase method: Study of acute Chagas disease, congenital form. Allergol Immunopathol (Madr) 14:509–513, 1986.

108. Latovitzki N, Abrams G, Clark C, Mayeux R, Ascherl G, and Sciarra D: Cerebral cysticercosis. Neurology 28:838–842, 1978.

109. Leblanc R, Knowles KF, Melanson D, MacLean JD, Rouleau G, and Farmer J: Neurocysticercosis: Surgical and medical management with praziquantel. Neurosurgery 18:419–427, 1986.

109a. Leiguarda R, Roncoroni A, Taratuto AL, et al: Acute CNS infection by *Trypanosoma cruzi* (Chagas' disease) in immunosuppressed patients. Neurology 40:850–851, 1990.

110. Leport C, Raffi F, Matheron et al: Treatment of central nervous system toxoplasmosis with pyrimethamine/sulfadiazine combination in 35 patients with the acquired immunodeficiency syndrome. Am J Med 84:94–100, 1988.

111. Lewis DW and Tucker SH: Central nervous system involvement in cat scratch disease. Pediatrics 77:714–721, 1986.

112. Lobel HO, Campbell CC, Schwartz IK, and Roberts JM: Recent trends in the importation of malaria caused by *Plasmodium falciparum* into the United States from Africa. J Infect Dis 152:613–617, 1985.

113. Lotz HO, Hewlett R, Alheit B, and Bowen R: Neurocysticercosis: Correlative pathomorphology and MR imaging. Neuroradiology 30:35–41, 1988.

114. Lumsden WHR: Chagas' disease—a survey of the present position. Tran R Soc Trop Med Hyg 70:121–122, 1976.

115. Lyon LW: Neurologic manifestations of cat scratch disease. Arch Neurol 25:23–27, 1971.

116. Maddison SE: The present status of serodiagnosis and seroepidemiology of schistosomiasis. Diagn Microbiol Infect Dis 7:93–105, 1987.

117. Mahmoud AA: Schistosomiasis. N Engl J Med 297:1329–1331, 1977.

118. Mahmoud AAF and Warren KS: Algorithms in the diagnosis and management of exotic disease. XI. African trypanosomiases. J Infect Dis 133:487–491, 1976.

118a. Marasco WA, Lester S, and Parsonnet J: Unusual presentation of cat scratch disease in a patient positive for antibody to the human immunodeficiency virus. Rev Infect Dis 11:793–803, 1989.

119. Margileth AM, Wear DJ, and English CK: Systemic cat scratch disease: Report of 23 patients with prolonged or recurrent severe bacterial infection. J Infect Dis 155:390–402, 1987.

120. Martinez AJ: Is *Acanthamoeba* encephalitis an opportunistic infection? Neurology 30:567–574, 1980.

121. Masdeu JC, Tantulavanich S, Gorelick PP, et al: Brain abscess caused by *Strongyloides stercoralis*. Arch Neurol 39:62–63, 1982.
122. Mason JC, Ordelheide KS, Grames GM, et al: Toxoplasmosis in two renal transplant recipients from a single donor. Transplantation 44:588–591, 1987.
123. Matson DO, Rouah E, Lee RT, Armstrong D, Parke JT, and Baker CJ: *Acanthameba* meningoencephalitis masquerading as neurocysticercosis. Pediatr Infect Dis J 7:121–124, 1988.
124. McCabe R and Remington J: The diagnosis and treatment of toxoplasmosis. Eur J Clin Microbiol 2:95–104, 1983.
125. McCabe R and Remington S: Toxoplasmosis: The time has come. N Engl J Med 318:313–315, 1988.
126. McCormick GF, Giannotta S, Zee C, and Fisher M: Carotid occlusion in cysticercosis. Neurology (Cleveland) 33:1078–1080, 1983.
127. McCormick GF, Zee C, and Heiden J: Cysticercosis cerebri. Arch Neurol 39:534–539, 1982.
127a. McDade JE: Ehrlichiosis—a disease of animals and humans. J Infect Dis 161:609–617, 1990.
128. McDade JE and Newhouse VF: Natural history of *Rickettsia rickettsii*. Annu Rev Microbiol 40:287–309, 1986.
129. Medina EA, Ventura FA, and Champalimaud JL: Computer-assisted tomographic findings in a patient with African trypanosomiasis. J Trop Med Hyg 89:75–77, 1986.
130. Mehren M, Burns PJ, Mamani F, Levy CS, and Laureno R: Toxoplasmic myelitis mimicking intramedullary spinal cord tumor. Neurology 38:1648–1650, 1988.
131. Mendelson MH, Finkel LJ, Meyers BR, Lieberman JP, and Hirschman SZ: Pulmonary toxoplasmosis in AIDS. Scand J Infect Dis 19:703–706, 1987.
132. Miller B, Grinnell V, Goldberg MA, and Heiner D: Spontaneous radiographic disappearance of cerebral cysticercosis: Three cases. Neurology (Cleveland) 33:1377–1379, 1983.
132a. Miller KD, Greenberg AE, and Campbell CC: Treatment of malaria in the United States with a continuous infusion of quinidine gluconate and exchange transfusion. N Engl J Med 321:65–70, 1989.
133. Mineura K and Mori T: Sparganosis of the brain. J Neurosurg 52:588–590, 1980.
133a. Mitchell A, Scheithauer BW, Kelly PJ, Forbes GS, and Rosenblatt JE: Cerebral sparganosis. J Neurosurg 73:147–150, 1990.
134. Mitchell WG and Crawford TO: Intraparenchymal cerebral cysticercosis in children: Diagnosis and treatment. Pediatrics 82:76–82, 1988.
134a. Moser DR, Kirchhoff LV, and Donelson JE: Detection of *Trypanosoma cruzi* by DNA amplification using the polymerase chain reaction. J Clin Microbiol 27:1477–1482, 1989.
135. Most H: Trichinosis—preventable yet still with us. N Engl J Med 298:1178–1180, 1978.
136. Most H: Treatment of parasitic infections of travelers and immigrants. N Engl J Med 310:298–304, 1984.
137. Most H and Abeles MM: Trichiniasis involving the nervous system. Arch Neurol Psychiatry 37:589–616, 1937.
138. Most H, Kane CA, Lavietes PH, et al: Schistosomiasis japonica in American military personnel: Clinical studies of 600 cases during the first year after infection. Am J Trop Med Hyg 30:239–299, 1950.
138a. Nahmias AJ: The TORCH complex. Hosp Prac May:65–72, 1974.
139. Naot Y, Desmonts G, and Remington JS: IgM enzyme-linked immunosorbent assay test for the diagnosis of congenital toxoplasma infection. J Pediatr 98:32–36, 1981.
140. Nash TE and Neva FA: Recent advances in the diagnosis and treatment of cerebral cysticercosis. N Engl J Med 311:1492–1496, 1984.

141. Navia BA, Petito CK, Gold JWM, Cho E, Jordan BD, and Price RW: Cerebral toxoplasmosis complicating the acquired immune deficiency syndrome clinical and neuropathological findings in 27 patients. Ann Neurol 19:224–238, 1986.

142. Neefe LI, Pinilla O, Garagusi VF, and Bauer H: Disseminated strongyloidiasis with cerebral involvement. Am J Med 55:832–838, 1973.

143. Nelson GS: More than a hundred years of parasitic zoonoses: With special reference to trichinosis and hydatid disease. J Comp Pathol 98:135–151, 1988.

143a. Nelson J, Frost JL, and Schochet SS Jr: Unsuspected cerebral toxocara infection in a fire victim. Clin Neuropathol 9:106–108, 1990.

144. Ofori-Kwakye SK, Sidebottom DG, Herbert J, Fischer ED, and Visvesvara GS: Granulomatous brain tumor caused by Acanthamoeba. J Neurosurg 64:505–509, 1986.

145. Oh SJ: Roentogen findings in cerebral paragonimiasis. Radiology 90:292–299, 1968.

145a. Regenery RL, Olson JG, Perkins BA, et al: Serological response to Rochlimaea henselae antigen in suspected cat-scratch disease. Lancet 339:1443–1445, 1992.

146. Orbison JA, Reeves N, Leedham CL, and Blumberg JM: Amebic brain abscess. Medicine (Baltimore) 30:247–282, 1951.

147. Oster CN, Burke DS, Kenyon RH, Ascher MS, Harber P, and Pedersen CE Jr: Laboratory-acquired Rocky Mountain spotted fever. N Engl J Med 197:859–863, 1977.

148. Owor R and Wamukota WM: A fatal case of strongyloidiasis with Strongyloides larvae in the meninges. Trans R Soc Trop Med Hyg 70:497–499, 1976.

149. Ozgen T, Erbengi A, Bertan V, Saglan S, Gurcay O, and Pirnar T: The use of computerized tomography in the diagnosis of cerebral hydatid cysts. J Neurosurg 50:339–342, 1979.

149a. Panisko DM and Keystone JM: Treatment of malaria—1990. Drugs 39:160–189, 1990.

149b. Pau A, Perria C, Turtas S, Brambilla M, and Viale G: Long-term follow-up of the surgical treatment of intracranial coenurosis. Br J Neurosurg 4:39–44, 1990.

150. Pearl M, Kotsillimbos DG, Lehrer HZ, Rao AH, Fink H, and Zaiman H: Cerebral echinococcosis, a pediatric disease: Report of two cases with one successful five-year follow-up. Pediatrics 61:915–920, 1978.

151. Percy AK, Byrd SE, and Locke GE: Cerebral cysticercosis. Pediatrics 66:967–971, 1980.

151a. Peter JB: Use and Interpretation of Tests in Medical Microbiology, Ed 2. Specialty Laboratories, Santa Monica, CA, 1990, pp. 3–4.

152. Petru AM, Azimi PH, Cummins SK, and Sjoerdsma A: African sleeping sickness in the United States. Am J Dis Child 142:224–228, 1988.

153. Potasman I, Resnick L, Luft BJ, and Remington JS: Intrathecal production of antibodies against Toxoplasma gondii in patients with toxoplasmic encephalitis and the acquired immunodeficiency syndrome (AIDS). Ann Intern Med 108:49–51, 1988.

154. Powell SJ, MacLeod I, Wilmot AJ, and Elsdon-Dew R: Metronidazole in amoebic dysentery and amoebic liver abscess. Lancet 2:1329–1331, 1966.

154a. Punyagupta S, Bunnag T, and Juttijudata P: Eosinophilic meningitis in Thailand. J Neurol Sci 96:241–256, 1990.

155. Punyagupta S, Bunnag T, Juttijudata P, and Rosen L: Eosinophilic meningitis in Thailand. Am J Trop Med Hyg 19:950–958, 1970.

156. Punyagupta S, Juttijudata P, Bunnag T, and Comer DS: Two fatal cases of eosinophilic myeloencephalitis, a newly recognized disease caused by Gnathostoma spinigerum. Trans R Soc Trop Med Hyg 62:801–809, 1968.

157. Quinn TC, Jacobs RF, Mertz GJ, Hook EW III, and Locklsey RM: Con-

genital malaria: A report of four cases and a review. J Pediatr 101:229–232, 1982.

158. Ramos OM, Stiebel-Chin G, Altman N, and Duchowny M: Diagnosis of neurocysticercosis by magnetic resonance imaging. Pediatr Infect Dis 5:470–473, 1986.

158a. Relman DA, Loutit JS, Schmidt TM, et al: The agent of bacillary angiomatosis. N Engl J Med 23:1573–1580, 1990.

159. Remington JS: Toxoplasmosis in an adult. Bull N Y Acad Med 50:211–227, 1974.

160. Remington JS and Desmonts G: Toxoplasmosis. In Remington JS, Klein JO (eds): Infectious Diseases of the Fetus and Newborn Infant. WB Saunders, Philadelphia, 1983, pp 191–332.

161. Report of the Committee on Infectious Disease, Ed. 21: Malaria. Peter G, Hall CB, Lepow ML, and Phillips CF (eds), American Academy of Pediatrics, 1988, pp 268–276.

162. Report of the Committee on Infectious Disease, Ed. 21: Primary amebic meningoencephalitis. Peter G, Hall CB, Lepow ML, and Phillips CF (eds), American Academy of Pediatrics, 1988, pp 120–121.

163. Report of the Committee on Infectious Disease, Ed. 21: Strongyloidiasis. Peter G, Hall CB, Lepow ML, and Phillips CF (eds), American Academy of Pediatrics, 1988, pp 398–400.

163a. Report of the Committee on Infectious Disease, Ed. 22: Malaria. Peter G, Lepow ML, McCracken GH, and Phillips CF (eds), American Academy of Pediatrics, 1991, pp 303–304.

164. Reyes VA, Yogore MG, and Pardo LP: Studies on cerebral schistosomiasis. J Philip Med Assoc 40:88–100, 1964.

165. Rolston KVI and Hoy J: Role of clindamycin in the treatment of central nervous system toxoplasmosis. Am J Med 83:551–554, 1987.

166. Rosas N, Sotelo J, and Nieto D: ELISA in the diagnosis of neurocysticercosis. Arch Neurol 43:353–356, 1986.

167. Ruskin J and Remington JS: Toxoplasmosis in the compromised host. Ann Intern Med 84:193–199, 1976.

168. Salgo MP, Telzak EE, Currie B, et al: A focus of Rocky Mountain spotted fever within New York City. N Engl J Med 318:1345–1348, 1988.

168a. Savva D, Morris JC, Johnson JD, and Holliman RE: Polymerase chain reaction for detection of Toxoplasma gondii. J Med Microbiol 32(1):25–31, 1990.

169. Schantz PM and Glickman LT: Toxocaral visceral larva migrans. N Engl J Med 298:436–439, 1978.

170. Scharf D: Neurocysticercosis. Arch Neurol 45:777–780, 1988.

170a. Marasco WA, Lester S, and Parsonnet J: Unusual presentation of cat scratch disease in a patient positive for antibody to the human immunodeficiency virus. Rev Infect Dis 11:793–803, 1989.

170b. Schochet SS: Human Toxocara canis encephalopathy in a case of visceral larva migrans. Neurology 17:227–229, 1967.

171. Scowden EB, Schaffner W, and Stone WJ: Overwhelming strongyloidiasis: An unappreciated opportunistic infection. Medicine 39:527–544, 1978.

171a. Seidel JS, Harmatz P, Visvesara GS, et al: Successful treatment of primary amoebic meningoencephalitis. N Engl J Med 306:346–348, 1982.

172. Selby G and Walker GL: Cerebral arteritis in cat-scratch disease. Neurology 29:1413–1418, 1979.

173. Sexton DJ: Rocky Mountain spotted fever. Arch Intern Med 145:2173, 1985.

174. Shanley JD and Jordan C: Clinical aspects of CNS cysticercosis. Arch Intern Med 140:1309–1313, 1980.

175. Shih Y, Ch'en Y, and Chang Y: Paragonimiasis of central nervous system. Chin Med J 77:10–19, 1958.

176. Sica RE, Filipini D, Panizza M, et al: Involvement of the peripheral sensory nervous system in human chronic Chagas disease. Medicina (B Aires) 46:662–668, 1986.

177. Singcharoen T, Rawd-Aree P, and

Baddeley H: Computed tomography findings in disseminated paragonimiasis. Br J Radiol 61:83–86, 1988.

178. Snider WD, Simpson DM, Nielsen S, Gold JWM, Metroka CE, and Posner JB: Neurological complications of acquired immune deficiency syndrome: Analysis of 50 patients. Ann Neurol 14:403–418, 1983.

179. Sotelo J, Escobedo F, Rodriguez-Carbajal J, Torres B, and Rubio-Donnadieu F: Therapy of parenchymal brain cysticercosis with praziquantel. N Engl J Med 319:1001–1007, 1984.

180. Sotelo J, Escobedo F, and Penagos P: Albendazole vs praziquantel for therapy for neurocysticercosis. Arch Neurol 45:532–534, 1988.

181. Sotelo J, Guerrero V, and Rubio F: Neurocysticercosis: A new classification based on active and inactive forms. Arch Intern Med 145:442–445, 1985.

182. Sotelo J and Marin C: Hydrocephalus secondary to cysticercotic arachnoiditis. J Neurosurg 66:686–689, 1987.

183. Sotelo J, Rosas N, and Palencia G: Freezing of infested pork muscle kills cysticerci. JAMA 256:893–894, 1986.

184. Sotelo J, Torres B, Rubio-Donnadieu F, Escobedo F, and Rodriguez-Carbajal J: Praziquantel in the treatment of neurocysticercosis: Long-term follow-up. Neurology 35:752–755, 1985.

185. Sotelo-Avila C, Taylor FM, and Ewing CW: Primary amebic meningoencephalitis in a healthy 7-year-old boy. J Pediatr 85:131–136, 1974.

186. Special Programme for Research and Training in Tropical Diseases, World Health Organization: The African trypanosomiases. In Tropical Disease Research: Seventh Programme Report, Avignon, France, Imprimerie A Barthelemy, 1985, p 5/3.

187. Spencer HC Jr, Gibson JJ, Brodsky RE, and Schultz MG: Imported African trypanosomiasis in the United States. Ann Intern Med 82:633–638, 1975.

188. Spina-Franca A: [American trypanosomiasis (Chagas disease) and the nervous system]. Bull Soc Pathol Exot Filiales 81:645–649, 1988.

189. Stagno S: Congenital toxoplasmosis. Am J Dis Child 134:635–637, 1980.

190. Stagno S, Reynolds DW, Amos CS, et al: Auditory and visual defects resulting from symptomatic and subclinical congenital cytomegaloviral and toxoplasma infections. Pediatrics 59:669–678, 1977.

191. Stepien L: Cerebral cysticercosis in Poland: Clinical symptoms and operative results in 132 cases. J Neurosurg 19:505–513, 1962.

192. Stern WE: Neurosurgical considerations of cysticercosis of the central nervous system. J Neurosurg 55:382–389, 1981.

193. Stevens H: Cat scratch fever encephalitis. Am J Dis Child 84:218–222, 1952.

194. Stray-Pedersen B: A prospective study of acquired toxoplasmosis among 8043 pregnant women in the Oslo area. Am J Obstet Gynecol 136:399–406, 1980.

195. Sumaya CV and Ench Y: Epstein-Barr virus infectious mononucleosis in children. Pediatrics 75:1003–1010, 1985.

196. Suss RA, Maravilla KR, and Thompson J: MR imaging of intracranial cysticercosis: Comparison with CT and anatomopathologic features. AJNR 7:235–242, 1986.

196a. Swisher C, et al: Neurologic function in treated congenital toxoplasmosis. Ann Neurol 32:448, 1992.

197. Taelman H, Schechter PJ, Marcelis L, et al: Difluoromethylornithine, an effective new treatment of gambian trypanosomiasis: Results in five patients. Am J Med 82:607–613, 1987.

198. Taylor MRH, O'Connor P, Keane CT, Mulvihille E, and Holland C: The expanded spectrum of toxocaral disease. Lancet 1:692–694, 1988.

199. Thompson DE, Bundy DAP, Cooper ES, and Schantz PM: Epidemiologi-

cal characteristics of Toxocara canis zoonotic infection of children in a Carribean community. Bull World Health Organ 64:283–290, 1986.

200. Tillman AJB: Schistosomiasis japonica with cerebral manifestations. Arch Intern Med 79:36–61, 1947.

201. Townsend JJ, Wolinsky JS, Baringer JR, and Johnson PC: Acquired toxoplasmosis. Arch Neurol 32:335–343, 1975.

202. Udaka F, Okuda B, Okada M, Tsuji T, and Kameyama M: CT findings of cerebral paragonimiasis in the chronic state. Neuroradiology 30:31–34, 1988.

203. Vazquez JL, Jung H, and Sotelo J: Plasma levels of praziquantel decrease when dexamethasone is given simultaneously. Neurology 37:1561–1562, 1987.

203a. Waikagul J: Serodiagnosis of paragonimiasis by enzyme-linked immunosorbent assay and immunoelectrophoresis. Southeast Asian J Trop Med Public Health 20:243–251, 1989.

204. Walker DH, Burday MS, and Folds JD: Laboratory diagnosis of Rocky Mountain spotted fever. South Med J 73:1443–1446, 1980.

205. Walker DH, Cain BG, and Olmstead PM: Laboratory diagnosis of Rocky Mountain spotted fever by immunofluorescent demonstration of *Rickettsia rickettsii* in cutaneous lesions. Am J Clin Pathol 69:619–623, 1978.

206. Walker DH, Lesesne HR, Varma VA, and Thacker WC: Rocky Mountain spotted fever mimicking acute cholecystitis. Arch Intern Med 145:2194–2196, 1985.

207. Walsh JA: Problems in recognition and diagnosis of amebiasis: Estimation of the global magnitude of morbidity and mortality. Rev Infect Dis 8:228–238, 1986.

207a. Wang SS and Feldman HA: Isolation of *Hartmannella* species from human throats. N Engl J Med 277:1174–1179, 1967.

208. Warwick WJ: Cat-scratch syndrome, many diseases or one disease? Prog Med Virol 9:256–301, 1967.

209. Wear DJ, Malaty RH, Zimmerman LE, Hadfield TL, and Margileth AM: Cat scratch disease bacilli in the conjunctiva of patients with Parinaud's oculoglandular syndrome. Ophthalmology 92:1282–1287, 1985.

210. Wear DJ, Margileth AM, Hadfield TL, Fischer GW, Schlagel CJ, and King FM: Cat scratch disease: A bacterial infection. Science 221:1403–1405, 1983.

211. Wellings FM, Amuso PT, Chang SL, and Lewis AL: Isolation and identification of pathogenic *Naegleria* from Florida lakes. Appl Environ Microbiol 34:661–667, 1977.

212. Williamson J: Chemotherapy of African trypanosomiasis. Trans R Soc Trop Med Hyg 70:117–119, 1976.

213. Willis J and Rosman NP: The Aicardi syndrome versus congenital infection: Diagnostic considerations. J Pediatr 96:235–239, 1980.

214. Willett KC: The "trypanosome chancre" in Rhodesian sleeping sickness. Trans R Soc Trop Med Hyg 60:689–690, 1966.

215. Wilson CB, Remington JS, Stagno S, and Reynolds DW: Development of adverse sequelae in children born with subclinical congenital toxoplasma infection. Pediatrics 66:767–774, 1980.

215a. Wilson LB and Chowning WM: Studies in pyroplasmosis hominis ("spotted fever" or "tick fever" of the Rocky Mountains). J Infect Dis 1:31–57, 1904.

216. Wilson M, Ware DA, and Walls KW: Evaluation of commercial serodiagnostic kits for toxoplasmosis. J Clin Microbiol 25:2262–2265, 1987.

217. Woo PTK and Soltys MA: Animals as reservoir hosts of human trypanosomes. J Wildl Dis 6:313–322, 1970.

218. Woodruff AW, Bisseru B, and Bowe JC: Infections with animal helminths as a factor in causing poliomyelitis and epilepsy. Br Med J 1:1576–1579, 1966.

219. Woodward TE, Pedersen CE, Oster CN, Bagley LR, Romberger J, and Snyder MJ: Prompt confirmation of Rocky Mountain spotted fever: Identification of rickettsiae in skin tissue. J Infect Dis 134:297–301, 1976.

220. World Health Organization: The use of DNA probes for malaria diagnosis. Memorandum from a WHO meeting. Bull World Health Organ 64:641–652, 1986.

221. World Health Organization: Severe and complicated malaria. Trans R Soc Trop Med Hyg 80:3–50, 1986.

222. Wright SW and Trott AT: North American tick-borne diseases. Ann Emerg Med 17:964–972, 1988.

223. Wyler DJ: Malaria—resurgence, resistance, and research. N Engl J Med 308:875–878, 1983.

224. Yoshida M, Moritaka K, Kuga S, and Angegawa S: CT findings of cerebral paragonimiasis in the chronic state. J Comput Assist Tomogr 6:195–196, 1982.

225. Zinkham WH: Visceral larva migrans. Am J Dis Child 132:627–633, 1978.

Chapter 13

ANTIBACTERIAL AND ANTIFUNGAL THERAPY FOR CNS INFECTIONS

William E. Bell, M.D., **and**
Gail A. McGuinness, M.D.

ANTIBACTERIAL THERAPY
ANTIFUNGAL THERAPY

ANTIBACTERIAL THERAPY

Any form of reasonable treatment for acute bacterial meningitis had to await the ability to identify the illness in life, a milestone achieved by Quincke's introduction of the technique of lumbar puncture in 1891. The first effective method of treatment of bacterial meningitis was with antimeningococcal horse serum, introduced in 1906 almost simultaneously by Flexner[81] in the United States and Jochmann[116] in Germany. Although cumbersome and hazardous, serum therapy did significantly reduce the death rate from meningococcal meningitis, then referred to as "epidemic spinal meningitis." The next major advances were the introduction of sulfonamides in 1935 and of penicillin in 1941. Over the ensuing years, numerous other antimicrobials were discovered, and other refinements in the treatment of bacterial meningitis were developed. Currently, one may choose from many antibiotics available for the treatment of central nervous system (CNS) bacterial infections. Proper use of these antimicrobials requires knowledge of the spectrum of antibacterial activity of each, as well as

their pharmacokinetic characteristics and possible adverse effects. The availability of new antibiotics undoubtedly represents progress in the treatment of CNS infections, but rapid diagnosis and accurate prediction of the most likely bacterial causes remain the cornerstones of successful therapy.

For optimal treatment of bacterial meningitis, the antibiotic chosen should be bactericidal and achieve cerebrospinal fluid (CSF) levels well in excess of the minimum bactericidal concentration for the causative organism. Combinations of antimicrobials are avoided that might be antagonistic relative to the organism that is isolated. For example, chloramphenicol antagonizes the bactericidal action of penicillin or ampicillin against *Streptococcus pneumoniae* and group B streptococci. Chloramphenicol also interferes with the bactericidal action of gentamicin against certain Gram-negative enteric rods. There is also evidence of in vitro inactivation in infusion fluids when certain beta-lactam antibiotics are mixed with aminoglycosides, and, therefore, these drugs should be given independently.[112] It is important to remember that antimicrobial agents can only eradicate infection in the CSF if they can gain entrance into the infected site. For most antibiotics, except for chloramphenicol, CSF penetration is dependent on the presence of meningeal and meningovascular inflammation.

The use of corticosteroids in acute bacterial meningitis has been controversial for a number of years. There is concern that they may suppress leukocyte phagocytic function and that their reduction of the inflammatory response might compromise antibiotic penetration into CSF. Also, among those acute cases of meningitis that later are found to be viral or tuberculous in origin, early initiation of corticosteroids might accelerate the dissemination of the process.

Recent investigations, however, indicate that corticosteroids may have salutary effects upon acute bacterial meningitis, especially when begun early in the illness and with moderately high dosage.[143,144] To this date, the majority of the data pertain to acute *Haemophilus influenzae* meningitis in children. Experimental work by McCracken and Lebel[166] has shown that bacterial cell products in meningitis stimulate the production of cytokines, especially cachectin and interleukin 1, which have adverse effects on capillary cell walls and cerebral blood flow. These effects disturb cerebral perfusion, contribute to cerebral swelling, and stimulate the inflammatory process. The beneficial effect of dexamethasone is attributed to a decrease in the production of these injury-provoking cytokines. Clinical studies suggest that dexamethasone in a dosage of 0.6 mg/kg per day in divided doses has beneficial effects on CSF chemistries, results in reduction in CSF lactic acid content, and improves outcome, including a reduction in the incidence of hearing loss.[143,144] The evidence compiled to date of the benefits of dexamethasone supports its use for acute bacterial meningitis in children beyond the newborn period and begun simultaneous to the initiation of antibiotic therapy. Dexamethasone is given in a dosage of 0.6 mg/kg per day intravenously in divided doses every 6 hours, up to a total of 24 mg/day, and continued for 4 days.

The importance of the use of bactericidal antibiotics is related to the concept that CSF represents a regional site of impaired host resistance against infection.[208,229] Immunoglobulin and complement contents are low in infected CSF compared to serum, and, for this reason, opsonic activity is impaired in CSF. Encapsulation of bacteria inhibits opsonization in serum and CSF; most cases of sepsis-induced meningitis in previously healthy persons are caused by encapsulated organisms, including *Haemophilus influenzae* type b, *Streptococcus pneumoniae,* and *Neisseria meningitidis.* Conversely, unencapsulated bacteria are much less common causes of meningitis unless the infection is secondary to an infected indwelling foreign body such as a ventricular shunt or to a complication of a neurosurgical procedure, an open head injury, or a CSF fistula.

In the past 2 decades, there have been major advances in the development of new antibiotics for treatment of meningitis, and investigative efforts have yielded a broader comprehension of the pharmacokinetics of the available drugs in various age groups. Relatively new additions important in select instances include the extended-spectrum penicillins, referred to as the acylampicillins (piperacillin, mezlocillin, and azlocillin), and the third-generation cephalosporins, including cefotaxime, ceftriaxone, and ceftazidime. Relatively new uses of "old" drugs have been developed for vancomycin, rifampin, and metronidazole. Vancomycin can play a role in certain cases of methicillin-resistant staphylococcal infections, enterococcal group D streptococcal infections, *Flavobacterium meningosepticum* meningitis, and penicillin-resistant strains of *Streptococcus pneumoniae,* or in persons infected with *S. pneumoniae* who are allergic to the penicillins. Rifampin is now the drug of choice for meningococcal and *Haemophilus influenzae* prophylaxis, in the treatment of tuberculous meningitis, and, with vancomycin, for certain cases of resistant *Staphylococcus* meningitis and for *Flavobacterium*

Table 13–1 MOST COMMON CAUSES OF ACUTE BACTERIAL MENINGITIS RELATIVE TO AGE AND PREDISPOSING FACTORS

Birth to 6 weeks
  Escherichia coli, other Gram-negative organisms
  Group B streptococci
6 weeks to 3 months
  Escherichia coli
  Group B streptococci
  Listeria monocytogenes
  Streptococcus pneumoniae
  Salmonella species (especially foreign countries)
  Haemophilus influenzae, type b
3 months to 3 years
  Haemophilus influenzae, type b
  Streptococcus pneumoniae
  Neisseria meningitidis
Older than 3 years and adults
  Streptococcus pneumoniae
  Neisseria meningitidis
  Listeria monocytogenes
  Escherichia coli and other Gram-negative organisms (trauma, postneurosurgical)
Meningitis complicating intraventricular shunts
  Staphylococcus species (75%–80%)
  Gram-negative bacilli
Meningitis complicating CSF fistulas
  Intracranial—*Streptococcus pneumoniae* (85%)
  Spinal—mostly Gram-negative bacilli and *Staphylococcus* species
Meningitis complicating splenectomy
  Streptococcus pneumoniae (75%–80%)
  Haemophilus influenzae, type b

upon a number of factors. In children, the primary considerations are the age of the child, which is a predictor of the most probable cause, and whether or not other factors, such as a ventricular shunt or a prior history of splenectomy, predispose to infection with certain specific bacteria (Table 13–1). In older children or adults, meningitis that complicates neurosurgical procedures or follows open head injuries is more likely to be caused by Gram-negative pathogens than by those usually seen with primary septic meningitis. Nontraumatic brain abscess or meningitis resulting from dental sepsis, chronic sinusitis and mastoid disease, or intra-abdominal sepsis is more likely to be from anaerobic bacteria. Physical signs, such as a rash characteristic of meningococcemia, and the results of the Gram stain of CSF or latex agglutination on CSF also influence the selection of the initial antibiotic regimen (Table 13–2). Once the organism is isolated and sensitivities are known or predictable, the regimen is altered; the

meningosepticum meningitis. Metronidazole has an undeniable role in the treatment of brain abscess and the rare cases of meningitis caused by a number of anaerobic organisms. Sulfonamides, the oldest of the antimicrobials and long of value for treatment of meningococcal and pneumococcal disease, are now largely relegated to the treatment of *Nocardia* infections. Nocardiosis, mainly seen in the immunocompromised patient, is usually responsive to sulfonamides in a dose required to achieve peak serum levels of 12 to 15 mg/dL. Trimethoprim-sulfamethoxazole is an acceptable alternative, and amikacin or ampicillin is sometimes added in unyielding cases.[41,54]

The choice of antibiotics for the treatment of pyogenic meningitis depends

Table 13–2 INITIAL ANTIBIOTIC SELECTIONS FOR MENINGITIS PENDING SENSITIVITIES (2,3,4 = ALTERNATIVE REGIMENS)

Meningitis (birth to 6 weeks)—unspecified
  1. Ampicillin and cefotaxime
  2. Ampicillin and ceftriaxone
  3. Ampicillin and gentamicin
Meningitis (over 6 weeks)—unspecified
  1. Ampicillin and cefotaxime
  2. Ampicillin and chloramphenicol
  3. Ceftriaxone
Meningitis (anaerobic)—unspecified
  1. Penicillin and metronidazole
  2. Penicillin and chloramphenicol
Meningitis (posttrauma or operative)—unspecified
  1. Ceftriaxone and nafcillin
Group B streptococci
  1. Penicillin
  2. Ampicillin and gentamicin
  3. Ceftriaxone
Haemophilus influenzae, type B
  1. Ampicillin and cefotaxime
  2. Ampicillin and chloramphenicol
Neisseria meningitidis
  1. Penicillin
  2. Cefotaxime
  3. Chloramphenicol   (*continued*)

Table 13–2—*Continued*

Streptococcus pneumoniae
1. Penicillin G
2. Ceftriaxone
3. Vancomycin

Bacteroides fragilis
1. Metronidazole
2. Chloramphenicol
3. Piperacillin

Escherichia coli
1. Cefotaxime and ampicillin
2. Ampicillin and gentamicin
3. Ceftriaxone and aminoglycoside

Klebsiella pneumoniae
1. Cefotaxime and gentamicin
2. Piperacillin and aminoglycoside
3. Ceftriaxone and aminoglycoside

Pseudomonas aeruginosa
1. Ceftazidime and aminoglycoside
2. Piperacillin and aminoglycoside
3. Carbenicillin and gentamicin

Flavobacterium meningosepticum
1. Vancomycin and rifampin

Acinetobacter species
1. Ceftazidime and aminoglycoside
2. Cefotaxime and gentamicin
3. Ampicillin and gentamicin

Salmonella species
1. Ceftriaxone
2. Ampicillin
3. Chloramphenicol

Proteus mirabilis
1. Ampicillin

Indole-positive *Proteus* species
1. Ceftriazone and gentamicin
2. Carbenicillin and gentamicin

Group D streptococci (enterococcal)
1. Ampicillin and gentamicin
2. Vancomycin and gentamicin
3. Mezlocillin and gentamicin

Group D streptococci (nonenterococcal)
1. Penicillin

Staphylococcus species
1. Nafcillin
2. Vancomycin
3. Vancomycin and rifampin
4. Regimen 1 or 2 with intraventricular gentamicin

Listeria monocytogenes
1. Ampicillin
2. Penicillin
3. Regimen 1 or 2 with gentamicin

specific antibiotic regimen most reasonable for the organism is chosen, and dosages are selected on the basis of established criteria (Tables 13–3, 13–4, and 13–5).

Although antimicrobial agents are the cornerstone of effective treatment of acute bacterial meningitis, there are numerous other important considerations. These include the control of hyperthermia; the control of convulsions, which increase metabolic requirements of the brain and can compromise both respiratory function and cerebral venous drainage; the maintenance of an adequate blood volume; the maintenance of an adequate airway; and the control of marked increase in intracranial pressure. A severe convulsion with airway obstruction or a shock episode with compromised cerebral perfusion, especially in the highly febrile patient, can lead to irreversible necrotizing changes in the brain that will result in either death or permanent sequelae.

Penicillins

Penicillin is the prototype of the beta-lactam antibiotics, which include penicillins, cephalosporins, monobactams, and carbapenems. All have a beta-lactam ring and have bactericidal activity resulting from their ability to inhibit bacterial cell-wall synthesis.[68,174] With the exception of certain of the semisynthetic preparations, the penicillins are inactivated by beta-lactamase, which causes opening of the beta-lactam ring. In addition to aqueous penicillin G, the available preparations for invasive infections include the semisynthetic penicillinase-resistant penicillins and the so-called extended-spectrum penicillins (Table 13–6). Like penicillin G, those in the extended-spectrum group are inactivated by beta-lactamase.

The electrolyte content of the penicillin preparations varies and can be important in patients receiving large doses. The potassium salt of benzylpenicillin contains 1.7 mEq of potassium per million units and is not a significant factor unless a large amount is given by rapid intravenous injection. Hypokalemia is an infrequent complication of several of the penicillins, however, including sodium penicillin G, nafcillin, carbenicillin, and piperacillin. Large doses of sodium-containing penicillin preparations can be hazardous in pa-

Table 13–3 ANTIBIOTIC DOSAGES FOR BACTERIAL MENINGITIS (BIRTH TO 2 MONTHS)

Ampicillin	150–200 mg/kg per day, IV (q8h)
Penicillin G	
Less than 1 week	150,000 units/kg per day, IV (q8h)
1 week to 2 months	150,000–250,000 units/kg per day, IV (q6h)
Group B streptococci	250,000–400,000 units/kg per day, IV (q6h)
Methicillin	100 mg/kg per day, IV (q8h)
Nafcillin	100 mg/kg per day, IV (q8h)
Carbenicillin	300 mg/kg per day, IV (q8h)
Ticarcillin	200 mg/kg per day, IV (q8h)
Piperacillin	200 mg/kg per day, IV (q8h)
Kanamycin	
Less than 1 week	20 mg/kg per day, IM, IV (q12h)
1 week to 2 months	30 mg/kg per day, IM, IV (q8h)
Gentamicin	
Less than 1 week	5 mg/kg per day, IM, IV (q12h)
1 week to 2 months	7.5 mg/kg per day, IM, IV (q8h)
Tobramycin	
Less than 1 week	5 mg/kg per day, IM, IV (q12h)
1 week to 2 months	7.5 mg/kg per day, IM, IV (q8h)
Amikacin	
Less than 1 week	15 mg/kg per day, IM, IV (q12h)
1 week to 2 months	22.5 mg/kg per day, IM, IV (q8h)
Cefotaxime	
Birth to 7 days	100 mg/kg per day, IV (q12h)
7 days to 2 months	150 mg/kg per day, IV (q8h)
Ceftriaxone	
Birth to 1 week	75 mg/kg per day, IV (once daily)
1 week to 2 months	100 mg/kg per day, IV (q12h)
Ceftazidime	100 mg/kg per day, IV (q8h)
Vancomycin	
Birth to 1 week	30 mg/kg per day, IV (q12h)
1 week to 2 months	30 mg/kg per day, IV (q8h)
Metronidazole	15 mg/kg per day, IV (q12h)
Chloramphenicol	
Premature (birth to 1 month)	25 mg/kg per day, IV (q12h)
Full term (first 7 days)	25 mg/kg per day, IV (q12h)
Full term (7 to 30 days)	50 mg/kg per day, IV (q8h)
Full term (1 to 2 months)	50–100 mg/kg per day, IV (q6h)

Key: IM = intramuscularly; IV = intravenously; q8h = every 8 hours, q6h = every 6 hours, etc.

tients with advanced cardiac or renal disease.

BENZYLPENICILLIN G

Penicillin G is the drug of choice for meningitis caused by group A and group B streptococci, *Streptocococcus pneumoniae, Neisseria meningitidis,* and the rare cases caused by *Pasteurella multocida* as well as *Actinomyces* species. *Neisseria gonorrhoeae* meningitis is a rarely encountered disorder that can be treated with penicillin if the organism is sensitive or with ceftriaxone if it is penicillin-resistant. Penicillin is effective against most anaerobic bacteria except for *Bacteroides fragilis* and certain other *Bacteroides* species and is active for most strains of nonenterococcal group D streptococci. Ampicillin is commonly given for treatment of meningitis due to beta-lactamase–negative *Haemophilus influenzae, Listeria monocytogenes, Proteus mirabilis,* and some *Salmonella* species. Ampicillin in combination with an aminoglycoside is synergistic for meningeal infections caused by sensitive

Table 13–4 ANTIBIOTIC DOSAGES FOR BACTERIAL MENINGITIS (OLDER THAN 2 MONTHS AND BODY WEIGHT UP TO 40 kg)

Ampicillin	300–400 mg/kg per day, IV (q4h)
Penicillin G	250,000 units/kg per day, IV (q4h)
Methicillin	200–300 mg/kg per day, IV (q4h)
Nafcillin	200 mg/kg per day, IV (q4h)
Carbenicillin	400–600 mg/kg per day, IV (q4h)
Ticarcillin	300–400 mg/kg per day, IV (q4h)
Piperacillin	300 mg/kg per day, IV (q4h)
Chloramphenicol	75–100 mg/kg per day, PO, IV (q6h)
Gentamicin	4 mg/kg per day, IM, IV (q8h)
Tobramycin	4 mg/kg per day, IM, IV (q8h)
Amikacin	15 mg/kg per day, IM, IV (q8h)
Cefotaxime	150 mg/kg per day, IV (q4h)
Ceftriaxone	150 mg/kg per day, IV (q12h)
Ceftazidime	150 mg/kg per day, IV (q6h)
Rifampin	20 mg/kg per day, PO (q8h) (up to 600 mg)
Streptomycin	20–30 mg/kg per day, IM (q12h) (up to 1 g)
Vancomycin	45 mg/kg per day, IV (q6h)
Sulfadiazine	150 mg/kg per day, IV (q8h)
Metronidazole	40 mg/kg per day, PO (q8h)
	30 mg/kg per day, IV (q6h)
Intrathecal agents—administered daily or every second day (dose depends on ventricular capacity)	
Gentamicin	1–3 mg
Amikacin	2–5 mg
Methicillin	10–25 mg
Vancomycin	2–10 mg

Key: IM = intramuscularly; IV = intravenously; PO = per os (by mouth); q4h = every 4 hours, q6h = every 6 hours, etc.

Enterobacteriaceae and enterococcal group D streptococci.[121] Nafcillin is the drug of choice for treating sensitive penicillinase-producing staphylococcal infections. Carbenicillin, in combination with an aminoglycoside, has been recommended for meningitis caused by *Pseudomonas* species and indole-positive *Proteus* species, although ceftazidime with an aminoglycoside is now preferred by most.

Penicillin G undergoes rapid renal excretion, resulting in a short serum half-life following intravenous administration. The half-life correlates inversely with postnatal age and creatinine clearance. In neonates younger than 6 days of age, the penicillin half-life is approximately 3.2 hours.[165] In infants older than 14 days, the half-life is 1.4 hours, and in older children and adults, it is in the range of 30 minutes. Because of its rapid renal excretion, penicillin G should be administered intravenously over approximately 20 minutes at intervals of 4 hours, except in the newborn period. The half-life of penicillin can be markedly prolonged with renal failure and requires caution in the dosage or frequency of administration in

Table 13–5 ANTIBIOTIC DOSAGES FOR BACTERIAL MENINGITIS IN ADULTS

Ampicillin	8–12 g/day (IV)
Penicillin G	12–24 million units/day (IV)
Methicillin	8–12 g/day (IV)
Nafcillin	8–12 g/day (IV)
Carbenicillin	18–30 g/day (IV)
Ticarcillin	12–20 g/day (IV)
Piperacillin	10–15 g/day (IV)
Chloramphenicol	4–6 g/day (IV)
Gentamicin	200 mg/day (IM, IV)
Tobramycin	200 mg/day (IM, IV)
Amikacin	750 mg/day (IM, IV)
Cefotaxime	8–10 g/day (IV)
Ceftriaxone	8–10 g/day (IV)
Ceftazidime	8 g/day (IV)
Streptomycin	1 g/day (IM)
Rifampin	600 mg/day (PO)
Vancomycin	2.5 g/day (IV)
Metronidazole	1.5 g/day (IV)

Key: IM = intramuscularly; IV = intravenously; PO = per os (by mouth).

Table 13–6 PENICILLINS

Natural penicillins
  Penicillin G
  Penicillin V
Semisynthetic penicillinase-resistant penicillins
  Methicillin
  Nafcillin
  Oxacillin
  Dicloxacillin
Extended-spectrum penicillins
  Ampicillin
  Amoxicillin
  Carbenicillin
  Ticarcillin
  Piperacillin
  Mezlocillin
  Azlocillin

such patients. Penicillin G is transported from serum to CSF poorly under normal conditions, reaching CSF concentrations only 1% to 2% of those in the serum.[184] Meningeal inflammation, however, considerably enhances CSF penetration of penicillin. With intravenous doses of penicillin of 250,000 units/kg per day for children with meningitis, Hieber and Nelson[109] found mean CSF concentrations of 0.8 μg/mL, 0.7 μg/mL, and 0.3 μg/mL on the first, fifth, and tenth day of treatment, respectively. These levels represented 18.4%, 9.9%, and 3.4% of the simultaneous serum levels.

Allergic reactions manifested by various types of skin eruptions, fever, and hematologic changes are the most commonly encountered adverse effect of penicillin, estimated to occur in 1% to 10% of persons receiving the drug[233,249] (Table 13–7). Acute anaphylaxis is an unusual but life-threatening reaction that usually occurs soon after the initial dose of penicillin. Hematologic or nephrotoxic reactions are uncommon with penicillin G, although neutropenia, thrombocytopenia, and Coombs-positive hemolytic anemia have been described.[182] Interstitial nephritis, well known with methicillin therapy, is an unusual complication from penicillin G.[203] Neurotoxic reactions to penicillin are infrequent and have been recorded with the use of high doses (usually over 25 million units/day) in patients with renal failure.[22,25,43] Decreased respon-

siveness, myoclonus, generalized seizures, confusion, and hallucinations have been the characteristic clinical features of penicillin-induced toxic encephalopathy.

PENICILLINASE-RESISTANT PENICILLINS

Methicillin, introduced in 1959, was the first available penicillin effective against penicillinase-producing *Staphylococcus* species. Initially, methicillin-resistant staphylococci were infrequently isolated, but their prevalence gradually increased,[178] and currently most strains of *Staphylococcus epidermidis* are resistant. Methicillin is rapidly eliminated by renal excretion, with a serum half-life ranging from 2.8 to 3.1 hours in premature infants younger than 2 weeks of age and 1.1 hours in term infants 3 to 6 weeks of age.[196] The half-life is shorter in older children and adults with normal renal function. Little is known regarding penetration of methicillin into CSF with meningitis, although available information suggests that the concentrations achieved are usually less than or barely equal to the minimal inhibitory concentration (MIC) for penicillinase-producing staphylococci.[176]

Methicillin can cause side effects like those of penicillin G but has a greater predisposition to induce a nephropathy

Table 13–7 ADVERSE EFFECTS OF PENICILLINS

Allergic reactions: Skin eruptions
  (maculopapular rash, urticaria, erythema
  multiforme)
Acute anaphylaxis
Bleeding due to altered platelet function
  (extended-spectrum penicillins)
Neutropenia
Thrombocytopenia
Hemolytic anemia
Diarrhea
Hypokalemia
Drug fever
Toxic encephalopathy (high serum levels)
Interstitial nephritis (especially with methicillin)
Soft tissue necrosis following subcutaneous
  extravasation (nafcillin)

manifested by hematuria, which can be associated with fever, rash, and eosinophilia.[195] Renal tubular dysfunction with renal salt wasting, impaired ability to excrete potassium, and tubular acidosis is a less common form of renal toxicity.[42]

Nafcillin differs from other penicillins in that 20% or less undergoes renal excretion, and the major fraction is excreted by the biliary system. Renal failure does not significantly affect its half-life.[62] For this reason, nafcillin is usually the drug of choice in azotemic patients who require a penicillinase-resistant agent. Conversely, the use of nafcillin in patients with hepatic insufficiency requires dosage adjustments to avoid excessively high serum levels. The half-life of nafcillin in older infants and children with normal liver function is 0.76 hours.[79] Nafcillin gains entrance into the CSF better than other penicillinase-resistant penicillins and even enters the CSF in measurable amounts when the meninges are uninflamed.[83]

Subcutaneous extravasation of nafcillin during intravenous administration can result in soft tissue necrosis.[228] Neutropenia is an occasional side effect of nafcillin,[96] as with other penicillins. Nephropathy can occur but is less common than with methicillin.

EXTENDED-SPECTRUM PENICILLINS

Ampicillin is the most widely used extended-spectrum penicillin for treatment of suppurative meningitis because of its relatively broad spectrum of action. Strains of *Haemophilus influenzae* type b were once believed to be consistently sensitive to ampicillin, but the discovery in 1974 of resistant isolates compromised the usefulness of the drug as the sole, initial method of treatment of meningitis in patients beyond the neonatal period. At the present time in many communities, 20% to 40% of *Haemophilus influenzae* type b isolates are resistant to ampicillin. Ampicillin results in higher peak serum

concentrations in premature than in full-term infants and has a half-life in serum of 4 hours in infants from birth to 7 days of age, 2.8 hours in infants from 8 to 14 days of age, and 1.7 hours in infants 15 to 30 days of age.

Ampicillin is at least as allergenic as natural penicillin. Whereas the most common type of rash associated with benzylpenicillin is urticarial, the usual ampicillin rash is a maculopapular erythema. The occurrence of this type of rash raises concern about the possibility of drug allergy with future exposures but is not necessarily a contraindication for the future use of ampicillin or other penicillins, especially when it occurs in a patient with a viral illness, in particular infectious mononucleosis.[125] Interstitial nephritis secondary to ampicillin is far less common than with methicillin.[193]

Carbenicillin has a spectrum similar to that of ampicillin except for its greater activity against *Pseudomonas aeruginosa* and indole-positive *Proteus* species.[23,172] Because of a synergistic effect of carbenicillin with gentamicin against *Pseudomonas aeruginosa*, both drugs are recommended for infections caused by this organism. Most strains of *Klebsiella* species are resistant to carbenicillin. Carbenicillin half-life in adults with normal renal function is approximately 1 hour following intravenous administration.[111] Renal failure markedly prolongs the serum half-life, resulting in elevated serum levels. Little information is available regarding the CSF penetrability of carbenicillin.

Possible complications of carbenicillin therapy include granulocytopenia, hepatotoxicity, metabolic acidosis, hypokalemia, and clinical bleeding secondary to disturbed platelet activity. Clinical bleeding due to altered platelet function can occur with any of the penicillins, but the risk is greater with the extended-spectrum penicillins than with other members.[75]

Ticarcillin is similar to carbenicillin, including its pharmacokinetics, but it has greater activity against *Pseudomonas aeruginosa*.[173]

Piperacillin is a monosodium, semi-synthetic, extended-spectrum penicillin with chemical and biologic similarities to carbenicillin and ticarcillin, but with greater activity against certain Gram-negative pathogens. It is inactivated by beta-lactamase and is cleared primarily by renal excretion. Piperacillin, like mezlocillin, contains only about one third the sodium content of carbenicillin, a factor of possible importance in patients with renal or cardiac failure.[246] Like other penicillins, possible adverse effects include eosinophilia, diarrhea, drug fever, neutropenia, and rash. Piperacillin can produce a defect in platelet aggregation and prolongation of the bleeding time, as occurs with carbenicillin and ticarcillin.[89]

The major attribute of piperacillin is its increased effectiveness against *Klebsiella pneumoniae* and *Pseudomonas* species compared with carbenicillin, although all isolates are not susceptible to piperacillin.[70] The anti-*Pseudomonas* activity of piperacillin is enhanced by the addition of an aminoglycoside.[205] It is also effective against *Serratia marcescens*, *Bacteroides fragilis* and other Gram-negative anaerobes, and other members of the family Enterobacteriaceae.[248] Piperacillin has been found to penetrate well into CSF when meninges are inflamed. Dickinson and colleagues[63] administered the drug by continuous intravenous infusion and found the mean CSF concentration in 24 hours to be 32% of the serum level.

Mezlocillin is another member of the acylampicillins and has characteristics similar to piperacillin. Mezlocillin is also broadly effective against Gram-negative bacilli but has less activity than piperacillin against *Pseudomonas* species, although the difference is probably insignificant. Mezlocillin is effective against certain strains of enterococcal group D streptococci. Neither drug should be used alone for treatment of invasive infection because of the rapid emergence of resistant organisms.

Third-Generation Cephalosporins

The initially developed cephalosporins were penicillinase-resistant antimicrobials with very poor CSF penetrability. The first-generation cephalosporins were important for their effectiveness against Gram-positive organisms and were not of value for CNS infections. The second-generation preparations added extended activity against some Gram-negative organisms but also were of little value for CNS infections. The third-generation cephalosporins have added an entirely new dimension to the treatment of CNS infections in all age groups, because of their markedly improved ability to penetrate CSF, their excellent tolerance by most patients, their resistance to beta-lactamase, and their high antimicrobial activity against many Gram-negative organisms. Some preparations are highly active against certain Gram-positive pathogens. Despite the broad spectrum of action of these antimicrobials, *Listeria monocytogenes*, *Clostridium difficile*, and enterococcal group D streptococci are resistant. The third-generation cephalosporins of greatest importance for use against CNS infections include cefotaxime, ceftriaxone, and ceftazidime.

CEFOTAXIME

Cefotaxime was the first of the third-generation cephalosporins of value for treatment of CNS infections. Cefotaxime has some degree of activity against certain Gram-positive cocci, but its major virtue is its bactericidal action against *Escherichia coli*, *Klebsiella*, *Proteus*, and *Serratia* species. It is also active against *Neisseria meningitidis* and *Haemophilus influenzae*, with studies showing it to be more active than ampicillin against *Haemophilus influenzae*.[55] The drug penetrates CSF well, with an adult intravenous dosage of 8 to 12 g/day resulting in CSF levels of 5 to 13 μg/mL. Such CSF levels have been estimated to be 40 to 500 times the minimum bactericidal concentration for most *Escherichia coli* and *Klebsiella* strains.[138] Cefotaxime has also been found to enter CSF quite well in neonates and children with meningitis.[5,119]

The half-life of cefotaxime in adults with normal renal function is approximately 1 hour.[114] In low–birth-weight and full-term neonates, mean peak serum levels following a 10-minute infusion of 50 mg/kg of cefotaxime were found to be 116 and 132 μg/mL, respectively. The mean half-lives in these neonates were 4.6 and 3.4 hours.[169] For sensitive organisms, cefotaxime is the preferred third-generation cephalosporin in neonates because of its extensive use in this age group in the past and its lack of effect on bilirubin-albumin binding. Cefotaxime is excreted in the urine, both in unchanged form and in the form of its major metabolite, deacetylcefotaxime. In patients with severe reduction in creatinine clearance, it is recommended that the dosage be reduced by half.

The high level of activity against many Gram-negative rods and its excellent CSF penetrability make cefotaxime an important antibiotic for treatment of neonatal Gram-negative meningitis, as well as for Gram-negative meningitis complicating head injuries or neurosurgical procedures in adults. Because cefotaxime is weakly effective against group B streptococci and ineffective against *Listeria monocytogenes* and group D streptococci, it should not be used as monotherapy in neonatal meningitis. A combination of cefotaxime with ampicillin or an aminoglycoside, depending upon in vitro sensitivities of the isolate, is more effective than previously used regimens for infants or adults with Gram-negative bacillary meningitis. It has an important role in the management of *Haemophilus influenzae* meningitis when the organism is resistant to ampicillin and can also be considered an effective alternative to penicillin for treatment of meningococcal meningitis when penicillin cannot be used.

Table 13–8 ADVERSE EFFECTS OF THIRD-GENERATION CEPHALOSPORINS

Phlebitis at administration site
Rash
Hematologic effects
   Eosinophilia
   Thrombocytosis (ceftriaxone)
   Coagulation defects
Biliary pseudolithiasis (ceftriaxone)
Drug fever
Diarrhea
Pseudomembranous colitis
CNS effects (rare)

The clinical importance of the cross-reactivity between the penicillins and cefotaxime is yet uncertain but is not usually a major factor. Side effects are infrequent but include phlebitis at the administration site, rash, eosinophilia, drug fever, pseudomembranous colitis, and, rarely, CNS effects such as vertigo and disorientation[212] (Table 13–8).

CEFTRIAXONE

Ceftriaxone differs from the previously available third-generation cephalosporins because of its extended spectrum against Gram-positive and Gram-negative bacteria and because of its uniquely prolonged serum and CSF half-life.[218] In addition to its superior antibacterial activity against members of the family Enterobacteriaceae, *Haemophilus influenzae*, and *Neisseria meningitidis*, ceftriaxone reaches serum and CSF concentrations far in excess of that needed for effective treatment for infections caused by *Streptococcus pneumoniae*, group B streptococci, and many *Salmonella* species. Ceftriaxone thus is effective against all the common causes of bacterial meningitis in the newborn infant, as well as in the older child. Like the other newer cephalosporins, it is not active against group D streptococci and *Listeria monocytogenes*, however. Drugs in this class are not considered adequate antistaphylococcal agents. Although not of primary neurologic interest, ceftriaxone also has an important place in the treatment of *Neisseria gonorrhoeae,* now frequently penicillin-resistant; chancroid caused by *Haemophilus ducreyi;* and, perhaps, certain cases of syphilis when penicillin cannot be used.[146]

Ceftriaxone is eliminated by both renal and hepatic mechanisms, so that impairment of function of either organ does not markedly alter drug excretion. With compromise in the excreting mechanism of either the kidneys or the liver, the other will increase its excretory function, resulting in little drug accumulation. The half-life of ceftriaxone in young children is approximately 6.5 hours and is still longer in adults, in the range of 7 to 9 hours.[15,222] Ceftriaxone is highly protein bound and does compete with bilirubin for albumin binding, thus raising concern about its use in jaundiced neonates.[80] The prolonged half-life, the dual mechanism of elimination, the low incidence of adverse effects, and the readily achievable serum and CSF levels that are many times higher than the MICs of all the common bacteria that cause meningitis in infants and children[153] make ceftriaxone a serious consideration for clinical use for these infections. Although it has not achieved "drug of choice" popularity, ceftriaxone can be accepted as a strong alternative for treatment of meningitis caused by *Haemophilus influenzae, Streptococcus pneumoniae,* or *Neisseria meningitidis* when the standard antibiotics cannot be used because of intolerance to the drugs or because of resistant bacterial strains.[44]

CEFTAZIDIME

Ceftazidime has some degree of activity against certain Gram-positive bacteria, but it should not be thought of as clinically important against these organisms or for anaerobic infections. The greatest value of ceftazidime is for treatment of aerobic, Gram-negative invasive infections, especially those caused by *Pseudomonas aeruginosa.*[104,159] It appears to be more effective against *Pseudomonas* species and

against many isolates of *Acinetobacter* species than other third-generation cephalosporins. In addition, it is highly effective against *Haemophilus influenzae* and *Neisseria meningitidis* but not against *Campylobacter* species, most isolates of *Bacteroides fragilis,* or *Staphylococcus aureus.*

Ceftazidime is less than 20% proteinbound in serum, the least of the available third-generation cephalosporins. It is little metabolized and is largely excreted by glomerular filtration. Thus, the dose of ceftazidime must be reduced in patients with significant impairment of renal glomerular function. The serum half-life in the adult with normal glomerular function is approximately 1.8 hours.

CSF penetration of ceftazidime depends upon the presence of meningeal inflammation. Among patients with meningitis, the degree of CSF penetration of ceftazidime is adequate for treatment of sensitive organisms,[82] and, like the penicillins, is greater during the first 3 days of therapy.[104]

Ceftazidime is generally well tolerated. Possible adverse effects include hypersensitivity reaction with rash and diarrhea. Because of its striking activity against many Gram-negative organisms and its inactivity against *Clostridium difficile,* intestinal superinfection can occur. Ceftazidime has limited indications for treatment of CNS infections but is considered to be the drug of choice, with an aminoglycoside, for meningitis or brain abscess due to *Pseudomonas aeruginosa* and perhaps for CNS infections caused by *Acinetobacter* species. At the present time, ceftazidime is a valuable antimicrobial, and its use should be restricted to absolute indications to avoid the development of widespread resistance.

Aminoglycosides

Although the aminoglycosides still have a role in the treatment of CNS infections caused by certain Gram-negative organisms, their use has been reduced with the development of the third-generation cephalosporins and certain new extended-spectrum penicillins. Aminoglycoside antibiotics in common use include streptomycin, kanamycin, gentamicin, tobramycin, and amikacin.

The aminoglycosides are characterized by a narrow margin between therapeutically effective and toxic serum concentrations, low protein binding in the serum, relatively poor CSF penetration with parenteral doses in the safe range, and potential ototoxic and nephrotoxic properties (Table 13–9). With continued administration, the aminoglycosides accumulate in renal tissue to a greater extent than in other tissues. Morphologic changes in patients with renal nephrotoxicity are primarily located in the proximal renal tubules, even though glomerular dysfunction is the usual clinical abnormality.[145] With adherence to the standard recommendations for dosage and monitoring of peak and trough serum levels, complete functional reversibility of aminoglycoside nephrotoxicity is the rule. The combined use of an aminoglycoside with vancomycin is believed to worsen the nephrotoxic effects of each. Unlike aminoglycoside nephrotoxicity, ototoxicity is frequently irreversible. Total aminoglycoside dose and duration of therapy are among the factors associated with the development of ototoxicity.[161]

The aminoglycosides are largely excreted by glomerular filtration; serum levels will become elevated in patients with impaired renal function unless the dose is appropriately reduced.[210] These antibiotics are well absorbed after intramuscular injection. When given intravenously, they should be infused over a 20-minute period and not be mixed in the same infusion bottle with penicillin preparations. The aminoglycosides have less bactericidal activity in an acid medium, a factor that may reduce their effectiveness in the treatment of acute meningitis, in which the CSF pH characteristically declines secondary to an increase in the CSF lactic-acid content. This factor partially explains why bactericidal levels of aminoglycosides are higher in CSF than in vitro.

Gentamicin is effective against most members of the Enterobacteriaceae, most strains of *Pseudomonas aeruginosa,* and many isolates of *Serratia marcescens.*[1] It is synergistic with carbenicillin, ticarcillin, or piperacillin against *Pseudomonas aeruginosa* and is synergistic with ampicillin against *Listeria monocytogenes.* Enhanced bacterial killing of group B streptococci, enterococcal group D streptococci, and *Escherichia coli* has been claimed with gentamicin in combination with ampicillin, presumably due to penicillin-induced injury to the bacterial cell wall, which increases the permeability to the aminoglycoside. Gentamicin is not metabolized and is excreted by glomerular filtration. Peak serum levels are achieved 30 to 60 minutes following intramuscular injection. The mean half-life in serum is approximately 5 hours in neonates younger than 72 hours of age and may be considerably longer in low–birth-weight neonates.[164] In infants older than 7 days of age with normal renal function, the mean half-life of gentamicin is approximately 3 hours,[163] and it is shorter in older persons.

Because of the poor penetration of gentamicin into CSF in the dose range that can safely be used, direct intrathecal or intraventricular injection of the drug has been attempted but has not improved the outcome in infants with Gram-negative meningitis.[167,168] Concentrations of gentamicin within the ventricular system that are consider-

Table 13–9   ADVERSE EFFECTS OF AMINOGLYCOSIDES

Nephrotoxicity—reversible
Ototoxicity—frequently irreversible
Neuromuscular blockade
Rash
Drug fever

ably higher than the MIC of sensitive organisms can be obtained by direct intraventricular instillation. The disadvantages of intraventricular therapy include the difficulty entering the lateral ventricle by transfontanel tap in the infant and the need for a burr hole or the placement of a ventricular reservoir after the fontanel has closed. Intraventricular injection of an antibiotic is less complicated in the shunted child, in whom the shunt allows ready access to the ventricular system. Gentamicin continues to have an important role in treatment of infected shunts when the infection is not rapidly cleared by systemic therapy and the organism is sensitive.

Tobramycin has a spectrum of activity similar to that of gentamicin and is also excreted almost entirely by glomerular filtration. Optimal peak serum levels, as with gentamicin, are 4 to 10 μg/mL. Certain isolates of *Pseudomonas* species are more sensitive to tobramycin than to gentamicin. Tobramycin is less nephrotoxic than gentamicin,[133,201,213] and, for this reason, may be a better selection among patients with preexisting renal disease.

Amikacin is a semisynthetic aminoglycoside with pharmacokinetic properties similar to kanamycin. It is equally as effective as gentamicin against gentamicin-sensitive Enterobacteriaceae and *Pseudomonas* species and is equally ototoxic and nephrotoxic.[139] Peak serum concentrations are achieved 30 to 60 minutes after intramuscular injection. Because of considerable individual variation, peak and trough serum levels should be monitored. The desired therapeutic peak serum level of amikacin is 15 to 20 μg/mL, and the trough level is 3 to 8 μg/mL. Penetration of amikacin from serum into CSF through uninflamed meninges is poor, a trait common to all aminoglycosides. Intrathecal or intraventricular administration of amikacin has been described in several instances in patients with multiply resistant organisms, especially for the treatment of meningitis following head injuries or neurosurgical procedures.[101,211]

Chloramphenicol

The use of chloramphenicol for treatment of CNS infections has diminished considerably since the development of the third-generation cephalosporins and with the recognition of the value of metronidazole for anaerobic infections. Chloramphenicol still has a role in treatment of CNS infections in select instances. Its metabolic characteristics and its unique pharmacokinetics make it one of the most interesting of the antibiotics.

Chloramphenicol sodium succinate and chloramphenicol palmitate are biologically inactive materials and must be hydrolyzed in vivo, forming the free, or biologically active, compound. Hydrolysis of the succinate ester administered intravenously occurs primarily in the liver and kidneys. The rate of hydrolysis is variable in different individuals, and in some, a considerable amount of chloramphenicol succinate is excreted unchanged in the urine and thus is not available in the free or active form. For this reason, it is not possible to accurately predict the serum level that will be achieved following a given intravenous dose. Conversely, the oral preparation, chloramphenicol, palmitate, is hydrolyzed by pancreatic enzymes in the proximal gastrointestinal lumen to free chloramphenicol, which is well absorbed into the systemic circulation. Accordingly, the bioavailability is greater with the oral preparation of chloramphenicol than with the intravenous succinate ester.[123] For this reason, the oral dose often must be less than the intravenous dose to achieve the same serum levels. The use of the oral preparation and its bioavailability have been incompletely studied in the neonate, although it appears that intestinal hydrolysis is less predictable at this age. Treatment of serious infections by the oral route is acceptable after 3 to 4 days of intravenous therapy, assuming that compliance is assured, oral preparations are tolerated, and serum levels can be obtained. The peak serum level occurs approximately 2 hours after oral ingestion of the drug. The half-life of chloramphenicol has been found to be 1.6 to 3.3 hours in adults; in children it is more variable, with a mean just short of 6 hours.[85,134] It is little affected by renal compromise but is prolonged with liver failure.[130]

Chloramphenicol in concentrations readily achievable in tissues and body fluids is bactericidal against *Haemophilus influenzae, Neisseria meningitidis* and, to a lesser extent, *Streptococcus pneumoniae.*[187] Chloramphenicol is extensively metabolized within the body, so that only a small amount of the unchanged drug is excreted in the urine, although this varies from patient to patient. Hepatic glucuronide conjugation results in the principal metabolite, which is then excreted by the kidneys. The presence of hepatic dysfunction can diminish the rate of conjugation, possibly leading to elevated blood levels of the antimicrobial.

Chloramphenicol readily penetrates brain and CSF. CSF penetration of chloramphenicol occurs with or without meningeal inflammation, a feature important in patients with localized parenchymal or meningeal suppurative lesions (see Chapter 87). It is generally stated that the CSF concentration of chloramphenicol is at least one half the simultaneous serum level, although variation occurs from patient to patient. A theoretical advantage of chloramphenicol over the penicillins, cephalosporins, and aminoglycosides is the higher degree of intracellular penetration of chloramphenicol.[245] Killing of intracellular bacteria should be more rapid with such an agent, although the clinical importance of this factor is uncertain.

Chloramphenicol remains an acceptable alternative for the treatment of meningitis caused by beta-lactamase–positive *Haemophilus influenzae,* as well as for patients with *Haemophilus influenzae* meningitis who are allergic to the penicillins, although most now prefer one of the third-generation cephalosporins. It can also be used for meningitis or intracranial abscesses caused by penicillin-resistant anaerobic infections, especially *Bacteroides fragilis,* although metronidazole is preferable for this purpose. It remains the drug of choice in children with Rocky Mountain spotted fever, due to the potential adverse effects of tetracyclines in this age group. Chloramphenicol is bacteriostatic against Gram-negative enteropathogens and antagonizes the bactericidal activity of gentamicin against certain Gram-negative rods.[177] The dose of chloramphenicol is that amount required to obtain peak serum levels in the safe and therapeutic range of 15 to 25 μg/mL.

DRUG INTERACTIONS

There are significant drug interactions between chloramphenicol and certain anticonvulsants.[129,132] Phenobarbital enhances the hepatic metabolism of chloramphenicol, resulting in lower serum levels of the antimicrobial. The concurrent administration of chloramphenicol and phenytoin can inhibit metabolism of either, thus elevating serum levels of both. Because of these interactions, periodic blood levels of chloramphenicol and the anticonvulsants should be obtained whenever they are used simultaneously. Hepatic enzyme induction by rifampin significantly reduces chloramphenicol serum levels,[124] although these drugs are seldom used together. Acetaminophen causes a prolongation of chloramphenicol half-life and thereby elevates serum levels.[32]

ADVERSE EFFECTS

The use of chloramphenicol has been restricted largely on the basis of its toxic reactions, more dramatic than frequent (Table 13–10). Unlike the penicillins, chloramphenicol is not recognized as a cause of anaphylaxis. Drug

Table 13–10 ADVERSE EFFECTS OF CHLORAMPHENICOL

Hematologic effects
  Bone marrow suppression—dose-related, reversible
  Aplastic anemia—idiosyncratic
  Neutropenia
Gray baby syndrome—related to serum level:
  Peripheral vascular collapse
  Myocardial suppression
Toxic delirium (rare)
Optic neuropathy (chronic use)

fever and drug eruptions are quite unusual. In past years, chronic use of chloramphenicol was associated with optic nerve damage and visual loss.[40,113] Toxic delirium with mental confusion has also been described[147] but is rare.

Chloramphenicol's reputation for toxicity is primarily because of three different types of adverse actions that it may produce. The first is a dose-related, reversible type of bone marrow suppression, mainly of erythropoiesis. The second is idiosyncratic aplastic anemia, and the third is an acute, serum-level–related type of peripheral vascular collapse and myocardial suppression referred to as the "gray baby syndrome."

Most recipients of a treatment course of chloramphenicol develop some degree of dose-related, reversible bone marrow suppression. The first evidence of this process is usually reticulocytopenia and vacuolation of erythroblasts in bone marrow. Hemoglobin content will subsequently decline and, if the drug is continued, thrombocytopenia can follow. It is for this reason that hemoglobin, platelets, white blood cell count, and reticulocyte count should be determined prior to starting chloramphenicol therapy and repeated every 4 days during the treatment course.

Idiosyncratic aplastic anemia due to chloramphenicol is unrelated to the dose or serum level and is estimated to occur in 1 in 25,000 to 40,000 treatment courses.[239] The complication can develop soon after the drug exposure or may be delayed for weeks or months. Once believed to be limited to oral administration of the drug, aplastic anemia is now known to be a possible adverse effect of its parenteral use as well.[243]

The gray baby syndrome is an acute, life-threatening disorder directly related to markedly elevated serum levels of chloramphenicol. It was first described almost simultaneouly in 1959 by Sutherland[225] in Cincinnati and Burns and coworkers[34] in Los Angeles. The condition has been seen primarily in neonates, in whom maturational factors limit the hepatic metabolism of the drug. It can, however, occur at any age when large doses are administered to a patient with hepatic dysfunction. Currently, most examples stem from errors in calculation of the dose. The mechanism of the toxic effect is believed to be inhibition of electron transport within mitochondria by high serum levels of chloramphenicol. Clinical signs begin within hours or up to 2 to 4 days after the drug is started and consist of lethargy, poor feeding, vomiting, abdominal distention, hypothermia, and an ashen-gray appearance, followed by overt manifestations of shock. Chloramphenicol blood levels at onset of symptoms are over 50 μg/mL and usually are much higher. Peripheral vascular collapse occurs in conjunction with reduced myocardial contractility, leading to a high mortality rate.[21,86] Charcoal-column hemoperfusion has been the most effective form of treatment.[84,154]

Metronidazole

Metronidazole (Flagyl) was introduced in 1959 for treatment of *Trichomonas vaginalis* infections and was later shown to be effective against *Entamoeba histolytica, Giardia lamblia*, and highly so with bactericidal activity against most obligate anaerobic organisms except certain non–spore-forming Gram-positive organisms.[192,226] *Actinomyces* species and *Propionibacterium* species are resistant. It is as active against *Clostridium difficile* as vancomycin. Its antibacterial effect is on the basis of disruption of bacterial deoxyribonucleic acid (DNA).[127] Metronidazole has been used successfully for the treatment of serious infections caused by *Bacteroides* species, *Fusobacterium* species, and other obligate anaerobic organisms. The drug is well absorbed after oral administration, with peak serum levels achieved between 1 and 2 hours, or within 30 minutes after intravenous administration. The average serum half-life is approximately 8 hours, and the drug is minimally protein bound.[188] It diffuses well into tissues and has excellent penetration into CSF. Because metronidazole is metabolized by the liver, it should be used with caution in patients with severe liver disease; reduction in dosage may be necessary.

For CNS infections, metronidazole is now widely accepted as a first-line antimicrobial for treatment in any age group of brain abscess, cerebritis, or meningitis caused by *Bacteroides fragilis, Bacteroides melaninogenicus, Fusobacterium* species, and a host of other susceptible anaerobic bacteria.[241] When these organisms are isolated or suspected, metronidazole is commonly combined with penicillin and sometimes with a third-generation cephalosporin, because of the common polymicrobial nature of such infections. Clindamycin is not useful for CNS anaerobic infections, as it does not gain entrance into CSF.

Most strains of *Bacteroides fragilis* have MICs of 6 μg/mL or lower for metronidazole, a level readily achieved in blood and CSF. The dosage of metronidazole for treatment of invasive neurologic infections when used by oral administration in adults is 1500 to 2000 mg/day given in divided doses every 6 to 8 hours. An oral pediatric dosage of 30 to 40 mg/kg per day in divided doses every 6 to 8 hours would be expected to result in CSF levels of greater than 10 μg/mL. The intravenous preparation has been used in the newborn with a loading dose of 15 mg/kg followed by 15 mg/kg per day, given in divided doses

Table 13-11 ADVERSE EFFECTS OF METRONIDAZOLE

Nausea, vomiting
Metallic taste
Peripheral neuropathy (usually reversible)
Prolongation of prothrombin time (with warfarin)
Neutropenia
Toxic encephalopathy (high dose, intravenous)
   Mental confusion
   Seizures
   Cerebellar signs
Disulfiram-like reaction
Pancreatitis

every 12 hours.[115] The intravenous dosage for older infants, children, and adults is 30 mg/kg per day, in divided doses every 6 hours, infused over 1 hour.

Metronidazole is well tolerated, and serious adverse effects are infrequent (Table 13-11). Nausea, vomiting, and a metallic taste can occur but do not usually restrict its use. Peripheral neuropathy is one of the more concerning adverse reactions, although it is reversible in most instances after therapy is stopped.[26,49] High-dose metronidazole given intravenously can produce a toxic encephalopathy with mental confusion, seizures, and cerebellar signs.[8] The drug also potentiates the effect of warfarin, with prolongation of the prothrombin time.

Rifampin

Rifampin is a derivative of the rifamycins, a group of antimicrobials that are products of *Nocardia mediterranei*. The antibacterial action of rifampin stems from its inhibition of bacterial ribonucleic acid (RNA) synthesis.[242] Rifampin is supplied as an oral preparation that is well absorbed[56] and has a serum half-life of 1.5 to 5 hours. The drug is deacetylated in the liver and excreted via the biliary tract, the primary clearance mechanism. Renal insufficiency does not significantly alter the serum level of the drug. Rifampin penetrates tissues reasonably well; in patients with tuberculous meningitis, CSF concentrations have been found to be approximately 20% of the serum concentration.[67]

Rifampin is important in the treatment of various types of tuberculosis and is included in the regimen for tuberculous meningitis. It is also the drug of choice for chemoprophylaxis of household and other intimate contacts of a patient with meningococcal disease and *Haemophilus influenzae* meningitis. Rifampin and vancomycin are also selected for treatment of methicillin-resistant staphylococcal infections in some instances, although there is controversy over the role of rifampin in this setting.[3,191] Rifampin also has antifungal activity, with synergism with amphotericin B against a number of organisms,[155] although its clinical role as an antifungal agent is not yet determined. Rifampin is not given as monotherapy for active infection of any type because of the rapid emergence of resistant bacteria when it is given alone.

Rifampin is a potent inducer of hepatic enzymes, leading to important interactions with many drugs if given concomitantly. In most instances, drugs that interact with rifampin will require a dosage increase to maintain a therapeutic blood level. Rifampin can enhance the metabolism of warfarin, oral contraceptives, glucocorticoids, digitoxin, barbiturates, and chloramphenicol.[124]

A number of complications and adverse effects of rifampin therapy need to be closely monitored (Table 13–12). Rifampin has been assumed to be hepatotoxic, largely because of its common use with isoniazid for tuberculosis, the latter being well known for its liver toxicity. Recent observations have questioned the degree of hepatotoxicity stemming from the use of rifampin,[99] but because it must be metabolized and excreted by the liver, one should be cautious of its use in patients with liver disease.

An influenzalike syndrome secondary to rifampin is the result of the formation of antigen-antibody complexes

Table 13–12 ADVERSE EFFECTS OF RIFAMPIN

Nausea, vomiting
Thrombocytopenia
Hemolytic anemia
Influenza-like syndrome (intermittent therapy):
    Fever, chills
    Myalgia, arthralgia
    Headache
Acute encephalopathy (rare)
Orange discoloration of urine and CSF
Hepatotoxicity

and is mainly seen with intermittent therapy, such as once-per-week administration.[99] Symptoms include fever, chills, myalgia, arthralgia, and headache, usually occurring after several months of exposure to the drug. Nausea and vomiting may also occur secondary to rifampin administration, in addition to more serious hematologic complications including thrombocytopenia and hemolytic anemia. An acute encephalopathy has been described, with confusion and disorientation,[186] although it is rare. An interesting and potentially serious side effect of an acute overdose of the drug is referred to as the "red man syndrome," characterized by a cutaneous orange appearance and an orange-brown discoloration of secretions including urine, tears, and sweat.[175] Among patients receiving rifampin, the CSF may acquire a pale-orange or xanthochromic staining.[148] Rifampin in large doses can have certain immunosuppressive effects measurable by laboratory methods but not believed to be of clinical significance.[99]

Vancomycin

Vancomycin became available in 1956 and was used from the start for treatment of penicillinase-producing staphylococcal infections. Its importance as a primary antibiotic for this purpose was displaced by the introduction in 1960 of methicillin, which seemingly had fewer side effects. The value of vancomycin has again emerged with the increasing incidence of infections caused by methicillin-resistant *Staphylococcus* species, especially those caused by *Staphylococcus epidermidis.*

Vancomycin is poorly absorbed from the gastrointestinal tract and must be given intravenously for invasive infections. It is approximately 50% to 60% protein-bound, is excreted by the kidneys, and has a half-life of about 6 hours in adults with normal renal function. The antibacterial action of vancomycin is on the basis of inhibition of synthesis of peptidoglycan, a cell wall component. Vancomycin does not gain entrance into CSF in the absence of meningeal inflammation. With meningeal inflammation, its entrance into CSF has been found to range from 7% to 21% of the serum level, with a mean of 14%.[198] Penetration into ventricular fluid was found to be 18% of the serum level in a subsequent study.[199]

Vancomycin has bactericidal activity mainly against Gram-positive organisms, but most Gram-negative bacteria are resistant. Sensitive organisms include most *Staphylococcus* species, *Streptococcus pneumoniae,* and certain other *Streptococcus* species. Vancomycin alone is not highly active against the enterococcus, but it becomes bactericidal in combination with an aminoglycoside. Given orally, it is the treatment of choice for *Clostridium difficile* enterocolitis, although metronidazole is probably equally effective.

Vancomycin has its most important role in the treatment of sepsis, meningitis, or shunt infections caused by methicillin-resistant *Staphylococcus* species.[100,105] *Staphylococcus aureus* and *Staphylococcus epidermidis* are the most common causes of shunt infections and the latter organism has become the most common cause of nosocomial neonatal sepsis among low-birth-weight neonates in most neonatal intensive care units. The sharp increase in methicillin resistance among *Staphylococcus epidermidis* isolates in the past decade has been associated with a dramatic escalation in the use of vancomycin in this setting. Although most *Staphylococcus* species isolates are sensitive to vancomycin, resistant strains have been recovered.[204] Vancomycin alone is often recommended for shunt infections. It is sometimes used with an aminoglycoside and less often is used in combination with rifampin.[237] Among intractable cases, treatment sometimes requires the intraventricular injection of vancomycin or gentamicin, in addition to systemic therapy.

CNS infections resulting from group D enterococci *(Streptococcus faecalis, Streptococcus faecium)* are not common and, when encountered, are treated initially with penicillin and an aminoglycoside. Vancomycin plus an aminoglycoside is the optimal alternative regimen when the organism is not penicillin-sensitive or when the patient is intolerant to penicillin.[10] Additional uses of vancomycin include the treatment of pneumococcal infection in persons who cannot be given penicillin or when the organism is penicillin-resistant. The rare ventricular shunt infection with *Corynebacterium* species (when resistant to penicillin)[45] and the infrequent cases of vancomycin-sensitive *Flavobacterium meningosepticum* meningitis are still other uses of vancomycin.

ADVERSE EFFECTS

In the early years after the introduction of vancomycin, nephrotoxicity and ototoxicity were recognized to be its most significant toxic effects (Table 13–13). Nephrotoxicity is now much less common than before, in part because of greater purification of the compound and in part because of greater attention to dosage and the monitoring of serum levels. Interstitial nephritis remains a potential hazard of vancomycin therapy, especially when used in combination with aminoglycosides, but it is believed to be reversible with discontinuation of the drugs.[19] Ototoxicity is a major adverse effect and is probably serum-level related, indicating the importance of serum level determinations, with peak levels kept below 30

Table 13-13 ADVERSE EFFECTS OF VANCOMYCIN

Phlebitis at site of infusion
Red man (red neck) syndrome:
   Intense pruritus
   Erythema of face, neck, upper torso
   Systemic hypotension in some cases
Interstitial nephritis—reversible (more common
   when combined with aminoglycosides)
Ototoxicity (related to serum level)
Neutropenia, thrombocytopenia
Drug fever
Hypersensitivity rash

μg/mL.[108] Phlebitis at the site of infusion is a common problem, and neutropenia can occur but is unusual.

A peculiar but not infrequent adverse effect of vancomycin has been called the "red man" (or "red neck") syndrome, manifested by the abrupt onset of intense pruritis; erythema of the face, neck, and upper torso; and systemic hypotension in some instances. It can occur in any age group including neonates and in unusual instances will be associated with a shocklike reaction.[136,185] Some aspects of the disorder are thought to be secondary to acute histamine release and in some is associated with rapid infusion of the drug.

DOSAGE

Because of the relationship of side effects of vancomycin to dose and serum levels, the dosage of the drug should be carefully determined, serum levels should be obtained at appropriate intervals, and, with the initial infusion, the patient should be observed and blood pressure recorded at frequent intervals. The recommended dosage of vancomycin for CNS infections in infants up to 2 months of age is 30 mg/kg per day given in divided fashion every 12 hours in the first week of life, and every 8 hours from 1 week to 2 months of age. After age 2 months, the dosage is 45 mg/kg per day, in divided doses at 6-hour intervals. For adults, the total daily dose is 2.5 g given in divided doses every 6 hours. Each intravenous infusion should extend over at least 60 minutes.

In some, these doses may result in serum levels that are higher than desired, requiring a reduction in the dose. Peak serum levels obtained 30 to 60 minutes after the end of the infusion should not exceed 30 μg/mL, and trough levels obtained just before the next infusion should be in the range of 10 μg/mL.

Various doses have been recommended for intraventricular or intrathecal vancomycin. The most common dose selected for intraventricular injection is 5 mg, with a range from 2 to 10 mg depending on ventricular capacity. The trough ventricular-fluid level obtained from CSF collected 24 hours after the previous dose should be less than 20 μg/mL. Vancomycin can be given intraventricularly at daily intervals, but this may need to be reduced to every second day depending on the CSF levels obtained. Intraventricular vancomycin is well tolerated in most instances. In one reported case, an infant received 45 mg of vancomycin inadvertently by intraventricular injection without obvious adverse effects.[179]

Specific Types of Bacterial Meningitis and Their Treatment

NEONATAL MENINGITIS AND GRAM-NEGATIVE BACILLARY MENINGITIS IN OLDER CHILDREN AND ADULTS

Among Gram-positive organisms causing meningitis in the neonate, group B streptococci are the most common, and *Listeria monocytogenes*, *Streptococcus pneumoniae*, and group D streptococci account for a much smaller percentage of cases. Penicillin G in a dosage of 250,000 units/kg per day given every 8 hours is the treatment of choice for neonatal group B streptococcus and *Streptococcus pneumoniae* meningitis. The importance of the synergism between ampicillin and gentamicin[46] against group B streptococci is uncertain, although the combination is used in patients that relapse during therapy or that do not respond adequately to penicillin alone. Ampicillin is the optimal therapy for the term neonate with *Listeria monocytogenes* meningitis. Enterococcal group D streptococci often exhibit multiple antibiotic resistance, including resistance to penicillin. Sensitivity testing determines the most appropriate therapy, which usually includes the synergistic combination of penicillin or ampicillin and gentamicin,[12] or vancomycin plus an aminoglycoside when penicillin cannot be used.[14] Nonenterococcal group D streptococci are generally sensitive to penicillin. In the adult, a relationship has been found between the occurrence of *Streptococcus bovis* sepsis or meningitis and intestinal carcinoma, an association that is sufficient to warrant studies to exclude bowel neoplasm whenever this type of infection is encountered.

Gram-negative bacillary meningitis has a well-defined clinical spectrum: it is seen predominantly in the neonate, following craniofacial or craniocerebral injuries, complicating neurosurgical operative procedures, and in older persons with alcoholism and other chronic debilitating diseases. *Escherichia coli* is the most common offender among such patients, followed by *Klebsiella pneumoniae, Citrobacter* species, *Acinetobacter calcoaceticus, Pseudomonas aeruginosa, Proteus* species, and *Serratia* species. These infections in the neonate continue to have high mortality, and high morbidity rates among survivors. With *Escherichia coli* meningitis in the neonate, for example, the mortality rate is still in the range of 26%.[162]

Treatment of Gram-negative bacillary meningitis has not had a uniformly accepted recommended approach. A combination of ampicillin and gentamicin has been the most commonly used regimen; however, many strains of the family Enterobacteriaceae are not sensitive to ampicillin, and rapid eradication of Gram-negative rods from CSF does not occur with ampicillin,

even among sensitive strains. Gentamicin penetrates CSF only in limited quantities in doses safely used.

The third-generation cephalosporins have found application in the treatment of most types of Gram-negative bacillary meningitis, regardless of age group. For neonatal Gram-negative meningitis and for Gram-negative bacillary meningitis in older persons, cefotaxime in combination with ampicillin is an appropriate initial regimen. If the isolate is resistant to ampicillin but sensitive to aminoglycosides, then gentamicin, tobramycin, or amikacin is used in place of ampicillin. If the isolate is of *Klebsiella* species, ampicillin is not used, as most strains are resistant. Cefotaxime, ceftriaxone, or piperacillin are considered, depending on sensitivities. Lack of a favorable response with progressive worsening of CSF abnormalities may warrant intraventricular gentamicin therapy. For *Pseudomonas* species meningitis, whether ceftazidime and gentamicin or carbenicillin and gentamicin will be optimal therapy will depend upon the sensitivity studies. An alternative approach is the combination of piperacillin and gentamicin, agents also with a synergistic effect against many *Pseudomonas* species. The length of therapy of *Pseudomonas* meningitis often must be prolonged compared with certain other types;[82] it may require at least 3 weeks.

Acinetobacter calcoaceticus is a Gram-negative organism previously designated *Herellea vaginicola, Bacterium anitratum,* or *Mima polymorpha.* Invasive infections with this organism are most often seen in debilitated hospitalized patients or following instrumentation or invasive procedures.[92] It has become an increasingly important cause of acute meningitis following craniocerebral trauma or neurosurgical operative procedures.[20] *Acinetobacter* species commonly show resistance to multiple antibiotics, including penicillin, ampicillin, and chloramphenicol. Selection of antibiotic therapy is best determined by sensitivity testing. Most strains are susceptible to aminoglycosides, and ceftazidime is often the most active of the third-generation cephalosporins. *Bacteroides fragilis* is an unusual cause of neonatal CNS infection but is well known as a cause of meningitis or brain abscess complicating chronic otitis or sinusitis, intra-abdominal sepsis, or following open craniocerebral trauma. The organism is a Gram-negative anaerobe that is usually relatively resistant to penicillin, but the majority of isolates are sensitive to metronidazole.

Neutropenia both predisposes to Gram-negative septic infections and is associated with a higher mortality rate therefrom. Granulocyte transfusions, usually at 12-hour intervals, have been used in the septic neonate to attempt to improve the host defense mechanisms. Irradiated granulocytes are used to avoid the graft-versus-host reaction. This approach to therapy is still controversial, in part because of concern about adverse effects, but studies thus far tend to show a favorable and beneficial result.[35,38,140]

HAEMOPHILUS INFLUENZAE MENINGITIS

Haemophilus influenzae type b is the single most common cause of bacterial meningitis in the United States, accounting for an estimated 8000 to 10,000 cases per year. The importance of the disorder is reflected by its mortality rate of 3% to 5%, and neurologic sequelae in 15% to 30% of survivors. *Haemophilus influenzae* meningitis is primarily a disease of infants and young children, with its highest incidence between 6 and 12 months of age. It is less frequently seen in patients older than 2 years of age. *Haemophilus influenzae* has long been considered to be an unusual cause of invasive disease in adults but has become more prevalent in recent years, especially due to non-encapsulated (non-type b) organisms.[53] Persons with chronic pulmonary or other debilitating diseases are predisposed to this illness, but previ-

ously healthy adults can also be affected. *Haemophilus influenzae* meningitis has likewise increased in adults in recent years, usually in association with predisposing factors such as sinusitis, otitis, pneumonia, tracheobronchitis, or head injury.[215]

Treatment of *Haemophilus influenzae* meningitis, like other types of acute suppurative meningitis, requires intravenous antibiotics as well as constant attention to supportive measures. Marked hyperthermia should be prevented, and adequate ventilation is mandatory to prevent hypercapnia and hypoxia, which can lead to ischemic cerebral injury or to internal herniation. Intermittent intravenous doses of mannitol are sometimes indicated when intracranial hypertension is believed to be contributing to the child's downhill course and when increased pressure is not the result of subdural fluid collections. Because of the high frequency of inappropriate antidiuretic-hormone secretion in the early stages of the illness,[78] fluid intake should be mildly restricted for the first 24 to 48 hours unless the child is significantly dehydrated or in shock at the time of hospital admission. The presence of hypotension or shock requires immediate expansion of the blood volume with either crystalloid (isotonic saline or lactated Ringer's) or colloid (Plasmanate). As mentioned earlier, it is now recommended to begin dexamethasone therapy intravenously at the time antibiotics are initiated. As a result of the emergence of ampicillin-resistant organisms, ampicillin and cefotaxime are now the recommended initial treatment of acute meningitis in the infant or child yet to be diagnosed etiologically, or for the child with proven *Haemophilus influenzae* meningitis. Ten days is the usual duration of therapy for *Haemophilus influenzae* meningitis unless the illness is complicated by septic arthritis, infected subdural effusions, or other problems that prolong treatment.

During the course of treatment of children with *Haemophilus influen-*

zae meningitis, fever will recur in 20% to 30% a few days into the regimen, after subsiding on the second or third day of therapy.[9] Relapse of fever (so-called secondary fever) has many possible causes, but when the organism is sensitive to the antibiotic being used and when the dosage is appropriate, recurrence of fever is not usually the result of unyielding or relapsing meningitis. More common explanations include otitis media, pneumonitis, an infected cutdown or intravenous infusion site, septic arthritis, infected subdural effusions or subdural abscess, or a hospital-acquired viral illness with a short incubation period. Drug fever is often considered but is probably an overestimated cause. Infrequent sources of recurrent fever include pericarditis and brain abscess.

Nasopharyngeal carriage of *Haemophilus influenzae* type b has been shown to increase dramatically among household contacts of an infected patient, and outbreaks of meningitis have been described among persons within an enclosed population. Ward and associates[240] have calculated that the risk of severe illness in the next 30 days among household contacts of a patient with *Haemophilus influenzae* meningitis is 585 times greater than the age-adjusted risk in the general population. The risk, therefore, is almost as great as that of household contacts of a patient with meningococcal disease and warrants antimicrobial prophylaxis.[94] Household contacts younger than 4 years of age are at greatest risk of invasive disease from *Haemophilus influenzae,* but all children and adults in the household should receive rifampin therapy for 4 days when the household contains another child younger than 4 years of age. Older children and adults are included because they may be nasopharyngeal carriers of the organism and might reinfect susceptible children subsequent to the prophylactic regimen. In addition, the index case should be started on rifampin therapy at the termination of the conventional antibiotic regimen. Rifampin is given in a dosage of 20 mg/kg per day (up to 600 mg) for those older than 12 months, and 10 mg/kg per day for infants younger than 12 months. It is given in divided doses twice per day and is continued for 4 days. Rifampin is not recommended during pregnancy.

MENINGOCOCCAL MENINGITIS

Penicillin G administered intravenously is the treatment of choice for meningococcal sepsis and meningitis. Because of the potential danger of rapid deterioration that may accompany this disease, an effective antibiotic blood level should be achieved as rapidly as possible when the diagnosis is suspected. This can be accomplished by administering half the calculated daily dosage intravenously over 30 to 60 minutes at the initiation of treatment. The dosage of penicillin G for meningococcal meningitis in patients without renal impairment is 250,000 units/kg per day, up to 20 million units per day, given intravenously every 4 hours over a 20-minute period. In persons allergic to penicillin, cefotaxime, ceftriaxone, or chloramphenicol are adequate alternatives. Seven days of antibiotic therapy are usually sufficient.

Management of fulminating meningococcemia with endotoxic shock continues to be a debatable subject. Appropriate antibiotic therapy is critical, and restoration of blood volume with correction of electrolyte deficits may be necessary if vomiting or diarrhea have occurred. Intravenous fluids may be adequate, but in certain instances, plasma expanders or fresh whole blood may be needed. Bicarbonate therapy in conjunction with measures to correct dehydration is useful if metabolic acidosis is present. Central venous and arterial catheters for pressure monitoring facilitate fluid and drug administration if hypotension or shock is present. Dopamine can be used for treatment of septic shock, but with caution and dosage adjustments in patients who have been taking monoamine oxidase inhibitors. Because it is inactivated in alkaline solution, dopamine should not be mixed with sodium bicarbonate. The value of corticosteroids in septic shock has been a topic of debate, although they are often incorporated into the regimen.

Laboratory evidence of intravascular coagulation is considered by some to be an indication for heparin therapy, but reports of its effectiveness have been quite variable.[90] Corrigan[47] has recommended initial treatment with appropriate antishock measures and antibiotics without the addition of heparin. Should laboratory evidence of consumption coagulopathy persist despite these measures, and especially if accompanied by bleeding, heparin is then given in an attempt to abolish intravascular consumption. The duration of heparin therapy required is determined by clinical judgment plus evidence of improvement of laboratory data regarding blood clotting factors and platelets. In bleeding patients, it is important to replace depleted clotting factors by transfusions of platelets, cryoprecipitate, or plasma. In addition, plasma infusions provide antithrombin III (heparin cofactor), a protein that is consumed during intravascular coagulation and that is necessary for optimal therapeutic effects of heparin.

In certain cases of meningococcal meningitis, the course is rapidly progressive, leading to deep coma in the absence of systemic hypotension or shock. Severe cerebral swelling results in high-grade increase in intracranial pressure, which will eventually lead to transtentorial herniation, brainstem compression, and death. Immediate recognition of the importance of intracranial hypertension in such cases can be difficult, but survival depends on control of the intracranial pressure. Fluid restriction and mannitol infusions may be sufficient in some; others require aggressive treatment. The placement of a subdural bolt or intraventricular catheter to provide a continuous measurement of the intracranial pressure greatly simplifies the development of the most appropriate treatment regimen.

The importance of prophylactic treatment among household contacts and others who have been in intimate contact with a patient with meningococcal disease has been emphasized because such persons are at risk, with an attack rate at least 500 to 800 times that of the general population. Rifampin is the drug of choice and is given to all household members of the index case and to persons who have been in intimate contact with the patient. Rifampin is administered orally every 12 hours for 4 doses.

Meningococcal vaccines are not recommended for routine use among the population generally but are selected for the control of local outbreaks and for high-risk groups such as military recruits. There is now a quadrivalent meningococcal vaccine containing capsular polysaccharides of groups A, C, Y, and W-135. Group B polysaccharide preparations are not immunogenic in adults, and a satisfactory vaccine against this serogroup has not been developed. Antibody responses resulting from group C vaccine administration to infants younger than 2 years of age are less than in older children, and group C vaccine is not recommended in this age group. Adverse reactions to the vaccine are more common in infants than in older persons.[180]

PNEUMOCOCCAL MENINGITIS

Penicillin administered intravenously is the treatment of choice for *Streptococcus pneumoniae* meningitis. Treatment is continued for a minimum of 2 weeks and occasionally longer. Among cases, especially in early infancy, when the illness is associated with severe necrotizing cerebral changes in the early stages, one should continue therapy for 3 weeks and watch closely for possible relapse for several days thereafter. Viable pneumococci can persist in infarcted brain tissue despite adequate therapy. This can bring about a relapse of meningitis early after the discontinuation of therapy, or brain abscess many weeks later. For those who are allergic to the penicillins, or those with pneumococcal isolates found to be resistant to penicillin, vancomycin and ceftriaxone are acceptable alternatives. Because of possible antagonism, penicillin and chloramphenicol should not be used together for infections caused by pneumococci.

Streptococcus pneumoniae is the most common cause of meningitis in patients with CSF fistulas, with sickle cell disease, with hyposplenism, and following splenectomy, as well as being the most common cause of primary, septic-borne meningitis in children older than 2 years of age and in adults. Anatomic defects with CSF leakage must be considered and searched for in all patients with recurrent meningitis. The possibility of a predisposing cause should be entertained whenever the pneumococcus is the cause of meningitis, even in the absence of previous attacks. This is especially true in older children or adults with congenital deafness or after craniofacial trauma with fractures.

A 23-valent pneumococcal vaccine is now available. The duration of protection provided by the vaccine is uncertain, but it is believed that elevated antibody titers will persist for at least 2 years after immunization. Recommendations are that reimmunization be considered in 5 years.[110] Pneumococcal vaccine is not recommended for children younger than 2 years of age because of the poor antibody responses in infancy to certain pneumococcal antigens within the vaccine.[48] The vaccine is recommended for children with sickle-cell disease and for patients following splenectomy or with functional asplenia. Immunization is also advised for children older than 2 years of age and for adults with certain chronic disease, including malignant disorders, immune deficiency states, diabetes

mellitus, and conditions with impaired renal or hepatic function, in which there is an increased risk of pneumococcal infection.[91] Antibody response to pneumococcal vaccine is impaired in patients with Hodgkin's disease when the vaccine is administered during or soon after treatment with irradiation and chemotherapeutic agents.[158] For this reason, it is recommended that such patients be immunized before initiation of the therapeutic regimen.

ANTIFUNGAL THERAPY

Prior to the mid-1960s, fungal infections of the CNS could largely be equated with cryptococcosis and coccidioidomycosis, and treatment (after 1956) was limited to amphotericin B. The latter remains the cornerstone of therapy, but with advances in technology and expanding methods of medical treatment, the spectrum of fungal infections and the age groups affected have changed dramatically. One of the first observed departures regarding CNS fungal infections was the capacity for members of the *Zygomycetes* to cause paranasal sinus and carotid artery invasion in the diabetic and in other conditions with acute metabolic acidosis. Improved survival in persons with leukemia and lymphoma, as well as the profound alteration of immune competence required for organ transplantation, was followed by invasive infections caused by *Candida* species, *Aspergillus* species, and other fungi.[72,190,202,209] Prolonged use of intravascular catheters in conjunction with antibiotics for a variety of disorders in the neonatal period enlarged the susceptible age range for invasive fungal infections, especially with *Candida* species. Since 1981, the novel defect in cell-mediated immunity generated by the human immunodeficiency virus type 1 has become associated with numerous types of CNS infections, including those due to *Cryptococcus neoformans* and *Histoplasma capsu-*

latum[2,65,71] (see Chapter 3). With the gradual elaboration of the many causes of prolonged immunosuppression and the abundant use of antibiotics and corticosteroids, the list of fungal species that can provoke CNS infection in such patients has grown to include many that are extremely rare in the normal individual (Table 13–14).

Fungi in tissue or in culture on artificial media occur in two forms, referred to as yeasts and molds. Yeasts are unicellular organisms, often encapsulated, as is the case with *Cryptococcus neoformans* and *Blastomyces dermatitidis*. *Candida* species are yeastlike organisms in which reproductive blastospore formation results in elongated structures resembling filments, referred to as pseudohyphae. The filamentous structures characteristic of molds are called hyphae and may be of variable diameter, branched or unbranched, and septate or nonseptate. *Aspergillus* species hyphae are thin, branched, and septated; those of the *Zygomycetes* are generally broader and nonseptated. Certain disease-producing fungi can assume one form in tissue and the other in culture; these

Table 13–14 FUNGI CAUSING CNS INFECTION (FROM MOST TO LEAST COMMON)

PREVIOUSLY NORMAL HOST
Cryptococcus neoformans
Coccidioides immitis
Histoplasma capsulatum
Blastomyces dermatitidis
Sporothrix schenckii

IMMUNOSUPPRESSED HOST
Candida species
Aspergillus species
Zygomycetes (Phycomycetes)
Cryptococcus neoformans
Coccidioides immitis
Histoplasma capsulatum
Blastomyces dermatitidis
Pseudallescheria (Petriellidium) boydii
Sporothrix schenckii
Fusarium species
Hansenula species
Dematiaceous fungi
    Cladosporium species
    Drechslera (Curvularia) species

Table 13–15 PATHOLOGIC REACTIONS OF CNS TISSUE TO FUNGAL INVASION

Meningitis (acute, subacute, chronic)
Granulomatous meningoencephalitis
Abscess (solitary, multiple, microabscess)
Granuloma (microgranuloma, mass lesions)
Infarction secondary to vascular thrombosis
Cavernous sinus and orbital apex syndromes

so-called dimorphic fungi include *Histoplasma capsulatum*, *Coccidioides immitis*, and *Sporothrix schenckii*.

The tissue reaction within the central nervous system to fungal infection is quite variable with different organisms but also can differ somewhat from case to case with the same organism[16] (Table 13–15). *Cryptococcus neoformans* usually results in a multifocal granulomatous encephalitis in concert with meningitis to some extent. *Coccidioides immitis* gives rise to an intense granulomatous meningeal inflammatory reaction, especially at the base of the brain, in association with multifocal parenchymal lesions with a pathognomonic microscopic pattern. *Aspergillus* species are best known to cause multifocal cerebral granulomas and large, focal, hemorrhagic infarcts that reflect the organism's ability to invade vascular structures, leading to thrombosis. The *Zygomycetes* (Phycomycetes) likewise have a decided predisposition to invade vascular structures, including major vessels such as the carotid arteries, resulting in an infarctional type of pathologic lesion. Meningitis, parenchymal microgranulomas, and abscesses of variable size are found with neurologic infection due to *Candida* species, and macroabscesses are the customary reaction to infection with *Pseudallescheria (Petriellidium) boydii* and the pigmented fungi, *Cladosporium* species. Meningitis is the predominant reaction to the rare CNS invasion that occurs with *Histoplasma capsulatum* and *Sporothrix schenckii*. With any type of CNS fungal infection with injury to the ependyma or with granulomatous meningeal inflammation, progressive hydrocephalus is a common complication and is an important therapeutic consideration.

Antifungal Antimicrobials

Unlike the dozens of antibiotics for bacterial infections, there are only a few effective antifungal antimicrobials for invasive infections. Amphotericin B became available in 1956 and has remained, without rival, the most useful of the antifungal preparations. The introduction of flucytosine (5-fluorocytosine) in 1972 added new treatment dimensions for a limited number of fungal infections, especially those due to yeast or yeastlike organisms. The more recent addition of the imidazoles (miconazole, ketoconazole, fluconazole) adds a further dimension to the available treatment methods, although their precise role and indications for CNS fungal infections are yet to be defined. Among these preparations, only flucytosine and fluconazole have ready access into CSF, and most have notable adverse side effects.

Other drugs with antifungal activity have had limited roles in select instances but currently are of no importance for CNS infections. Potassium iodide has been known to be effective for cutaneous sporotrichosis for almost 100 years. Stilbamidine at one time showed promise for treatment of blastomycosis until its use was curtailed because of its cranial nerve neurotoxicity. Its successor was hydroxystilbamidine, a drug better tolerated but now infrequently used. Nystatin, a polyene antibiotic like amphotericin B, became available in 1950[106] and remains useful for gastrointestinal and cutaneous candidiasis but is of no value for invasive infections. Sulfonamides have a suppressive effect on *Histoplasma capsulatum* and have been used extensively for paracoccidioidomycosis but have now been replaced for that purpose by ketoconazole. Rifampin has been shown to have a synergistic effect with amphotericin B, probably due to the increased uptake of rifampin by the fungal cell because of altered membrane function brought about by the polyene.[155] Synergism has been found when both drugs have been used for infections caused by *Cryptococcus neoformans, Histoplasma capsulatum,* and certain *Aspergillus* species, although the clinical applicability remains uncertain. An alternative approach to treatment with the use of transfer factor, a dialyzable extract of immune white blood cells capable of transferring cellular immunity, has been used for infections with a number of fungi but with variable results.[77,98,219]

The antifungal drugs are beset with the disadvantage of narrow therapeutic-to-toxic ratios, with the most important adverse reactions being upon the kidneys, hematopoietic system, the gastrointestinal tract, and, to a lesser degree, the liver (see Tables 13–17 to 13–21). Because side effects are common, their possible occurrence should be anticipated by obtaining periodic laboratory studies including hemoglobin content, white blood cell count, reticulocyte count, urinalysis, renal function tests, serum electrolytes, and liver function tests. These should be done two or three times per week during the course of treatment. Periodic CSF examinations are also important, as the results often provide the best estimate of the response to therapy. With specified infections, serial cryptococcal polysaccharide antigen titers or *Coccidioides immitis* complement fixation titers in CSF as well as in serum may reflect the degree of response to treatment. Because of the long-term treatment regimen required for most CNS fungal infections, the ability to monitor the course as well as possible adverse effects of the drugs is facilitated by daily recording of the daily dose, total accumulated dose of amphotericin B, laboratory test results, and repeated CSF findings on a well-designed flow sheet (Table 13–16).

Table 13–16 SAMPLE FLOW SHEET—TREATMENT WITH AMPHOTERICIN B

[Name of patient]
Age: 38 years
Weight in kilograms: 70
Date of onset of treatment: 15 May 1991

	Amph. B (mg/Dose IV)	Amph. B (mg Total to Date)	Urinalysis	BUN-Cr	Serum Electrolytes	Hb–Plat. Count	CSF	CSF Cryptococcal Antigen
June 1	35	500	Cells 0 Protein 0	18–1.6	Na 140 Cl 102 K 4	14–200,000		
June 2	35	535	Cells 4 Protein 0	20–1.6			OP 180 Cells 60 Protein 250 Glucose 30 India ink(−)	1/8
June 3	35	570	Cells 4 Protein trace	22–2.0	Na 136 Cl 102 K 3.8	14–200,000		
June 4								
June 5								

Key: Amph. B = amphotericin B; BUN-Cr = blood urea nitrogen–creatinine; Hb–Plat. Count = hemoglobin–platelet count; OP = opening pressure.

AMPHOTERICIN B

Amphotericin B is the only member of the large group of antimicrobials called the polyenes that is suitable for systemic administration for treatment of invasive fungal infections. Its antifungal effect is based on the ability of the drug to bind with ergosterol, the principal steroid of fungal cell membranes, resulting in increased permeability of the cell membrane. As a result, there is leakage of potassium, glucose, and other essential constituents from the fungal cell, ultimately leading to its death.

Amphotericin B is poorly absorbed from the gastrointestinal tract. Solubilized with sodium deoxycholate and phosphate buffer, amphotericin B forms a colloid in glucose solution that can be given systematically. It should not be mixed with saline but is administered with 5% dextrose in water, with a drug concentration no greater than 1 mg per 10 mL of fluid. The preparation should be used promptly after compounding but undergoes little decomposition over the usual 4- to 6-hour infusion period and need not be shielded from customary room light, as is sometimes claimed.

A new investigational drug-delivery system utilizing liposome-encapsulated amphotericin B has recently been devised, which minimizes the toxicity of the drug and shows promise to be an important advance in future treatment of invasive fungal infections, at least with extraneural involvement.[149,227] Compared with the conventional amphotericin B preparation, liposome-encapsulated amphotericin B in mice has been shown to have increased antifungal activity and decreased toxicity.[150] The liposome-encapsulated preparation given intravenously is distributed mainly to reticuloendothelial-laden tissues, including the liver, lung, bone marrow, and kidney, sites commonly infected in disseminated fungal infection.[244] The dose of amphotericin B that can be safely administered is greater with this system, and the infusion time of 10 to 15 minutes per dose is shorter than is the case with the conventional amphotericin B preparation. Although the advantages of this delivery system are obvious for systemic, extraneural infections, it has not been shown to play a role in the treatment of CNS infections.

What happens to amphotericin B following its intravenous injection has long been a point of controversy and speculation. The route of excretion, where and to what degree tissue storage occurs, and how much metabolic conversion there is to other, yet-unidentified products have been unresolved issues. Earlier studies indicated that a certain component of the drug was excreted in the urine and by the biliary system, but the fate of 60% to 70% of the drug given intravenously was uncertain.[6,52] Protein binding of the drug in serum ($>$ 90%) in part accounts for the low urine excretion. Atkinson and Bennett[6] predicted the elimination half-life of amphotericin B in adults to be approximately 15 days, which they felt reflected slow release of the drug from binding sites in tissue compartments. Because of these metabolic characteristics, these authors stated that serum amphotericin B concentrations would not be expected to increase appreciably with impaired renal function and that renal compromise, therefore, would not be an indication to reduce the dosage.

More recent investigations have clarified these problems to some extent, although many questions remain. With repeated daily infusions of amphotericin B, only about 5% of an intravenous dose appears daily in the urine, but continued urine excretion occurs for 3 or more weeks after termination of therapy. With the improved technique of high-performance liquid chromatography to assay the serum and body-fluid concentration of amphotericin B, Christiansen and coworkers[39] have provided evidence that the liver is the major site of storage of the drug, followed by the spleen, kidneys, and lung. They found little evidence for metabolism of the drug and that biliary excretion is probably the major route of elimination. Pharmacokinetic studies in infants and children by Starke and colleagues[217] have revealed that children older than 3 months of age have a more rapid clearance of amphotericin B than adults and thus achieve lower serum concentrations with equal per-kilogram doses, perhaps explaining why infants and children appear to be more tolerant than adults to the drug.

Fungi sensitive to amphotericin B have been found to be inhibited in vitro by serum levels of somewhat less than 1.0 μg/mL.[6,69] The correlation between serum or other body-fluid concentrations of amphotericin B and clinical effectiveness is unclear, however. Using the customary dosage, serum levels somewhat greater than 1.0 μg/mL can usually be achieved by the third day of therapy, but such levels do not approach those of many antibacterial antibiotics, which are 40 to 100 times the MIC against the organism being treated. Starke's group[217] found that in neonates receiving a 1.0 mg/kg per day dosage, the serum amphotericin B level varied from 0.31 to 2.08 μg/mL. In both infants and children, they determined that an amphotericin B dosage of 0.75 mg/kg per day was sufficient to rapidly achieve levels equal to or above the MIC for the offending organism in virtually all cases studied. A team led by Koren[128] administered amphotericin B to children in an initial dose of 0.5 mg/kg per day over 4 to 6 hours for 2 days, followed by subsequent doses of 1.0 mg/kg per day. By day 3 of treatment, all serum levels were greater than 0.3 μg/mL throughout the 24 hours. With the 1.0 mg/kg per day dose, the serum levels became higher, with a mean of 2.5 μg/mL and with a general tendency toward increasing serum concentrations with continued treatment. The authors advised periodic therapeutic drug monitoring among patients in the pediatric age group receiving amphotericin B, with the possible need for reduction in daily dosage during the course of therapy to minimize side effects. Data regarding CSF levels following intravenous amphotericin B are limited. CSF penetration is known to be poor, estimated at approximately $\frac{1}{40}$ that of serum.[231]

Adverse Effects. Adverse side effects are among the most characteristic features of amphotericin B and occur in some fashion in a high percentage of persons who receive prolonged therapy with the drug (Table 13–17). Efforts to minimize toxic effects have included the use of a minute initial test dose to identify those susceptible to idiosyncratic reactions such as anaphylaxis or urticaria; use of a low-dose regimen combined with flucytosine, when the latter is appropriate therapy; development of the lipsome-encapsulated preparation; frequent monitoring of laboratory data during the treatment regimen; and use of accurate methods of monitoring amphotericin B serum levels to avoid unnecessarily high serum concentrations.

Possible acute reactions that occur during or immediately after intravenous infusion of amphotericin B include an anaphylactic reaction, chills, fever, nausea, vomiting, myalgia, and cardiac arrhythmias. The occurrence of arrhythmias is generally related to the rate of infusion and acute hyperkalemia and is minimized by prolonging the infusion time to 4 to 6 hours.[51] Cardiac arrhythmias can also occur secondary to hypokalemia from renal tubular potassium loss during the course of therapy. Acute febrile reactions, sometimes to high levels and with shaking chills, are seen repeatedly with each infusion in certain patients. This is primarily a

Table 13–17 ADVERSE REACTIONS TO THE SYSTEMIC USE OF AMPHOTERICIN B

Chills, fever, nausea, vomiting, myalgia
Nephrotoxicity
Hypokalemia, hypomagnesemia
Anemia, neutropenia, thrombocytopenia
Anaphylaxis
Convulsions
Cardiac arrhythmia
Hepatotoxicity

matter of discomfort in most but can be compromising in critically ill patients. Giving diphenhydramine or hydrocortisone 30 minutes before starting the amphotericin B infusion is beneficial in some but not in others. Intravenous meperidine[33] or dantrolene sodium[97] have been reported to control such acute reactions in some instances. Phlebitis at the site of infusion is a frequent complication and is managed by the addition of heparin to the amphotericin B infusion.

Anemia is a common complication of amphotericin B therapy but only infrequently requires blood replacement. Anemia is usually normocytic and normochromic and without a compensatory reticulocyte response. A decrease in hematocrit of greater than 10 has been found in 76% of amphotericin B treatment courses and does not correlate with the degree of azotemia.[232] Decline in hematocrit levels will stabilize in most cases despite continued administration of the drug. Amphotericin B–induced anemia is believed to be due to suppression of bone marrow erythropoiesis and in one study was associated with inhibition of erythropoietin production.[151]

Leukopenia can also occur secondary to amphotericin B therapy but does not usually create a major problem in management. Neutrophil phagocytic and killing capacity have been found to be suppressed by in vitro exposure to amphotericin B[152] and could, perhaps, be a compromising factor on the patient's own immune attack against the infection. Amphotericin B has also been reported to provoke acute, severe pulmonary reactions manifested by dyspnea, hypoxia, and interstitial infiltrates in patients who receive leukocyte transfusions.[250] The presumed mechanism of this reaction is lysis of transfused leukocytes trapped in the pulmonary microvasculature, with the release of lung-damaging proteases. This complication has not yet been substantiated but deserves caution.

Since its introduction over 3 decades ago, amphotericin B has been widely recognized for its nephrotoxic effects. In early studies, over 80% of patients receiving the drug developed evidence of renal compromise.[232] With refinements in methods of use of the drug, largely related to the use of lower doses, more recent data show rates of azotemia to be as low as 26% during the course of therapy.[216] Renal tubular dysfunction reflecting tubular structural changes[232] results in potassium wasting with potentially dangerous degrees of hypokalemia, which can require supplemental potassium administration. Magnesium wasting is less widely recognized.[11] Magnesium depletion is usually mild but in some instances also will require replacement therapy.

The mechanism of glomerular dysfunction caused by amphotericin B has not yet been clarified. Renal vasoconstriction has been postulated by some,[189] leading to therapeutic attempts with dopamine and saralasin. Improvement or correction of glomerular dysfunction by prevention of salt depletion or use of sodium chloride supplementation has suggested that the recently identified tubuloglomerular feedback mechanism may be a factor in causation of abnormal glomerular function.[28,107] Tubuloglomerular feedback is a physiologic response by which failure of proximal tubular function resulting in an increased delivery of sodium and chloride ions to the distal tubule precipitates local vasoconstriction, which reduces formation of the glomerular filtrate. Although this explanation for compromised glomerular function brought about by amphotericin B remains speculative, the available evidence warrants careful attention to fluid and electrolyte metabolism in persons receiving amphotericin B and prevention of hyponatremia with the use of salt supplementation as required.

Intrathecal amphotericin B is restricted to absolute indications, primarily because of the frequent poor tolerance to this route of administration and because of the common complications with an intraventricular catheter attached to a subcutaneous reservoir through which the drug is injected. Arachnoiditis resulting from repeated intrathecal injections of amphotericin B is clinically associated with radicular signs, cranial nerve deficits, and signs of spinal cord dysfunction. Direct damage to the spinal cord, even at cord levels well removed from the site of injection of amphotericin B, has also been described.[36]

FLUCYTOSINE

Flucytosine (5-fluorocytosine) is a fluorinated pyrimidine that was originally synthesized as a potential antineoplastic drug. It is well absorbed from the gastrointestinal tract after oral administration and reaches peak serum levels 2 to 4 hours after oral ingestion. The half-life in persons with normal renal function is approximately 3 hours, but it can become markedly prolonged in those with renal compromise.[57] Flucytosine has excellent CSF penetration, yielding CSF concentrations approximately 50% to 75% of the simultaneous serum level. The drug is little metabolized, and approximately 90% of an orally administered dose is excreted unchanged in the urine. Because of this high level of renal excretion by glomerular filtration, renal compromise can result in unacceptably high serum levels of the drug unless the dose or frequency of administration is appropriately reduced. Blood level determinations are important so that the oral dose can be adjusted to maintain serum levels in the range of 60 to 80 μg/mL. The usual oral dose of flucytosine is 100 to 150 mg/kg per day given in four divided doses in infants, children, and adults with normal renal function.

Flucytosine enters the fungal cell by nature of the effect of an enzyme, cytosine permease. Therein, the drug is deaminated to 5-fluorouracil by enzymatic action of cytosine deaminase. Flucytosine is only effective against fungi that contain cytosine deaminase. 5-Fluorouracil is metabolized to 5-fluorouridine, and the formation of this metabolite along with 5-fluorodeoxyuridine probably explains the antifungal mechanism of action of the drug. It is believed that these metabolites are incorporated into fungal-cell RNA and DNA,[238] thus inhibiting nucleic acid biosynthesis and leading to the eventual death of the cell. Some degree of conversion of flucytosine to 5-fluorouracil may also occur in human cells and has been considered to be a possible factor causing certain toxic manifestations.[61]

Flucytosine has a narrow spectrum of antifungal activity and is primarily effective against certain yeasts. Sensitive organisms can include *Cryptococcus neoformans, Candida* species, *Torulopsis glabrata,* certain of the dematiaceous fungi such as *Cladosporium trichoides* and *Phialophora* species, and, to a lesser degree, certain *Aspergillus* species.[76,126,157,236]

Good evidence supports the combined use of amphotericin B and flucytosine therapy among patients with cryptococcal meningoencephalitis, especially those who are more than mildly ill or those who have had renal transplants, have renal compromise unrelated to the infection, or are receiving potentially nephrotoxic drugs such as cyclosporine.[18,66,102] The advantages of combined therapy include the synergism between the two drugs, in part the result of increased permeability of the fungal cell membrane to flucytosine due to the membrane-damaging effect of amphotericin B; the ability to use reduced doses of amphotericin B, thus minimizing its side effects; and the rapid achievement of effective CSF levels of one drug, flucytosine, in the initial stages of the treatment regimen, while the dose of amphotericin B is gradually being escalated. For patients not immunocompromised, with good renal function, and who are only mildly ill, some continue to use amphotericin B alone, mainly to avoid potential side effects of the second drug.

Among *Candida* species, up to 50% are resistant to flucytosine de novo, and sensitive strains often rapidly become resistant after exposure to the drug when it is used alone. For this reason, flucytosine is not used as the sole therapy for fungal infections. In recent years, the incidence of invasive *Candida* species infections has increased sharply in neonates, especially among low–birth-weight newborn infants. The available studies provide support for combined amphotericin B and flucytosine therapy in this group,[117] in some instances showing rapid sterilization of CSF with combined treatment after unsuccessful amphotericin B therapy alone.[73] The importance of flucytosine in combating systemic candidiasis depends to some degree on the sensitivity of the organism, although synergism between amphotericin B and flucytosine has been demonstrated among *Candida* isolates that were highly resistant to flucytosine alone.[160] Flucytosine appears to be well tolerated in both premature and full-term neonates.

Cladosporium trichoides, a pigmented fungus with a high predisposition to cause brain abscess formation, is difficult to eradicate and should be treated with surgical therapy when possible, with combined treatment with amphotericin B and flucytosine. Most *Aspergillus* species are minimally sensitive or resistant to flucytosine, and the latter has little role in the management of patients with CNS *Aspergillus* species infections.

Adverse Effects.   In the early period following the introduction of flucytosine, the drug was claimed to have few side effects and only rare serious toxicity. Experience has shown that it is not as innocuous as originally thought, but it is generally tolerated better than amphotericin B and can be given to low–birth-weight neonates as well as to older individuals. In a recent study involving 194 patients treated with antifungal drugs,[216] 38% had one or more toxic reactions to flucytosine (Table 13–18). Bone marrow suppression manifested by leukopenia or thrombocytopenia occurred in 22%. Diarrhea developed in 13% and evidence of hepatic dysfunction in 7%.

Table 13–18 ADVERSE REACTIONS TO FLUCYTOSINE

Nausea, vomiting, diarrhea
Abdominal pain
Anemia, neutropenia, thrombocytopenia
Confusion, disorientation
Hepatotoxicity

Bone marrow suppression is the most concerning toxic effect of flucytosine and has been shown to be related to the serum level of the drug.[122] In most instances, bone marrow suppression is reversible with reduction of the dosage or discontinuation of the drug, although fatal aplastic anemia has been reported.[31,156] Because it is believed that serum levels over 100 µg/mL increase susceptibility to bone marrow toxicity and other side effects, it is recommended that serum levels be monitored during therapy and the oral dose adjusted to maintain the level between 60 and 80 µg/mL. Because flucytosine is usually given in conjunction with amphotericin B, which so often leads to reduced glomerular filtration, one can anticipate the need to reduce the oral dosage of flucytosine depending on the creatinine clearance and the flucytosine serum concentration.

Nausea, vomiting, and diarrhea are troublesome adverse side effects, partly because of patient discomfort but also because such complications can limit the oral dosing and, in the case of diarrhea, may compromise the intestinal absorption. In addition, there are unusual descriptions of flucytosine-induced diarrhea leading to intestinal perforation.[102] Hepatotoxicity is generally in the form of alteration of liver function tests and elevation of liver enzyme levels, but frank toxic hepatitis can also occur.

MICONAZOLE

Miconazole is a synthetic imidazole preparation with broad antifungal activity, but it enjoys only very selective use in clinical practice. The drug is sparingly soluble in water, 90% to 95% protein-bound in serum[221] and gains entrance into CSF quite poorly. Elimination of miconazole is little dependent on renal function and dosages usually need not be adjusted with renal compromise.

The mechanism of antifungal action of miconazole is believed to be the result of alterations in the permeability of the cell membrane of sensitive cells, resulting in leakage of potassium and phosphate-containing compounds from the cell.[24,235] These cell membrane alterations are believed to be the result of interference with lipid synthesis in the fungal cell by the antimicrobial agent.

With one exception, miconazole is not considered to be a primary drug used alone for any invasive fungal infection. Its role is mainly to treat sensitive invasive fungal infections that have not responded to an adequate trial with amphotericin B or to be used when amphotericin B cannot be used further because of intolerance. As an alternative drug, miconazole has been used in the treatment of coccidioidal and cryptococcal meningitis. Miconazole is active against many strains of *Cryptococcus neoformans, Coccidioides immitis, Candida* species, and *Histoplasma capsulatum.* Most, but not all, isolates of *Pseudallescheria* (Petriellidium) *boydii* are sensitive to miconazole, and some consider it the drug of choice for infections caused by this organism,[142,181] especially among those in whom the isolate exhibits in vitro resistance to amphotericin B. CNS infection with this organism is usually in the form of focal abscess formation, however, and favorable outcome is, perhaps, more determined by surgical drainage than by the antimicrobial agent chosen.[17]

Following intravenous administration of miconazole, the CSF concentration rarely achieves or exceeds the MIC of the infecting organism.[59] For this reason, treatment of CNS fungal infection with miconazole usually requires intrathecal or intraventricular injection of the drug. The recommended intravenous dosage of miconazole is 30 mg/kg per day, given over 30 to 60 minutes in divided doses every 8 hours. On the first day of therapy, it is often advised to give one fifth of the full dose, again in three divided doses, to determine the patient's tolerance to the drug. Electrocardiogram monitoring during the first few infusions is advisable, as rare instances of cardiac dysfunction have occurred. Miconazole can be administered into the lumbar subarachnoid space, via the cisterna magna, or directly into the lateral ventricle through a ventricular reservoir. The usual *adult* intrathecal or intraventricular dose of miconazole is 20 mg, initially given daily or every second day. Subsequent frequency of dosing and duration of therapy will depend on the clinical and laboratory response to treatment and the patient's tolerance to the drug. In infants and small children, the intrathecal dose is 1 to 5 mg, which is diluted in 1 to 2 mL of 5% dextrose in water and instilled slowly. In older children, the dose is 10 to 20 mg, depending on the size of the child and the ventricular capacity, if it is to be injected directly into the ventricle.

Adverse Effects. Phlebitis at the site of intravenous administration is one of the most common problems with miconazole[221] (Table 13–19). This sometimes requires the use of a central venous catheter, which may increase the risk of bacterial infection. Nausea, vomiting, and malaise can occur with each administration of miconazole but are not usually as severe as can occur with amphotericin B. Toxic encephalopathy is not common but can be dramatic, with tremor, dizziness, confusion, hallucinations, and seizures.[118] Hyponatremia is a recognized complication and can be secondary to repeated vomiting, to inappropriate antidiuretic hormone release,[59] or as a component of

Table 13–19 ADVERSE REACTIONS TO MICONAZOLE

Nausea, vomiting
Anemia, thrombocytopenia, thrombocytosis
Skin eruption
Phlebitis
Confusion, disorientation, convulsions
Hyponatremia
Hyperlipidemia

the syndrome referred to as pseudohyponatremia explained by the presence of hyperlipidemia. The hyperlipidemia found in persons receiving miconazole is ascribed to the polyethoxylated castor-oil vehicle used to increase the solubility of the preparation. Anemia and thrombocytosis may occur during therapy. Cardiac toxicity from miconazole is unusual with the recommended dosage but is a danger with drug overdosage. Kanarek and Williams[120] described a low–birth-weight neonate who received three times the recommended daily dose, which resulted in lethargy, bradycardia, and an ectopic atrial rhythm with delayed atrioventricular conduction.

KETOCONAZOLE

Ketoconazole was approved in 1981 for treatment of coccidioidomycosis, chromomycosis, histoplasmosis, paracoccidioidomycosis, and selected forms of candidiasis. It is an imidazole preparation that is well absorbed when given orally and is dispensed in a 200-mg tablet. In addition to its antifungal effects, ketoconazole has been found to be a potent inhibitor of gonadal and adrenal steroid synthesis and thus has potential value in the treatment of conditions in which suppression of gonadal and adrenal steroid hormones has beneficial effects. Studies indicate a possible role for ketoconazole in the treatment of patients with prostatic cancer, for Cushing's disease, and for certain patients with Cushing's syndrome secondary to ectopic adrenocorticotropic hormone (ACTH)-producing tumors.[74,207,214] Inhibition of cholesterol synthesis by ketoconazole, resulting in reduction in serum cholesterol and low-density lipoproteins, is an additional metabolic effect of the drug,[131] which has been considered as a possible mode of treatment of hypercholesterolemia.

Ketoconazole is believed to be extensively metabolized by the liver, with the elimination of the unchanged drug and its metabolites via the biliary system.[29] Renal insufficiency is not expected to alter its serum levels significantly, although serum levels can rise with hepatic failure. Significant hepatic disease is a contraindication to its use in most cases.

After oral intake, peak serum levels of ketoconazole are reached in approximately 2 hours. With a single oral dose of 200 mg, the 2-hour serum level is in the range of 3 to 4 μg/mL. With 400 mg, the mean peak level achieved is 6.2 μg/mL, and with 800 mg, the mean peak serum level is 9.2 μg/mL.[13,170] Ketoconazole absorption was found to be reduced in acquired immunodeficiency syndrome (AIDS) patients with gastric hypochlorhydria,[137] said to be common among this group. Absorption was corrected by the oral administration of hydrochloric acid with the drug, an approach recommended when ketoconazole is given to such patients.[137] In serum, ketoconazole is over 90% protein-bound, which, in part, accounts for its poor CSF penetration. Among patients without meningeal disease, the drug remains undetectable in CSF, but investigators[50] were able to measure levels of ketoconazole in CSF of patients with fungal meningitis after oral doses of 800 and 1200 mg. The CSF level was considerably higher in CSF obtained from the lumbar area than in that obtained from the ventricles and was no longer detectable 24 hours after an oral dose. The antifungal mechanism of action of ketoconazole is the result of inhibition of synthesis of ergosterol in the fungal cell membrane.

There is some evidence that ketoconazole and amphotericin B, used in combination, may be antagonistic, especially if the imidazole is given immediately prior to amphotericin B.[200,223] Although this antagonism has not been established to be applicable to all invasive fungi, it is advisable to avoid use of the two drugs together, unless the combined use is with intrathecal amphotericin B.

Ketoconazole has reasonably certain applicability in special instances for the treatment of nonmeningitic fungal infections that include a number of the superficial mycoses, paracoccidioido-mycosis, histoplasmosis, blastomyco-sis, and coccidioidomycosis.[27,37,87,171] Its role in the treatment of CNS fungal in-fections is still ill-defined. Probably its only useful role in the treatment of neu-rologic infections is its use for chronic suppressant therapy in patients with coccidioidal meningitis. Even for this role it may be replaced by the triazoles, discussed later. Several reports have described the use of ketoconazole for fungal meningitis, mainly for coccidi-oidal meningitis.[50,93] Craven and co-workers[50] gave chronic "high-dose" ke-toconazole, 800 to 1200 mg/day, to adults with coccidioidal meningitis and generally found favorable results when compared to the problems associated with long-term amphotericin B treat-ment. Oral ketoconazole in combina-tion with intraventricular miconazole has been used in children with menin-gitis caused by *Coccidioides immitis,* also with favorable responses.[103,206]

Adverse Effects. Ketoconazole is generally well tolerated in doses of 400 mg/day in adults but has had more side effects at 800 mg/day. Anorexia, nau-sea, and vomiting occurred in 16.9% of patients receiving 400 mg/day and in 42.9% of those given 800 mg/day.[170] Pruritus, rash, and dizziness are addi-tional occasional unpleasant side ef-fects (Table 13–20).

DeFelice and associates[58] reported gynecomastia and breast tenderness in men receiving ketoconazole in 1981. This observation led to the discovery of the drug's capacity to inhibit gonadal androgen and adrenal glucocorticoid

Table 13–20 ADVERSE REACTIONS TO KETOCONAZOLE

Anorexia, nausea, vomiting, diarrhea
Asymptomatic elevation in liver function tests
Hepatotoxicity
Vertigo, dizziness
Drowsiness
Hair thinning
Gonadal and adrenal steroid synthesis inhibition
  (gynecomastia, impotence, adrenal
  insufficiency)

synthesis. Although the once-per-day dosage of ketoconazole allows "escape" of these endocrine-suppressive ef-fects,[30] clinical manifestations of adre-nal insufficiency may occur.[230]

ITRACONAZOLE

In a fashion analogous to the classi-fication of the cephalosporins, the im-idazoles have been assigned to a "gen-eration."[234] Miconazole, clotrimazole, and others synthesized in 1967 are considered first-generation azoles. Ke-toconazole is classified as a second-generation member, and the triazoles, itraconazole and fluconazole, are re-ferred to as third-generation azoles. Like the earlier imidazoles, the mecha-nism of antifungal activity of itracona-zole is the inhibition of ergosterol bio-synthesis. The half-life of itraconazole after an oral dose is approximately 15 hours, almost twice that of ketocona-zole. As it has not been shown to inhibit gonadal or adrenal steroidogenesis, it is administered twice per day. Dosage of itraconazole has not yet been entirely defined for invasive mycoses, although doses recommended for adults are be-tween 100 and 400 mg/day.[88,141,183]

Itraconazole has antifungal activity against paracoccidioidomycosis, coc-cidioidomycosis, histoplasmosis, can-didiasis, cryptococcosis, sporotricho-sis, aspergillosis, and certain of the superficial mycoses.[88,141,197] For most sensitive fungi, studies with itracona-zole have found it to be substantially more effective and better tolerated than ketoconazole. Its potential effective-ness against certain *Aspergillus* spe-cies and for sporotrichosis may ulti-mately prove to be its greatest antifungal virtue.

There is little information thus far re-garding CSF penetration by itracona-zole, although preliminary studies in-dicate that it is probably poor.[88] It is possible that if higher doses of the drug than have been used to date are found to be tolerated, entry into CSF may be improved, as was found with ketocona-zole. At the present time, itraconazole is a promising new imidazole for a number of nonneurologic fungal infections, perhaps with a future role in the treatment in select instances of patients with aspergillosis and sporotrichosis. Its future importance, if any, in the treatment of CNS fungal infections remains to be defined.

FLUCONAZOLE

Fluconazole, another triazole, has a number of characteristics that should allow it to emerge as the most useful of the imidazoles for CNS fungal infections.[64] It is more water-soluble than ketoconazole or itraconazole, and unlike those agents, fluconazole is only approximately 11% protein-bound. As a result, it has remarkably favorable penetration into CSF, with levels reaching 70% to 80% of simultaneous serum levels.[4]

Fluconazole is well absorbed after oral administration, has a prolonged half-life of almost 30 hours[194] (which allows once per day dosing), and is generally well tolerated, at least in dosages thus far utilized. Its most common side effects have been nausea, vomiting, abdominal discomfort, and increase in liver enzyme levels (Table 13–21).

Clinical studies with fluconazole have been mainly related to its use as chronic suppressive therapy for patients with AIDS with disseminated cryptococcosis.[220,224] The drug shows promise in this fashion, but additional investigation is needed to clarify the optimal regimen, its spectrum of antifungal activity, and its value as an adjunctive therapeutic agent for CNS fungal infection.

Table 13–21 ADVERSE REACTIONS TO FLUCONAZOLE

Anorexia, nausea, vomiting
Abdominal discomfort
Rash
Asymptomatic elevation in liver function tests
Hepatotoxicity
Bone marrow suppression (infrequent)

Design of the Treatment Regimen for Fungal Meningitis

CNS fungal infections in most cases require long-term treatment with constant attention to the effects of the drug regimen on the infectious process, possible adverse effects of the antimicrobial agents, and complications of the illness itself. Daily physical examination (often overlooked or minimized with chronic illnesses) and daily charting on a flow sheet of the progress of the treatment regimen and the laboratory data are indispensable for optimal management of such patients (see Table 13–16). Neurosurgical intervention can play a critical role in fungal CSF infections and must be considered at intervals during the course of therapy.[251] Many fungal meningeal infections, like tuberculous meningitis, result in a granulomatous exudate within the basilar cisterns that can disrupt CSF flow, leading to hydrocephalus. Symptoms therefrom are often obscured by the symptoms of the illness itself, but the process can be identified by computed tomography (CT) or magnetic resonance imaging (MRI) at intervals of 1 to 2 weeks. All patients who develop ventricular enlargement do not require shunting, but those who develop symptoms such as lethargy or papilledema may show decided improvement after ventriculoperitoneal shunting. A ventricular shunt connected to a subcutaneous reservoir is also required for direct intraventricular injection of amphotericin B or miconazole in select instances. Fungal granulomas or abscesses, located either in the brain parenchyma or in the epidural space, may require excision or aspiration. In general, corticosteroids should not be used to treat cerebral swelling with CNS fungal infections except in unusual instances.

Amphotericin B is the cornerstone of treatment of CNS fungal infection. It is used as monotherapy in many instances and is combined with one of a limited number of antimicrobial agents in other situations. Among patients moderately ill or immunosuppressed who have *Cryptococcus neoformans* or *Candida* species meningitis, amphotericin B is usually given in combination with flucytosine. Rifampin and amphotericin B are synergistic against some isolates of *Cryptococcus neoformans, Candida* species, and *Aspergillus* species and can be considered when the clinical course is unfavorable despite conventional therapy. In practice, rifampin is rarely used in the treatment of CNS fungal infections. Miconazole is restricted to use against sensitive organisms in which intrathecal therapy seems advised, but amphotericin B cannot be given. The primary role of miconazole is for CNS infection caused by *Pseudallescheria (Petriellidium) boydii* when the isolate shows definite in vitro resistance to amphotericin B.

Amphotericin B is given intravenously for the majority of CNS fungal infections, with intrathecal or intraventricular therapy reserved for those instances in which the response to treatment is poor or repeated relapse occurs. Coccidioidal meningitis usually requires intravenous and intrathecal therapy almost from the onset. Recommendations vary for the initial dosage of amphotericin B, the rate of increase in the dose, the ultimate daily dosage achieved, the number of days per week the drug is administered, and the total cumulative dose to achieve. An intravenous test dose of 1.0 mg in the adult (less in the child and not usually given in the neonate) can be followed a few hours later by the initial therapeutic dose of approximately 0.25 mg/kg intravenously over a 4- to 6-hour period. The daily dose is increased at periodic intervals, with the rate of increase depending on the patient's tolerance to the drug and the degree of illness. For example, amphotericin B may be given in an intravenous dosage of 0.25 mg/kg on day 1 and day 2 of therapy, to be increased to 0.5 mg/kg on day 3 and day 4, and increased further to 0.75 mg/kg

by day 5. In adults, this is frequently a satisfactory ultimate dose, and in infants and children, it is commonly raised to 1.0 mg/kg per day, at least for 10 to 14 days. The maximum daily dose of amphotericin B is 1.0 mg/kg, but not over 50 mg/day. With organisms sensitive to flucytosine, the amphotericin B dose can be maintained between 0.5 and 0.75 mg/kg per day, thus diminishing the chances of toxic effects.

During the initial stages of treatment, amphotericin B should be given daily, although sometimes this will eventually need to be altered to every-second-day administration. The total cumulative dose of amphotericin B that constitutes the course of treatment will vary from patient to patient depending upon several factors, including the rate and degree of clinical recovery, the patient's tolerance of the treatment, and the fungal organism being treated. A general guideline is that the total cumulative dose should be in the range of 1500 to 2000 mg of amphotericin B per 1.7 m^2 of body surface area for cryptococcal meningitis and others similar to it, which are known to be difficult to eradicate. Approximately 5 to 6 weeks are usually required to deliver this amount. With *Candida* species meningitis, 2 to 3 weeks of therapy may be sufficient, depending on the clinical and CSF responses.

Coccidioidal meningitis is the only type of fungal meningitis that is routinely treated from the outset with intrathecal amphotericin B. For other types of fungal meningitis, the intrathecal use of amphotericin B or, less frequently, miconazole is reserved for special circumstances. The initial intrathecal injection of amphotericin B should be a test dose of 0.1 mg or less. Thereafter, the intrathecal dose of amphotericin B in the older child or adult is gradually increased to 0.25 to 0.50 mg mixed in 5 to 10 mL of distilled water or CSF and administered slowly every other day. Once improvement occurs, the frequency of intrathecal treatment is gradually decreased to twice per week and later to once per week. Side effects can be minimized by adding the semi-succinate salt of hydrocortisone to the mixture. This is useful in patients who experience immediate but transient reactions to the intrathecal infusion. Labadie and Hamilton[135] have used amphotericin B by cisternal injection for coccidioidal meningitis in doses of 1 to 1.5 mg mixed with 25 to 50 mg of crystalline hydrocortisone succinate. Experience with this high-dose regimen is otherwise limited but might be considered with infections unyielding to the more conventional approach. Intrathecal amphotericin B itself can result in a chemical meningitis manifested by CSF pleocytosis and elevation of the protein content.[247] Among patients treated with intrathecal or intraventricular amphotericin B, CSF analysis for cells and protein content cannot usually be depended on as a guide to the presence or absence of improvement; other parameters such as cultures, antibody studies, and clinical findings must be resorted to.

Among patients who develop posterior fossa obstruction, amphotericin B administered in the lumbar or cisternal region will not gain entrance into the intracranial space. Direct intraventricular injection of amphotericin B via a ventricular reservoir is generally reserved for patients with enlarged ventricles in whom technical difficulty has been encountered with the other sites for injection, or for those with intraventricular obstruction, in which case the lumbar intrathecal route is not effective. When a ventriculoperitoneal shunt has previously been inserted before intraventricular therapy is decided upon, the rapid diversion of the antimicrobial agent from the ventricle via the shunt will diminish its antifungal effect. The development of hydrocephalus in the patient who may require intraventricular antifungal therapy is better managed by the placement of a ventricular reservoir without a shunt and maintaining ventricular decompression by twice-per-day tapping of the reservoir. The reservoir can then be used for intraventricular therapy as indicated. There are many complications with ventricular reservoirs used for intraventricular antifungal therapy, however.[60,95] Dislodgment of the ventricular end of the catheter, intraluminal obstruction of the catheter, bacterial infection of the CSF with colonization of the apparatus, subcutaneous CSF leak, and bleeding are sufficiently common that this approach should only be used when clearly indicated.

Treatment of coccidioidal meningitis is often associated with a variety of problems because of the usual suboptimal response of the infection to therapy and the need for very prolonged systemic and intrathecal treatment. Amphotericin B is the preferred therapy, but because of intolerance to the drug or the inability to successfully continue its direct injection into the CSF, it ultimately must be terminated in many instances. Ketoconazole can be used in these occasional instances and may suppress the infectious process for a lengthy period. Later, relapse might again respond to amphotericin B. When both systemic and intrathecal amphotericin B must be stopped in the patient with coccidioidal meningitis, oral ketoconazole can be supplemented by the intraventricular administration of miconazole, if necessary.

Management of the patient with a fungal CNS infection in most instances is best done in a medical center equipped with many resources, skilled physicians in a variety of disciplines, and the dedicated nurses and attendants customarily found in such institutions. In addition to the patient's primary physician, ongoing cooperative assistance is often needed from persons trained in neurology, infectious disease, ophthalmology, neuroradiology, neurosurgery, and sometimes others. Prior experience with the treatment of such illness and with the use of the antifungal antimicrobial agents is a decided advantage for optimal patient care. Although many persons will take part in critical decisions, it is nevertheless important that a single physician direct the day-to-day care and be responsible for the many details of the treatment regimen.

REFERENCES

1. Appel GB and Neu HC: Gentamicin in 1978. Ann Intern Med 89:528–538, 1978.

2. Anaissie E, Fainstein V, Samo T, Bodey GP, and Sarosi GA: Central nervous system histoplasmosis. An unappreciated complication of acquired immunodeficiency syndrome. Am J Med 84:215–217, 1988.

3. Archer GL, Tenenbaum MJ, and Haywood HB III: Rifampin therapy of *Staphylococcus epidermidis*. Use in infections from indwelling artificial devices. JAMA 240:751–753, 1978.

4. Arndt CA, Walsh TJ, McCully CL, Balis FM, Pizzo PA, and Poplack DG: Fluconazole penetration into cerebrospinal fluid. Implications for treating fungal infections of the central nervous system. J Infect Dis 157:178–180, 1988.

5. Asmar BI, Thirumoorthi MC, Buckley JA, Kobos DM, and Dajani AS: Cefotaxime diffusion into cerebrospinal fluid of children with meningitis. Antimicrob Agents Chemother 28:138–140, 1985.

6. Atkinson AJ Jr, and Bennett JE: Amphotericin B pharmacokinetics in humans. Antimicrob Agents Chemother 13:271–276, 1978.

7. Axline SH, Yagge SJ, and Simon HJ: Clinical pharmacology of antimicrobials in premature infants. II. Ampicillin, methicillin, oxacillin, neomycin, and colistin. Pediatrics 39:97–107, 1967.

8. Bailes J, Willis J, Priebe C, and Strub R: Encephalopathy with metronidazole in a child. Am J Dis Child 137:290–291, 1983.

9. Balagtas RC, Levin S, Nelson KE, and Gotoff SP: Secondary and prolonged fevers in bacterial meningitis. J Pediatr 77:957–964, 1970.

10. Barriere SL, Lutwick LI, Jacobs RA, and Conte JE: Vancomycin treatment for enterococcal meningitis. Arch Neurol 42:686–688, 1985.

11. Barton CH, Pahl M, Vaziri ND, and Cesario T: Renal magnesium wasting associated with amphotericin B therapy. Am J Med 77:471–474, 1984.

12. Bavikatte K, Schreiner RL, Lemons JA, and Gresham EL: Group D streptococcal septicemia in the neonate. Am J Dis Child 133:493–496, 1979.

13. Baxter JG, Brass C, Schentag JJ, and Slaughter RL: Pharmacokinetics of ketoconazole administered intravenously to dogs and orally as tablet and solution to humans and dogs. J Pharm Sci 75:443–447, 1986.

14. Bayer AS, Seidel JS, Yoshikawa TT, Anthony BF, and Guze LB: Group D enterococcal meningitis. Clinical and therapeutic considerations with report of three cases and review of the literature. Arch Intern Med 136:883–886, 1976.

15. Beam TR Jr: Ceftriaxone: A beta-lactamase stable, broad-spectrum cephalosporin with an extended half-life. Pharmacotherapy 5:237–253, 1985.

16. Bell WE and McCormick WF: Neurologic Infections in Children, Ed. 2. WB Saunders, Philadelphia, 1981.

17. Bell WE and Myers MG: *Allescheria (Petriellidium) boydii* brain abscess in a child with leukemia. Arch Neurol 35:386–388, 1978.

18. Bennett JE, Dismukes WE, Duma RJ, et al: A comparison of amphotericin B alone and combined with flucytosine in the treatment of cryptococcal meningitis. N Engl J Med 301:126–131, 1979.

19. Bergman MM, Glew RH, and Ebert TH: Acute interstitial nephritis associated with vancomycin therapy. Arch Intern Med 148:2139–2140, 1988.

20. Berk SL and McCabe WR: Meningitis caused by *Acinetobacter calcoaceticus* var *antitratus*. Ann Neurol 38:95–98, 1981.

21. Biancaniello T, Meyer RA, and Kaplan S: Chloramphenicol and cardiotoxicity. J Pediatr 98:828–830, 1981.

22. Bloomer HA, Barton LJ, and Maddock

RK Jr: Penicillin-induced encephalopathy in uremic patients. JAMA 200:121–123, 1967.

23. Bodey GP, Whitecar JP Jr, Middleman E, and Rodriquez V: Carbenicillin for *Pseudomonas* therapy. JAMA 218:62–66, 1971.

24. Borgers M: Mechanism of action of antifungal drugs, with special reference to the imidazole derivatives. Rev Infect Dis 2:520–534, 1980.

25. Borman JB and Eyal Z: Neurotoxic effects of large doses of penicillin administered intravenously. Arch Surg 97:662–665, 1968.

26. Bradley WG, Karlsson IJ, and Rassol CG: Metronidazole neuropathy. Br Med J 2:610–611, 1977.

27. Bradsher RW, Rice DC, and Abernathy RS: Ketoconazole therapy for endemic blastomycosis. Ann Intern Med 103:872–879, 1985.

28. Branch RA: Prevention of amphotericin B–induced renal impairment. A review on the use of sodium supplementation. Arch Intern Med 148:2389–2394, 1988.

29. Brass C, Galginni JN, Blaschke TF, Defelice R, O'Reilly RA, and Stevens DA: Disposition of ketoconazole, an oral antifungal, in humans. Antimicrob Agents Chemother 21:151–158, 1982.

30. Britton H, Shehab Z, Lightner E, and Chow D: Adrenal response in children receiving high doses of ketoconazole for systemic coccidioidomycosis. J Pediatr 112:488–492, 1988.

31. Bryan CS and McFarland JA: Cryptococcal meningitis. Fatal marrow aplasia from combined therapy. JAMA 239:1068–1069, 1978.

32. Buchanan N and Moodey GP: Interaction between chloramphenicol and paracetamol. Br Med J 2:307–308, 1979.

33. Burks LC, Aisner J, Fortner CL, and Wiernik PH: Meperidine for the treatment of shaking chills and fever. Arch Intern Med 140:483–484, 1980.

34. Burns LE, Hodgman JE, and Cass AB: Fatal circulatory collapse in premature infants receiving chloramphenicol. N Engl J Med 261:1318–1321, 1959.

35. Cario MS, Rucker R, Bennetts GA, et al: Improved survival of newborns receiving leukocyte transfusions for sepsis. Pediatrics 74:887–892, 1984.

36. Carnevale NT, Galgiani JN, Stevens DA, Herrick MK, and Langston JW: Amphotericin B-induced myelopathy. Arch Intern Med 140:1189–1192, 1980.

37. Catanzaro A, Einstein H, Levine B, et al: Ketoconazole for treatment of disseminated coccidioidomycosis. Ann Intern Med 96:436–440, 1982.

38. Christensen RD, Rothstein G, Anstall HB, and Bybee B: Granulocyte transfusions in neonates with bacterial infection, neutropenia, and depletion of mature marrow neutrophils. Pediatrics 70:1–6, 1982.

39. Christiansen KJ, Bernard EM, Gould JWM, and Armstrong D: Distribution and activity of amphotericin B in humans. J Infect Dis 152:1037–1043, 1985.

40. Cocke JG Jr, Brown RE, and Geppert LJ: Optic neuritis with prolonged use of chloramphenicol. Case report and relationship to fundus changes in cystic fibrosis. J Pediatr 68:27–31, 1966.

41. Cockerill FR III, Edson RS, Roberts GD, and Waldorf JC: Trimethoprim-sulfamethoxazole-resistant *Nocardia asteroides* causing multiple hepatic abscesses. Successful treatment with ampicillin, amikacin, and limited computed tomography–guided needle aspiration. Am J Med 77:558–560, 1984.

42. Cogan MC and Arieff AI: Sodium wasting, acidosis and hyperkalemia induced by methicillin interstitial nephritis. Evidence for selective distil tubular dysfunction. Am J Med 64:500–507, 1978.

43. Cohill DF, Pezzi PJ, Greenberg SR, and Frobese AS: Central nervous system toxicity secondary to massive doses of penicillin G in the treatment of overwhelming infections. Am J Med Sci 254:692–694, 1967.

44. Congeni BL, Bradley J, and Hammer-

schlag MR: Safety and efficacy of once daily ceftriaxone for the treatment of bacterial meningitis. Pediatr Infect Dis J 5:293–297, 1986.

45. Cook FV and Farrar WE Jr: Vancomycin revisited. Ann Intern Med 88:813–818, 1978.

46. Cooper MD, Keeney RE, Lyons SF, and Cheatle EL: Synergistic effects of ampicillin-aminoglycoside combinations on Group B streptococci. Antimicrob Agents Chemother 15:484–486, 1979.

47. Corrigan JJ: Heparin therapy in bacterial septicemia. J Pediatr 91:695–700, 1977.

48. Cowan MJ, Ammann AJ, Wara DW, et al: Pneumococcal polysaccharide immunization of infants and children. Pediatrics 62:721–727, 1978.

49. Coxon A and Pallis CA: Metronidazole neuropathy. J Neurol Neurosurg Psychiatry 39:403–405, 1976.

50. Craven PC, Graybill JR, Jorgensen JH, Dismukes WE, and Levine BE: High-dose ketoconazole for treatment of fungal infections of the central nervous system. Ann Intern Med 98:160–167, 1983.

51. Craven PC and Gremillion DH: Risk factors of ventricular fibrillation during rapid amphotericin B infusion. Antimicrob Agents Chemother 27:868–871, 1985.

52. Craven PC, Ludden TM, Drutz DJ, Rogers W, Haegele KA, and Skrdlant HB: Excretion pathways of amphotericin B. J Infect Dis 140:329–341, 1979.

53. Crowe HM and Levitz RE: Invasive *Haemophilus influenzae* disease in adults. Arch Intern Med 147:241–244, 1987.

54. Curry WA: Human nocardiosis. A clinical review with selected case reports. Arch Intern Med 140:818–826, 1980.

55. Dabernat HJ and Delmas C: Comparative activity of cefotaxime and selected β-lactam antibiotics against *Haemophilus influenzae* and aerobic Gram-negative bacilli. Rev Infect Dis 4(Suppl):401–405, 1982.

56. Dans PE, McGehee RF Jr, Wilcox C, and Finland M: Rifampin: Antibacterial activity in vitro and absorption and excretion in normal young men. Am J Med Sci 259:120–132, 1970.

57. Dawborn JK, Page MD, and Schiavone DJ: Use of 5-fluorocytosine in patients with impaired renal function. Br Med J 4:382–384, 1973.

58. DeFelice R, Johnson DG, and Galgiani JN: Gynecomastia with ketoconazole. Antimicrob Agents Chemother 19:1073–1074, 1981.

59. Deresinski SC, Lilly RB, Levine HB, Galgiani JN, and Stevens DA: Treatment of fungal meningitis with miconazole. Arch Intern Med 137:1180–1185, 1977.

60. Diamond RD and Bennett JE: A subcutaneous reservoir for intrathecal therapy of fungal meningitis. N Engl J Med 288:186–188, 1973.

61. Diasio RB, Lakings DE, and Bennett JE: Evidence for conversion of 5-fluorocytosine to 5-fluorouracil in humans: Possible factor in 5-fluorocytosine clinical toxicity. Antimicrob Agents Chemother 14:903–908, 1978.

62. Diaz CR, Kane JG, Parker RH, and Pelsor FR: Pharmacokinetics of nafcillin in patients with renal failure. Antimicrob Agents Chemother 12:98–101, 1977.

63. Dickinson GM, Droller DG, Greenman RL, and Hoffman TA: Clinical evaluation of piperacillin with observations on penetrability into cerebrospinal fluid. Antimicrob Agents Chemother 20:481–486, 1981.

64. Dismukes WE: Azole antifungal drugs: Old and new. Ann Intern Med 109:177–179, 1988.

65. Dismukes WE: Cryptococcal meningitis in patients with AIDS. J Infect Dis 157:624–628, 1988.

66. Dismukes WE, Cloud G, Gallis HA, et al: Treatment of cryptococcal meningitis with combination amphotericin B and flucytosine for four as compared with six weeks. N Engl J Med 317:334–341, 1987.

67. D'Oliveira JJG: Cerebrospinal fluid

concentrations of rifampin in meningeal tuberculosis. Am Rev Respir Dis 106:432–437, 1972.

68. Donowitz GR: Beta-lactam antibiotics. N Engl J Med 318:419–426, 490–500, 1988.

69. Drutz DJ, Spickard A, Rogers DE, and Koenig MG: Treatment of disseminated mycotic infections. A new approach to amphotericin B therapy. Am J Med 45:405–418, 1968.

70. Eliopoulos GM and Moellering RC Jr: Azlocillin, mezlocillin, piperacillin: New broad-spectrum penicillins. Ann Intern Med 97:755–760, 1982.

71. Eng RHK, Bishburg E, Smith SM, and Kapila R: Cryptococcal infections in patients with acquired immune deficiency syndrome. Am J Med 81:19–23, 1986.

72. Engelhard D, Marks MI, and Good RA: Infections in bone marrow transplant recipients. J Pediatr 108:335–346, 1986.

73. Faix RG: Systemic *Candida* infections in infants in intensive care nurseries: High incidence of central nervous system involvement. J Pediatr 105:616–622, 1984.

74. Farwell AP, Devlin JT, and Stewart JA: Total suppression of cortisol excretion by ketoconazole in the therapy of the ectopic adrenocorticotropic hormone syndrome. Am J Med 84:1063–1066, 1988.

75. Fass RJ, Copelan EA, Brandt JT, Moosehberger ML, and Ashton JJ: Platelet-mediated bleeding caused by broad-spectrum penicillins. J Infect Dis 155:1242–1248, 1987.

76. Fass RJ and Perkins RL: 5-Fluorocytosine in the treatment of cryptococcal and candida mycoses. Ann Intern Med 74:535–539, 1971.

77. Feigin RD, Shackelford PG, Eisen S, Spitler LE, Pickering LK, and Anderson DC: Treatment of mucocutaneous candidiasis with transfer factor. Pediatrics 53:63–70, 1974.

78. Feigin RD, Stechenberg BW, Chang MJ, et al: Prospective evaluation of treatment of *Hemophilus influenzae* meningitis. J Pediatr 88:542–548, 1976.

79. Feldman WE, Nelson JD, and Stanberry LR: Clinical and pharmacokinetic evaluation of nafcillin in infants and children. J Pediatr 93:1029–1033, 1978.

80. Fink S, Karp W, and Robertson A: Ceftriaxone effect on bilirubin-albumin binding. Pediatrics 80:873–875, 1987.

81. Flexner S: Experimental cerebrospinal meningitis and its serum treatment. JAMA 47:560–566, 1906.

82. Fong IW and Tompkins KB: Review of *Pseudomonas aeruginosa* meningitis with special emphasis on treatment with ceftazidime. Rev Infect Dis 7:604–612, 1985.

83. Fossieck BE Jr, Kane JF, Diaz CR, and Parker RH: Nafcillin entry into human cerebrospinal fluid. Antimicrob Agents Chemother 11:965–967, 1977.

84. Freundlich M, Cynamon H, Tamer A, Stecle B, Zilleruelo G, and Strauss J: Management of chloramphenicol intoxication in infancy by charcoal hemoperfusion. J Pediatr 103:485–487, 1983.

85. Friedman CA, Lovejoy FC, and Smith AL: Chloramphenicol deposition in infants and children. J Pediatr 95:1071–1077, 1979.

86. Fripp RR, Carter MC, Werner JC, et al: Cardiac function and acute chloramphenicol toxicity. J Pediatr 103:487–490, 1983.

87. Galgiani JN, Stevens DA, Graybill JR, Dismukes WE, and Cloud GA: Ketoconazole therapy of progressive coccidioidomycosis. Comparison of 400- and 800-mg doses and observations at higher doses. Am J Med 84:603–610, 1988.

88. Garner A, Arathoon E, and Stevens DA: Initial experience in therapy for progressive mycoses with itraconazole, the first clinically studied triazole. Rev Infect Dis 9:S77–S86, 1987.

89. Gentry LO, Jemsek JG, and Natelson EA: Effects of sodium piperacillin on platelet function in normal volunteers. Antimicrob Agents Chemother 19:532–533, 1981.

90. Gerald P, Moriau M, Bachy A, Malvaux P, and DeMeyer R: Meningococcal

purpura: Report of 19 patients treated with heparin. J Pediatr 82:780–786, 1973.

91. Giebink GS: Preventing pneumococcal disease in children. Recommendations for using pneumococcal vaccine. Pediatr Infect Dis J: 4:343–348, 1985.

92. Glew RH, Moellering RC, and Kunz LJ: Infections with *Acinetobacter calcoaceticus (Herellea vaginicola)*: Clinical and laboratory studies. Medicine 56:79–97, 1977.

93. Goodpasture HC, Hershberger RE, Barnett AM, and Peterie JD: Treatment of central nervous system fungal infection with ketoconazole. Arch Intern Med 145:879–880, 1985.

94. Granoff DM, Gilsdorf J, Gessert C, and Basden M: *Hemophilus influenzae* type b disease in a day care center: Eradication of carrier state by rifampin. Pediatrics 63:397–401, 1979.

95. Graybill JR and Ellenbogen C: Complications with the Ommaya reservoir in patients with granulomatous meningitis. J Neurosurg 38:477–480, 1973.

96. Greene GR and Cohen E: Nafcillin-induced neutropenia in children. Pediatrics 61:94–97, 1978.

97. Gross M, Fulkerson WJ, and Moore JO: Prevention of amphotericin B–induced rigors by dantrolene. Arch Intern Med 146:1587–1588, 1986.

98. Gross PA, Patel C, and Spitler LE: Disseminated cryptococcus treated with transfer factor. JAMA 240:2460–2462, 1978.

99. Grosset J and Leventis S: Adverse effects of rifampin. Rev Infect Dis 5:S440–S446, 1983.

100. Gump DW: Vancomycin for treatment of bacterial meningitis. Rev Infect Dis 3:S289–S292, 1981.

101. Hamory B, Ignatiadis P, and Sande MA: Intrathecal amikacin administration. Use in the treatment of gentamicin-resistant *Klebsiella pneumoniae* meningitis. JAMA 236:1973–1974, 1976.

102. Harder EJ and Hermans PE: Treatment of fungal infections with flucy-tosine. Arch Intern Med 135:231–237, 1975.

103. Harrison HR, Galgiani JN, Reynolds AF, Sprunger LW, and Friedman AD: Amphotericin B and imidazole therapy for coccidioidal meningitis in children. Pediatr Infect Dis J 2:216–221, 1983.

104. Hatch D, Overturf GD, Kovacs A, Forthal D, and Leong C: Treatment of bacterial meningitis with ceftazidime. Pediatr Infect Dis J 5:416–420, 1986.

105. Hawley HB and Gump DW: Vancomycin therapy of bacterial meningitis. Am J Dis Child 126:261–264, 1973.

106. Hazen EL and Brown R: Nystatin. Ann N Y Acad Sci 89:258–266, 1960.

107. Heidemann HTh, Gerkens JF, Spickard WA, Jackson EK, and Branch RA: Amphotericin B nephrotoxicity in humans decreased by salt repletion. Am J Med 75:476–481, 1983.

108. Hermans PE and Wilhelm WP: Vancomycin. Mayo Clin Proc 62:901–905, 1987.

109. Hieber JP and Nelson JD: A pharmacologic evaluation of penicillin in children with purulent meningitis. N Engl J Med 297:410–413, 1977.

110. Hilleman MR, Carlson AJ Jr, McLean AA, Vella PP, Weibel RE, and Woodhour AF: *Streptococcus pneumoniae* polysaccharide vaccine: Age and dose responses, safety, persistence of antibody, revaccination, and simultaneous administration of pneumococcal and influenzae vaccines. Rev Infect Dis 3(Suppl):31–42, 1981.

111. Hoffman TA, Cestero R, and Bullock WE: Pharmacodynamics of carbenicillin in hepatic and renal failure. Ann Intern Med 73:173–178, 1970.

112. Holm SE: Interaction between β-lactam and other antibiotics. Rev Infect Dis 8:S305–S314, 1986.

113. Huang NN, Harley RD, Promadhattavedi V, and Sproul A: Visual disturbances in cystic fibrosis following chloramphenicol administration. J Pediatr 68:32–44, 1966.

114. Ings RMJ, Fillastre J-P, Godin AL, Leroy A, and Humbert G: The pharmacokinetics of cefotaxime and its metabolites in subjects with normal

and impaired renal function. Rev Infect Dis 4(Suppl):379–391, 1982.

115. Jager-Roman E, Doyle PE, Baird-Lambert J, Cvejie M, and Buchanan N: Pharmacokinetics and tissue distribution of metronidazole in the newborn infant. J Pediatr 100:651–654, 1982.

116. Jochmann G: Versuche zur serodiagnostik und serotherapie der epidemischen genickstarre. Dtsch Med Wochenschr 32:788, 1906.

117. Johnson DE, Thompson TR, Green TP, and Ferrieri P: System candidiasis in very low-birth weight infants (< 1,500 grams). Pediatrics 73:138–143, 1984.

118. Jordan WM, Bodey GP, Rodriquez V, Ketchel SJ, and Henney J: Miconazole therapy for treatment of fungal infections in cancer patients. Antimicrob Agents Chemother 16:792–797, 1979.

119. Kafetzis DA, Brater DC, Kapiki AN, Papas CV, Dellagrammaticas H, and Papadatos CJ: Treatment of severe neonatal infections with cefotaxime. Efficacy and pharmacokinetics. J Pediatr 100:483–489, 1982.

120. Kanarek KS and Williams PR: Toxicity of intravenous miconazole overdosage in a premature infant. Pediatr Infect Dis J 5:486–488, 1986.

121. Kaplan JM, McCracken GH Jr, Horton LJ, Thomas ML, and Davis N: Pharmacologic studies in neonates given large doses of ampicillin. J Pediatr 84:571–577, 1974.

122. Kauffman CA and Frame PT: Bone marrow toxicity associated with 5-fluorocytosine therapy. Antimicrob Agents Chemother 11:244–247, 1977.

123. Kauffman RE, Thirumoorthi MC, Buckley JA, Aravind MK, and Dajani AS: Relative bioavailability of intravenous chloramphenicol succinate and oral chloramphenicol palmitate in infants and children. J Pediatr 99:963–967, 1981.

124. Kelly HW, Couch RC, Davis RL, Cushing AH, and Knott R: Interaction of chloramphenicol and rifampin. J Pediatr 112:817–820, 1988.

125. Kerns DL, Shira JE, Go S, Summers RJ, Schwab JA, and Plunket DC: Ampicillin rash in children. Relationship to penicillin allergy and infectious mononucleosis. Am J Dis Child 125:187–190, 1973.

126. Kim RC, Hedge CF Jr, Lamberson HV Jr, and Weiner LB: Traumatic introcerebral implantation of *Cladosporium trichoides*. Neurology 31:1145–1148, 1981.

127. Knight RC, Skolimowski IM, and Edwards DI: The interaction of reduced metronidazole with DNA. Biochem Pharmacol 27:2089–2093, 1978.

128. Koren G, Lau A, Klein J, et al: Pharmacokinetics and adverse effects of amphotericin B in infants and children. J Pediatr 113:559–563, 1988.

129. Koup JR, Gilbaldi M, McNamara P, Hilligoss DM, Colburn WA, and Bruck E: Interactions of chloramphenicol with phenytoin and phenobarbital. Clin Pharmacol Ther 24:571–575, 1978.

130. Koup JR, Lau AH, Brodsky B, and Slaughter RL: Chloramphenicol pharmacokinetics in hospitalized patients. Antimicrob Agents Chemother 15:651–657, 1979.

131. Kraemer FB and Pont A: Inhibition of cholesterol synthesis by ketoconazole. Am J Med 80:616–622, 1986.

132. Krasinski K, Kusmiesz H, and Nelson JD: Pharmacologic interactions among chloramphenicol, phenytoin and phenobarbital. Pediatr Infect Dis J 1:232–235, 1982.

133. Kumin GD: Clinical nephrotoxicity of tobramycin and gentamicin. A prospective study. JAMA 244:1808–1810, 1980.

134. Kunin CM, Glazko AJ, and Finland M: Persistence of antibiotics in blood of patients with acute renal failure. II. Chloramphenicol and its metabolic products in the blood of patients with severe renal disease or hepatic cirrhosis. J Clin Invest 38:1498–1509, 1959.

135. Labadie EL and Hamilton RH: Survival improvement in coccidioidal meningitis by high-dose intrathecal amphotericin B. Arch Intern Med 146:2013–2018, 1986.

136. Lacouture PG, Epstein MF, and Mitch-

ell AA: Vancomycin-associated shock and rash in newborn infants. J Pediatr 111:615–616, 1987.

137. Lake-Bakaar G, Tom W, Lake-Bakaar D, et al: Gastropathy and ketoconazole malabsorption in the acquired immunodeficiency syndrome (AIDS). Ann Intern Med 109:471–473, 1988.

138. Landesman SG, Corrado ML, Shah PM, Armengaud M, Barza M, and Cherubin CE: Past and current roles for cephalosporin antibiotics in treatment of meningitis. Emphasis on use in gram-negative bacillary meningitis. Am J Med 71:693–703, 1981.

139. Lane AZ, Wright GE, and Blair DC: Ototoxicity and nephrotoxicity of amikacin. An overview of phase II and phase III experience in the United States. Am J Med 62:911–918, 1977.

140. Laurenti F, Ferro R, Isacchi G, et al: Polymorphonuclear leukocyte transfusion for the treatment of sepsis in the newborn infant. J Pediatr 98:118–123, 1981.

141. Lavalle P, Suchil P, De Ovando F, and Reynoso S: Itraconazole for deep mycoses. Preliminary experience in Mexico. Rev Infect Dis 9:S64–S70, 1987.

142. Lazarus HS, Myers JP, and Brocker RJ: Post-craniotomy wound infection caused by Pseudallescheria boydii. J Neurosurg 64:153–154, 1986.

143. Lebel MH, Freij BJ, Syrogiannopoulis GA, et al: Dexamethasone therapy for bacterial meningitis. Results of two double-blind, placebo-controlled trials. N Engl J Med 319:964–971, 1988.

144. Lebel MH, Hoyt MJ, Waagner DC, Rollins NK, Finitzo T, and McCracken GH Jr: Magnetic resonance imaging and dexamethasone therapy for bacterial meningitis. Am J Dis Child 143:301–306, 1989.

145. Leitman PS and Smith CR: Aminoglycoside nephrotoxicity in humans. Rev Infect Dis 5:S284–S292, 1983.

146. LeSaux N and Ronald AR: Role of ceftriaxone in sexually transmitted diseases. Rev Infect Dis 11:299–309, 1989.

147. Levine PH, Regelson W, and Holland JF: Chloramphenicol-associated encephalopathy. Clin Pharmacol Ther 11:194–199, 1970.

148. Liggett SB, Berger JR, and Hush J: Cerebrospinal fluid xanthochromia with rifampin. Ann Neurol 12:228–229, 1982.

149. Lopez-Berestein G: Liposomal amphotericin B in the treatment of fungal infections. Ann Intern Med 105:130–131, 1986.

150. Lopez-Berestein G, Mehta R, Hopfer RL, et al: Treatment and prophylaxis of disseminated infection due to Candida albicans in mice with liposome-encapsulated amphotericin B. J Infect Dis 147:939–945, 1983.

151. MacGregor RR, Bennett JE, and Erslev AJ: Erythropoietin concentration in amphotericin B–induced anemia. Antimicrob Agents Chemoth 14:270–273, 1978.

152. Marmer DJ, Fields BT Jr, France GL, and Steele RW: Ketoconazole, amphotericin B, and amphotericin B methyl ester: Comparative in vitro and in vivo toxicologic effects on neutrophil function. Antimicrob Agents Chemother 20:660–665, 1981.

153. Martin E, Koup JR, Paravicini V, and Stoeckel K: Pharmacokinetics of ceftriaxone in neonates and infants with meningitis. J Pediatr 105:475–481, 1984.

154. Mauer SM, Chavers BM, and Kjellstrand CM: Treatment of an infant with severe chloramphenicol intoxication using charcoal-column hemoperfusion. J Pediatr 96:136–139, 1980.

155. Medoff G: Antifungal action of rifampin. Rev Infect Dis 5(Suppl 3):614–619, 1983.

156. Meyer R and Axelrod JL: Fatal aplastic anemia resulting from flucytosine. JAMA 228:1573, 1974.

157. Middleton FG, Jurgenson PF, Utz JP, Shadomy S, and Shadomy HJ: Brain abscess caused by Cladosporium trichoides. Arch Intern Med 136:444–448, 1976.

158. Minor DR, Schiffman G, and McIntosh LS: Response of patients with Hodgkin's disease to pneumococcal vaccine. Ann Intern Med 90:887–892, 1979.

159. Moellering RC: Ceftazidime: A new broad spectrum cephalosporin. Pediatr Infect Dis J 4:390–393, 1985.

160. Montgomerie JZ, Edwards JE Jr, and Guze LB: Synergism of amphotericin B and 5-fluorocytosine for *Candida* species. J Infect Dis 132:82–86, 1975.

161. Moore RD, Smith CR, and Lietman PS: Risk factors for the development of auditory toxicity in patients receiving aminoglycosides. J Infect Dis 149:23–30, 1984.

162. Mulder CJJ, van Alphen L, and Zanen HC: Neonatal meningitis caused by *Escherichia coli* in the Netherlands. J Infect Dis 150:935–940, 1984.

163. McCracken GH Jr: Clinical pharmacology of gentamicin in infants 2 to 24 months of age. Am J Dis Child 124:884–887, 1972.

164. McCracken GH Jr: Pharmacological basis for antimicrobial therapy in newborn infants. Am J Dis Child 128:407–419, 1974.

165. McCracken GH Jr, Ginsberg C, Chrane DF, Thomas ML, and Horton LS: Clinical pharmacology of penicillin in newborn infants. J Pediatr 82:692–698, 1973.

166. McCracken GH Jr and Lebel MH: Dexamethasone therapy for bacterial meningitis in infants and children. Am J Dis Child 143:287–289, 1989.

167. McCracken GH Jr and Mize SG: A controlled study of intrathecal antibiotic therapy in gram-negative enteric meningitis of infancy. J Pediatr 89:66–72, 1976.

168. McCracken GH Jr, Mize SG, and Threlkeld N: Intraventricular gentamicin therapy in gram-negative bacillary meningitis of infancy. Report of the second neonatal meningitis cooperative study group. Lancet 1:787–791, 1980.

169. McCracken GH, Threlkeld NE, and Thomas ML: Pharmacokinetics of cefotaxime in newborn infants. Antimicrob Agents Chemother 21:683–684, 1982.

170. National Institute of Allergy and Infectious Diseases Mycoses Study Group: Treatment of blastomycosis and histoplasmosis with ketoconazole. Results of a prospective randomized clinical trials. Ann Intern Med 103:861–872, 1985.

171. Negroni R, Robles AM, Arechavala A, Tuculet MA, and Galimberti R: Ketoconazole in the treatment of paracoccidioidomycosis and histoplasmosis. Rev Infect Dis 2:643–649, 1980.

172. Nelson JD: Carbenicillin—a major new antibiotic. Am J Dis Child 120:382–383, 1970.

173. Nelson JD, Kusmiesz H, Shelton S, and Woodman E: Clinical pharmacology and efficacy of ticarcillin in infants and children. Pediatrics 61:858–863, 1978.

174. Neu HC: β-lactam antibiotics. Structural relationships affecting in vitro activity and pharmacologic properties. Rev Infect Dis 8:S237–S259, 1986.

175. Newton RW and Forrest ARW: Rifampin overdosage—"the red man syndrome." Scott Med J 20:55–56, 1975.

176. Oppenheimer S, Beaty HN, and Petersdorf RG: Pathogenesis of meningitis. VIII. Cerebrospinal fluid and blood concentrations of methicillin, cephalothin, and cephaloridine in experimental pneumococcal meningitis. J Lab Clin Med 73:535–543, 1969.

177. Paisley JW and Washington JA II: Susceptibility of *Escherichia coli* K1 to four combinations of antimicrobial agents potentially useful for treatment of neonatal meningitis. J Infect Dis 140:183–191, 1979.

178. Parker MT and Hewitt JH: Methicillin resistance in *Staphylococcus aureus.* Lancet 1:800–804, 1970.

179. Pau AK, Smego RA, and Fisher MA: Intraventricular vancomycin: Observations of tolerance and pharmacokinetics in two infants with ventricular shunt infections. Pediatr Infect Dis J 5:93–96, 1986.

180. Peltola H, Kayhty H, Kuronen T, Hague N, Sarna S, and Makela P: Meningococcus group A vaccine in children three months to five years of age. J Pediatr 92:818–822, 1978.

181. Perez RE, Smith M, McClendon J, Kim J, and Eugenio N: *Pseudallescheria boydii* brain abscess. Complication of an intravenous catheter. Am J Med 84:359–362, 1988.

182. Petz LD and Fudenberg HH: Coombs-positive hemolytic anemia caused by

penicillin administration. N Engl J Med 274:171–178, 1966.

183. Phillips P, Fetchick R, Weisman I, Foshee S, and Graybill JR: Tolerance and efficacy of itraconazole in treatment of systemic mycoses: Preliminary results. Rev Infect Dis 9:S87–S93, 1987.

184. Plorde J, Garcia M, and Petersdorf RG: Studies on the pathogenesis of meningitis. IV. Penicillin levels in the cerebrospinal fluid in experimental meningitis. J Lab Clin Med 64:960–969, 1964.

185. Polk RE, Healy DP, Schwartz LB, Rock DT, Garson ML, and Roller K: Vancomycin and the red-man syndrome: Pharmacodynamics of histamine release. J Infect Dis 157:502–507, 1988.

186. Pratt TH: Rifampin-induced organic brain syndrome. JAMA 241:2421–2422, 1979.

187. Rahal JJ Jr and Simberkoff MS: Bactericidal and bacteriostatic action of chloramphenicol against meningococcal pathogens. Antimicrob Agents Chemother 16:13–18, 1979.

188. Ralph ED, Clarke JT, Libke RD, Luthy RP, and Kirby WMM: Pharmacokinetics of metronidazole as determined by bioassay. Antimicrob Agents Chemother 6:691–696, 1974.

189. Reiner NE and Thompson WL: Dopamine and saralasin antagonism of renal vasoconstriction and oliguria caused by amphotericin B in dogs. J Infect Dis 140:564–575, 1979.

190. Rifkind D, Marchiaro TL, Schneck SA, and Hill RB: Systemic fungal infections complicating renal transplantation and immunosuppressive therapy. Am J Med 43:28–38, 1967.

191. Ring JC, Cates KL, Belani KK, Gaston TL, Sveum RJ, and Marker SC: Rifampin for CSF shunt infections caused by coagulase-negative staphylococci. J Pediatr 95:317–319, 1979.

192. Rosenblatt JE and Edson RS: Metronidazole. Mayo Clin Proc 62:1013–1017, 1987.

193. Ruley EJ and Lisi LM: Interstitial nephritis and renal failure due to ampicillin. J Pediatr 84:878–881, 1974.

194. Sagg MS and Dismukes WE: Azole antifungal agents: Emphasis on new triazoles. Antimicrob Agents Chemother 32:1–8, 1988.

195. Sanjad SA, Haddad GG, and Nassar VH: Nephropathy, an underestimated complication of methicillin therapy. J Pediatr 84:873–877, 1974.

196. Sarff LD, McCracken GH Jr, Thomas ML, Horton LJ, and Threlkeld N: Clinical pharmacology of methicillin in neonates. J Pediatr 90:1005–1008, 1977.

197. Saul A, Bonifaz A, and Arias I: Itraconazole in the treatment of superficial mycoses: An open trial of 40 cases. Rev Infect Dis 9:S100–S103, 1987.

198. Schaad VB, McCracken GH Jr, and Nelson JD: Clinical pharmacology and efficacy of vancomycin in pediatric patients. J Pediatr 96:119–126, 1980.

199. Schaad VB, Nelson JD, and McCracken GH Jr: Pharmacology and efficacy of vancomycin for staphylococcal infections in children. Rev Infect Dis 3:S282–S288, 1981.

200. Schaffner A and Frick PG: The effect of ketoconazole on amphotericin B in a model of disseminated aspergillosis. J Infect Dis 151:902–910, 1985.

201. Schentag JJ, Plaut ME, and Cerra FB: Comparative nephrotoxicity of gentamicin and tobramycin: Pharmacokinetic and clinical studies of 201 patients. Antimicrob Agents Chemother 19:859–866, 1981.

202. Schober R and Herman MM: Neuropathology of cardiac transplantation. Survey of 31 cases. Lancet 1:962–967, 1973.

203. Schrier RW, Bulger RJ, and Van Arsdel PP Jr: Nephropathy associated with penicillin and homologues. Ann Intern Med 64:116–127, 1966.

204. Schwalbe RS, Stapleton JT, and Gilligan PH: Emergence of vancomycin resistance in coagulase-negative staphylococci. N Engl J Med 316:927–931, 1987.

205. Shah PP, Briedis DJ, Robson HG, and Conterato JP: In vitro activity of piperacillin compared to that of carbenicillin, ticarcillin, ampicillin, cephalothin, and cefamandole against *Pseudomonas aeruginosa*

and Enterobacteriaceae. Antimicrob Agents Chemother 15:346–350, 1979.

206. Shelab ZM, Britton H, and Dunn JH: Imidazole therapy of coccidioidal meningitis in children. Pediatr Infect Dis J 7:40–44, 1968.

207. Shepherd FA, Hoffert B, Evans WK, Emergy G, and Trachtenberg J: Ketoconazole. Use in the treatment of ectopic adrenocorticotropic hormone production and Cushing's syndrome in small-cell lung cancer. Arch Intern Med 145:863–864, 1985.

208. Simberkoff MS, Moldover NH, and Rahal JR Jr: Absence of detectable bactericidal and opsonic activities in normal and infected human cerebrospinal fluids. A regional host defense deficiency. J Lab Clin Med 95:362–372, 1980.

209. Singer C, Kaplan MH, and Armstrong D: Bacteremia and fungemia complicating neoplastic disease. A study of 364 cases. Am J Med 62:731–742, 1977.

210. Sirinavin S, McCracken GH Jr, and Nelson JD: Determining gentamicin dosage in infants and children with renal failure. J Pediatr 96:331–334, 1980.

211. Sklaver AR, Greenman RL, and Hoffman RA: Amikacin therapy of gram-negative bacteremia and meningitis. Treatment in diseases due to multiple resistant bacilli. Arch Intern Med 138:713–716, 1978.

212. Smith CR: Cefotaxime and cephalosporins: Adverse reactions in perspective. Rev Infect Dis 4(Suppl):481–488, 1982.

213. Smith CR, Lipsky JJ, Laskin OL, et al: Double-blind comparison of the nephrotoxicity and auditory toxicity of gentamicin and tobramycin. N Engl J Med 302:1106–1109, 1980.

214. Sonio N: The use of ketoconazole as an inhibitor of steroid production. N Engl J Med 317:812–818, 1987.

215. Spagnuolo PJ, Ellner JJ, Lerner PI, et al: *Haemophilus influenzae* meningitis: The spectrum of disease in adults. Medicine 61:74–85, 1982.

216. Stamm AM, Diasio RB, Dismukes WE, et al: Toxicity of amphotericin B plus flucytosine in 194 patients with cryptococcal meningitis. Am J Med 83:236–242, 1987.

217. Starke JR, Mason EO Jr, Kramer WG, and Kaplan SL: Pharmacokinetics of amphotericin B in infants and children. J Infect Dis 155:766–774, 1987.

218. Steele RW: Ceftriaxone: Increasing the half-life and activity of third generation cephalosporins. Pediatr Infect Dis J 4:188–191, 1985.

219. Steele RW, Sieger BE, McNitt TR, Gentry LO, and Moore WL Jr: Therapy for disseminated coccidioidomycosis with transfer factor from a related donor. Am J Med 61:283–286, 1976.

220. Stern JJ, Hartman BJ, Sharkey P, et al: Oral fluconazole therapy for patients with acquired immunodeficiency syndrome and cryptococcosis: Experience with 22 patients. Am J Med 85:477–480, 1988.

221. Stevens DA, Levine HB, Deresinski SC: Miconazole in coccidioidomycosis. II. Therapeutic and pharmacologic studies in man. Am J Med 60:191–202, 1976.

222. Stoeckel K: Pharmacokinetics of Rocephin, a highly active new cephalosporin with an exceptionally long biological half-life. Chemotherapy 27(Suppl):42–46, 1981.

223. Sud IJ and Feingold DS: Effect of ketoconazole on the fungicidal action of amphotericin B in *Candida albicans*. Antimicrob Agents Chemother 23:185–187, 1983.

224. Sugar AM and Saunders C: Oral fluconazole as suppressive therapy of disseminated cryptococcosis in patients with acquired immunodeficiency syndrome. Am J Med 85:481–489, 1988.

225. Sutherland JM: Fatal cardiovascular collapse of infants receiving large amounts of chloramphenicol. Am J Dis Child 97:761–767, 1959.

226. Tally FP, Sutter VL, and Finegold SM: Treatment of anaerobic infections with metronidazole. Antimicrob Agents Chemother 7:672–675, 1975.

227. Taylor RL, Williams DM, Craven PC, Graybill JR, Drutz DJ, and Magee WE: Amphotericin B in liposomes: A novel

therapy for histoplasmosis. Am Rev Respir Dis 125:610–611, 1982.

228. Tilden SJ, Craft JC, Cano R, and Daum RS: Cutaneous necrosis associated with intravenous nafcillin therapy. Am J Dis Child 134:1046–1048, 1980.

229. Tofte RW, Peterson PK, Kim Y, and Quie PG: Opsonic activity of normal human cerebrospinal fluid for selected bacterial species. Infect Immun 26:1093–1098, 1979.

230. Tucker WS, Snell BB, Island DP, and Gregg CR: Reversible adrenal insufficiency induced by ketoconazole. JAMA 253:2413–2414, 1985.

231. Utz JP: Chemotherapy for the systemic mycoses: The prelude to ketoconazole. Rev Infect Dis 2:625–632, 1980.

232. Utz JP, Bennett JE, Brandriss MW, Butler WT, and Hill GJ: Amphotericin B toxicity. Ann Intern Med 61:334–354, 1964.

233. Van Arsdel PP Jr: Allergic reactions to penicillin. JAMA 191:172–173, 1965.

234. Van Cutsem J, Van Gerven F, and Janssen PAJ: Activity of orally, topically, and parenterally administered itraconazole in the treatment of superficial and deep mycoses: Animal models. Rev Infect Dis 9:S15–S32, 1987.

235. Van den Bossche H: Biochemical effects of miconazole on fungi. I. Effects on the uptake and/or utilization of purines, pyrimidines, nucleosides, amino acids and glucose by Candida albicans. Biochem Pharmacol 23:887–899, 1974.

236. Vandevelde AG, Mauceri AA, and Johnson JE III: 5-Fluorocytosine in the treatment of mycotic infections. Ann Intern Med 77:43–51, 1972.

237. Vichyanond P and Olson LC: Staphylococcal CNS infection, treated with vancomycin and rifampin. Arch Neurol 41:637–639, 1984.

238. Waldorf AR and Polak A: Mechanism of action of 5-fluorocytosine. Antimicrob Agents Chemother 23:79–85, 1983.

239. Wallerstein RO, Condit PK, Kasper CK, Brown JW, and Morrison FR: Statewide study of chloramphenicol therapy and fatal aplastic anemia. JAMA 208:2045–2050, 1969.

240. Ward JI, Fraser DW, Baraff LJ, and Plikaytis BD: Haemophilus infuenzae meningitis. A national study of secondary spread in household contact. N Engl J Med 301:122–126, 1979.

241. Warner JF, Perkins RL, and Cordero L: Metronidazole therapy of anaerobic bacteremia, meningitis, and brain abscess. Arch Intern Med 139:167–169, 1979.

242. Wehrli W: Rifampin: Mechanisms of action and resistance. Rev Infect Dis 5:S407–S411, 1983.

243. West BC, DeVault GA Jr, Clement JC, and Williams DM: Aplastic anemia associated with parenteral chloramphenicol. Review of 10 cases, including the second case of possible increased risk with cimetidine. Rev Infect Dis 10:1048–1051, 1988.

244. Wiebe VJ and DeGregorio MW: Liposome-encapsulated amphotericin B: A promising new treatment for disseminated fungal infections. Rev Infect Dis 10:1097–1101, 1988.

245. Wilson CB, Jacobs RF, and Smith AL: Cellular antibiotic pharmacology. Sem Perinatol 6:205–213, 1982.

246. Wilson CB and Koup JR: Clinical pharmacology of extended-spectrum penicillins in infants and children. J Pediatr 106:1049–1054, 1985.

247. Winn WA: The treatment of coccidioidal meningitis. California Medicine 101:78–89, 1964.

248. Winston DJ, Murphy W, Young LS, and Hewitt WL: Piperacillin therapy for serious bacterial infections. Am J Med 69:255–261, 1980.

249. Wright AJ and Wilkowske CJ: The penicillins. Mayo Clin Proc 58:21–32, 1983.

250. Wright DG, Robichaud KJ, Pizzo PA, and Deisseroth AB: Lethal pulmonary reactions associated with the combined use of amphotericin B and leukocyte transfusions. N Engl J Med 304:1185–1189, 1981.

251. Young RF, Gade G, and Grinnell V: Surgical treatment for fungal infections in the central nervous system. J Neurosurg 63:371–381, 1985.

INDEX

A "T" following a page number indicates a table; an "F" indicates a figure.

355